NEOPLASM IMMUNITY

DEVELOPMENTS IN CANCER RESEARCH

NEOPLASM IMMUNITY: EXPERIMENTAL AND CLINICAL

Proceedings of a Chicago Symposium, Chicago, Illinois, U.S.A., September 13–15, 1978

Editor:

RAY G. CRISPEN
Director of ITR Biomedical Research
904 W. Adams, University of Illinois, Chicago, Illinois, U.S.A.

Sponsored by:

University of Illinois at the Medical Center and Illinois Cancer Council

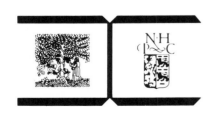

N·H
P～C

ELSEVIER/NORTH-HOLLAND
NEW YORK • AMSTERDAM • OXFORD

© 1980 by Elsevier North Holland, Inc.

Published by:

Elsevier North Holland, Inc.
52 Vanderbilt Avenue, New York, New York 10017

Sole distributors outside of the United States and Canada:

Elsevier/North-Holland Biomedical Press
335 Jan van Galenstraat, P.O. Box 211
Amsterdam, The Netherlands

Library of Congress Cataloging in Publication Data

Main entry under title:

Neoplasm immunity, experimental and clinical.

    Bibliography: p.
    Includes index.
    1. Cancer—Immunological aspects—Congresses. I. Crispen, Ray G.
    II. University of Illinois at the Medical Center. III. Illinois Cancer Council.
    IV. American Cancer Society. Chicago Unit. [DNLM: 1. Immunotherapy—
    Congresses. 2. Neoplasms—Immunology—Congresses. QZ200 N4365 1978]
RC268.3.N44   616.99′4079   80-16593
ISBN 0-444-00433-5
ISSN 0163-6146

Manufactured in the United States of America

TABLE OF CONTENTS

vi

IMMUNOLOGIC ASPECTS OF THERAPY

EDITOR'S NOTE

The symposium was very informative and demonstrated recent advancements made in our understanding of the role of the immune system, the role of tumor antigens and the importance of measuring immunologic parameters in clinical trials.

Dr. Fidler has shown that the pathogenesis of metastasis is a complex biological phenomenon which is highly selective. His results suggest that in a weakly immunogenic tumor system the constant interaction of tumor cells with syngeneic lymphocytes may lead to tumor growth and spread. Metastasis occurs when these unique tumor cells can evade the host's defense mechanisms. Dr. Kollmorgen demonstrated that a fat diet in animals allows progression of tumor growth and may be related to the carcinogenicity of various antigens when they are covalently linked with lipid moieties.

The integration of viral DNA into human neoplastic cells was illustrated by the research work of Dr. Kit. The fact that viral c-type particles can have a normal physiologic function during gestation in addition to their pathogenic role was investigated. Dr. Panem demonstrated that an antigen which reacts with antisera prepared to the placenta antigen can also be found during the pathogenesis of systemic lupus erythematosus. And the isolation of tumor-related proteins in the urine of cancer patients by Dr. Rudman may shed new light on the relation between proteolysis and tumorigenesis.

Many studies have demonstrated that tumor-associated antigens and tumor-associated immune responses are present in all experimental animal and human tumors. These responses include cell-mediated and humoral immunity as well as nonspecific host defense mechanisms. A model for selectively stimulating cellular immunity without stimulating detectable antibody formation was presented by Dr. Hunter and cell-mediated immunity assays for breast cancer were reported by Dr. McCoy. The relationship of tumor induced cellular immunity and cellular suppression in tumor bearing animals, as well as, passive transfer of tumor immunity using *in vitro* sensitized cells were explored.

Immunologic manipulation of the host has laid the foundation for clinical immunotherapy, and the necessity for the immune monitoring of the patient. In 1964 Professor Georges Mathé proposed one of the first clinical trials of systemic immunotherapy. He reported on its efficacy in the maintenance of chemotherapy induced remissions in patients with leukemic lymphosarcomas, resulting in enhanced survival. Currently he is conducting experiments on second generation immune adjuvants searching for those which do not induce suppressor cells and at the same time possess the favorable effects of BCG for antitumor activity. Various approaches to immunotherapy including immunization with tumor cells or tumor antigen, and immunorestorative immunotherapy with thymic hormones and levamisole are presented.

It is apparent that this conference has clearly demonstrated the large experimental basis for establishing immunotherapy programs in humans and gives a better understanding of the mechanisms involved in manipulating the immune system.

NEOPLASM IMMUNITY

TUMOR ANTIGENS AND MODULATORS OF IMMUNITY

Effect of Syngeneic Lymphocytes on the Vascularity, Growth and Induced Metastasis of the B16 Melanoma*

Isaiah J. Fidler[1]
D.M. Gersten[2]

SUMMARY—We investigated the possible mechanism(s) by which syngeneic lymphocytes participate in the establishment and growth of experimental metastases. In the weakly immunogenic B16 melanoma system, host lymphocytes can increase the arrest of circulating tumor emboli in pulmonary capillaries. In the present studies we wished to determine whether syngeneic lymphocytes also can affect the process of cancer metastasis at steps which occur after tumor cell arrest. Lung metastases were produced in C57BL/6 mice by injecting B16 melanoma cells i.v. Fewer lung metastases resulted from the injection of tumor cells into immunosuppressed mice than normal syngeneic mice. The mice were immunosuppressed by adult thymectomy and sublethal (450R) whole-body X-irradiation (ATX mice). Normal and ATX mice were also injected i.v. with a single dose of 10^7 syngeneic lymphocytes at 24 hr before, or 24 or 48 hr after the i.v. injection of tumor cells. All mice were killed 3 weeks after tumor cell injection and the number of artificial metastases was determined. The data demonstrated that a) the number of pulmonary metastases in ATX mice was significantly lower than in normal mice; b) reconstitution of ATX mice with 10^7 lymphocytes reversed this decrease; and c) the enhancement of metastasis in ATX mice by the injection of 10^7 lymphocytes occurred at all times of reconstitution. Even in ATX mice injected with lymphocytes 48 hr after tumor cell arrest had already taken place, and tumor cells invaded the parenchyma, a dramatic increase in metastases was observed. In subsequent studies the B16 melanoma was injected s.c. into normal and immunosuppressed mice which were or were not reconstituted with the i.v. injection of 10^7 syngeneic lymphocytes 24 hr before tumor cell injection. Tumor growth and vascularity were monitored and found to be significantly decreased in the ATX mice. In lymphocyte-reconstituted ATX mice, however, tumor growth and vascularity were pronounced and indistinguishable from control groups. Therefore, the present studies indicate that lymphocyte enhancement of metastasis can occur at several steps of the process which follow initial tumor cell arrest.

[1]Head, Biology of Metastasis, Cancer Biology Program, NCI Frederick Cancer Research Center, Frederick, Maryland.
[2]Department of Pathology, Georgetown University School of Medicine and Dentistry, Washington, D.C.
*Research sponsored by the National Cancer Institute (NCI) under contract NO1-CO-75380 with Litton Bionetics, Inc.

3

INTRODUCTION

Since the initial proposal by Prehn(1) that the immune response could play both a stimulatory and inhibitory role in the progression of tumor growth, several investigations on the participation of immune factors in experimental metastasis have been reported (2-4). Two types of evidence suggest that lymphocytes may have a profound effect on the outcome of experimental metastasis in mice. First, injection of lymphocyte:tumor cell aggregates containing varying ratios of lymphocytes to tumor cells altered the number of lung colonies formed by constant numbers of tumor cells. The extent and direction of the alteration was dependent both on the immune status of the lymphocytes and their number. Second, lymphocyte depletion of animals by thymectomy and X-irradiation prior to i.v. injection of weakly immunogenic tumor cells produced a significant decrease in the number of lung colonies, which could be reversed by reconstitution of mice with syngeneic lymphocytes 24 hr prior to i.v. tumor cell injection. Again, the number of metastases was dependent on the source and number of syngeneic lymphocytes (2).

The mere presence of tumor cells in the circulation does not constitute metastasis. Metastases must result from the arrest of circulating tumor cells in a capillary bed, extravasation into the organ parenchyma and subsequent growth of tumor cells into visible colonies. Since tumor cell arrest in the microvasculature must precede the subsequent development of tumor cells, the formation of an heterotypic circulating embolus of some critical size is a crucial event in the pathogenesis of metastasis. Since the formation of such an embolus would ensure the initial arrest of tumor cells in the capillary bed of an organ, such arrest would influence the ultimate number of visible metastases (5). To test this proposal, experiments evaluating the effects of lymphocytes on the initial arrest of radioisotopically labeled tumor cells injected i.v. in the lung as well as their subsequent kinetic distribution throughout the body were performed (6). The results of those studies demonstrated that the ultimate outcome of experimental metastasis could not be predicted from the initial arrest data of tumor cells. While the critical embolus size probably has a significant role in the initial arrest of circulating emboli and therefore some effect on their subsequent survival and growth, it was clear that additional factors were involved.

In the present study, we wished to determine whether lymphocytes could influence the outcome of metastasis by interacting with tumor cells at steps other than initial arrest in the sequence of experimental metastasis. Specifically we investigated the influence of normal and sensitized syngeneic lymphocytes on the vascularity surrounding tumors growing s.c., as well as on tumor growth s.c. and in the lungs. In addition, we asked whether the outcome of such interactions is influenced by properties of host lymphocytes and of the tumor cells themselves.

MATERIALS AND METHODS

Animals

Inbred C57BL/6 mice were obtained from the Animal Production Area, Frederick Cancer Research Center, Frederick, Maryland. At 4 wk of age, mice were either thymectomized or sham-thymectomized as described previously (6). One week later and 4 wk before the i.v. tumor cell injection these animals were given a single, acute exposure to 450R, whole body X-irradiation. The animals were given drinking water which contained 10 ppm chlorine (7).

Tumor Cells and Cell Culture

B16-F1 (with low metastatic potential) and B16-F10 (with high metastatic potential) tumor cells were isolated originally by sequential i.v. passage through C57BL/6 mice (1) and have been maintained in culture as described previously (8). The tumors were checked and found free of mycoplasma and pathogenic murine viruses including LDH virus.

Sensitization of C57BL/6 Mice to B16 Melanoma

C57BL/6 mice, 6 to 8 wk old, were given a s.c. injection of 100,000 viable B16 cells. Three weeks later when the tumors were 10 to 30 mm in diameter the animals were killed. Their lymph node and spleen lymphocytes were prepared as described below and designated as tumor-bearing lymphocytes.

Preparation of Normal and Sensitized Lymphocytes

Axillary, cervical, and mesenteric lymph nodes and spleens were collected aseptically from normal or tumor-bearing mice, placed in cold Hanks' balanced salt solution (HBSS) and forced through a wire mesh sieve. The resulting suspensions were filtered through a glass wool column and centrifuged, and the cellular pellets were resuspended in serumless complete minimum essential medium (CMEM). Erythrocytes were removed from the preparation by hypotonic lysis as described previously (6). Viability was about 95% as determined by the trypan exclusion test. Practically all cells were determined morphologically to be lymphocytes.

Procedures for Study of Experimental Metastasis

For studies of experimental metastasis we routinely harvested cells from nonconfluent monolayers by overlaying the cultures with a thin layer of 0.25% trypsin−0.02% EDTA for 1 min. The flask was tapped to facilitate removal of cells from the plastic, and fresh medium was immediately added. The cells were washed and resuspended in HBSS. Tumor cell viability as

5

determined by the trypan blue exclusion test usually exceeded 95%. The suspension was diluted to yield 5 x 10⁴ single cells/0.2 ml, the inoculum volume per mouse. This dose was selected because that number of cells could produce enough metastases to be easily counted.

Tumor cells were injected i.v. into the tail vein of C57BL/6 mice and mice were killed 18 days later. The number of resultant pulmonary tumor colonies was determined with the aid of a dissecting microscope by two independent observers.

Procedure for Study of Experimental Metastasis in Immunosuppressed C57BL/6 Mice with or without Lymphocyte Reconstitution

Mice were divided into three major groups: adult thymectomized X-irradiated (450R) (ATX); sham-thymectomized X-irradiated (STX) and normal mice. In addition, each of these groups was subdivided into four lymphocyte treatment groups: no lymphocyte reconstitution, (0); lymphocyte reconstitution 24 hr prior to i.v. tumor cell injection (−24); lymphocyte reconstitution 24 hr following i.v. tumor cell injection (+24); and lymphocyte reconstitution 48 hr following tumor cell injection (+48). Thus, each experiment represents a 3 x 4 array using 10 animals for each of the three experiments. The number of tumor cells injected i.v. was always 50,000 single viable cells. The number of i.v.-injected lymphocytes varied among the different experiments. We injected mice with either 1 x 10⁷ or 1 x 10⁸ lymphocytes from either normal or tumor-bearing mice. All mice were killed 18 days following the i.v. injection of tumor cells, and the number of lung metastases was determined as described above.

Influence of Syngeneic Lymphocytes on the Growth and Vascularization of Tumor Cells Injected Subcutaneously

The B16 melanoma F10 cell line was used throughout these experiments. Fifty thousand viable cells were injected in 0.1 ml HBSS s.c. lateral to the midline on the abdomen. The study included the following groups of mice (15/group): 1) normal mice; 2) ATX mice, and 3) STX mice. Each major group of mice consisted of three subgroups (5/group): 1) unirradiated unreconstituted, 2) irradiated (450R) unreconstituted, and 3) irradiated (450R) and lymphocyte-reconstituted (1 x 10⁷ normal C57BL/6 spleen and lymph node lymphocytes). Fourteen and 20 days later the mice were killed and the skin was reflected to expose s.c. implants and vessels in the flank (9). Tumor size was measured and the degree of vascularization surrounding the growing tumors was compared to that on the uninjected side and recorded as mild or pronounced.

Statistical Analysis

Statistical significance was analyzed using Colhran's modified t-test.

6

RESULTS

We have shown previously that the initial arrest of i.v.-injected tumor cells in the pulmonary vasculature does not correlate with the final number of visible metastases. However, both initial arrest and development of metastases can be altered by the interaction with host lymphocytes (6,10). The first experiment asks whether post-initial arrest events in the metastatic process (see Discussion) can be affected by the presence of tumor-bearing lymphocytes. In Table 1 it is shown that, as reported previously (2), ATX significantly reduced the number of tumors following the i.v. injection of an equal number of B16-Fl cells from 42 ± 5 to 16 ± 2 ($p < 0.01$). Prior injections (-24 hr) of recipients with 10^7 tumor-bearing lymphocytes (so that lymphocytes were present at the time of tumor cell injection) increased the number of tumors to 246 ± 10 in the normal group, 239 ± 18 in the STX group and 166 ± 23 in the ATX group. This implies that 10^7 lymphocytes from tumor-bearing mice are sufficient to abrogate the decrease in the

Table 1—NUMBER OF LUNG TUMOR COLONIES IN CONTROL, THYMECTOMIZED X-IRRADIATED AND SHAM-THYMECTOMIZED X-IRRADIATED C57BL/6 MICE

Group of C57BL/6 Mice Given i.v. Injection	Av. No. of Pulmonary Metastases[a]			
		Lymphocyte-treated		
	Untreated	-24 hr	+24 hr	+48 hr
Normal Controls	42 ± 5[b]	246 ± 10	44 ± 4	55 ± 6
	(20 - 72)	(213 - 243)	(26 - 60)	(38 - 90)
Thymectomized X-Irradiated[c]	16 ± 2	166 ± 23	60 ± 11	39 ± 3
	(6 - 25)	(99 - 240)	(35 - 118)	(24 - 51)
Sham-thymectomized X-Irradiated	60 ± 11	239 ± 18	47 ± 8	90 ± 14
	(32 - 140)	(170 - 300)	(20 → 88)	(28 - 150)
Normal Mice Injected With Lymphocytes Alone	—	0	0	0

Mice were either Untreated or Treated Once by i.v. Injection of 10^7 Syngeneic Lymphocytes from Tumor-Bearing Donors at 24 hr prior to and 24 hr or 48 hr following i.v. Injection of 50,000 Viable B16-F1 Melanoma Cells.

[a]Ten mice/group; pulmonary metastases were counted 21 days after i.v. injection with the aid of a dissecting microscope.

[b]Mean $\pm$ SEM (Range).

[c]Thymectomized at 4-5 weeks of age; 450R total body irradiation given 10 days after surgery and 4 weeks prior to tumor cell injection.

number of lung tumor colonies observed in the ATX animals. In this and subsequent experiments, the number of lung tumor colonies observed in the STX group did not differ from normal mice. Therefore, since the surgery itself had no effect on the outcome of experimental metastasis, the STX and normal groups will be considered together.

Administration of lymphocytes at +24 hr and +48 hr had no significant effect on the number of pulmonary metastases observed in normal recipients, but did significantly increase the number of tumors in the ATX group ($p < 0.01$). These data suggested that lymphocytes may participate in phenomena other than initial arrest of circulating tumor cells in the lung, and prompted the next experiment.

The experiment shown in Table 2 agrees with previous experiments (2,6) which demonstrate that reconstitution at -24 hr with 10^8 syngeneic tumor-bearing lymphocytes has an inhibitory effect on both normal and ATX hosts. The extent of the inhibition appears to be greater for normal than ATX animals, reducing the number of tumors from 27 to 4 in the former case and 18 to 10 for the ATX. Injection of lymphocytes at 24 hr or 48 hr

Table 2—NUMBER OF LUNG TUMOR COLONIES IN CONTROL, THYMECTOMIZED X-IRRADIATED AND SHAM-THYMECTOMIZED X-IRRADIATED C57BL/6 MICE

Group of C57BL/6 Mice Given i.v. Injection	Av. No. of Pulmonary Metastases[a]			
		Lymphocyte-treated		
	Untreated	-24 hr	+24 hr	+48 hr
Normal Controls	27 ± 2[b] (17 - 32)	4 ± 1 (2 - 8)	15 ± 1 (12 - 19)	14 ± 3 (6 - 26)
Thymectomized X-Irradiated[c]	18 ± 3 (8 - 33)	10 ± 2 (4 - 16)	30 ± 6 (10 - 60)	43 ± 7 (14 - 70)
Sham-thymectomized X-Irradiated	32 ± 4 (20 - 49)	15 ± 3 (7 - 35)	16 ± 11 (15 - 112)	69 ± 14 (28 - 124)

Mice were either Untreated or Treated Once by i.v. Injection of 10^8 Syngeneic Lymphocytes from Tumor-Bearing Donors at 24 hr Prior to and 24 hr or 48 hr following i.v. Injection of 50,000 Viable B16-F1 Melanoma Cells.

[a]Ten mice/group; pulmonary metastases were counted 21 days after i.v. injection with the aid of a dissecting microscope.

[b]Mean ± SEM (Range).

[c]Thymectomized at 4-5 weeks of age; 450R total body irradiation given 10 days after surgery and 4 weeks prior to tumor cell injection.

8

following i.v. tumor cell injection again enhanced the number of metastases in ATX mice. These two experiments appear to confirm the earlier work (dealing only with reconstitution 24 hr prior to i.v. injection of tumor cells) that injection of 10^7 or 10^8 lymphocytes from tumor-bearing donors has either an enhancing or an inhibitory effect respectively in ATX animals (6).

We have previously reported that differences in tumor cell properties can also influence the outcome of experimental metastasis. It was shown that differences in the incidence of experimental metastasis between B16-F1 (low metastasis) and B16-F10 (high metastasis) were maintained irrespective of the nature of the host (6). For that reason, we repeated the above experiments, but used the highly metastatic B16-F10 (Table 3). In order to minimize the influence of specifically sensitized lymphocytes and to maximize the influence of tumor cell properties *per se*, we reconstituted the mice with lymphocytes obtained from normal donors. The injection of 10^7 normal lymphocytes 24 hr prior to i.v. injection of tumor cells into normal animals resulted in an increase incidence of metastasis ($p < 0.02$). However, lymphocyte injection at 24 hr or 48 hr following tumor cells had little effect

Table 3—NUMBER OF LUNG TUMOR COLONIES IN CONTROL, THYMECTOMIZED X-IRRADIATED AND SHAM-THYMECTOMIZED X-IRRADIATED C57BL/6 MICE

Group of C57BL/6 Mice Given i.v. injection	Av. No. of Pulmonary Metastases[a]			
		Lymphocyte-treated		
	Untreated	-24 hr	+24 hr	+48 hr
Normal Controls	125 ± 6[b]	181 ± 18	164 ± 19	125 ± 15
	(94 - 156)	(101 - 248)	(62 - 246)	(58 - 192)
Thymectomized	106 ± 18	96 ± 9	262 ± 32	205 ± 20
X-Irradiated[c]	(30 - 197)	(43 - 130)	(126 - 400)	(107 - 340)
Sham-thymectomized	194 ± 19	163 ± 16	175 ± 14	169 ± 15
X-Irradiated	(114 - 300)	(107 - 248)	(128 - 260)	(98 - 238)

Mice were either Untreated or Treated Once by i.v. Injection of 10^7 Syngeneic Lymphocytes from Tumor-Bearing Donors at 24 hr Prior to and 24 hr or 48 hr following i.v. Injection of 50,000 Viable B16-F10 Melanoma Cells

[a]Ten mice/group; pulmonary metastases were counted 21 days after i.v. injection with the aid of a dissecting microscope.
[b]Mean ± SEM (Range).
[c]Thymectomized at 4-5 weeks of age; 450R total body irradiation given 10 days after surgery and 4 weeks prior to tumor cell injection.

on the incidence of metastasis ($p < 0.05$; < 0.1). The prior reconstitution of ATX mice did not lead to a significant difference in metastases as compared to control mice. However, highly significant increases for both groups injected with lymphocytes at 24 hr or 48 hr post tumor cell injection were observed ($p < 0.002$) (Table 3).

It became apparent that one possible explanation for the increase in the incidence of metastasis shown in Table 1 could have been the inadvertent introduction of tumor cells mixed in with the lymphocyte preparation (from tumor-bearing mice). That is, if lymph node metastasis occurred in the tumor-bearing donors, then inoculation of 10^7 lymphocytes contaminated with 100 tumor cells, for example, could account for an observed increase of some metastases. As a separate control, a preparation of 10^7 lymphocytes alone from s.c. tumor-bearing donors was injected i.v., resulting in no lung metastases (Table 1).

Tumor cells were injected s.c. Tumor growth and size were monitored once weekly. Tumor size in all test groups except ATX mice at 20 days following the s.c. injection was similar, and ranged between 25-40 mm in diameter. In contrast, tumor size in ATX mice was smaller, ranging between 5-10 mm in diameter. No essential differences in the degree of vascularity were noted among the groups with one exception: ATX mice whose tumor was smaller than in all other test groups demonstrated little degree of vascularity (Figure 1H). However, ATX mice, which were injected i.v. with 10^7 normal lymphocytes 24 hr prior to tumor cell injection s.c., demonstrated patterns of tumor growth and vascularization that were similar to normal, control mice.

DISCUSSION

The complex process of metastasis consists of many sequential steps. It begins with the invasion of tissues and vessels by cells originating in the primary cancer. Following their entry into the circulation, many cells are arrested in the first capillary bed encountered, but some recirculate and are trapped in other organs. After their immediate arrest, tumor cells must invade the parenchyma, proliferate, establish a vascular supply, and escape host defense mechanisms in order to develop into secondary foci.

The initial arrest of i.v.-administered B16 melanoma cells in the lung can be affected by the recipient's immune status. But the initial arrest of circulating tumor cells in the pulmonary capillary bed does not correlate with the ensuing tumor cell survival kinetics and the ultimate number of lung colonies (6). We sought, therefore, to determine whether events in the metastatic cascade which occur after initial arrest and involve lymphocyte: tumor cell interaction could affect the ultimate number of experimental tumor colonies. We have performed two types of lymphocyte reconstitution

10

Figure 1—TUMOR GROWTH AND VASCULARITY FOLLOWING THE SUBCUTANEOUS INJECTION OF 50,000 VIABLE B16 MELANOMA CELLS

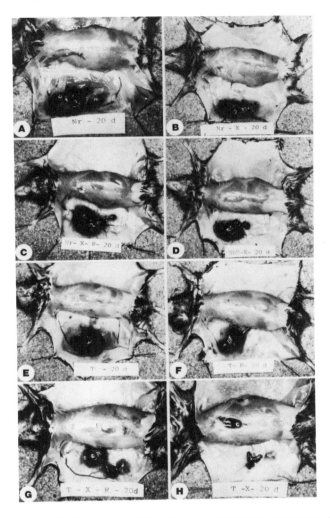

All mice were killed 20 days later and the skin was reflected to expose s.c. tumors and vessels in the flank as described previously in (9). Note appearance of tumors and dilatation of major vessels. A. Normal mice. B. Normal X-irradiated (450R). C. Normal X-irradiated, lymphocyte-reconstituted 24 hr prior to tumor cell injection. D. Sham-thymectomized X-irradiated. E. Thymectomized. F. Thymectomized, lymphocyte reconstituted. G. Thymectomized X-irradiated, lymphocyte-reconstituted. H. ATX mice. B16 tumor growth in ATX mice is decreased as compared to all other groups.

11

of ATX animals: prior reconstitution, when lymphocytes were administered 24 hr before tumor cell injection, and post-reconstitution, when lymphocytes were administered 24 hr or 48 hr following i.v. tumor cell injection.

The results shown in Tables 1 and 2 clearly demonstrate that post-reconstitution with i.v. injection of 10^7 and 10^8 lymphocytes from tumor-bearing donors enhanced the number of tumor colonies in lungs of lymphocyte-deficient ATX animals. Apparently, the injected lymphocytes influenced the outcome of experimental metastasis while interacting with tumor cells at stages of metastasis which followed initial arrest.

The data of Tables 2 and 3 indicate that the effects of lymphocytes injected following tumor cell arrest as observed above for B16-F1 cells are not seen for B16-F10 cells. This reaffirms the proposition that differences in tumor cell properties may profoundly affect the outcome of experimental metastasis.

There are no clear-cut explanations that account for the observed results. Two possibilities are most likely. First, studies on the kinetic distribution of labeled tumor cells in ATX and STX animals indicated that at 24-hr post-injection, a small number of viable originally injected B16-F1 and B16-F10 cells still remain in the circulation (6). Delayed interaction of the few circulating cells could account for the observed effects of reconstituting ATX with lymphocytes after i.v. injection of tumor cells. The use of labeled tumor cells is, unfortunately, not sensitive enough to detect differences in small numbers of circulating cells. However, since 64% of the i.v.-injected B16-F1 cells and 94% of the B16-F10 cells could be found in the lungs 2 min after injection, it could be that fewer B16-F10 cells would be available for late interaction. Therefore, increased tumor cell arrest of recirculating cells cannot be ruled out as the crucial event.

The alternative explanation is that syngeneic lymphocytes may be involved in steps of the metastatic process other than the initial arrest of tumor cells in the microvasculature. Many immunological and nonimmunological functions have been attributed to the immune system, in general and to the lymphocyte, in particular. The data concerning the "trephocytic" function of lymphocytes, i.e., serving as a source of essential growth substances for various organs, were reported as early as 1922 by Carrell (11). Several investigators have suggested that the lymphoreticular system regulates the growth of other normal tissue (12,13). Syngeneic lymphocytes were also shown to enhance the growth of mouse and rat tumors *in vitro* (14-19), but at present the exact mechanisms by which lymphocytes or their product (20, 21) may enhance tumor growth is unclear (22).

Recent reports have suggested that tumor angiogenesis (vascularity) in tumor-bearing mice could be induced by lymphocytes reacting either against the growing tumors or participating in a graft-versus-host reaction (23,24).

This lymphocyte-induced angiogenesis (LIA) is distinguished from tumor angiogenesis factor (TAF) described previously (25). In our current studies we have investigated the vascularization around tumors growing s.c. as correlated with tumor size. It was interesting to note that s.c. tumor growth of the weakly immunogenic B16 melanoma was retarded in ATX mice as compared to all other groups. Since tumor growth was unaffected in normal, X-irradiated recipients, or in STX recipients it appeared that neither irradiation nor surgery influenced the phenomenon. Further proof implicating immune depletion in the retardation of tumor growth and vascularity was obtained from ATX animals injected with normal lymphocytes 1 day prior to tumor challenge. As can be seen in Figure 1G, tumor growth in these animals was comparable to all other control groups.

Collectively the present results suggest that in a weakly immunogenic tumor system the interaction of tumor cells with syngeneic lymphocytes may lead to enhancement of tumor growth and spread. This is consistent with our earlier work (2) and that of Vaage (26) who surveyed the growth characteristics and host immune reactivity to 100 successive spontaneous mammary carcinomas of C3H mice. In his studies, the ability of tumor cells to grow in the lung (as metastases) after i.v. injection was directly correlated with their immunogenicity. In similar studies, Hager *et al.* reported that the metastatic potential of mammary tumor cells of BALB/CfC3H origin was associated with their ability to induce cell-mediated reactivity *in vitro* (27). Moreover, in the B16 system, tumor cells that have been selected *in vitro* for their resistance to lysis by syngeneic lymphocytes are less metastatic than their lymphocyte-susceptible parent lines (10).

Our present findings concern a tumor system that is weakly immunogenic. The immunostimulation hypothesis of Prehn and Lappe (28) predicts that in weakly immunogenic systems, host immunity may actually enhance tumor growth. Such is not the case in other tumor systems which are highly immunogenic, and in which immune suppression tends to increase tumor incidence or metastasis (13). The pathogenesis of metastasis is a complex biological phenomenon, which is highly selective. The ultimate growth of secondary tumors represents the end point of many destructive events (29). Metastasis does not succeed because tumor cells grow independently of their host. Rather the development of clinical metastases is the result of a constant interplay between the properties of tumor cells and their host in which the rules of "survival of the fittest" apply. Thus, metastasis occurs when unique tumor cells can either evade or overwhelm host defense mechanisms or even use normal host homeostatic mechanisms to their own gain (29).

ACKNOWLEDGMENT

We thank Zoa Barnes for valuable technical assistance; Charles Riggs and Lenita Thibault for statistical analysis.

REFERENCES

1. Prehn, R.T., "Perspectives in Oncogenesis: Does Immunity Stimulate or Inhibit Neoplasia?" *J. Reticuloendothel. Soc.* 10: 1-12, 1971.
2. Fidler, I.J., "Immune Stimulation-Inhibition of Experimental Cancer Metastasis." *Cancer Res.* 34: 491-498, 1974.
3. Weiss, L., Glaves, D., and Waite, D., "The Influence of Host Immunity on the Arrest of Circulating Cancer Cells and Its Modification by Neuraminidase." *Int. J. Cancer* 13: 850-862, 1974.
4. Wexler, H., Sindelar, W.F., and Ketcham, A.S., "The Role of Immune Factors in the Survival of Circulating Tumor Cells." *Cancer* 37: 1701-1706, 1976.
5. Liotta, L.A., Kleinerman, and Saidel, G.M., "The Significance of Hematogenous Tumor Cell Changes in the Metastatic Process." *Cancer Res.* 36: 889-894, 1976.
6. Fidler, I.J., Gersten, D.M., and Riggs, C., "Relationship of Host Immune Status to Tumor Cell Arrest, Distribution and Survival in Experimental Metastasis." *Cancer* 40: 46-55, 1977.
7. Fidler, I.J., "Depression of Macrophages in Mice Drinking Hyperchlorinated Water." *Nature* 270: 735-736, 1977.
8. Fidler, I.J., "Selection of Successive Tumor Lines for Metastasis." *Nature, New Biol.* 242: 148-149, 1973.
9. Coman, D.R., Sheldon, W.F., "The Significance of Hyperemia around Tumor Implants." *Am. J. Pathol.* 22: 821-831, 1946.
10. Fidler, I.J., Gersten, D.M., and Budmen, M.B., "Characterization *in vivo* and *in vitro* of Tumor Cells Selected for Resistance to Syngeneic Lymphocyte-Mediated Cytotoxicity." *Cancer Res.* 36: 3160-3165, 1976.
11. Carrel, A., "Growth Promoting Function of Leukocytes." *J. Exp. Med.* 36: 385-391, 1922.
12. Prehn, R.T., "The Immune Reaction as a Stimulator of Tumor Growth." *Science* 176: 170-171, 1972.
13. Prehn, R.T., "Immunostimulation of the Lymphodependent Phase of Neoplastic Growth." *J. Natl. Cancer Inst.* 59: 1043-1049, 1977.
14. Medina, D., Heppner, G., "Cell-mediated Immunostimulation induced by Mammary Tumor Virus Free BALB/c Mammary Tumors." *Nature* 242: 329-330, 1973.
15. Jeejeebhoy, H.F., "Stimulation of Tumor Growth by the Immune Response." *Int. J. Cancer* 13: 665-678, 1974.
16. Kall, M.A., Hellström, I., "Specific Stimulatory and Cytotoxic Effects of Lymphocytes Sensitized *in vitro* to Either Alloantigens or Tumor Antigens." *J. Immunol.* 114: 1083-1088, 1975.
17. Prehn, L.M., "Immunostimulation of Highly Immunogenic Target Tumor Cells by Lymphoid Cells *in vitro*." *J. Natl. Cancer Inst.* 56: 833-838, 1976.
18. Norbury, K.C., *"In vitro* Stimulation of Tumor Cell Growth Mediated by Different Lymphoid Cell Populations." *Cancer Res.* 37: 1408-1415, 1977.
19. Fidler, I.J., *"In vitro* Studies of Cellular-mediated Immunostimulation of Tumor Growth." *J. Natl. Cancer Inst.* 50: 1307-1312, 1973.
20. Ilfeld, D., Carnaud, C., Cohen, I.R., et al., *"In vitro* Cytotoxicity and *in vivo* Tumor Enhancement induced by Mouse Spleen Cells Autosensitized *in vitro*." *Int. J. Cancer* 12: 213-222, 1973.

14

21. Shearer, W.T., "Stimulation of Cells by Antibody." *Science* 182: 1357-1359, 1973.

22. Prehn, R.T., "Tumor Progression and Hemostasis." In: *Advances in Cancer Research,* Academic Press, NY, 203-236, 1976.

23. Sidkey, Y.A. and Auerback, R., "Lymphocyte Induced Angiogenesis: A Quantitative and Sensitive Assay of the Graft vs. Host Reaction." *J. Expt. Med.* 141: 1084-1100, 1975.

24. Sidkey, Y.A. and Auerback, R., "Lymphocyte-Induced Angiogenesis in Tumor-bearing Mice." *Science* 192: 1237-1238, 1976.

25. Folkman, J., "Tumor Angiogenesis." In: *Cancer: A Comprehensive Treatise,* F.F. Becker (ed.) Plenum Press, NY, Vol. 3, 355-388, 1975.

26. Vaage, J., "A Survey of the Growth Characteristics of and the Host Reactions to One Hundred C3H/He Mammary Carcinomas." *Cancer Res.* 38: 331-338, 1978.

27. Hager, J.C., Griswold, D.E., and Heppner, G.H., "Clinical and Immunological Behavior of Serially Transplanted Strain BALB/CfC3H Mouse Mammary Tumors." *Proc. AACR.* 19: 16, 1978.

28. Prehn, R.T. and Lappé, M.A., "An Immunostimulation Theory of Tumor Development." *Transplant Rev.* 7: 26-54, 1971.

29. Fidler, I.J., and Kripke, M.L., "Metastasis Results from Preexisting Variant Cells with a Malignant Tumor." *Science* 197: 793-795, 1977.

A Possible Role of MER in Protection Against DMBA-Induced Tumors in Rats Fed Different Rat Diets

G. Mark Kollmorgen[1]
W. Sansing[1]
G. Fischer[1]
D. Cunningham[1]
R. Longley[1]
A. Lehman[2]
M. King[3]
P. McCay[3]

SUMMARY—The incidence of mammary carcinoma in the Sprague-Dawley, female rat after exposure to DMBA was related to the quantity and quality of dietary fat. Rats fed a diet containing 20% polyunsaturated fat had the highest tumor incidence (about 100%), rats fed the 20% saturated fat diet had an incidence of about 70% and rats on the 2% low fat diet had the least incidence (about 35%). Immunization with MER prior to exposure to DMBA reduced the incidence and/or retarded the development of tumors. Protection was independent of diet, and measured by a reduced tumor incidence in the population, a reduction in the average number of tumors in tumor-bearing rats, and a reduction in tumor mass. The blastogenic activity of spleen lymphocytes in autologous serum after stimulation with con A correlated with tumor incidence. Rats on the low fat diet had the most reactive lymphocytes and the least incidence of tumor while rats on the high polyunsaturated fat diet had the least reactive lymphocyte and the highest incidence of tumor. Lymphocyte reactivity was limited by serum inhibitory factors. Immunization with MER minimized these factors and preserved lymphocyte function.

INTRODUCTION

A number of investigators have shown a positive correlation between the incidence of mammary cancer and intake of dietary fat in both humans (1-6) and animals (1, 7-9). In animals, the effects of dietary fat appear to be independent of caloric intake. More recent experiments (10-13) have shown that dietary fat increased the incidence of mammary tumors produced in

[1]Cancer Research Program, Oklahoma Medical Research Foundation, Oklahoma City, Oklahoma.
[2]Biometrics Unit, Oklahoma Medical Research Foundation, Oklahoma City, Oklahoma.
[3]Biomembrane Research Laboratory , Oklahoma Medical Research Foundation, Oklahoma City, Oklahoma.

17

rats by a single oral dose of 7, 12-dimethylbenz(α)anthracene (DMBA). For example, Carroll, et al. (10-12) reported that rats fed high fat diets, especially polyunsaturated fats, developed a greater number of tumors with a shorter latent period when compared to animals on low fat diets or saturated fat diets. The difference in incidence was independent of small differences in caloric intake. This observation was recently confirmed by King, et al. (13), who observed that tumor incidence in the population, number of tumors per rat, and rate of tumor growth were significantly higher in rats fed a high level of polyunsaturated fat compared to rats fed low fat diets. Rats fed high levels of saturated fats had intermediate values.

While the mechanism(s) by which high fat diets promote tumor formation is(are) not known, distribution and absorption of DMBA is apparently not altered by dietary fat (10, 14). In light of other data, it seems reasonable that high fat diets may promote tumor formation by suppression of immune responses. Several investigators have reported that injection or feeding of linoleic acid prolongs skin allograft survival in rodents (15-18).

Other reports indicate that polyunsaturated fatty acids may be beneficial as an adjunct to immunosuppressive therapy following renal transplantation (19-22). In addition, fatty acids (23-27) and lipoproteins (28) inhibit lymphocyte stimulation by lectins and by allogeneic lymphocytes.

While a number of factors and conditions inhibit immune responses, non-specific immunostimulants may preserve, restore or heighten immunological reactivity. Immunostimulants have been used almost exclusively as therapeutic agents and their role in tumor prevention has not been established.

Hence, a series of experiments was designed, using rats maintained on different fat diets, to determine: a) if immunization with MER prior to exposure to DMBA reduces the incidence of mammary carcinoma, and b) the relationship between lymphocyte function and tumor incidence.

MATERIALS AND METHODS

Animals

Sprague-Dawley female, albino, outbred rats were used for these studies. Weanlings (21 days old) were obtained from the Charles River Colony or from Charles River Breeders at the Oklahoma University Health Sciences Center. Upon arrival in our animal facility, rats were placed and subsequently maintained on one of three diets outlined in Table 1. Based on calories per gram of diet and the average amount of food consumed per day, it was estimated that all groups consumed about 70 calories per day. Growth curves indicated that none of the groups was significantly different.

Animals which were exposed to the carcinogen were given 10 mg of DMBA in 1 ml of corn oil via stomach tube on day 50. Animals which were

18

immunized with MER were given an intraperitoneal dose of 0.5 mg suspended in 0.2 ml of vehicle on days 28 and 35. Control animals were given 0.2 ml of vehicle, via the same route, which contained the following per ml of water: 9 mg sodium chloride, 5 mg sodium carboxymethylcellulose, 0.004 ml of polysorbate, and 0.009 ml of benzyl alcohol.

Animals were weighed and examined for tumors on a weekly basis. When animals were 220 to 250 days old, tumors were removed, and certified as carcinoma using histological techniques.

Table 1—CONTENT OF VARIOUS DIETS

	20% Poly- unsaturated Fat Diet	20% Saturated Fat Diet	2% Low Fat Diet
	gm	gm	gm
Casein	23	23	23
Fat	20[1]	20[2]	2[3]
Sucrose	46	46	64
Salt Mixture[4]	4	4	4
Alphacel (non nutrient bulk)	6	6	6
Vitamin Mixture[5]	1	1	1

[1]Corn Oil
[2]Coconut Oil, 18% + Linoleic Acid, 2%
[3]Linoleic Acid
[4]Salt Mixture (29)
[5]Vitamin Mixture (Vitamin Fortification Mixture of ICN Life Sciences Co., Cleveland, Ohio 44128)

Collection of Serum and Cell Samples

Animals were anesthetized with sodium nembutal (30 mg/Kg) and blood was taken via cardiac puncture. Serum was used immediately or stored at $-70°C$ until use.

Blood lymphocytes were obtained with a heparinized syringe and separated through a ficoll-hypaque column (density=1.077).

Spleens were excised and gently homogenized to provide a single cell suspension. Cells were washed in Hank's balanced salt solution, transferred to minimal essential medium (MEM), and cell aggregates and debris were removed. Cells were counted with a Coulter counter (Model ZBI), centrifuged and resuspended in MEM supplemented with antibiotics and appropriate serum using concentrations of 2.5% or 5.0%.

19

Lymphocyte Blastogenesis

Cells were pipetted into Micro-test plates (Falcon plastics) in 0.1 ml aliquots (5 x 10^5 cells per aliquot). An equal volume of appropriately diluted concanavalin A (con A; Calbiochem) or phytohemagglutinin-M (PHA; GIBCO) was added. For each mitogen concentration, triplicate reactions were performed. Unstimulated values, i.e., cells cultured without mitogens, were determined in 6 to 12 wells. Plates were incubated in a moist 5% CO_2 atmosphere for 72 hours. Twenty-four hours prior to harvesting, cells were exposed to 1 μCi of ^{3}H-thymidine (New England Nuclear; specific activity of 20 Ci/mMole). Cells were harvested onto glass-fibre filters using a multiple automated sample harvester (MASH-I; Microbiological Associates). The filters were allowed to air-dry prior to counting on a Beckman Liquid Scintillation Counter (model LS3155T). Values are expressed as net cpm, i.e., cpm for cells exposed to mitogens minus the cpm for cells cultured without mitogens or as a ratio of stimulated to unstimulated counts.

RESULTS

As shown in Figure 1, the incidence of DMBA-induced mammary carcinoma was dependent on the quantity and quality of fat in the diets on

Figure 1—PERCENT OF RATS WITH TUMOR VS. TIME

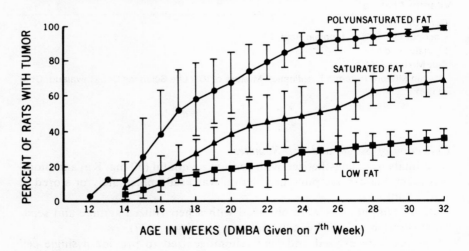

The percent of rats with tumor is shown as a function of the age of rats. Rats were maintained on one of three diets starting on day 21 and exposed to DMBA on day 50. Three experiments were done and each dietary group consisted of 30 to 32 rats per experiment. The data from 90 to 96 rats per dietary group is expressed as the mean tumor incidence of the three experiments ± the standard error.

20

which these rats were maintained. While the variability in tumor incidence from experiment to experiment was considerable during the early stages of tumor growth, all groups were more similar during the later stages of tumor growth.

Spleen and blood lymphocytes from rats (on the low fat diet and the saturated fat diet) which did not develop tumors were evaluated for their blastogenic response to con A and PHA. These data indicated that lymphocytes from either source were responsive to these mitogens only when taken from rats which had been maintained on the low fat diet and which were not exposed to DMBA (Figures 2 and 3). Lymphocytes were not responsive if they were taken from: a) rats on the low fat diet exposed to DMBA, or b) rats maintained on the saturated fat diet, but not exposed to

Figure 2—RESPONSE OF SPLEEN LYMPHOCYTES TO MITOGENS

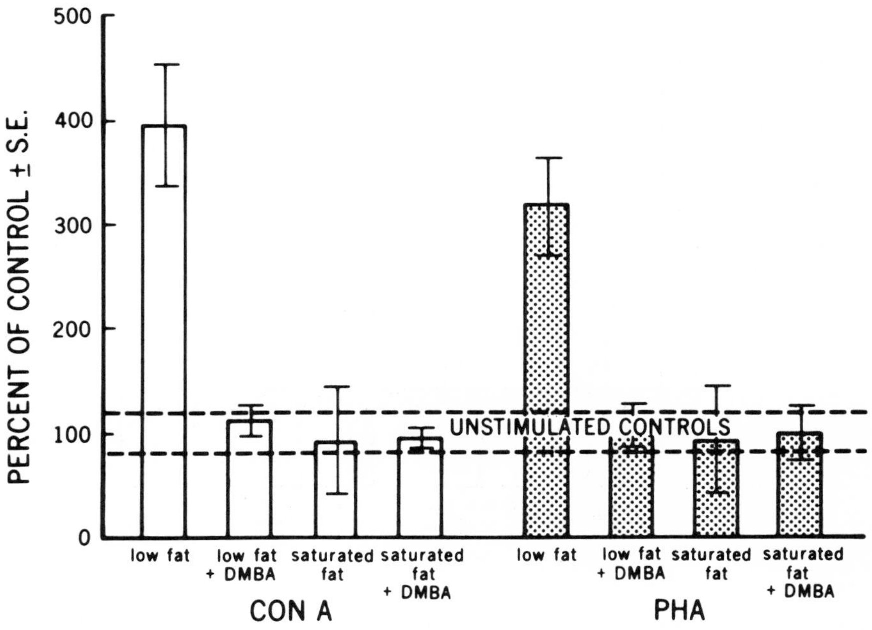

Some rats maintained on the low fat diet and the saturated fat diet did not develop tumor after exposure to DMBA. Spleen lymphocytes from these rats were cultured in autologous serum with con A and PHA and their response was compared to the response of lymphocytes taken from rats maintained on the same diet, but not exposed to DMBA. Rats were about one year old at the time of this study and each group contained from 6 to 12 rats.

Figure 3—RESPONSE OF BLOOD LYMPHOCYTES TO MITOGENS

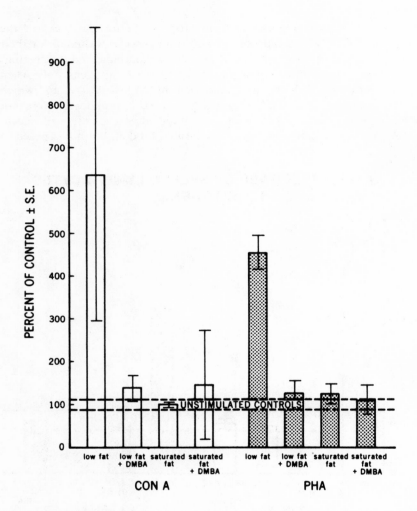

The blastogenic response of blood lymphocytes to con A and PHA, cultured in autologous serum, is shown for rats described in Figure 2. Each group consisted of 6 to 12 rats and these animals were about one year old at the time of this study.

DMBA. The combination of the saturated fat diet and DMBA also resulted in non-responsive lymphocytes.

22

Since lymphocytes from rats on the saturated fat diet were not responsive, studies were designed to determine if serum from these rats inhibited the blastogenic response of lymphocytes from rats on the low fat diet. Results, shown in Figure 4, indicated that when serum from animals on the saturated fat diet was diluted with serum from rats on the low fat diet, the response of the low fat lymphocyte increased. At the dilution of 1:16, the response was similar to that obtained using autologous serum or allogeneic serum from rats on the low fat diet. The possibility of serum deficiency was eliminated since both 2.5% and 5.0% low fat serum supported a good blastogenic

Figure 4—INDEX OF SERUM INHIBITION (LYMPHOCYTES FROM RATS ON LOW FAT DIET)

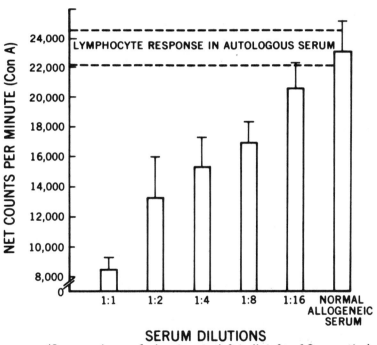

SERUM DILUTIONS
(Serum donor fed saturated fat diet for 10 months)

Spleen lymphocytes from rats on the low fat diet were cultured in autologous serum, allogeneic serum from rats on the low fat diet, and in serum from rats on the saturated fat diet which was diluted with allogeneic low fat serum. Triplicate cultures were done using two concentrations of con A. The mean of these six values ±the standard error is shown for all allogeneic serum. The range of values for six cultures is shown for autologous serum.

response, while the mixture of 2.5% low fat serum and 2.5% saturated fat serum inhibited the blastogenic response.

Figure 5 illustrates tumor incidence in rats immunized with MER or treated with vehicle prior to exposure to DMBA. Both groups were maintained on the polyunsaturated fat diet. The number of tumors in each of these groups is shown in Figure 6. These data indicate that MER reduced tumor incidence in the population and also limited the number of tumors in tumor-bearing rats.

Figure 5—PERCENT OF RATS WITH TUMOR VS. TIME AFTER DMBA (POLYUNSATURATED FAT DIET)

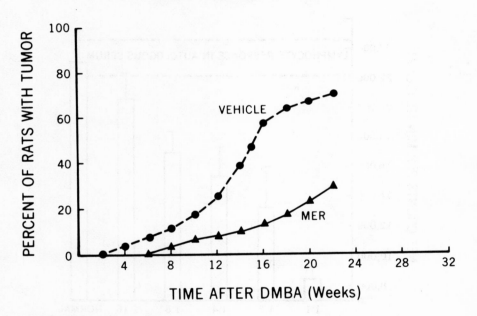

Percent of rats with tumor is shown as a function of time after exposure to DMBA. Rats were maintained on the 20% polyunsaturated fat diet starting on day 21 and immunized with MER or treated with vehicle on days 28 and 35. DMBA was given on day 50. Each group consisted of 30 to 32 rats.

A similar protective effect of MER was observed for rats maintained on the saturated fat diet. The percent of rats with tumor and the number of tumors per group were reduced in rats immunized with MER compared to rats treated with vehicle as shown in Figures 7 and 8.

24

Figure 6—TOTAL NUMBER OF TUMORS VS. TIME AFTER DMBA (POLYUNSATURATED FAT DIET)

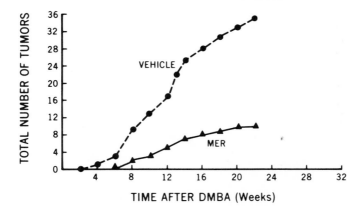

The number of tumors per group is shown as a function of time after exposure to DMBA. Rats were maintained on the 20% polyunsaturated fat diet starting on day 21 and immunized with MER or treated with vehicle on days 28 and 35. DMBA was given on day 50. Each group consisted of 30 to 32 rats.

Figure 7—PERCENT OF RATS WITH TUMOR VS. TIME AFTER DMBA (SATURATED FAT DIET)

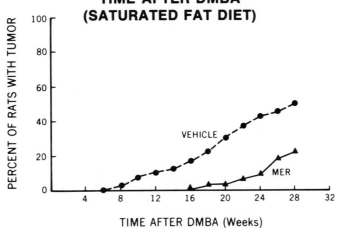

Percent of rats with tumor is shown as a function of time after exposure to DMBA. Rats were maintained on the 20% saturated fat diet starting on day 21 and immunized with MER or treated with vehicle on days 28 and 35. DMBA was given on day 50. Each group consisted of 30 to 32 rats.

25

Figure 8—TOTAL NUMBER OF TUMORS VS. TIME
AFTER DMBA
(SATURATED FAT DIET)

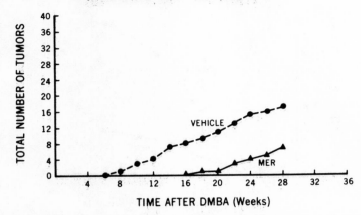

The number of tumors per group is shown as a function of time after exposure to DMBA. Rats were maintained on the 20% saturated fat diet starting on day 21 and immunized with MER or treated with vehicle on days 28 and 35. DMBA was given on day 50. Each group consisted of 30 to 32 rats.

Figure 9—PERCENT OF RATS WITH TUMOR VS.
TIME AFTER DMBA
(LOW FAT DIET)

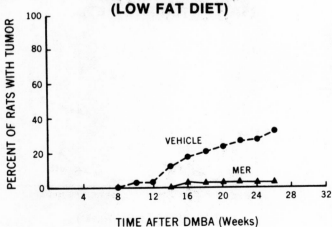

Percent of rats with tumor is shown as a function of time after exposure to DMBA. Rats were maintained on the 2% low fat diet starting on day 21 and immunized with MER or treated with vehicle on days 28 and 35. DMBA was given on day 50. Each group consisted of 30 to 32 rats.

26

In terms of an absolute effect, MER was most beneficial when given to rats on the low fat diet. A single tumor developed in only one of the MER-treated rats as illustrated in Figures 9 and 10.

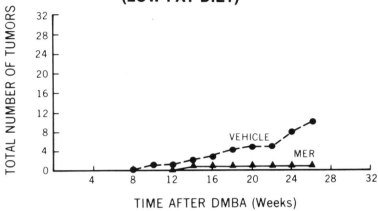

Figure 10—TOTAL NUMBER OF TUMORS VS. TIME AFTER DMBA (LOW FAT DIET)

The number of tumors per group is shown as a function of time after exposure to DMBA. Rats were maintained on the 2% fat diet starting on day 21 and immunized with MER or treated with vehicle on days 28 and 35. DMBA was given on day 50. Each group consisted of 30 to 32 rats.

Table 2 shows the distribution of tumor weight in tumor-bearing rats maintained on different diets. Tumors which appeared in the rats immunized with MER tended to be smaller when compared to tumors taken from rats treated with vehicle.

Table 2—DISTRIBUTION OF TUMOR WEIGHT

Diet	0-20 grams	20-40 grams	40-60 grams	60-80 grams	80-100 grams
Polyunsaturated					
MER	6	1	2	1	0
Vehicle	18	7	0	5	5
Saturated					
MER	7	0	0	0	0
Vehicle	3	5	5	3	1
Low Fat					
MER	1	0	0	0	0
Vehicle	3	4	1	0	0

27

The blastogenic response of spleen lymphocytes taken from rats on different diets is shown in Figure 11. Lymphocytes were cultured in autologous serum and stimulated with con A. These data suggested a relationship between lymphocyte function and tumor incidence. Rats on the polyunsaturated fat diet had the least functional lymphocytes and the highest incidence of tumors. Rats on the low fat diet had the most functional lymphocytes and the lowest incidence of tumors. Lymphocyte response was similar when autologous serum was compared to allogeneic serum taken from rats on the same fat diet.

Figure 11—EFFECT OF DIET ON MITOGEN INDUCED LYMPHOCYTE BLASTOGENESIS

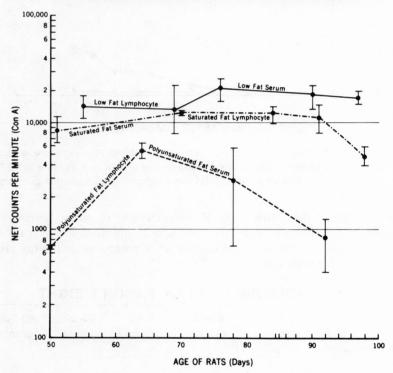

Lymphocytes from spleens of rats maintained on different diets were cultured in autologous serum and stimulated with con A using concentrations of 4 and 8 μg/ml. Triplicate cultures were done at each concentration. The average cpm of six non-stimulated cultures was substrated from the average value of the six stimulated cultures to determine the net cpm for a single rat. Three rats were used at each time point and the data is expressed as the average value and the range of response for each group of lymphocyte cultures.

28

However, when lymphocytes from rats on the polyunsaturated fat diet were cultured in allogeneic serum taken from rats on the low fat diet, responsiveness was increased. Figure 12 shows the response of poly-unsaturated fat lymphocytes in polyunsaturated fat serum and in low fat serum. While these lymphocytes responded better in low fat serum, they did

Figure 12—EFFECT OF HIGH POLYUNSATURATED FAT DIET ON MITOGEN INDUCED LYMPHOCYTE BLASTOGENESIS (NOT IMMUNIZED)

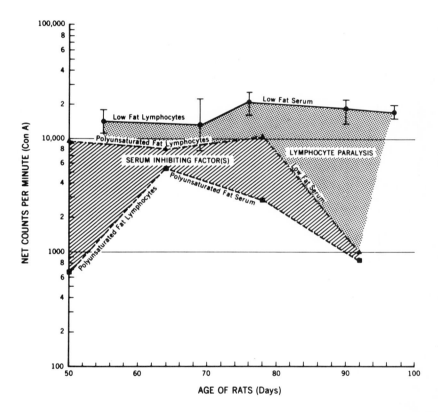

Lymphocytes from spleens of rats on the polyunsaturated fat diet were cultured in allogeneic serum and stimulated with con A using concentrations of 4 and 8 µg/ml. Allogeneic serum was taken from rats on the polyunsaturated fat diet and from rats on the low fat diet. These responses are compared to the response of lymphocytes from rats on the low fat diet cultured in allogeneic serum taken from rats on the low fat diet. Three rats were used at each time point and the data is expressed as the average value for each group of lymphocyte cultures.

29

Figure 13—EFFECT OF HIGH POLYUNSATURATED FAT DIET ON MITOGEN INDUCED LYMPHOCYTE BLASTOGENESIS (IMMUNIZED WITH MER)

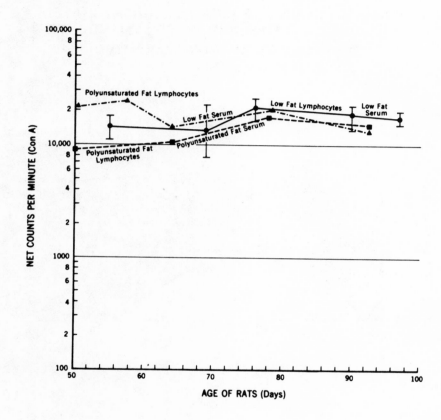

Rats were placed on the polyunsaturated fat diet on day 21 and immunized with MER on days 28 and 35. Lymphocytes from the spleens of these rats were cultured in allogeneic serum and stimulated with con A using concentrations of 4 and 8 μg/ml. Allogeneic serum was taken from immunized rats on the polyunsaturated fat diet and from non-immunized rats on the low fat diet. Responses of these lymphocytes are compared to the responses of lymphocytes from non-immunized rats on the low fat diet cultures in allogeneic serum taken from rats on the low fat diet. Three rats were used at each time point and the data is expressed as the average value for each group of lymphocyte cultures.

30

not respond as well as low fat lymphocytes in low fat serum. Collectively these data along with earlier observations suggested that lymphocyte response was limited by serum factors. Response was partially reversible in younger rats (less than 78 days old) and much less reversible in older rats (more than 78 days old).

In contrast to these observations, lymphocytes from immunized rats were highly responsive even though these rats were maintained on the polyunsaturated fat diet. Figure 13 illustrates that the response of lymphocytes from immunized rats maintained on the polyunsaturated fat diet was not improved by culturing in the low fat serum. Furthermore, the response of these lymphocytes in either serum compared favorably with the response of low fat lymphocytes in low fat serum.

In order to determine if immunization with MER minimized serum inhibiting factors, lymphocytes from rats on the low fat diet were cultured in serum from rats fed the 20% polyunsaturated fat diet which had been immunized with MER or treated with vehicle. Both 78 and 92 day serum was evaluated and compared to the response obtained in autologous serum. Results shown in Table 3 indicate that serum from immunized rats contained less inhibiting factor when compared to the non-immunized group.

Table 3—RESPONSE OF LOW FAT LYMPHOCYTES IN POLYUNSATURATED FAT SERUM*

78 DAY SERUM		92 DAY SERUM	
Rats Given Vehicle	Rats Given MER	Rats Given Vehicle	Rats Given MER
31	66	36	98
27	60	29	96
11	58	24	95

*Shown as percent response in autologous low fat serum. Serum from 3 rats was evaluated from each group at both time intervals.

DISCUSSION

Immunization with MER prior to exposure to DMBA reduced the incidence and/or retarded the development of mammary carcinoma in the Sprague-Dawley female rat. This observation was independent of the dietary state and consistent with results recently reported by Weislow, et al. (30) who were able to protect rats against this tumor using a Xenotropic type C virus. While both studies were done using the same model, neither study was designed to develop an optimal immunization schedule which would provide the maximum amount of protection. Based on results from therapeutic studies, it is clear that dose, route, and schedule are important factors in providing optimal benefit from immunostimulants (31-36). The data from Weislow, et al. is consistent with this view since the protective effect they observed was dependent on when virus was given. However, their data does not indicate whether the age of rats or the interval between immunization and exposure to DMBA was the critical factor.

While our data supports a correlation between lymphocyte reactivity and tumor incidence, we are not suggesting that loss of lymphocyte function is the critical or primary lesion of the immune system. Serum factors which inhibit lymphocytes may also inhibit other lymphoid cells or other lymphoid cells may be regulated by other factors (37). Preliminary studies done in collaboration with Dr. David Talmage (University of Colorado) indicate that macrophages were activated using serum from rats fed the low fat diet, but were not activated using serum from rats maintained on the high fat diets. Furthermore, the extent to which communication between macrophages and lymphocytes is inhibited by high fat diets is not known.

The observation that the responsiveness of lymphocytes depends on the source of serum, and that serum which does not promote blastogenesis is not deficient, supports the presence of suppressive factors whose influence was minimized by dilution. The responsiveness of polyunsaturated fat lymphocytes in low fat serum depended on when lymphocytes were studied. Lymphocytes taken from rats after prolonged exposure to the polyunsaturated fat diet were less responsive in low fat serum compared to lymphocytes taken after feeding this diet for a limited time. While it is not known if structural components of the lymphocyte membrane are changed with time, it is clear that the saturated fatty acids are important structural components of the lipids of the cell membrane (38-41). Hence, lack of lymphocyte function in serum from rats on the low fat diet may reflect changes in the structural components of the cell membrane.

While the relationship between serum suppressive factors and immunostimulants has not been established, our data indicate that suppressive factors were minimized in rats immunized with MER. Serum from these rats (maintained on the polyunsaturated fat diet) supported a good response of both autologous lymphocytes and lymphocytes from rats on the low fat diet. In addition, preliminary evidence indicates that non-immunized rats on the polyunsaturated fat diet had elevated levels of very low density lipoprotein in their serum when compared to immunized rats on the same diet and to rats on the low fat diet. While these lipoproteins have not been identified as the suppressive factor, other studies indicate that these lipoproteins inhibit lymphocyte response. Plasma from patients with type IV or type V hyperlipoproteinemia has elevated levels of very low density lipoprotein and this plasma inhibited lymphocyte stimulation by lectins and by allogeneic cells (42).

32

While elevated levels of lipoprotein and/or changes in the relative amount of each lipoprotein class may inhibit functions of lymphoid cells, other changes induced by MER are probably involved. Rats on the low fat diet apparently do not have changes in serum lipoproteins and yet are susceptible to DMBA induced tumors. The mechanism by which MER protects these animals is not known. MER may also elevate the number of lymphoid cells and thereby minimize the absolute cell killing which follows exposure to DMBA (43). Studies in progress are designed to determine how cell number and function are influenced by immunization with MER.

REFERENCES

1. Carroll, K.K., Gammal, E.B. and Plunkett, E.R., "Dietary Fat and Mammary Cancer." *Canad. Med. Ass. J.* 98: 590-594, 1968.
2. Drasar, B.S. and Irving, D., "Environmental Factors and Cancer of the Colon and Breast." *Brit. J. Cancer* 27:167-172, 1973.
3. Lea, A.J., "Dietary Factors Associated With Death-Rates From Certain Neoplasms in Man." *Lancet* ii: 332-333, 1966.
4. Lea, A.J., "Neoplasms and Environmental Factors." *Ann. Roy. Coll. Surg. Engl.* 41: 432-438, 1967.
5. Wynder, E.L., "Current Concepts of the Aetiology of Breast Cancer." In *Prognostic Factors in Breast Cancer, Proc. 1st Tenovus Symp.* Edited by Forrest and Kunkler, 32-49, Livingstone, Edinburgh 1968.
6. Wynder, E.L., "Identification of Women at High Risk from Breast Cancer." *Cancer, Philad.* 24: 1235-1240, 1969.
7. Tannenbaum, A., "The Genesis and Growth of Tumors. III. Effects of a High-Fat Diet." *Cancer Res.* 2: 468-475, 1942.
8. Tannenbaum, A., "The Dependence of Tumor Formation on the Composition of the Calorie-Restricted Diet as Well as on the Degree of Restriction." *Cancer Res.* 5: 616-625, 1945.
9. Silverstone, H. and Tannenbaum, A., "The Effect of the Proportion of Dietary Fat on the Rate of Formation of Mammary Carcinoma in Mice." *Cancer Res.* 10: 448-453, 1950.
10. Carroll, K.K. and Khor, H.T., "Effects of Dietary Fat and Dose Level of 7, 12-Dimethylbenz(α)Anthracene on Mammary Tumor Incidence in Rats." *Cancer Res.* 30: 2260-2264, 1970.
11. Carroll, K.K. and Khor, H.T., "Effects of Level and Type of Dietary Fat on Incidence of Mammary Tumors Induced in Female Sprague-Dawley Rats by 7, 12-dimethylbenz(α) Anthracene." *Lipids* 6: 415-420, 1971.
12. Gammal, E.B., Carroll, K.K. and Plunkett, E.R., "Effects of Dietary Fat on Mammary Carcinogenesis by 7, 12-Dimethylbenz(α)Anthracene in Rats." *Cancer Res.* 27: 1737-1742, 1967.
13. King, M.M., Bailey, D.M., Gibson, D.D., et al., "The Incidence and Growth of Mammary Tumor Induced by 7, 12-Dimethylbenz(α)Anthracene as Related to the Dietary Content of Fat and Antioxidant." Submitted to *J. Natl. Can. Inst.*
14. Gammal, E.B., Carroll, K.K. and Plunkett, E.R., "Effects of Dietary Fat on the Uptake and Clearance of 7, 12-Dimethylbenz(α)Anthracene by Rat Mammary Tissue." *Cancer Res.* 28: 384-385, 1968.

15. Mertin, J. and Hunt, R., "Influence of Polyunsaturated Fatty Acids on Survival of Skin Allografts and Tumor Incidence in Mice." *Proc. Natl. Acad. Sci., USA* 73: 928-931, 1976.

16. Mertin, J., "Effect of Polyunsaturated Fatty Acids on Skin Allograft Survival and Primary and Secondary Cytotoxic Response in Mice." *Transplantation* 21: 1-4, 1976.

17. Ring, J., Seifert, J., Mertin, J. and Brendel, W., "Prolongation of Skin Allografts in Rats by Treatment with Linoleic Acid." *Lancet* 2: 1331, 1974.

18. Hughes, D., Caspary, E.A. and Wisniewski, H.M., "Immunosuppression by Linoleic Acid." *Lancet* 2: 501-502, 1975.

19. Uldall, P.R., Wilkinson, R., McHugh, M.I., et al., "Linoleic Acid and Transplantation." *Lancet* 2: 128-129, 1975.

20. Uldall, P.R., Wilkinson, R., McHugh, M.I., et al., "Unsaturated Fatty Acids and Renal Transplantation." *Lancet* 2: 514, 1974.

21. Mertin, J., "Unsaturated Fatty Acids and Renal Transplantation." *Lancet* 2: 717, 1974.

22. McHugh, M.I., Wilkinson, R., Elliott, R.W., et al., "Immunosuppression with Polyunsaturated Fatty Acids in Renal Transplantation." *Transplantation* 24: 263-267, 1977.

23. Mertin, J., Hughes, D., Shenton, B.K. and Dickenson, J.P., "*In Vitro* Inhibition of Unsaturated Fatty Acids of the PPD- and PHA-Induced Lymphocyte Response." *Klin. Wochenschr.* 52: 248-250, 1974.

24. Mertin, J. and Hughes, D., "Specific Inhibitory Action of Polyunsaturated Fatty Acids in Lymphocyte Transformation Induced by PHA and PPD." *Int. Arch. Allergy Appl. Immunol.* 48: 203-210, 1975.

25. Offner, H. and Clausen, J., "Inhibition of Lymphocyte Response to Stimulants Induced by Unsaturated Fatty Acids and Prostaglandins." *Lancet* 2: 400-401, 1974.

26. Mertin, J., "Polyunsaturated Fatty Acids and Cancer." *Brit. Med. J.* 4: 357, 1973.

27. Weyman, C., Belin, J., Smith, A.D. and Thompson, R.H.S., "Linoleic Acid as an Immunosuppressive Agent." *Lancet* 2: 33, 1975.

28. Morse, J.H., Witte, L.D. and Goodman, D.S., "Inhibition of Lymphocyte Proliferation Stimulation by Lectins and Allogeneic Cells by Normal Plasma Lipoproteins." *J. Expt. Med.* 146: 1791-1803, 1977.

29. Hayward, J., *Cancer.* Springer-Verlag, New York, 1-149, 1970.

30. Weislow, O.S., Allen, P.T., Shepherd, R.E., et al., "Protection Against 7, 12-Dimethylbenz(α)Anthracene Induced Rat Mammary Carcinoma by Infection with Mouse Xenotropic Type C Virus." *J. Natl. Cancer Inst.* 61: 123-129, 1978.

31. Amiel, J.L. and Berardet, M., "Factor Time for Active Immunotherapy after Cytoreductive Chemotherapy." *Europ. J. Cancer* 10: 89-91, 1974.

32. Currie, G.A. and Bagshawe, K.D., "Active Immunotherapy with *Corynebacterium Parvum* and Chemotherapy in Murine Fibrosarcomas." *Brit. Med. J.* 1: 541-544, 1970.

33 Kollmorgen, G.M., Killion, J.J., Sansing, W.A., et al., "Immunotherapy with Neuraminidase-Treated Cells and Bacillus Calmette-Guerin." *Surgery* 79: 202-208, 1976.

34. Kollmorgen, G.M., Cox, D.C., Killion, J.J., et al., "Immunotherapy of EL4 Lymphoma with Reovirus." *Immunology and Immunotherapy* 1: 239-244, 1976.

35. Hawrylko, E. and Machaness, G.B., "Immunopotentiation with BCG: IV Factors Affecting the Magnitude of an Anti-tumor Response." *J. Natl. Cancer Inst.* 51: 1683-1688, 1973.

36. Zbar, B. and Tanaka, T., "Immunotherapy of Cancer: Regression of Tumors after Intralesional Injection of Living *Mycobacterium bovis.*" *Science* 172: 271-273, 1971.

37. Tomasi, T.B., Jr., "Serum Factors Which Suppress the Immune Response." In 11th Leukocyte Culture Conference entitled, *Regulatory Mechanisms and Lymphocyte Activation,* edited by D.O. Lucas, Academic Press, 219-250, 1977.

38. Walker, B.L. and Kummerow, F.A., "Dietary Fat and the Structure and Properties of Rat Erythrocytes. I. Effect of Dietary Fat on the Erythrocyte Lipids."*J. Nutr.* 81: 75-80, 1963.

39. Walker, B.L. and Kummerow, F.A., "Dietary Fat and the Structure and Properties of Rat Erythrocytes. III. Response of Erythrocyte Fatty Acids to Various Dietary Fats." *J. Nutr.* 82: 329-332, 1964.

40. Bloj, B., Morero, R.D., Farias, R.N. and Trucco, R.E., "Allosteric Behaviour of Erythrocyte Mg²ATPase, (NA⁺+K⁺)-ATPase and Acetylcholinesterase from Rats Fed Different Fat-Supplemented Diets." *Biochem. Biophys. Acta.* 311: 67-79, 1973.

41. Witting, L.A., Harvey, C.C., Century, B. and Horwitt, M.K., "Dietary Alterations of Fatty Acids of Erythrocytes and Mitochondria of Brain and Liver." *J. Lipid Res.* 2: 412-418, 1961.

42. Waddell, C.C., Taunton, O.D. and Twomey, J.J., "Inhibition of Lympho-Proliferation by Hyperlipoproteinemic Plasma." *J. Clin. Invest.* 58: 950-954, 1976.

43. Bansal, M.P., Kanwar, K.C. and Kalla, N.R., "Dimethylbenz(α)Anthracene—Radiation Synergism in the Induction of Leukemia in Mice: Biochemial Analysis of Leukemia Bone Marrow and Blast Cells." *Indian J. Exptl. Biology* 16: 145-147, 1978.

Serological Studies of Surface Antigens of Murine B16 Melanoma as Detected by Xenoantisera*

John J. Marchalonis[1]
D.M. Gersten[2]

SUMMARY—Melanomas are antigenic and induce the formation of antibodies in both syngeneic and xenogeneic species. The nature of melanoma-associated antigens remains problematic, however. We found that xenogeneic (goat) antiserum to the murine (C57BL/6) melanoma B16, following appropriate absorptions with nonmelanoma cells, showed specificity for melanoma-associated surface antigens of B16 and one other murine melanoma. The reactivity was shown using complement-dependent cytotoxicity assays and direct binding as assessed by use of radioiodinated *Staphylococcus aureus* protein A as the developing reagent. Studies with various tumor lines provided serological evidence that the antibody to B16 did not react with histocompatibility antigens, mouse-specific xenoantigens, viral antigens or melanin. The IgG fraction of the goat antibody was bound covalently to protein A-Sepharose using the cross-linker dimethyl-suberimidate. This immunoadsorbent was used to isolate antigens from culture fluid in which B16 cells had been grown and from detergent extracts of biosynthetically labeled (^{3}H-leucine) B16 cells. The immune-affinity purified antigen preparation contained two major components of apparent mass 60,000 and 50,000 daltons as assessed by polyacrylamide gel electrophoresis in sodium dodecyl sulfate-containing buffers and a minor component of approximate mass 20,000 daltons. Immunization of rabbits with immune-affinity purified B16 antigens induced antibodies in rabbits which bound specifically to B16 cells. Studies of the antigenic and structural properties of these molecules are in progress.

INTRODUCTION

Studies of both human (1-3) and murine (4) melanomas show that these tumors are immunogenic and possess antigens which can be demonstrated using syngeneic and xenogeneic antisera. The nature of the melanoma-associated antigens is problematic, however, and questions can arise whether or not such antigens are of viral origin (murine systems), are

[1]Head, Cell Biology and Biochemistry Section, Cancer Biology Program, NCI, Frederick Cancer Research Center, Frederick, Maryland.
[2]Department of Pathology, Georgetown University School of Medicine and Dentistry, Washington, D.C.
*Research sponsored by the National Cancer Institute under Contract No. NO1-CO-75380 with Litton Bionetics, Inc.

associated with markers of the histocompatibility complex, are oncofetal or are strictly associated with melanomas. In the present study we report results of serological and biochemical investigations using xenogeneic antiserum to the murine B16 melanoma. We provide evidence that appropriately absorbed antibody produced by immunized goats can recognize a melanoma-associated antigen or antigens which are serologically distinguishable from murine xenoantigens, histocompatibility complex antigens, viral antigens and melanin. In addition, we report partial characterization of antigenic proteins produced by the B16 melanoma.

MATERIALS AND METHODS

Animals, Cells and Cell Culture

Inbred C57BL/6 mice were obtained from the Experimental Animal Production Area, Frederick Cancer Research Center, Frederick, Maryland. Tumor cells, unless otherwise specified, were maintained as monolayer cultures or complete minimum essential medium supplemented with 10% fetal calf serum as described previously (5). The tumor cells used are as follows: B16 melanoma variants, FO, FO-U1, FO-U2, F10, F10^{Lr}, obtained from Dr. I.J. Fidler; melanoma 1735 Mel 8, ultraviolet light induced fibrosarcomas UV-112 and 2237, obtained from Dr. M.L. Kripke; AKR low-passage fibroblasts, AKR adenocarcinoma, and DMBAII fibrosarcoma, obtained from Dr. I.J. Fidler. The relevant characteristics of these cells are given in Table 1.

Goats and Immunization

The B16 melanoma, syngeneic to the C57BL/6 mouse, was grown *in vivo* following subcutaneous (s.c.) inoculation. When tumors reached a size of 1.5-2.5 cm they were removed aseptically, minced in cold Hanks' balanced salt solution (HBSS) and dispersed mechanically to prepare single cell suspension. Cell viability as measured by the trypan blue exclusion assay ranged from 25-35%. The cell suspension was mixed with Complete Freund's Adjuvant (CFA) at 4:1 ratio. Each goat was injected intradermally (i.d.) at 4 different sites with 0.5 ml of cell:CFA mixture. A total volume of viable cells injected per goat was 2 x 10^7. Two weeks later, the injection of 2 x 10^7 viable cells/goat was repeated without CFA. Seven days thereafter, each goat was injected intravenously (i.v.) with 1 x 10^6 viable cells and bled 2 weeks later. Thereafter goats were given a booster injection i.v. of 1 x 10^6 viable cells and were bled on alternate weeks (total of 3 bleedings). The serum was passed through a 0.2 μM Millipore filter and frozen in liquid nitrogen until absorption. This method is similar to that described for production of goat-anti-mouse macrophage serum (6).

38

Growth and Fixation of EL-4 Cells for Absorption of Antisera

EL-4 lymphoma cells, syngeneic to C57BL/6 mice, were grown at 37°C in specimen culture to early stationary phase in RPMI-1640 medium supplemented per liter with 100 ml fetal calf serum (Flow Labs, Rockville, MD), 10 ml sodium pyruvate, 10 ml nonessential amino acids, 10 ml penicillin-streptomycin, 10 ml glutamine, 20 ml MEM vitamins (Grand Island Biological, Grand Island, NY). The cells were harvested by centrifugation at 350 x g and washed 3 times in phosphate buffered saline (PBS) consisting of 0.145 M NaCl, .02 M phosphate, pH 7.4. The cells were then fixed with 0.5% glutaraldehyde in PBS for 1 hr at 4°C. Following the fixation, the cells were washed 3 times in PBS as above and stored until use in PBS + 0.1% NaN_3 at 4°C.

Absorption of Sera

A pellet of 1 x 10^9 glutaraldehyde-fixed EL-4 cells is prepared by being washed 3 times in a solution of 1 mg/ml fraction V bovine serum albumin (BSA) (Sigma Chemical Co., St. Louis, MO). Five ml of goat anti-B16 melanoma or goat anti-UV-112 fibrosarcoma was diluted with 20 ml of PBS and added to the EL-4 pellet. The suspension was incubated for 1 hr at 37°C then 2 hr at 4°C, centrifuged at 500 x g and the supernatant was retained for testing. This cycle was repeated until no anti-C57BL/6 erythrocyte activity (below) was observed. Two to four absorptions were routinely necessary.

Complement-Dependent Cytotoxicity

Once the absorbed antisera demonstrated no complement-dependent lysis of C57BL/6 erythrocytes, their specificity was assessed using the various tumor targets listed above. The cytotoxicity was determined using a Coulter counter assay described previously (7) and verified by a direct binding measurement described below.

Target cells were harvested by brief trypsinization from the monolayer, washed twice in HBSS (Grand Island Biological), and resuspended at a concentration of approximately 1 x 10^6/ml. One-tenth ml of cell suspension was mixed with 0.1 ml of antiserum appropriately diluted in PBS and incubated at 37°C in a 12 x 75mm polypropylene tube. The suspension was agitated every 10 min to prevent the cells from plating out on the walls of the tube. After 30 min, 0.02 ml of freshly thawed guinea pig complement was added and the incubation was continued for an additional 4-5 min. The interaction was terminated by moving the cells to an ice bath while maintaining the agitation at 10 min intervals. The cells were washed from the incubation tubes with 10 ml of counting electrolyte and the cell numbers were determined. The counting electrolyte was "Isoton" (Coulter Electronics, Hialeah, FL). The Coulter counter, model ZBI was fitted with an 100 μ aperture and the setting of the lower threshold descriminator was varied according to the target cell used. The data represent the means of duplicate observations of duplicate determinations of at least two separate experiments. Percent cytotoxicity was calculated by subtracting the number of cells remaining in the incubation tube following antiserum treatment from the number of cells in the PBS blank divided by the number of cells in the PBS blank.

Antibody Binding Assay

Goat IgG was purified from the absorbed serum by affinity chromatography on a column of protein A-Sepharose (Pharmacia Fine Chemicals, Piscataway, NJ) as described previously (8). B16-F10 or UV-112 were inoculated into a 96 well microtest plate (Falcon Plastics, Oxnard, CA) at a concentration of 1-10 x 10^3 cells/0.2 ml/2311 and allowed to grow to confluency. The wells were washed twice with PBS and the monolayers fixed to the plastic with glutaraldehyde according to the method of Segal and Klinman (9). The fixation solution was 0.1 M potassium phosphate buffer pH 7.0 to which glutaraldehyde was added to a final concentration of 0.15% (W/V). After 5 min incubation at room temperature, the wells were washed twice with a solution of fraction V BSA, 1.0 mg/ml containing 0.1% NaN_3. The plates were stored at 4°C until use.

Immediately prior to use, the plates were warmed to room temperature and the wells were washed twice with PBS to remove residual BSA and NaN_3. Fifty μl of appropriately diluted IgG were overlaid on the monolayer and incubated for 2 hr at room temperature. The wells were washed twice more with PBS and overlaid with 100 μl of protein A from *S. aureus* which had been prelabeled with ^{125}I by the chloramine T method (10). The protein A solution contained 100-200 mg protein A/ml in 1 mg/ml BSA. Following overnight incubation of the plates at 4°C, unbound radioactivity was removed by two washes in PBS. The monolayers were harvested and counted for radioactivity in a Searle model 1185 gamma counter equipped with a 2 x 2-inch well-type NaI (T1) detector.

Immunoadsorbents and Isolation of Antigen

The IgG fraction of normal goat serum, goat antiserum to UV-112 or absorbed antiserum to B16 was coupled covalently to a matrix of *S. aureus* protein A-Sepharose as described elsewhere (11). Briefly, 5 ml of serum was reacted with 3 ml of swollen protein A-Sepharose and washed exhaustively with PBS. The bound IgG was covalently coupled to the matrix using the cross-linker dimethylsumberimidate. The immunoadsorbent was used as a column. A sample was loaded and washed through with PBS until protein absorbance at A_{280} or ^{125}I-radioactivity fell to background levels. Specifically bound material was eluted with 0.01 *M* acetic acid/0.15 *M* NaCl. This immunoadsorbent was used in the isolation of melanoma-associated antigens from (a) "shed" surface material released *in vitro* by cells growing in monolayers, (b) Triton X-100 extracts of B16 cells in monolayers and (c)

40

Triton X-100 extracts of B16 cells biosynthetically labeled with ^{3}H-leucine. In the first case, 4 tissue culture flasks, each containing 15 x 10^6 cells, were washed to remove medium. Twenty-five ml serum-free Eagle's Minimal Essential Medium was added to each flask, and these were incubated 16 hr at 37°C. The supernatant was removed, dialyzed against distilled H$_2$O and lyophilized. Each cell layer was then extracted with 10 ml of 0.1% Triton X-100 in PBS for 1 hr at room temperature. Cell debris was removed by centrifugation. In the biosynthetic incorporation experiment, 8 x 10^6 cells as a subconfluent monolayer were incubated 24 hr at 37°C in the presence of 10 ml of leucine-free RPMI 1640 medium which contained 100 μCi ^{3}H-leucine and 2% fetal calf serum. The monolayer was extracted with 10 ml of 0.1% Triton X-100, as above. Control "shed" culture fluids and Triton X-100 extracts were prepared from cultures of the UV-induced fibrosarcoma UV-112. A control immunoadsorbent was prepared in a similar fashion using normal goat serum which had been absorbed with the lymphoma EL-4. In some experiments, the "shed" material was radio-iodinated with ^{125}I-iodide using the chloramine-T method (10) to allow rapid quantitative monitoring.

Immunization of Rabbits

Rabbits were immunized using the immune-affinity isolated melanoma antigen preparation isolated from material released into serum-free medium. The fraction was eluted from the immunoadsorbent using acetic acid (0.01 M)/saline (0.15 M), dialyzed against PBS and passed through protein A-Sepharose to remove γ-globulin which might have eluted from the matrix. Two rabbits were each given 2 injections consisting of 200 μg of purified antigen preparation. The first injection was given in complete Freund's adjuvant, the second was given 3 weeks later using incomplete Freund's adjuvant. Serum was obtained two weeks following the second injection. In addition, serum samples were prepared prior to immunization.

Polyacrylamide Gel Electrophoresis in Sodium Dodecyl Sulfate (SDS)-Containing Buffers

This was essentially the method of Laemmli and Favre (12) using conditions and standards described in detail previously (13).

RESULTS

Serological Demonstration of Antibodies to Melanoma Antigens

Goat antiserum to B16 melanoma was absorbed with fixed EL-4 lymphoma cells until no complement-dependent hemolysis was observed against C57BL/6 erythrocytes. The absorbed antiserum was then titrated for complement-dependent cytotoxic activity against B16 line F10 and against the syngeneic fibrosarcoma UV-112. As depicted in Figure 1, the antiserum showed strong lytic activity towards B16-F10 but no significant lysis of UV-112 was observed. A goat antiserum made against UV-112 and absorbed with EL-4 was used to control for the susceptibility of B16-F10 to lysis with goat serum. Less than 15% lysis was observed at any concentra-

Figure 1—CYTOTOXICITY ASSAY OF GOAT ANTISERUM TO MURINE MELANOMA B16.

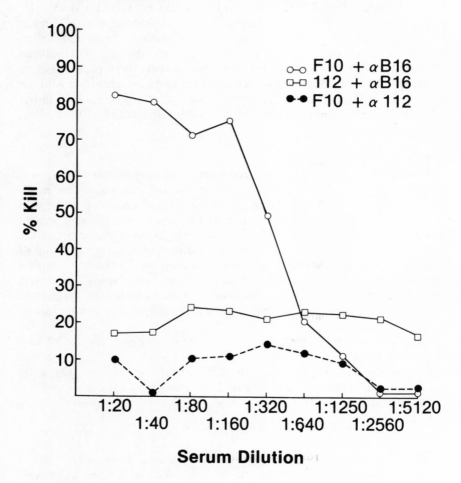

F10, B16 line F10; α B16, goat antiserum to B16, absorbed with the lymphoma EL-4; 112, fibrosarcoma UV-112, syngeneic to B16; α 112, goat antiserum to UV-112, absorbed with EL-4 cells. Assay was performed as described by Gately and Mayer (7).

tion. Based upon the titration curve in Figure 1, we chose an antiserum dilution of 1:100 in order to obtain further information regarding the specificity of the antiserum by assaying reactivity against various syngeneic, allogeneic and xenogeneic tumors. Table 1 presents cytotoxicity data obtained in these assays. Consistent with the titration data, only B16 lines are lysed by the antiserum. Although the UV-112 cells showed 11% lysis this is not a significant value because this tumor generally gives high background lysis which does not vary with antibody concentration. These data indicate that activity to B16 antigens is not directed against mouse-specific antigens, alloantigens or antigens specified by C-type viruses.

Table 1—SPECTRUM OF COMPLEMENT-MEDIATED CYTOTOXICITY AGAINST RODENT TARGETS BY GOAT ANTI-B16 MELANOMA ANTISERUM

Target Cell Designation (ref)	Strain of Origin	C-type[a] Virus	% Cyto-toxicity[b]
B16-F10 melanoma (5)	C57BL/6 mouse	positive	57 ± 6
B16-F10^{Lr-6} melanoma (18)	C57BL/6 mouse	positive	32 ± 3
UV-112 fibrosarcoma (19)	C57BL/6 mouse	negative	11 ± 2
UV-112 fibrosarcoma (19)	C57BL/6 mouse	positive	0 ± 0
UV-2237 fibrosarcoma (19)	C3H mouse	negative	3 ± 1
AKR low-passage fibroblasts (20)	AKR mouse	negative	4 ± 1
AKR adenocarcinoma (20)	AKR mouse	positive	0 ± 0
DMBAII fibrosarcoma (20)	F344 rat	negative	5 ± 1

[a]The presence of endogenous C-type virus (MuLV) was determined by radio-immune precipitation assay (20).

[b]Data represent mean ± standard error of pooled data of 2 experiments, each one carried out in triplicate. Data are rounded off to integral numbers.

To further refine quantitative assessment of the specificity of the goat antiserum to B16 melanoma, we devised a radioimmunoassay which measures directly the binding of IgG to the target cells. ^{125}I-labeled protein A of *S. aureus,* which recognizes the Fc portion of IgG molecules (14), was used to demonstrate bound antibody. As shown by the titration curve given in Figure 2, specific binding was observed with line B16-F10, but not with fibrosarcoma UV-112 (syngeneic to B16) or the allogenic fibrosarcoma UV-2237.

Further comparison data illustrating the capacity of several variant lines derived from B16 melanoma and melanoma 1735 syngeneic to the C3H mouse to bind goat anti-B16 melanoma antibodies are given in Table 2. All of the B16 sublines bound the antiserum, but quantitative variation was

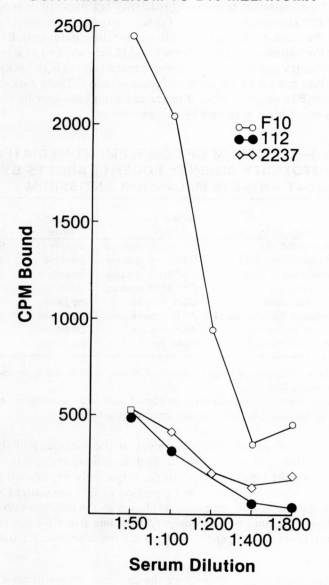

Figure 2—RADIOACTIVE BINDING ASSAY OF GOAT ANTISERUM TO B16 MELANOMA

F10
112
2237

Ordinate gives ¹²⁵I-radioactivity of Labeled *S. aureus* protein A used to detect the F_c region of cell-bound IgG. Absorbed α B16 was used. F10, B16 line F10; 112, UV-112, syngeneic to B16; 2237, UV-induced fibrosarcoma 2237, allogeneic (C3H) to B16.

apparent. For example, in three separate experiments the following quantitative order was observed: $F10 = F10^{Lr-6} > FO > FO - U_1 = FO - U_2$. Since $F_0 - U_1$ and $F_0 - U_2$ showed comparable binding and $F_0 - U_2$ is nonpigmented, it is unlikely that the antiserum is directed against melanin components. This result is consistent with the work of Cannon et al. (15) who report that extracts of melanotic and amelanotic melanoma cells give equal reactivity in cell-mediated immune reactions specific for human melanoma antigens. Binding, moreover, does not correlate with metastatic potential of B16 cells because F10 is highly metastatic, whereas $F10^{Lr-6}$ lacks the capacity to metastasize. Since line $F10^{Lr}$ is resistant to lysis by syngeneic lymphocytes and F10 is sensitive to killing by such lymphocytes, the possiblity arises that the goat antiserum, recognizes a murine melanoma surface determinant distinct from that to which syngeneic lymphocytes bind. Further evidence for this comes from the observation that the C3H melanoma 1735 bound a substantial quantity of antibody, whereas the C3H fibrosarcoma (UV-2237) exhibited no significant binding.

Table 2—BINDING OF GOAT ANTI-B16 MELANOMA ANTISERUM TO SURFACE OF MURINE MELANOMAS

Target Cell Designation	Origin	Description	CPM Bound[a]
B16-F0	C57BL/6	Parent tumor to which antiserum was raised, pigmented, low metastasis	1620 ± 40
B16-F0-U1	C57BL/6	Pigmented variant, low metastasis	1360 ± 130
B16-F0-U2	C57BL/6	Nonpigmented variant, low metastasis	1220 ± 130
B16-F10	C57BL/6	Selected *in vivo,* pigmented, high metastasis	2050 ± 180
B16-F10^{Lr}	C57BL/6	Selected *in vitro,* pigmented, resistant to lysis by syngeneic lymphocytes, low metastasis	1960 ± 180
UV-112	C57BL/6	Fibrosarcoma syngeneic to C57BL/6 mouse	330 ± 18
1735 Mel 8	C3H	Melanoma syngeneic to C3H mouse	1460 ± 170
UV-2237	C3H	Fibrosarcoma syngeneic to C3H mouse	405 ± 20

[a]Data represents mean ± S.E. of three observations in at least two separate experiments.

Partial Characterization of Melanoma-Associated Antigens

The preceding data indicated that goat antibodies to the B16 melanoma recognize melanoma-associated surface component(s) which are present on murine melanomas B16 and 1735. In order to obtain the melanoma-associated components for serological and biochemical characterization, we prepared immune-affinity reagents by coupling the IgG fraction of the goat antiserum to a Sepharose matrix. This was done by passing the antiserum through *S. aureus* protein A bound to Sepharose and then forming the covalent linkage using the cross-linking agent dimethylsuberimidate (11). Three preparations made from B16 and UV-112 cells were tested for the presence of components which bound specifically to the immunoadsorbent. In the first series of experiments, cells were washed free of fetal calf serum and allowed to shed membrane components into serum-free medium. The released material was dialyzed against distilled H_2O, freeze-dried and radioiodinated for binding studies. In a typical experiment using radioiodinated released material, no specific ^{125}I-labeled material was bound from the UV-112 preparation (830 cpm bound to the anti-B16 immunoadsorbent), whereas 1300 cpm bound to the normal goat IgG/protein A-Sepharose control. By contrast, 44,700 cpm from the B16 preparation bound to the anti-B16 immunoadsorbent, while 11,600 cpm bound to the normal goat IgG matrix. When analyzed by polyacrylamide gel electrophoresis under reducing conditions, three components were resolved in the specifically bound and eluted material as shown by both label and protein stain using the Comassie blue reagent. Figure 3 represents a polyacrylamide gel electrophoresis pattern of the stained antigen preparation isolated specifically from 17.2 mg of lyophilized B16 "shed" material. This pattern represents approximately 10 μg of antigen. The major component comprises two closely spaced bands having mobilities compatible with a mass of about 60,000 daltons. A minor bind of about 50,000 daltons is clearly present and a trace component is also seen in the vicinity of the 20,000-dalton marker. This preparation was used in studies involving immunization of rabbits (see below). No specific components were isolated from the UV-112 preparation (not shown).

The second preparation consisted of an unlabeled Triton X-100 lysate of B16 cells. As above, the major component specifically isolated showed a migration position compatible with a mass of 60,000-70,000 daltons. In the third series of experiments, B16 cells were cultured in the presence of ^{3}H-leucine to determine whether the putative melanoma-associated antigen was actually synthesized by the cells. B16 cells were incubated in media containing ^{3}H-leucine for 24 hr, washed and extracted with 0.1% Triton X-100. The lysate was reacted with the anti-B16 immuno-adsorbent and bound components were eluted with acetic acid/NaCl. The specifically eluted fraction contained two major components of approximate masses 68,000 and 48,000 daltons and a minor component of about 20,000 daltons. This result is consistent with those obtained above for the shed material and the cells extracted with Triton on a bulk basis.

In order to establish that the affinity-purified fraction contained specific B16-associated antigens, two rabbits were immunized with the putative

46

Figure 3—ANALYSIS BY POLYACRYLAMIDE GEL ELECTROPHORESIS IN SDS-CONTAINING BUFFER OF B16 MELANOMA-ASSOCIATED XENOANTIGEN PREPARATION ISOLATED BY IMMUNE AFFINITY CHROMATOGRAPHY ON GOAT ANTIBODY/SEPHAROSE FROM CULTURE FLUID OF *IN VITRO* GROWN B16 CELLS

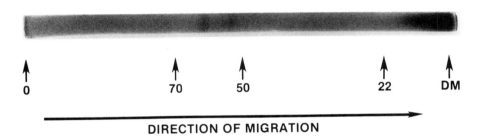

0, origin; 70, position of immunoglobulin μ chain standard (70,000 daltons); 50, position of immunoglobulin γ chain standard (50,000 daltons); 22, position of immunoglobulin light chain standard (22,000 daltons); DM, dye marker. In control experiments, (a) material from B16 culture fluid was reacted with an immunoadsorbent consisting of EL-4 absorbed normal goat IgG. No components were eluted, and (b) culture fluid of UV-112 was reacted at equal concentration with the goat α B16 immunoadsorbent. No detectable components were isolated.

47

Figure 4—BINDING TO B16 AND UV-112 TARGET CELLS OF RABBIT ANTISERA PRODUCED AGAINST THE MELANOMA-ASSOCIATED XENOANTIGEN PREPARATION ISOLATED USING GOAT ANTIBODIES

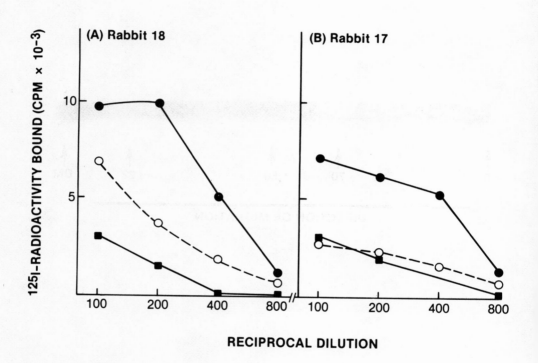

(A) Rabbit #18. ●————●, antiserum tested on B16 cells; ○———○, preimmunization serum tested on B16 cells; ■————■, antiserum tested on UV-112 cells. (B) rabbit #17. ●————●, antiserum tested on B16 cells; ○———○, preimmunization serum tested on B16 cells; ■————■, antiserum tested on UV-112 cells. ^{125}I-labeled *S. aureus* A protein was used to detect bound IgG. All sera were absorbed with UV-112 cells to remove activity directed against mouse-specific xenoantigens.

48

antigen fraction isolated from shed material using the anti-B16 immunoadsorbent. Samples of serum were also taken from the rabbits prior to immunization to serve as a control for naturally occurring antibodies. Both preimmune sera and antisera were absorbed with UV-112 cells to remove anti-mouse activity and then titrated for binding to B16 and UV-112 cells. As shown in Figure 4, immunization with the specifically purified antigen fraction induced antibodies binding to B16, but not to UV-112 cells. Rabbit 18 possessed some specific activity against B16 cells prior to immunization, but binding to B16 was substantially increased by immunization.

DISCUSSION

We have used a two stage xenoimmunization approach to prepare antisera specific for surface antigens of B16 melanoma. Goat antiserum produced against intact melanoma cells and absorbed exhaustively with murine lymphoma cells detected a melanoma specific antigen shared by B16 and an allogeneic murine melanoma 1735. Comparison studies of binding to various tumors showed that the component(s) detected were apparently not mouse-specific xenoantigens, histocompatibility antigens, viral antigens or melanin. An immunoadsorbent made with the IgG immunoglobulin of this goat antiserum was used to isolate an antigen-containing fraction from shed surface components and detergent lysates of the B16 melanoma. As assessed by polyacrylamide gel electrophoresis in SDS-containing buffers, the antigen fraction contained a major component with an apparent mass of 60,000-68,000 daltons, a second component of approximate mass 50,000 daltons and a minor component of about 20,000 daltons. The fact that this immune-affinity purified preparation contained B16-specific antigens was demonstrated by immunizing rabbits with the purified fraction. The rabbits produced antibodies directed against B16 cells. We have not yet tested the purified antigen fraction for its capacity to protect C57BL/6 mice against B16 melanoma.

It is noteworthy that the major component of the melanoma-specific surface antigen preparation is comparable in size to tumor surface antigens recently isolated from methylcholanthrene-induced sarcomas (16, 17) and 4-dimethylamino-azobenzene-induced hepatomas (16). Studies are in progress to determine whether all the components in the immune-affinity isolated preparation specify melanoma antigens and to ascertain their relationship to one another. Considerable effort must still be expended to obtain detailed biochemical characterization of the purified antigens of various tumors and to allow precise comparisons among the structural properties of the antigens.

ACKNOWLEDGMENT

We wish to thank Mss. Lisa Santucci and Deanna Willard for expert technical assistance.

REFERENCES

1. McCabe, R.P., Ferrone, S., Pellegrino, M.A., et al., "Purification and Immunologic Evaluation of Human Melanoma-Associated Antigens." *J. Natl. Cancer Inst.* 60: 773-777, 1978.
2. Dent, P.B., Liao, S.K., McCullock, P.B., et al., "Characterization of Human Malignant Melanoma Cell Lines. III. Membrane Immunofluorescence Reactivity with Sera from Patients with Melanoma." *Cancer Immunol. Immunother.* 3: 239-246, 1978.
3. Sorg, C., Briiggen, J., Seibert, E. and Macher, E., "Membrane-Associated Antigens of Human Malignant Melanoma. IV. Changes in Expression of Antigens on Cultured Melanoma Cells." *Cancer Immunol. Immunother.* 3: 259-271, 1978.
4. Bystryn, J.C., "Antibody Response and Tumor Growth in Syngeneic Mice Immunized to Partially Purified B16 Melanoma-Associated Antigens." *J. Immunol.* 120: 96-101, 1978.
5. Fidler, I.J., "Selection of Successive Tumor Lines for Metastasis." *Nature, New Biol.* 242: 148-149, 1973.
6. Peterson, D.E., Bucana, C.D. and Fidler, I.J., "Immunologic Specificity and Reactivity of Goat Anti-Guinea Pig and Goat Anti-Mouse Macrophage Sera." *J. Reticuloendothel. Soc.* 21: 119-130, 1977.
7. Gately, M.K. and Mayer, M.M., "The Molecular Dimensions of Guinea Pig Lymphotoxin." *J. Immunol.* 112: 168-177, 1974.
8. Marchalonis, J.J., Atwell, J.L. and Goding, J.W., "7S Immunoglobulins of a Monotreme, the Echidna *Tachyglossus aculeatus:* Two Distinct Isotypes Which Bind a Protein of *Staphylococcus aureus.*" *Immunology* 34: 97-103, 1978.
9. Segal, G.P. and Klinman, N.R., "Defining the Heterogeneity of Anti-Tumor Antibody Responses." *J. Immunol.* 116: 1539-1545, 1976.
10. Greenwood, F.C., Hunter, W.M. and Glover, J.S., "The Preparation of ^{131}I-Labelled Human Growth Hormone of High Specific Activity." *Biochem. J.* 89: 114-123, 1963.
11. Gersten, D.M. and Marchalonis, J.J., "A Rapid, Novel Method for the Solid Phase Derivatization of IgG Antibodies for Immune-Affinity Chromatography." *J. Immunol. Meth.,* in press.
12. Laemmli, U.K. and Favre, M., "Maturation of the Head of Bacteriophage T4. I. DNA Packaging Events." *J. Mol. Biol.* 80: 575-599, 1973.
13. Atwell, J.L. and Marchalonis, J.J., "Phylogenetic Emergence of Immunoglobulin Classes Distinct from IgM." *J. Immunogenetics* 1: 367-391, 1975.
14. Grey, H.M., Hirst, J.W. and Cohn, M., "A New Mouse Immunoglobulin: IgG3." *J. Exp. Med.* 133: 289-304, 1971.
15. Cannon, G.B., McCoy, J.L., Connor, R.J., et al., "Use of the Leukocyte Migration Inhibition Assay to Evaluate Antigenic Differences in Human Breast Cancers and Melanomas." *J. Natl. Cancer Inst.* 60: 969-978,
16. Baldwin, R.W., Price, M.R. and Moore, V.E., "Biochemical and Immunological Characteristics of Tumor Specific Antigens on Chemically-Induced Rat Tumors." In *Biological Markers of Neoplasia: Basic and Applied Aspects,* R.W. Ruddon (ed.), Plenum Press, New York, in press.
17. Appella, E., Dubois, G.C., Natori, T., et al., "Histocompatibility Antigens and Tumor-Specific Transplantation Antigens of a Methylcholanthrene-Induced Sarcoma." In *Biological Markers of Neoplasia: Basic and Applied Aspects,* R.W. Ruddon (ed.), Plenum Press, New York, in press.
18. Fidler, I.J., Gersten, D.M. and Budmen, M.B., "Characterization *in vivo* and *in vitro* of Tumor Cells Selected for Resistance to Syngeneic Lymphocyte-Mediated Cytotoxicity." *Cancer Res.* 36: 1360-1365, 1976.
19. Kripke, M.L., "Latency Histology and Antigenicity of Tumors Induced by Ultraviolet Light in Three Inbred Mouse Strains." *Cancer Res.* 37: 1395-1400, 1977.
20. Fidler, I.J., "Recognition and Destruction of Target Cells by Tumoricidal Macrophages." *Isr. J. Med. Sci.* 14: 177-191, 1978.

Crispen (ed.): Neoplasm Immunity: Experimental and Clinical

Immunobiological and Biochemical Characterization of Murine Tumor-Specific Transplantation Antigens

Neal R. Pellis[1]
H. Yamagishi[1]
M. Mokyr[2]
B. Kahan[1]

SUMMARY—The immune response to tumor specific transplantation antigens (TSTA) extracted from a methylcholanthrene induced fibro-sarcoma, MCA-F, of C3H/HeJ mice was studied by direct challenge with viable tumor cells and by local adoptive transfer assays (LATA). Optimal, but not supraoptimal, doses of crude solubilized antigen (CSA) induced specific resistance to neoplastic cell challenge. When assayed by LATA using spleen cells from donors pretreated with various doses of CSA, the dose-response was the same as that of primary hosts. Depletion of adherent cells from the transferred populations not only increased the tumor neutralizing capacity of spleen cells from hosts treated with optimal doses of CSA, but also revealed potently cytotoxic, non-adherent cells in mice sensitized with supraoptimal doses. Thus adherent cells may suppress the cytotoxic activity of lymphoid cells in mice treated with solubilized TSTA. Cells mediating CSA-induced resistance were sensitive to antithymocyte serum and inactivated by x-irradiation suggesting the participation of T lymphocytes. Sequential LATA performed 2, 6, 9, 12 and 15 days after an optimal dose of CSA treatment revealed progression of spleen cell activity through brief period of tumor facilitation (6 to 9 days) followed by a neutralization phase at (days 9-12). A relationship between these opposing activities and the chemical composition of CSA was suggested by the isolation of two fractions from CSA by preparative isoelectric focusing. Proteins which focused at pl 6.00 induced resistance to viable tumor cell challenge while materials at pl 2.00 to 3.6 facilitated neoplastic outgrowth. These results suggest that 1) separate components in CSA are responsible for the induction of resistance and tumor growth facilitation and 2) separate cell populations mediate these two effects, and 3) the net response induced by crude tumor antigen preparations may be the vectorial outcome of these several different responses.

---

[1]Departments of Surgery, and Biochemistry and Molecular Biology, The University of Texas Medical School, Houston, Texas.
[2]Department of Microbiology, University of Illinois Medical Center, Chicago, Illinois.

51

INTRODUCTION

An important consideration in the immunotherapy of neoplastic disease is a thorough understanding of the host response to antigens associated with the tumor cell surface. Among the galaxy of antigens displayed by tumor cells, those which induce protective immune responses in otherwise susceptible hosts have been the object of intense investigation. Elucidation of the immunoprotective antigens in human neoplasia has been difficult owing to the inability to perform transplantation tests in patients. However, in experimental animals these antigens have been operationally defined by their ability to induce specific resistance to engraftment with viable neoplastic cells. Elucidation of the immunobiological and biochemical characteristics of the tumor specific transplantation antigens (TSTA) of experimental animal tumors may provide insight into the complexity of the host response to neoantigens expressed by cancer cells and suggest methods by which immunoprotective antigens may be prepared from human neoplastic tissues. Indeed, purified, chemically-modified tumor antigens may serve as suitable reagents in the therapy of neoplastic disease.

To these aims we have established a model employing methylcholanthrene induced fibrosarcomas in C3H/HeJ mice (1). The objectives of the experiments in this model are to a) solubilize, purify, and characterize the cell surface antigens responsible for the induction of tumor specific resistance, and b) study the immunobiology of solubilized and purified tumor antigens. This communication presents results which demonstrate the immunoprotective activity and antigenicity of solubilized tumor antigens, characterization of the responding lymphoid cell populations, and a preliminary purification of TSTA.

MATERIALS AND METHODS

Induction and propagation of neoplasms, extraction of tumor antigens, and performance of the immunoprotection tests and local adoptive transfer assays (LATA) are described in detail elsewhere (1). Briefly, the methylcholanthrene induced fibrosarcoma, MCA-F, was serially propagated in syngeneic C3H/HeJ mice. Tumor nodules were excised and single cell suspensions prepared by treatment of minced tissue with 0.25% trypsin solution. Cell suspensions were used for serial propagation of tumors, challenge of immunized hosts, target cells for LATA, and as source materials for the extraction of TSTA. Crude solubilized extracts (CSA) of MCA-F cells were prepared by the 3M KCl procedure (2). Extracts were ultracentrifuged at 165,000 g to remove particulate membrane debris.

Fractionation of crude extracts was performed by preparative isoelectric focusing in a slab of Sephadex G-75 (3,4). Proteins in CSA were segregated in an ampholyte gradient (pH 3.5-10.0). The thirty-one fractions which spanned the entire gradient were eluted, concentrated, dialyzed, and assessed for TSTA activity by the immunoprotection test.

Immunogenic activity was assessed by subcutaneous (SC) administration of serial CSA dosages (0.0-2.0 mg protein) to groups of ten mice. Ten days later normal and treated mice were challenged SC with 10^4 MCA-F cells. Resultant tumor growth was monitored by serial measurements of tumor volume. Additionally, extract treated hosts served as spleen cell (SpC) donors for the local adoptive transfer assay (LATA). SpC were routinely harvested 10 days after treatment of donor mice with solubilized TSTA (5). Tumor cells were admixed with SpC from normal or extract-treated mice at a ratio of $10^4:10^7$, respectively, in a final volume of 0.2 ml and then injected and then inoculated SC into normal syngeneic recipients (10/group).

Fractionation of spleen cell populations were performed by three sequential incubation in 10 cm plastic petri dishes to remove adherent cells. Thymus dependent lymphocytes were removed by treatment of spleen cells with rabbit anti-mouse thymocyte serum and guinea pig complement. Efficacy of this latter treatment was confirmed by a 90% reduction in the proliferative response of the spleen cell populations to concanavalin A.

RESULTS AND DISCUSSION

Documentation of the antigenic activity of crude tumor cell extracts was demonstrated by the induction of tumor specific resistance in syngeneic murine hosts. Extracts of fibrosarcoma MCA-F induced a resistant state such that subsequent challenge with 100 times the minimum tumorigenic dosage (MTD) failed to grow as rapidly as the inoculum in normal mice (Table 1). This was evidenced by a 75% reduction in the mean tumor diameter, a 60% reduction in the number of palpable neoplasms, and significant increase in the survival of extract treated hosts. That this activity was related to the presence of tumor specific transplantation antigens in the CSA of MCA-F was evidenced by its inability to alter any of the tumor growth parameters for a challenge with the syngeneic but antigenically different MCA-C fibrosarcoma. Similar results for SV40 virus induced tumors (6) and for chemically induced guinea pig hepatomas (7) have been reported by other laboratories.

Of critical importance to the assertion that CSA-induced tumor resistance was the consequence of TSTA was 1) assessment of the dose response and 2) demonstration that CSA-induced protection was mediated by lymphoid cells. Table 2 illustrates, as reported previously (8), that resistance can be induced with usually 0.5 mg CSA and that twice this dosage often leads to failure to elicit protection upon direct challenge. Interestingly, the unusual

Table 1—INDUCTION OF TUMOR SPECIFIC RESISTANCE BY 3M KC1 EXTRACTS OF MCA-F CELLS[a]

Treatment	Challenge Cells	Mean Tumor Diameter on day 28 (mm)[b]	% Tumor Bearers (day 35)[c]	ST 50 (days)[d]
None	MCA-F	17.1±3.0	100	42
	MCA-C	20.2±2.8	100	35
0.5 mg CSA from MCA-F	MCA-F	4.8±2.5[e]	40[e]	500[e]
	MCA-C	19.1±3.2	100	35

[a]Crude extracts of MCA-F were administered SC to groups of 10 mice. Ten days later extract treated and parallel groups of normal mice were challenged with 10^4 MCA-F and MCA-C cells.
[b]Diameter measurements made with vernier calipers.
[c]Percent mice bearing a palpable neoplasm.
[d]50% survival time—Day on which half the mice in each group were dead.
[e]Significantly different from control at probability < 0.001 by Student's t-test, chi square, and linear regression analysis.

dose response also occurred when activity was assessed by LATA. These results suggest that soluble TSTA are weak antigens, and therefore induce resistance only within a narrow dose range. The mechanisms by which high doses of tumor antigens fail to induce resistance remains unclear. Nevertheless the unresponsiveness is apparently an active process of a subpopulation of cells in the lymphoreticular system. Indeed when the transferred SpC populations were fractionated by adherence to plastic petri dishes the tumor neutralizing capacity of the nonadherent fraction was significantly increased (Table 3). Not only did depletion of adherent cells potentiate the neutralizing activity of SpC from donors treated with 0.5 mg CSA but also it revealed that hosts pretreated with the supraoptimal dose (1.0 mg CSA) possess cytotoxic lymphoid cells. These results suggest that adherent cells exert a strong suppression upon the activity of lymphocytes in CSA-treated hosts. Poupon et al. (9) showed that splenic macrophages from tumor bearing mice were shown to suppress the *in vitro* lymphoproliferative response to mitogens and Glaser et al (10) described a similar splenic subpopulation which inhibited the *in vitro* secondary response to tumor cells. It may be that the suppression reported herein is due to activation of suppressor macrophages or lymphocytes which remained in the culture vessel during incubation.

Table 2—DOSE DEPENDENT TUMOR RESISTANCE INDUCED BY 3M KC1 EXTRACTS IN PRIMARY HOSTS AND IN LATA RECIPIENTS[a]

Assay	Dose of CSA (MCA-F)	Tumor Incidence %	p[b]
Direct Challenge	0.0	81	—
	0.5	40	0.02
	1.0	90	NS
LATA	0.0	85	—
	0.5	40	0.01
	1.0	90	NS

[a]Groups of 25 mice were pretreated with the various doses of CSA from MCA-F. Ten days later 10-15 mice from each group were challenged SC with 10^4 viable MCA-F cells. The remaining mice in each group were used as spleen cell donors for the LATA. Adoptive transfer hosts received a SC inoculation of a mixture containing 10^7 spleen cells and 10^4 MCA-F cells.

[b]Significance determined by chi square analysis.

Table 3—SUPPRESSION OF CRUDE EXTRACT INDUCED TUMOR RESISTANCE BY ADHERENT CELLS IN THE SPLEEN[a]

Dose of MCA-F (mg) CSA	Fraction of Spleen Cells	Tumor Growth[b] (% of Control)	p[c]
0.5	UN	50	0.02
1.0	UN	100	NS
0.5	NA	0	0.001
1.0	NA	11	0.005

[a]Spleen cell donors were pretreated with saline, 0.5 mg CSA, and 1.0 mg CSA. Ten days later spleen cells were harvested and either left unfractionated (UN) or depleted of adherent cells by incubation in plastic petri dishes and the non-adherent (NA) fraction assessed for tumor neutralization by LATA.

[b]Tumor growth was assessed by diameter measurements performed 30 days after inoculation of the spleen·cell-tumor cell mixture into groups of 10 normal syngeneic recipients.

[c]Significant by chi square analysis.

The lymphoid cells mediating tumor neutralization were characterized with respect to radiosensitivity and sensitivity to treatment with rabbit antithymocyte serum and complement. Spleen cells obtained 10 days after treatment of donors with 0.5 mg CSA were exposed to 5500 rads of x-irradiation or to antithymocyte serum and complement for 1 hr at 37°C (Table 4). Tumor neutralizing activity was completely obviated by both treatments, suggesting that the effector cell was probably a non-adherent, thymus-dependent lymphocyte.

Table 4—CHARACTERIZATION OF SPLEEN CELL POPULATIONS MEDIATING CRUDE EXTRACT INDUCED TUMOR RESISTANCE[a]

Donor Pretreatment	Spleen Cell Treatment	Tumor Incidence (%)	p[b]
None	None, Irradiation, or ATS	84	—
0.5 mg CSA (MCA-F)	None	40	0.01
	Irradiation	85	NS
	ATS	82	NS

[a]In the setting of the LATA spleen cells from extract and untreated donors were subjected to 5500 rads of x-irradiation or antithymocyte serum and complement prior to admixture with MCA-F cells and implantation into secondary hosts.
[b]Chi square analysis.

The LATA was used to study the progression of the immune response to MCA-F, 0.5 mg CSA by harvesting spleen cells at various times after pretreatment of donor mice. Parallel groups of normal spleen cell donors were used as controls to determine the percent reduction or facilitation of lymphoid cells from CSA-treated donors. Table 5 illustrates that SpC obtained 2 to 6 days after treatment of donors with 0.5 mg extract possess weak, insignificant neutralizing activity (25%). At 6 to 9 days SpC facilitated tumor growth by nearly 80%. By 9-12 days after CSA pretreatment SpC displayed significant neutralizing activity (nearly 60%). Neutralizing activity was insignificant by day 15. These results illustrate the sinusoidal evolution of tumor immunity suggested by Small and Trainin (11) using an *in vitro* cocultivation of tumor and lymphoid cells. Since by direct challenge maximum protection is observed at 10 days (unpublished data) it is possible that the two phase response may be due to more than one component of crude extract.

56

Table 5—PROGRESSION OF THE IMMUNE RESPONSE TO CRUDE EXTRACTS OF MCA-F FIBROSARCOMA CELLS[a]

Days After Treatment With CSA	Total No. SpC Donors	Total No. Recipients	Tumor Neutralizing Activity (%)[b]	p[c]
2-6	6	20	25± 7	NS
6-9	13	42	− 79± 16	0.01
9-12	22	73	59± 4	0.02
15	6	20	− 15± 10	NS

[a]Sequential LATA performed 2, 6, 9, 12, and 15 days after treatment of SpC donors with 0.5 mg CSA from MCA-F. Spleen cells were admixed with MCA-F cells and inoculated SC into syngeneic recipients.
[b]Neutralizing activity of SpC was determined by calculation of the percent change in tumor growth effected by SpC from treated donors over that of normal SpC. Positive values donate tumor neutralization; negative values indicate growth facilitation.
[c]Significance as determined by Student's t-test comparison with normal SpC recipients. NS-not significant.

In an attempt to purify the components in CSA responsible for the induction of tumor resistance the individual components which induced tumor resistance and facilitation were separated. Fractionation of CSA by preparative isoelectric focusing separated proteins in a linear pH gradient according to their respective isoelectric points. Of thirty fractions obtained over a pH gradient 3.5 to 10.0 two fractions, pI 3.6 and pI 6.0 displayed significant activity when assessed for immunobiologic activity by direct challenge of fraction-treated hosts (Figure 1). Proteins focusing at pI 6.0 induced resistance to challenge with viable MCA-F cells, reducing tumor growth by more than 50% ($p < 0.01$) when compared to control mice. On the other hand, materials which focused in the poorly resolved acidic region significantly facilitated tumor growth increasing tumor diameter by more than 40% ($p < 0.01$). The results suggest that antigens inducing tumor resistance may be partially purified by preparative isoelectric focusing, and that their activity may be nullified by a separate facilitating factor. Indeed, the wavelike progression of the immune response in Table 5 may be due to superimposed reactivities of these two moieties, each possessing unique kinetics; the facilitating antigen inducing a response by adherent cells which is maximal at day 6-9 and the resistance antigen inducing a response by non-adherent T-cells which is maximal at day 12. Separation of the immunoprotective antigens from tumor facilitating components of crude extracts may provide materials suitable for active immunotherapeutic protocols.

Figure 1—FRACTIONATION OF CSA FROM MCA-F BY PREPARATIVE ISOELECTRIC FOCUSING IN SEPHADEX G-75

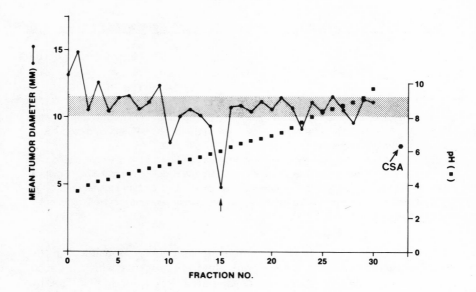

160 mg CSA was admixed with carry ampholyte solution and electrofocused at 8 watts constant power. The gel bed was cut into 30 zones and each eluted, dialyzed and concentrated. All fractions were assessed for immunoprotective activity in syngeneic mice. Twenty-five days after challenge tumor diameters (•) were measured and compared with parallel control hosts.

REFERENCES

1. Pellis, N.R. and Kahan, B.D., "Methods to Demonstrate the Immunogenicity of Soluble Tumor Specific Transplantation Antigens: The Immunoprophylaxis Assay." *Meth. Cancer Res.* 13: 291-330, 1976.
2. Reisfeld, R.A. and Kahan, B.D., "Biological and Chemical Characterization of Human Histocompatibility Antigens." *Fed. Proc. Fed. Amer. Soc. Exp. Biol.* 29: 2034-2040, 1970.
3. Radola, B.J., "Isoelectric Focusing in Layers of Granulated Gels. II. Preparative Isoelectric Focusing." *Biochem. Biphys. Acta* 386: 181-185, 1974.
4. Pellis, N.R., Yamagishi, H., Wiseman, F.C., et al., "Fractionation of 3M KCl Extracts from the Methylcholanthrene Induced Fibrosarcoma, MCA-F." *Fed. Proc. Fed. Amer. Soc. Exp. Biol.* 37: 1562, 1978.
5. Pellis, N.R. and Kahan, B.D., "Methods to Demonstrate the Immunogenicity of Soluble Tumor Specific Transplantation Antigens. II. The Local Adoptive Transfer Assay." *Meth. Cancer Res.* 14: 29-54, 1978.

6. Meltzer, M.J., Leonard, E.J., Hardy, A.S. and Rapp, H. J., "Protective Tumor Immunity Induced by Potassium Chloride Extracts of Guinea Pig Hepatomas." *J. Natl. Cancer Inst.* 54: 1349-1354, 1975.

7. Drapkin, M.S., Appella, E. and Law, L.W., "Immunogenic Properties of a Soluble Tumor Specific Transplantation Antigen Induced by Simian Virus 40." *J. Natl. Cancer Inst.* 52: 259-264, 1974.

8. Pellis, N.R. and Kahan, B.D., "Specific Tumor Immunity Induced with Soluble Materials." *J. Immunol.* 115: 1717-1722, 1975.

9. Poupon, M-F., Kolb, J-P. and Lespinats, G., "Evidence of Suppressor Cells in C3H/He, T-Cell Deprived C3H/He, and Nude Mice Bearing a 3-Methylcholanthrene Induced Fibrosarcoma." *J. Natl. Cancer Inst.* 57: 1241-1247, 1976.

10. Glaser, M., Kirchner, H., Holden, H.T. and Herberman, R.B., "Inhibition of Cell Mediated Cytotoxicity Against Tumor Associated Antigens by Suppressor Cells from Tumor Bearing Mice." *J. Natl. Cancer Inst.* 56: 865-867, 1976.

11. Small, M. and Trainin, N., "Separation of Populations of Sensitized Lymphoid Cells into Fractions Inhibiting and Fractions Enhancing Syngeneic Tumor Growth *in vivo.*" *J. Immunol.* 116: 292-297, 1976.

Interaction of Immune Complexes and Suppressor T-Cells in the Inhibition of Cytophilic Antibody Receptors on Macrophages

Malcolm S. Mitchell[1,2]
V. S. Rao[1]

SUMMARY—Administration of soluble immune complexes composed of hyperimmune (IgG_2) antibody to leukemia L1210 and L1210 antigens to allogeneic (C3H) mice inhibits receptors for cytophilic antibodies on their peritoneal macrophages. Macrophages from mice thus treated ("suppressed mice") are small and inactive appearing and fail to attach L1210 cells even in the presence of cytophilic antibodies to L1210. The inhibition is specific, in that cytophilic antibodies to sheep RBC or leukemia EL4 are not prevented from attaching to the same population of macrophages. Interestingly, if the Fc portion of antibody is removed, the complexes are rendered incapable of effecting suppression. The suppression is dependent upon suppressor T cells. Thymectomized, irradiated, bone marrow-reconstituted (T cell-deficient, or "B") mice are resistant to inhibition of their peritoneal macrophages, whereas sham-thymectomized mice are susceptible. Furthermore, adoptive transfer of syngeneic naive thymocytes into suppressed mice reinforces suppression, antagonizing the restorative effects of normal bone marrow cells. However, if syngeneic thymocytes are either exposed to an unrelated antigen after transfer to suppressed hosts, or are derived from donors who received an unrelated antigen 1 to 7 days before transfer, the thymocytes do not act as suppressor cells but rather reverse suppression. Suppressor T cells generated in mice given immune complexes can be adoptively transferred into normal syngeneic recipients, where they induce receptor-specific suppression of macrophages without the need for further L1210 antigens. If "B" mice are used as recipients for thymocytes containing suppressor cells, suppression of macrophages does not occur, unless normal thymocytes are admixed. Thus cooperation with (recruitment from, or a helper effect by) normal thymocytes is essential to the development of fully functional suppressor cells. It is suggested that immune complexes elicit suppressor T cells by stimulation of Fc receptor-bearing naive thymocytes, creating initiator cells which then generate functional suppressor cells after interaction with additional normal thymocytes.

INTRODUCTION

The importance of macrophage mediated cytotoxicity, through extracellular and phagocytic mechanisms, in the rejection of murine ascites

[1]Departments of Medicine and Pharmacology, Yale University School of Medicine, New Haven, Connecticut.
[2]Present Address: Department of Medicine, Los Angeles County-University of Southern California Medical Center, Los Angeles, California.

leukemias has been elucidated within the past decade, although there is a considerable variation among tumors in their susceptibility to destruction by macrophages (1). Cytophilic antibodies from B-lymphocytes, and their counterpart, specific macrophage arming factor from T-lymphocytes (2,3), permit the macrophage to identify foreign cells, in the initial phase of the rejection process. The first such antibodies were described in the attachment of sheep erythrocytes to guinea pig macrophages (4,5), but they have been found in the serum of mice immunized against allografted tumors as well as on peritoneal macrophages of the immunized animals (6,7), and in man at various stages of melanoma, acute leukemia and breast cancer (8,9). These cytophilic antibodies are usually found in IgG_2 globulin fraction of antiserum.

Immunological escape of neoplasms in syngeneic hosts in spite of the host's immune response has been well documented (10,11). Specific blocking factors noted in the serum of tumor-bearing animals of human beings have been considered by many investigators to be an important mechanism by which antigenic tumors may escape immunological destruction. Soluble tumor antigens (12,13), antigen-antibody complexes (14,16) or other immunosuppressive factors (17) all have blocking or immunoregulatory activity. Another regulatory entity which may also be important in the blocking of immunity to transplanted, and perhaps syngeneic, tumors is the suppressor T-cell (18,19).

While investigating the effects of hyperimmune antibody to murine leukemia L1210 on the rejection of leukemia L1210 *in vivo,* we noted a complete inhibition of spleen cell-mediated immunity produced by antibody given before L1210 cells (20). In addition, the mice given antibody and tumor cells lacked enlarged activated macrophages. Instead, their peritoneal macrophages were small monocytes with few stainable acid phosphatase granules. These cells failed to attach L1210 cells even in the presence of proved cytophilic anti-L1210 (21). They could, however, form rosettes with sheep erythrocytes or EL4 leukemia cells in the presence of the appropriate specific cytophilic antibody.

Since both antibody and antigen (tumor cells) are required to produce inhibition of macrophages, we have suspected that circulating immune complexes formed *in vivo* from soluble L1210 antigen and IgG antibody were responsible for such suppression of macrophages. The present studies were designed to examine this possibility and to determine the importance of the Fc portion of the antibody moiety in the suppression. Since we had considerable indirect evidence for involvement of suppressor T-cells, e.g. that the suppression of macrophages required an intact thymus (22), we have also attempted here to demonstrate conclusively the presence of suppressor T-cells induced by immune complexes, through adoptive transfer to normal syngeneic hosts. Our results indicate not only that suppressor T-cells are involved as intermediaries but also that a T-T cell interaction is required to generate functional suppressor cells.

MATERIALS AND METHODS

Animals

C3H/HeJ(H-2^k), BALB/C(H-2^d) (Microbiological Associates, Bethesda, Maryland), C57BL/6(H-2^b) (Charles River Laboratories, Wilmington, Massachusetts), and BDF$_1$ (C57BL/6 x DBA/2) (H-2^b x H-2^d) (The Jackson Laboratory, Bar Harbor, Maine) mice of 10-12 weeks old were used in the present studies.

Tumors

L1210 leukemia (H-2^d) was maintained in ascites form in BDF$_1$ male mice and EL4(H-2^b) leukemia was similarly passed in C57B/6 mice. The P815Y (H-2^d) mastocytoma and H-129 hepatoma (H-2^k) were cultivated in RPMI 1640 medium supplemented with antibiotics and 10% horse serum.

Antibody

Hyperimmune antibody to each leukemia was prepared with 7 to 8 weekly injections of 5 x 10^6 tumor cells i.p. into C57BL/6 mice (for L1210) or into BALB/C (for EL-4). One week after the last injection of the tumor cells, 0.5 ml of complete Freund's adjuvant was injected i.p. twice, 5 days apart. A week later, immune ascites fluid was collected, centrifuged and titrated for cytotoxicity as previously described (23). All the batches that led to significant lysis of 50% at a 1:16 to 1:64 dilution against L1210 or P815Y (for L1210 Ab), or EL-4 (for EL-4 Ab) target cells with guinea pig complement (absorbed) were pooled and used throughout these studies. This material was also found to have a cytophilic antibody titer of 1:256 or more and was also used as the source of cytophilic antibody in tests for rosette formation. The antibody-rich ascites is referred as anti-L1210 or anti-EL-4 in this paper.

Anti-SRBC[2] serum was prepared in C3H mice by 2 weekly injections of 5 x 10^8 SRBC (sheep red blood cells) and the antibody titer was determined with ^{51}Cr labeled SRBC in the presence of guinea pig complement.

Preparation of Antibody Classes

Various classes of immunoglobulin were obtained from anti-L1210 by Sephadex G-200 column chromatography (5 x 60 cm), eluting with PBS (phosphate buffered saline), 80 mM ionic strength, pH 7.2. IgM was eluted in peak I while IgG was eluted in peak II. The fractions were rechromatographed and concentrated and their antibody activity was tested as detailed earlier.

Preparation of F(ab¹)₂ Fragments from IgG Antibody

F(ab¹)₂ fragments were prepared as described by Feldmann and Diener (24) with slight modification. Anti-L1210 was treated with saturated ammonium sulfate to a concentration of 33%. The immunoglobulin fraction in 0.01M PB, pH 7.5 was loaded on a DEAE-cellulose column (2.5 x 40 cm) (DE-52, Whatman, Conn.) and the column was washed with the same buffer.

IgG was eluted from the column by a PBS gradient of 0.01 to 0.2M, pH 7.5. The cytotoxic activity of IgG was treated as detailed earlier.

IgG at a concentration of 30 mg per ml was digested with 1 mg of pepsin (Sigma Chemicals) (2 mg of pepsin per 100 mg of IgG) at 37° C for 20 hours. The digested mixture was adjusted to pH 8.0 with 5N NaOH to stop the reaction and dialyzed against PBS, pH 7.2 (to remove all the small polypeptides of the Fc fragment). The dialyzed material was chromato-graphed on a Sephadex G-150 (1.5 x 90 cm). Five ml fractions of different peaks were pooled, concentrated and checked for antibody activity. Peak 1 (undigested IgG) showed a significant complement-dependent cytotoxicity at 1:128 dilution, whereas peak No. 2 lacked the activity. F(ab¹)₂ fragments (peak 2) on rechromatography showed no IgG contamination. F(ab¹)₂ fragments prepared from IgG were tested for functional integrity (binding of antigen) and freedom from contamination with Fc fragments (lack of complement fixation).

Preparation of Fc Fragments from IgG

Fc fragments from IgG of anti-L1210 were prepared as described earlier (25). IgG (100 mg) was digested with mercury papain (Sigma Chemicals) (1.5 mg) in 5 ml of 0.1M sodium phosphate buffer, pH 7.2 containing 0.01M cysteine and 2 mM EDTA, at 37° C for 16 hours. The material after dialyzing against 0.01M acetate buffer was loaded onto a carboxymethyl cellulose (CM-52, Whatman, Conn.) column equilibrated with 0.01M sodium acetate buffer, pH 5.5. The papain digest was eluted with a sodium acetate gradient of 0.1M-0.9M, pH 5.5 and 2.5 ml fractions of each peak were pooled and concentrated to a convenient volume. Peaks I and II correspond to Fab, whereas peak III represents the Fc fragment. Fc fragments from IgG of normal C57 mice were prepared as controls.

Preparation of Soluble Antigen

Soluble antigen was prepared from L1210 leukemia cells by the 3M KCl extraction technique (26). Soluble antigens from leukemia EL-4, hepatoma H-129 and C57 spleen cells were prepared by the same method. The protein content of these soluble antigens was determined by the method of Lowry, et al. (27). The soluble antigenic extract of L1210 (SA-L1210) was concen-trated using PM10 DIAFLO membranes (Amicon Corporation, Lexington,

Massachusetts), precipitated with equal volume of 4M (NH4)₂ SO₄ and redissolved to its volume in 0.1M PBS, pH 7.2. The redissolved precipitate was applied to a Sephadex G-200 column (2.5 x 90 cm) and was eluted with PBS (80 mM ionic strength), pH 7.2, in the cold. Fractions were concentrated and the protein content of each fraction was estimated. The maximum antigenic activity was found in fractions eluted well after the peak in the protein profile corresponding to a molecular weight around 40,000 to 60,000 daltons. A 3-fold purification was achieved by gel filtration with 30% loss of activity.

Antigenic activity of SA-L1210 was determined by the inhibition of the cytotoxicity of anti-L1210, with P815Y or L1210 target cells (12). Anti-L1210 diluted to 1:32, which had killed 70-80% of the target cells, was used in experiments on antigenic activity. The percentage of inhibition of cytotoxicity was calculated using the equation:

$$\% \text{ Inhibition} = [\ 1 - \frac{\% \text{ stained cells in presence of SA}}{\% \text{ stained cells in absence of SA}}\ ] \times 100$$

Preparation of Immune Complexes

Antibody was incubated at 37° C for 1 hour with frequent shaking with SA-L1210 in PBS, pH 7.2. The amount of SA-L1210 added was slightly more than that required to inhibit cytotoxicity completely.

Preparation of Thymocytes and Spleen Cells from Suppressed Mice

C3H mice were injected with a single i.p. dose of 0.4 ml of anti-L1210, and with 5 x 10⁶ L1210 cells 1 day later, or with 0.8 ml of immune complexes (0.1 ml antibody to L1210 and 40 mg of SA-L1210) on four consecutive days. These mice are referred to as hereafter as "suppressed" mice. Ten days after the last injection thymocytes were prepared from the suppressed mice and adjusted to a concentration of 2 x 10⁸ viable cells per ml. These thymocytes are termed "suppressor thymocytes" for simplicity in this paper. Splenocytes from suppressed mice were processed and adjusted to 1.5 x 10⁸ cells per ml of suspension. These spleen cells are referred to as "suppressor spleen cells".

Fractionation of Spleen Cells

The suppressor spleen cells were fractionated on a nylon wool column, by methods described previously (28). The non-adherent cells were collected by adding to the column 25 ml of warm PBS, pH 7.2 (5% FCS) dropwise. The adherent cells were removed from the nylon wool with RPMI medium by squeezing, a process that was repeated twice with fresh RPMI medium. Both nylon non-adherent and adherent cells were washed 3 times and adjusted to 2 x 10⁸ cells per ml. The yields were reproducible, ranging from

25-30% of total spleen cells for non-adherent cells and 40-45% for the adherent cells.

Treatment of Thymocytes and Spleen T-Cells with Anti-Thymocyte Serum

Rabbit antimouse thymocyte serum (ATS) (Microbiological Associates, Bethesda, Md.) was absorbed twice with C57 BL/6 mouse or C3H mouse liver homogenate (6 ml of 1/3 dilution of ATS with 1 ml of packed liver homogenate) for 30 minutes at 25° C. The absorbed ATS was diluted to 1/30 with Fischer's medium. The treatment of thymocytes or spleen T-cells with ATS was done as detailed earlier (23).

"B" Mice (T-Cell Deprived Mice)

Four 6 week old C3H mice were thymectomized according to the method of Miller (29). The thymus was removed by suction through an incision in the neck and thoracic wall along the midline of the sternum, extending to the level of the second rib. Three weeks later, the thymectomized mice were lethally irradiated (750R) and within 24 hr they were reconstituted with 2 x 10^7 syngeneic bone marrow cells (i.v.). These mice were given food and water supplemented with penicillin and streptomycin and were watched for 20 days to note infection or deaths. Lethally irradiated, unreconstituted mice usually succumbed between 10 to 12 days after irradiation. The thymectomized, lethally irradiated, bone marrow-reconstituted mice are referred to as T-cell deprived or "B" mice.

In vivo Assay for Integrity of Cytophilic Antibody Receptors

Our previously described *in vivo* method for integrity of cytophilic antibody receptors was used (23). Briefly, each mouse whose peritoneal macrophages were to be tested was given an injection of 0.3 ml cytophilic antibody (present in hyperimmune ascites fluid) and 2.5 x 10^6 L1210 tumor cells i.p. sequentially. Four hours later, the mice were sacrificed and their peritoneal cavity was lavaged with 5 ml Fischer's medium. After centrifugation at 600 rpm for 5 minutes and resuspension of the pellet in saline containing 25% mouse serum, the percentage of macrophages forming rosettes with leukemic cells was determined by examination of a droplet by phase contrast microscope. Results were given a score of 0 to 4+ after recording the percentage of rosettes (monocytes surrounding a tumor cell or *vice versa*). The appearance of the tumor cells and the macrophages (size, presence of refractile granules or spherules, degree of vacuolation, etc.) and the presence or absence of clumping were also recorded. A score of < 10% of peritoneal macrophages with attached cells, usually one to two macrophages per tumor cell; 1+ = 10 to 30% of macrophages with attachment, with 2 to 4 cells per macrophage or *vice versa;* 2+ = 30 to 50% with rosettes of 2 to 6 cells/macrophage or *vice versa;* 3+ = 50 to 75% with four or more

66

cells per macrophage; $4+$ = 75 to 100% with rosettes of six or more cells/macrophage.

Each experimental group had three to four mice, and two slides were examined for each mouse. Experiments were performed three times with similar results in each.

In vitro *Assay for Cytophilic Antibody Receptors on Macrophages*

This method is essentially the same as described earlier (21). The peritoneal exudate cells (PEC) collected from mice were washed and adjusted to 5×10^5 per ml in Fischer's medium. 0.1 ml containing 5×10^4 PEC was added to each Lab-Tek chamber (Lab-Tek Products, Division Miles Laboratory, Inc., Illinois) containing 0.3 ml medium supplemented with 10% fetal calf serum (FCS) and the cells were incubated at 37° C for 60 minutes to form a monolayer on the glass slide. After removing the non-adherent cells by repeated washings with the medium containing 10% FCS, the adherent macrophages were incubated with 0.4 ml (1:10 dilution) of cytophilic antibody at 25° C for 60 minutes. The cells were washed gently with the medium and were incubated again with 5×10^5 L1210 cells at 25° C for 60 minutes. The cells were washed with medium without disturbing the rosettes. After removing the plastic chambers from the glass slide, the rosettes were examined under phase contrast microscopy and were scored as described for *in vivo* assay.

RESULTS

Inhibition of Cytophilic Antibody Receptors on Macrophages by Soluble Specific Immune Complexes

Complexes prepared *in vitro* were injected into various groups of mice. As shown in Table 1, mice in groups 1, 2 and 3 were treated with single injections of various doses of immune complexes. Mice of groups 4 and 5 received four daily injections of immune complexes composed of IgG or IgM antibodies, respectively, and SA-L1210. The peritoneal macrophages collected from mice given sufficient amounts of immune complexes containing whole antibody or IgG had inhibited cytophilic antibody receptors on their surface. Fewer than 10% of them formed rosettes with L1210 cells. In contrast, low doses of immune complexes (group 1 and 2) or IgM-containing immune complexes (group 5) were ineffective in inhibiting cytophilic antibody receptors (36-43% rosettes). Peritoneal macrophages collected from immunized mice (group 7) receiving only L1210 cells, were large and morphologically activated. More than 80% formed rosettes with L1210 cells. "Immune complexes" prepared by incubating NAF (Normal Ascites Fluid) with SA-L1210 were used as controls (group 6) and caused no inhibition.

67

Table 1—INHIBITION OF CYTOPHILIC ANTIBODY RECEPTORS OF MACROPHAGES BY SOLUBLE IMMUNE COMPLEXES

Group	Treatment[a]	Rosettes on Day 10 Mean (%) ± S.E.	Score
1	Ab-SA L1210 (0.4 ml)	35.8 ± 1.3	2+
2	Ab-SA L1210 (0.8 ml)	40.2 ± 2.1	2+
3	Ab-SA L1210 (1.6 ml)	9.0 ± 0.9	0
4	IgG-SA L1210 (3.2 ml)	8.5 ± 0.6	0
5	IgM-SA L1210 (3.2 ml)	42.8 ± 3.7	2+
6	NAF-SA L1210 (1.6 ml)	43.1 ± 3.5	2+
7	5×10^6 L1210 cells	92.8 ± 3.8	4+

[a]Immune complexes were prepared with SA-L1210 and whole anti-L1210 or antibody classes, as detailed in Materials and Methods. Group 1 mice received a single dose of 0.4 ml (0.1 ml antibody and 10 mg of SA-L1210 in 0.3 ml) of soluble immune complexes on day 0. Groups 2 and 3 mice received a single dose of 0.8 ml and 1.6 ml of immune complexes, respectively, on day 0. Mice of groups 4 and 5 received 0.8 ml IgG-SA-L1210 or IgM-SA-L1210 immune complexes, respectively (0.1 ml IgG or IgM and 40 mg SA-L1210 in 0.7 ml) on days (-3) to 0. Group 6 mice were injected with 1.6 ml NAF-SA L1210 in a single dose, and group 7 mice received Mitomycin-C treated 5×10^6 L1210 cells. Assays for rosette formation were performed 10 days after the last injection of immune complexes. Ab: Antibody to L1210; NAF: Normal Ascites Fluid.

Fractions of antibody classes prepared from the whole antibody were reconstituted to the original volume of the unfractionated antibody before injection.

Specificity of Inhibition of Cytophilic Antibody Receptors

The specificity of inhibition elicited by immune complexes was tested by injecting either complexes composed of antibody to L1210 and SA-L1210, or of antibody to leukemia EL4 and SA-EL4 (soluble antigen from EL4 cells), intraperitoneally into C3H mice. Ten days later we determined the ability of peritoneal macrophages to attach the corresponding or noncorresponding leukemia cells *via* the homologous cytophilic antibody. As shown in Table 2, macrophages from mice given anti-L1210-SA-L1210 complexes could not fix cytophilic antibody to L1210 (Group 1), but could attach antibody to EL4 or to SRBC (Groups 2 and 3). In the reciprocal experiment, mice given EL4-containing immune complexes could not attach EL4 cells in the presence of cytophilic antibody to EL4 (group 4), but could nonetheless attach L1210 (Group 5) or SRBC (Group 6) *via* their corresponding cytophilic antibody. These experiments affirmed the specificity of inhibition produced by antibody and specific antigen, which appears to be limited to receptors for the antibody contained in the immune complexes used as pretreatment.

Table 2—SPECIFICITY OF INHIBITION OF CYTOPHILIC ANTIBODY RECEPTORS OF MACROPHAGES BY SOLUBLE IMMUNE COMPLEXES BY *IN VITRO* ASSAY

Group	Treatment[a]	Monocytes Tested with:[b]	Rosettes on Day 10 Mean (%) ± S.E.	Score
1	Ab-SA L1210	anti-L1210 + L1210	10.8 ± 0.8	0
2	Ab-SA L1210	anti-EL + EL4	32.6 ± 2.4	2+
3	Ab-SA L1210	anti-SRBC + SRBC	40.7 ± 2.7	2+
4	Ab-SA EL4	anti-EL4 + EL4	11.2 ± 0.8	0
5	Ab-SA EL4	anti-L1210 + L1210	31.6 ± 2.8	2+
6	Ab-SA EL4	anti-SRBC + SRBC	45.2 ± 3.4	2+
7	NAF-SA EL4	anti-EL4 + EL4	33.1 ± 2.5	2+
8	5 x 10^6 EL4 cells	anti-EL4 + EL4	75.3 ± 3.9	3+

[a]Immune complexes were prepared *in vitro* with antibody to L1210 and SA-L1210 or with antibody to EL4 and SA-EL4. Groups 1, 2 and 3 mice received a single dose of L1210 immune complexes, 1.6 ml (0.4 ml Ab and 1.2 ml SA-L1210). Groups 4, 5 and 6 received the same dose of immune complexes of EL4. Group 7 mice were injected with 1.6 ml of NAF-SA EL4 and Group 8 mice were sensitized with EL4 cells. Ab: antibody to L1210 (in groups 1, 2 and 3) or to EL4 (groups 4, 5 and 6).

[b]Peritoneal monocytes from groups 1 and 5 mice were collected 10 days after the treatment and were tested for rosettes *in vitro* in the presence of cytophilic antibody to L1210 and L1210 cells. Monocytes collected from groups 2, 4, 7 and 8 were tested 10 days after treatment for rosette formation with EL 4 cells via cytophilic antibody to EL 4. Monocytes collected from groups 3 and 6 were tested for their ability to form rosettes with SRBC in the presence of cytophilic antibody to SRBC.

Effect of Immune Complexes of F(ab¹)₂-SA-L1210, or Fc Fragments on Inhibition of Cytophilic Antibody Receptors·

F(ab¹)₂ fragments from IgG antibody were prepared by pepsin digestion followed by Sephadex G-150 gel filtration. F(ab¹)₂ immune complexes with SA-L1210 were prepared *in vitro*. As shown in Table 3, mice given F(ab¹)₂ immune complexes, at a dose 4- to 6-fold higher than the effective dose of whole IgG (Groups 2 and 3), or given F(ab¹)₂ and subsequent SA-L1210 (Groups 5 and 6) did not show inhibition of their macrophages, which formed rosettes normally after the addition of specific antibody and L1210. In contrast, mice that received IgG containing complexes (Group 1) or IgG and SA-L1210 sequentially (Group 4) had monocytic cells with inhibited

69

cytophilic antibody receptors. Mice that received $F(ab^1)_2$ and 5 x 10^6 tumor cells (Group 7) had activated macrophages and >80% rosette formation, rather than suppression.

Table 3—EFFECT OF $F(ab^1)_2$ IMMUNE COMPLEXES OF IgG ANTIBODY ON CYTOPHILIC ANTIBODY RECEPTORS OF MACROPHAGES *IN VIVO*

A: *Treatment With Immune Complexes*

Group	Immune Complexes[a] Antibody Class	Dose (ml)	Rosettes on Day 10 Mean (%) ± S.E.	Score
1	IgG	0.3	8.7 ± 0.9	0
2	$F(ab^1)_2$	1.2	40.0 ± 3.9	2+
3	$F(ab^1)_2$	1.8	39.7 ± 4.2	2+

B: *Treatment With Antibody and SA-L1210 Sequentially*

Group	Antibody[b] Class Dose (ml)	Dose (mg)	SA-L1210[c] Mean (%)	Rosettes on Day 10 ± S.E.	Score
4	IgG	0.1	12	9.0 ± 1.0	0
5	$F(ab^1)_2$	0.4	48	38.5 ± 5.7	2+
6	$F(ab^1)_2$	0.6	72	37.2 ± 4.1	2+
7	$F(ab^1)_2$	0.6	5 x 10^6 Cells[d]	85.2 ± 2.0	4+
8	Nil	Nil	5 x 10^6 Cells	90.5 ± 2.2	4+

[a]Immune complexes prepared with IgG of $F(ab^1)_2$ and SA-L1210 were injected i.p. into different groups of mice as indicated. Each group received four injections of immune complexes (days -3 to "0"). 0.3 ml of immune complex injected to group 1 mice contained 0.1 ml IgG and 0.2 ml SA-L1210 (32 mg). The other doses of immune complexes given to groups 2 and 3 mice contained proportionally more $F(ab^1)_2$ and SA-L1210.

[b]IgG or $F(ab^1)_2$ antibody of different concentrations was given to other groups (4, 5, 6 and 7) in four injections i.p. starting on day (-4).

[c]On day "0" different concentrations of SA-L1210 were injected i.p. as shown in the table. One ml of SA-L1210 contained 160 mg progein.

[d]Irradiated 5 x 10^6 L1210 cells (5000R) in 0.2 ml were given i.p. to C3H mice.

NOTE: There was no difference in the effects on macrophages caused by several injections of $F(ab^1)_2$ fragments from that of a single injection.

Table 4 demonstrates the effect of Fc fragments *in vivo* on inhibition of cytophilic antibody receptors on macrophages. Fc fragments were prepared from IgG of anti-L1210, by papain digestion, followed by carboxymethyl

70

cellulose chromatography. These fragments were injected into various groups of animals with or without antigen and the peritoneal macrophages were tested for rosette forming capacity on day 10. Even Groups 3 and 4, which received 4- to 6-fold more Fc fragments than IgG, did not show any inhibition of receptors for cytophilic antibody on peritoneal macrophages. The 4- to 6-fold excess of Fc fragments was used in order to compensate for the known high excretion of these fragments *in vivo*. Aggregated Fc fragments when injected i.p. into mice did not cause inhibition of cytophilic antibody receptors of macrophages *in vivo* and the macrophages formed 30-50% rosettes with L1210 cells, the same as controls (results not presented).

Table 4—EFFECT OF Fc FRAGMENTS ON CYTOPHILIC ANTIBODY RECEPTORS OF MACROPHAGES *IN VIVO*

| Group | Antibody[a] | | L1210[b] | Rosettes on Day 10 | |
	Class	Dose (ml)	Dose (X10⁶)	Mean (%) ± S.E.	Score
1	IgG	0.1	Nil	41.3 ± 4.6	2+
2	IgG	0.1	5	9.2 ± 1.1	0
3	Fc	0.4	5	90.2 ± 2.3	4+
4	Fc	0.6	5	84.9 ± 4.6	4+
5	Fc	0.6	Nil	38.6 ± 4.2	2+
6	Nil	Nil	5	90.5 ± 2.0	4+

[a]Groups 1 and 2 mice received four injections of IgG i.p. starting on day -4 to -1. Groups 3, 4 and 5 received four daily injections of Fc fragments of various concentrations as indicated starting on day -4. The Fc fragments used were reconstituted to the original volume of IgG antibody.
[b]On day "0", groups 2, 3, 4 and 6 were given a single injection of 5 x 10⁶ L1210 cells i.p.

Transfer of Suppression of Macrophages by Suppressor T-cells:

C3H mice were injected with immune complexes or sequentially with anti-L1210 and L1210 cells. Ten days later thymocytes from these mice (putative suppressor thymocytes) were collected and tested for their ability to transfer suppression of macrophages to normal syngeneic mice. In Table 5, mice of groups 3 and 4 were given 4 or 5 x 10⁷ suppressor thymocytes (i.v.) and their peritoneal macrophages were collected 4 days later. These cells failed to fix cytophilic antibody to L1210, with fewer than 10% of them forming rosettes with L1210 cells. Two x 10⁷ or fewer suppressor thymocytes failed to transfer suppression (Groups 1 and 2), nor did 5 x 10⁷ ATS treated thymocytes (Group 5). Peritoneal macrophages from these mice were able to form rosettes to the same degree as controls receiving normal thymocytes

(Group 6). These results obtained by the *in vivo* assay were confirmed by the *in vitro* method.

Table 5—SUPPRESSION OF CYTOPHILIC ANTIBODY RECEPTORS ON MACROPHAGES BY ADOPTIVE TRANSFER OF THYMOCYTES FROM SUPPRESSED TO NORMAL MICE

Group	Thymocytes		Injected	Rosettes on day 4 after transfer[c]	
	Type		Number (1x10⁷)	Mean ± S.E.	Score
1	Suppressed[a]		1	36.2 ± 1.8	2+
2	Suppressed		2	40.1 ± 2.1	2+
3	Suppressed		4	8.6 ± 0.8	0
4	Suppressed		5	8.0 + 0.9	0
5	Suppressed (ATS +C)[b]		5	42.3 ± 2.8	2+
6	Normal		5	35.4 ± 3.0	2+

[a]C3H mice were injected with immune complexes i.p. on four consecutive days. Ten days later, the thymocytes from the suppressed mice were processed and injected I.V. into normal C3H mice.
[b]Suppressor thymocytes were treated with ATS and complement. One ml ATS (1:30 dil) was used per 1 x 10⁷ thymocytes.
[c]Four days after transfer of suppressor thymocytes into normal C3H mice, the peritoneal monocytes of these mice were tested for rosetting *in vivo* in the presence of L1210 *via* the cytophilic antibody to L1210.

NOTE: Similar results were observed with suppressor thymocytes obtained from mice suppressed with anti-L1210 (0.4 ml) and 4 x 10⁶ L1210 cells.

Spleen cells from suppressed mice (suppressor spleen cells) were fractionated on a nylon wool column, from which both nylon non-adherent and adherent cells were collected. These cells were tested separately for their ability to transfer suppression of macrophages to normal syngeneic mice (Figure 1). Four x 10⁷ non-adherent suppressor spleen cells were able to induce the suppression of macrophages in the recipients. In contrast, even 5 x 10⁷ nylon adherent splenocytes failed to inhibit the cytophilic antibody receptors on peritoneal macrophages, 35-45% of which formed rosettes with L1210 cells *via* cytophilic antibody. Treatment with ATS and complement abolished the suppressive activity of the non-adherent cells confirming their identity as T-cells (Figure 1).

Figure 1—INDUCTION OF MACROPHAGE SUPPRESSION (INHIBITION OF CYTOPHILIC ANTIBODY RECEPTOR ON THE MACROPHAGE) IN NORMAL MICE BY TRANSFER OF SUPPRESSOR SPLENIC T-CELLS

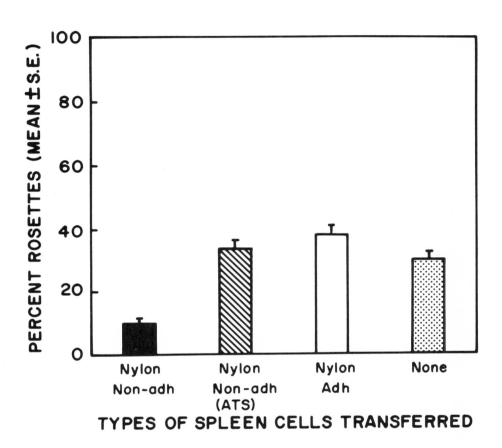

C3H mice were suppressed with immune complexes (anti-L1210—SA-L1210) as detailed in Materials and Methods. Ten days later, the suppressor spleen cells were fractionated on nylon column. Both nylon non-adherent (T-cell) and nylon adherent (non T-cell) fractions were injected I.V. into different groups of normal C3H mice. Four days later, their peritoneal macrophages were tested for the ability to form rosettes with L1210 cells in the presence of cytophilic antibody to L1210. Degree of macrophage suppression is indicated in recipient mice which received various fractions of suppressor spleen cells by adoptive transfer: ■ : 4 x 10⁷ nylon non-adherent spleen cells (nylon non-adh.); ▨ : 5 x 10⁷ ATS-treated nylon non-adherent spleen cells (nylon non-adh. (ATS)): ☐ : 5 x 10⁷ nylon adherent spleen cells (nylon adh.); and ▨ : no cells.

73

These results indicate that suppression of macrophages, i.e. inhibition of their receptors for cytophilic antibody, can be induced by adoptive transfer of thymocytes or peripheral (splenic) T-cells from donors that were suppressed by immune complexes.

Kinetics of Suppression after Adoptive Transfer
The degree of inhibition of cytophilic antibody receptors found at various times after transfer of suppressor thymocytes was studied. As shown in Figure 2, inhibition of the cytophilic antibody receptors of the peritoneal

Figure 2—TIME COURSE OF THE INHIBITION OF CYTOPHILIC ANTIBODY RECEPTORS INDUCED BY ADOPTIVE TRANSFER OF SUPPRESSOR THYMOCYTES

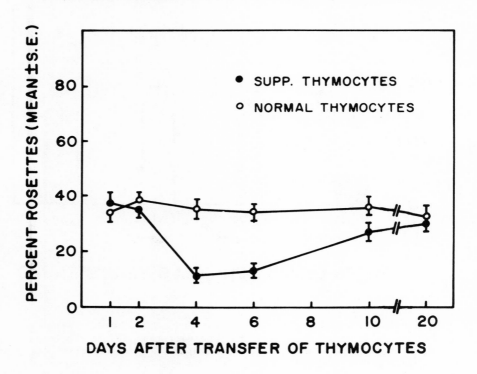

C3H mice were treated i.p. with immune complexes (anti-L1210—SA-L1210). Ten days later, the 4 x 10⁷ thymocytes from the suppressed mice (suppressor thymocytes) were injected I.V. into different groups of C3H mice. Peritoneal macrophages were tested at various times thereafter for their ability to form rosettes with L1210 cells *via* cytophilic antibody to L1210.

74

macrophages was observed 4 to 6 days after the transfer of 4×10^7 suppressor thymocytes. Ten to 15% of the peritoneal macrophages collected from recipients formed rosettes in the presence of cytophilic antibody to L1210, whereas macrophages collected on days 1, 2 and 20 after the cell transfer showed little or no difference from normal macrophages in their ability to form rosettes (30-40%).

Apparent Specificity of Macrophage Suppression by Suppressor T-Cells

C3H mice were treated with L1210 immune complexes. Ten days later, their thymocytes were injected (i.v.) to normal syngeneic mice (4×10^7 per mouse). Four days afterward the recipient's peritoneal monocytes were tested for their ability to form rosettes with L1210 in the presence of cytophilic antibody to L1210, and with antigenically unrelated cells such as EL4 and SRBC, in the presence of their respective cytophilic antibodies (Table 6). Recipients of suppressor T-cells from L1210-suppressed mice had monocytes that failed to fix cytophilic antibody to L1210 (Group 1), but formed rosettes normally with EL4 or SRBC (Groups 2 and 3). Seventy to 80% of activated macrophages from mice given L1210 cells alone formed rosettes; these served as a positive control (Group 5).

Table 6—SPECIFICITY OF INHIBITION OF CYTOPHILIC ANTIBODY RECEPTOR ON MACROPHAGE BY SUPPRESSOR THYMOCTYES

Group	Cells Injected Type	Number (x10⁷)	Monocytes Tested with[c]	Rosettes on Day 4 after Transfer Mean ± S.E.	Score
1	Suppressed Thy[a]	4	Anti L1210 + L1210	10.8 ± 0.9	0
2	Suppressed Thy	4	Anti EL4 + EL-4	40.2 ± 2.7	2+
3	Suppressed Thy	4	Anti SRBC + SRBC	35.3 ± 2.1	2+
4	Nil	Nil	Anti L1210 + L1210	37.4 ± 1.9	2+
5	L1210[b]	5	Anti L1210 + L1210	85.5 ± 3.5	4+

[a]C3H mice were treated with immune complexes as detailed in Materials and Methods. Ten days later, the thymocytes from the suppressed mice were injected I.V. on day zero into normal C3H mice.

[b]5×10^7 irradiated L1210 (5000R) were injected i.p. into C3H mice on day (-4).

[c]4 days after the transfer of suppressor thymocytes, the peritoneal monocytes were tested *in vivo* for rosetting with L1210 and/or EL4 and/or SRBC, *via* the corresponding antibody.

Interaction of Suppressor and Normal T-Cells in Suppression of Macro-
phages

Groups of T-cell depleted mice ("B" mice) were injected (i.v.) with 6×10^7 suppressor thymocytes. Four days later, their peritoneal macrophages were tested for uptake of cytophilic antibody and subsequent rosette formation. Thirty to 40% of the macrophages formed rosettes with L1210 (Table 7— groups 1, 2 and 3), i.e., no suppression was demonstrable. Similar results were obtained with suppressor splenic T-cells in "B" mice (Groups 4 and 5). In contrast, 4×10^7 suppressor thymocytes (Group 6) or splenic T-cells (Group 7) injected into syngeneic normal mice were able to suppress the cytophilic antibody receptors of their macrophages.

Table 7—LACK OF MACROPHAGE SUPPRESSION BY SUPPRESSOR THYMOCYTES IN "B" MICE (T-cell Deficient)

Group	Cells Injected[a]		Recipient (C3H Mice)	Rosettes on Day 4 After Transfer	
	Type	Dose ($\times 10^7$)		Mean ± S.E.	Score
1	Supp Thy	2	B-mice[b]	43.0 ± 2.9	2+
2	Supp Thy	4	B-mice	32.5 ± 2.1	2+
3	Supp Thy	6	B-mice	30.1 ± 2.5	2+
4	Supp Spl T-cell	4	B-mice	42.5 ± 3.1	2+
5	Supp Spl T-cell	6	B-mice	31.5 ± 2.4	2+
6	Supp Thy	4	Normal	9.2 ± 0.7	0
7	Supp Spl T-cell	4	Normal	11.3 ± 1.1	0

[a]C3H mice were immune suppressed with anti-L1210 and L1210 cells as detailed in the text. Ten days later, the thymocytes from the suppressed mice were used as suppressor thymocytes (Supp Thy). Spleen cells from the suppressed mice were fractionated on nylon column. The nylon non-adherent cells were used as suppressor spleen T-cells (Supp Spl T-cells).

[b]Thymectomized, lethally irradiated and bone-marrow reconstituted C3H mice ("B" mice) or T-cell depleted mice.

As shown in Table 8, interaction of the suppressor T-cells with normal T-cells was essential for the induction of suppression. Groups of "B" mice were injected with 4×10^7 suppressor T-cells admixed with various doses of normal T-cells, ranging from 2.5 to 20×10^6 cells and, 4 days later, their peritoneal macrophages were tested for the integrity of their cytophilic antibody receptors. Groups 3 and 4, which received 10×10^6 and 20×10^6

Table 8—COOPERATION OF SUPPRESSOR AND NORMAL T-CELLS IN MACROPHAGE SUPPRESSION IN "B" MICE

Group	Supp Cells Injected[a] (4 x 10^7)	Normal Cells Injected Type	Number (x10^6)	Recipient	Rosettes on Day 4 After Transfer Mean ± S.E.	Score
1	Supp Thy	Nor Thy	2.5	B-mice[c]	35.4 ± 2.4	2+
2	Supp Thy	Nor Thy	5	B-mice	37.2 ± 2.4	2+
3	Supp Thy	Nor Thy	10	B-mice	13.1 ± 1.2	0
4	Supp Thy	Nor Thy	20	B-mice	9.8 ± 0.8	0
5	Supp Thy	Nor Spl T-cell[b]	5	B-mice	42.8 ± 2.8	2+
6	Supp Thy	Nor Spl T-cell	10	B-mice	12.1 ± 1.0	0
7	Supp Thy	Nor Spl T-cell	20	B-mice	13.8 ± 1.1	0
8	Supp Thy	Supp Spl T-cell	20	B-mice	34.2 ± 2.5	2
9	Supp Thy	Nil	Nil	B-mice	39.2 ± 2.6	2+
10	Supp Thy	Nil	Nil	Normal	10.4 ± 0.9	0

[a]C3H mice were immune suppressed with immune complexes and/or anti-L1210 and SA-L1210 as detailed in the text. Ten days later, the thymocytes from the suppressed mice were used as suppressor thymocytes (Supp Thy).

[b]Spleen cells from normal C3H mice were fractionated on nylon wool column and the nylon non-adherent splenocytes were used as normal splenic T-cells (nor spl T-cell).

[c]Thymectomized, lethally irradiated and bone-marrow reconstituted mice.

normal thymocytes, respectively, in addition to suppressor thymocytes (4 x 10^7) showed suppression of macrophages to a degree comparable with normal recipients receiving 4 x 10^7 suppressor thymocytes alone (Group 10). The admixture of 4 x 10^7 suppressor thymocytes with 5 x 10^6 or fewer normal T-cells failed to inhibit macrophages in T-cell depleted recipients (Groups 1 and 2). Normal spleen T-cells could also be used by suppressor thymocytes for T-T cooperation to induce macrophage suppression in recipient mice (Groups 6 and 7). In contrast, the suppressor thymocytes did not cooperate with the splenic T-cells from suppressed mice, and the macrophages of the recipients of this mixture were not suppressed (Group 8).

These results suggest that the suppressor T-cells from donor mice need the presence of a considerable number of syngeneic normal T-cells in order to effect suppression upon adoptive transfer. Normal T-cells provided an essential element since even large numbers of suppressor T-cells alone failed to cause suppression in mice lacking T-cells.

DISCUSSION

In this paper, evidence is presented that soluble immune complexes are capable of inducing suppression of macrophage receptors for cytophilic antibody and that the Fc portion of immunoglobulin in the complex plays an essential role. Mice treated with both whole antibody (anti-L1210), and antigen (SA-L1210), but not either alone, elicited macrophages that were incapable of fixing cytophilic antibody to L1210 and failing to form rosettes with L1210 cells. The inhibition of receptors for cytophilic antibody to L1210 was immunologically specific, since the same macrophages were able to form rosettes normally with the antigenically unrelated leukemia EL4. Complementary results were obtained in reciprocal experiments where EL4-containing immune complexes inhibited only receptors for EL4 antibodies and not cytophilic anti-L1210.

The presence of different and distinct receptors on the macrophage for the Fc portion of immunoglobulin has been emphasized by several investigators (4,30,31). Walker (31) has demonstrated two types of receptors for Fc on mouse peritoneal macrophages which bound separately to IgG_{2a} and IgG_{2b} myeloma proteins. In the guinea pig, receptors for Fc on macrophages have been shown to bind guinea pig IgG_2 but not IgG_1. Inchley, et al. (32) found a disparity in the ability of subclasses of human myeloma proteins to bind to macrophages. Notably, even within a subclass (specifically, IgG), there was considerable variation in the degree of binding of immunoglobulins from different sources. Thus, while no one has shown that receptors for the Fc portion can distinguish among antibodies of the same class differing only in their idiotype, as our evidence suggests, published

78

data clearly show differences among such receptors for the allegedly "invariable" Fc portion of immunoglobulin.

Sinclair and his associates have emphasized the importance of the Fc portion of antibody in the feedback suppression of antibody synthesis. Although $F(ab^1)_2$ fragments had some suppressive activity, they were often 1000-fold less potent than intact immunoglobulin (33,34). The rapid excretion of $F(ab^1)_2$ fragments did fully account for the discrepancy, since several injections of the fragments to compensate for excretion failed to overcome the difference in suppression (34). In fact, augmented rather than diminished immunity has sometimes been observed with $F(ab^1)_2$ like fragments (35). Our inability to produce suppression of macrophages with $F(ab^1)_2$ immune complexes given at compensatorily high dosage (36), supports the concept that the Fc portion is a necessary component to produce suppression. The Fc portion alone was not sufficient; it must be part of an intact immunoglobulin molecule to constitute the signal that initiates suppression of macrophages *in vivo*.

The present study also demonstrates the ability of thymocytes or splenic T-cells from "suppressed" mice (pretreated with immune complexes) to transfer this specific suppression of macrophages adoptively to normal mice without the need for additional antigen. Suppression could not be transferred to T-cell depleted mice ("B" mice) unless normal T-cells were admixed.

The role of T-cells as regulators of the immune response has heretofore been explored mainly *in vitro*, through the generation of suppressor T-cells (37,38) by a high concentration of antigen. In most of the studies, however, the presence of suppressor T-cells was also demonstrated *in vitro* by adding a large number of educated cells to normal spleen cells (39). Reinisch, et al. (40) were able to generate suppressor T-cells *in vivo* with complete Freund's adjuvant, which suppressed the production of cytotoxic cells *in vitro*. The present study represents an *in vivo* demonstration of suppressive activity by suppressor T-cells, generated *in vivo* by immune complexes. The Fc portion of the antibody (36) and an intact thymus of the recipient (22) are both essential in the induction of the inhibition of cytophilic antibody receptors on macrophages. The presence of receptors for the Fc portion of antibody (Fc receptors, FcR) on the surface of T-cells has been substantiated in a number of studies (41,42). Stout and Herzenberg utilizing the fluorescence-activated cell sorter have demonstrated the presence of Fc receptors on the surface of a distinct subpopulation of murine T-lymphocytes, different from antigen-specific helper cells. These two subpopulations of T-lymphocytes, FcR^+ and FcR^- T-cells, also respond differently to various mitogens (43). It is most likely that immune complexes bind to FcR^+ T-lymphocytes, perhaps mainly in the thymus where naive cells may predominate, and induce suppressor T-cells. Since the binding of cytophilic anti-L1210 to its receptor was specifically prevented here, as in earlier studies (21,36), the influence of suppressor T-cells appears to be directed against the binding of the idiotype of antibody used to generate them. The specific suppressor signal to the T-cells probably requires binding of the immune complexes both to the antigen receptor and FcR sites of thymocytes (44). The transmittal of the signal could conceivably be solely through the FcR if a specific rearrangement of the immunoglobulin occurred as a result of its interaction with antigen.

The requirement of normal T-lymphocytes for the suppressor T-lymphocytes to elicit suppression of macrophages in "B" mice (Table 8) emphasizes the need for some type of T-T cell cooperation (45). Cooperation between subclasses of T-lymphocytes has been shown in the generation of mature cytotoxic lymphocytes (46,47). Cantor and Boyse (47) have in

Figure 3—SCHEMA OF THE INHIBITION OF CYTOPHILIC ANTIBODY RECEPTORS ON MACROPHAGES BY IMMUNE COMPLEXES THROUGH FUNCTIONAL SUPPRESSOR T-CELLS

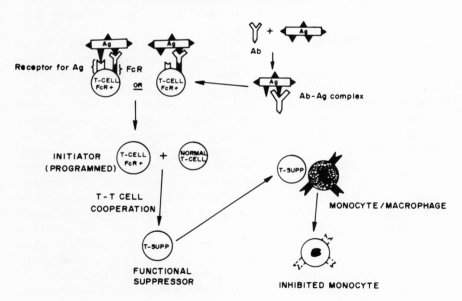

The functional suppressor T-cells may result from the interaction of initiator suppressor cells (specific to antigen) generated by immune complexes and normal T-cells. Ab: antibody; Ag: antigen; Ab-Ag complex: antibody-antigen complex; FcR+: Fc receptor-positive; T-Supp: suppressor T-cell.

80

particular shown that T-lymphocytes of the Ly1 phenotype enhance the generation of cytotoxic lymphocytes from the Ly2 cytotoxic precursor pool. Stout, et al. (48) have reported similar T-T cooperation in the induction of cytotoxicity. An analogy is suggested between the role of helper T-cells involved in the differentiation of mature antibody-producing cells (49,50), and that of "amplifier" T-cells involved in the generation of cell-mediated lympholysis (48). Cantor, et al. (51) have also shown that T-helper cells (Ly1) can induce cells of another T-cell subset (Ly 123[+]) to exert potent suppressive activity (as Ly23 suppressor cells).

In our system, (Figure 3) T-lymphocytes from the suppressed mice (immune complex-treated mice) may act as initiators, to recruit functional suppressor cells from the population of normal T-cells. Alternatively the "programmed", yet apparently non-functional, T-cells from the donor mice might interact with normal Ly 123 T-cells and thereby acquire full functional capacity as suppressor cells. The two possibilities are not exclusive, since once created the functional suppressor cells might later recruit more suppressors from normal T-cells. Studies characterizing the phenotypes of the subpopulations of donor and recipient T-lymphocytes that cooperate here and the nature of their interaction, are in progress.

REFERENCES

1. Amos, D.B., "Possible Relationship between Cytotoxic Effects of Isoantibody and Host Cell Function". *Ann. N.Y. Acad. Sci.* 87:273, 1960.
2. Piessens, W.F., Churchill, W.H., and David, J.R., "Macrophages Activated *in vitro* with Lymphocyte Mediators Kill Neoplastic but Normal Cells". *J. Immun.* 114:293, 1975.
3. Schmidt, M.F., Douglas, S.D., and Rubins, A.D., "Human Monocyte Activation by Supernatants from Conconavalin A (con A) Stimulated Lymphocytes". *Cell Immunol.* 9:45, 1973.
4. Berken, A., and Benecerraf, B., "Properties of Antibodies Cytophilic for Macrophages". *J. Exp. Med.* 123:119, 1966.
5. Boyden, S.V., "Cytophilic Antibody in Guinea Pig with Delayed Type Hypersensitivity". *Brit. Med. Bull.* 23:15, 1967.
6. Granger, G.A., Rubins, J., and Wieser, R.S., "The Role of Cytophilic Antibody in Immune Macrophage-Target Cell Interaction". *J. Reticuloendothel. Soc.* 3:354, 1966.
7. Bennet, B., Old, L.J., and Boyse, E.A., "Opsonization of Cells by Isoantibody *in vitro*". *Nature* 198:10, 1963.
8. Mitchell, M.S., Mokyr, M.B., Aspnes, G.T., and McIntosh, S., "Cytophilic Antibodies in Man". *Ann. Inter. Med.* 79:333, 1973.
9. Marti, J.H., Grosser, N., and Thomson, D.M.P., "Tube Leukocyte Adherence Assay for the Detection of Anti-Tumor Immunity. II. Monocyte Reacts with Tumor Antigen in a Cytophilic Anti-Tumor Antibody". *Int. J. Cancer* 18:48, 1976.
10. Hellström, K.E., and Hellström, I., "Lymphocyte-Mediated Cytotoxicity and Blocking Serum Activity to Tumor Antigens". *Adv. Immunol.* 18:209, 1974.
11. Baldwin, R.W., and Price, M.R., "Tumor Antigens and Tumor Host Relationships". *Ann. Rev. Medicine* 27:151, 1976.
12. Rao, V.S., Bagai, R., and Bonavida, B., "Specific Enhancement of Tumor Growth and

Depression of Cell Mediated Immunity following Sensitization to Soluble Tumor Antigens". *Cancer Res.* 36:1384, 1976.

13. Rao, V.S., and Bonavida, B., "Detection of Soluble Tumor-Associated Antigens in Serum of Tumor-Bearing Rats and Their Immunological Role *in vivo*". *Cancer Res.* 37:3385, 1977.

14. Baldwin, R.W., Price, N., and Robins, R., "Blocking of Lymphocyte Mediated Cytotoxicity for Rat Hepatoma Cells by Tumor Specific Antigen-Antibody Complexes". *Nature New Biol.* 238:185, 1972.

15. Sjogren, H.O., Hellstŕom, I., Bansal, S.C. and Hellström, K.E., "Suggestive Evidence that the Blocking Antibodies of Tumor Bearing Individuals may be Antigen-Antibody Complexes". *Proc. Natl. Acad. Sci.* 68:1272, 1971.

16. Rao, V.S., and Mitchell, M.S., "Suppression of Macrophage Mediated Immunity to Leukemia L1210 by Immune Complexes". *Proc. Amer. Assoc. Cancer Res.* 18:63, 1977.

17. Nimberg, R.B., Glasgow, A.H., Menzaian, J.O., et al., "Isolation of an Immunosuppressive Peptide Fraction from the Serum of Cancer Patients." *Cancer Res.* 35:1489, 1975.

18. Kall, M.A., Hellström, I., and Hellström, K.E., "Different Responses of Lymphoid Cells from Tumor Specific Bearing as Compared to Tumor Immunized Mice when Sensitized to Tumor Specific Antigens *in vitro*". *Proc. Natl. Acad. Sci.* 73:5086, 1975.

19. Green, M.I., Fujimoto, S., and Sehon, A.H., "Regulation of the Immune Response to Tumor Antigens III. Characterization of Thymic Suppressor Factor(s) Produced by Tumor Bearing Hosts". *J. Immunol.* 119:757, 1977.

20. Mitchell, M.S., "Central Inhibition of Cellular Immunity to Leukemia L1210 by Isoantibody." *Cancer Res.* 32:825, 1972.

21. Mitchell, M.S., and Mokyr, M.B., "Specific Inhibition of Receptors for Cytophilic Antibody on Macrophages by Isoantibody". *Cancer Res.* 32:832, 1972.

22. Gershon, R.K., Mokyr, M.B., and Mitchell, M.S., "Activation of Suppressor T-Cells by Tumor Cells and Specific Antibody". *Nature* 250:594, 1974.

23. Rao, V.S., Mokyr, M.B., Gershon, R.K., and Mitchell, M.S., "Specific T-Cell-Dependent, Antigen-Antibody Mediated Suppression of Macrophages: Abrogation by Non-Specifically Stimulated T-Cells". *J. Immunol.* 118:2117, 1977.

24. Feldmann, M., and Diener, E., "Antibody-Mediated Suppression of the Immune Response *in vitro*". *J. Immunol.* 108:93, 1971.

25. Porter, R.R., "The Hydrolysis of Rabbit-γ-globulin and Antibodies with Crystalline Papain". *Biochem. J.* 73:119, 1959.

26. Rao, V.S., Bonavida, B., Zighelboin, J., and Fahey, J.L., "Preferential Induction of Serum Blocking Activity and Enhancement of Skin Allograff by Soluble Alloantigen". *Transplantation* 17:568, 1974.

27. Lowry, O.H., Rosenbrough, N.J., Farr, A.L., and Randall, R.J., "Protein Measurement with the Folin Phenol Reagent". *J. Biol. Chem.* 193:265, 1951.

28. Trizio, D., and Cudkowicz, G., "Separation of T and B Lymphocytes by Nylon Wool Columns: Evaluation of Efficacy by Functional Assay *in vivo*". *J. Immunol.* 113:1093, 1974.

29. Miller, J.F., "Studies on Mouse Leukaemia: The Role of the Thymus in Leukaemogenesis by Cell-Free Leukaemic Filtrates". *Brit. J. Cancer* 14:93, 1960.

30. Unkeles, J.C., and Eisen, H.N., "Binding of Monomeric Immunoglobulins to Fc Receptors of Mouse Macrophages". *J. Exp. Med.* 142:1520, 1975.

31. Walker, W.S., "Separate Fc Receptors for Immunoglobulins IgG 2_a and IgG 2_b on an Established Cell Line of Mouse Macrophages". *J. Immunol.* 116:911, 1976.

32. Inchley, C., Grey, H.M., and Uhr, J.W., "The Cytophilic Activity of Human Immunoglobulins". *J. Immunol.* 105:362, 1970.

33. Sinclair, N.R., Lee, R.K., Chan, P.L., and Khan, R.H., "Regulation of the Immune Response. II. Further Studies on Differences in Ability of F(ab¹)₂ and 7S Antibodies to Inhibit an Antibody Response". *Immunology* 19:105, 1970.

34. Sinclair, N.R., Lee, R.K., Chan, P.L., and Khan, R.H., "Regulation of the Immune

Response. II. Further Studies on Differences in Ability of F(ab¹)₂ and 7S Antibodies to Inhibit an Antibody Response". *Immunology* 19:105, 1970.

35. Kulberg, A.J., Evnin, D.N., and Tarkhanova, I.A., "Enhancement of the Immune Response by a Catabolic Product of Normal Rabbit IgG: Effects of F(ab¹)₂-like fragment". *Immunology* 30:715, 1976.

36. Rao, V.S., Grodzicki, R.L., and Mitchell, M.S., "Specific *in vivo* Inhibition of Macrophage Receptors for Cytophilic Antibody by Soluble Immune Complexes". *Cancer Res.* 1978 (in press).

37. Gershon, R.K., "Immunoregulation by T Cells". In *Molecular Approaches to Immunology*, edited by E.E. Smith and D.W. Ribbons, Academic Press, New York, 267-288, 1975.

38. Gershon, R.K., "A Disquisition on Suppressor T-Cells". *Transplantation Rev.* 26:170, 1975.

39. Eardley, D.D., and Gershon, R.K., "Induction of Specific Suppressor T-Cells *in vitro*". *J. Immunol.* 117:313, 1976.

40. Reinisch, C.L., Andrew, S.D., and Schlossman, S.F., "Suppressor Cell Regulation of Immune Response to Tumors: Abrogation by Adult-thymectomy". *Proc. Natl. Acad. Sci.* 74:2989, 1977.

41. Anderson, C.L., and Grey, H.M., "Receptors for Aggregated IgG on Mouse Lymphocytes: Their Presence on Thymocytes, Thymus Derived and Bone Marrow-Derived Lymphocytes". *J. Exp. Med.* 139:1175, 1974.

42. Stout, R.D., and Herzenberg, L.A., "The Fc Receptor on Thymus-Derived Lymphocytes I. Detection of a Subpopulation of Murine T-Lymphocytes Bearing the Fc Receptor". *J. Exp. Med.* 142:611, 1975.

43. Stout, R.D., and Herzenberg, L.A., "The Fc Receptor on Thymus-Derived Lymphocytes II. Mitogen Responsiveness of T-Lymphocytes Bearing the Fc Receptor". *J. Exp. Med.* 142:1041, 1975.

44. Sinclair, N.R., and Chan, P.L., "Regulation of the Immune Response. IV. The Role of the Fc Fragment in Feedback Inhibition by Antibody". In *Morphological and Fundamental Aspects of Immunity*, Lindahl-Kiessling Alm. and Hanna (Eds.), Plenum Press, N.Y., 609, 1971.

45. Rao, V.S., and Mitchell, M.S., "Suppressor T-Cells Can Adoptively Transfer the Suppression of Macrophages Induced by Immune Complexes". *Proc. Assoc. Cancer Res.* 19:33, 1978.

46. Tigelaar, R.E. and Asofsky, R., "Synergy Among Lymphoid Cells Mediating the Graft-Versus-Host Response: V. Derivation by Migration in Lethally Irradiated Recipients of Two Interacting Subpopulation of Thymus-Derived Cells". *J. Exp. Med.* 137:239, 1973.

47. Cantor, H. and Boyse, E.A., "Functional Subclasses of T-Lymphocytes Bearing Different Ly Antigens. II. Cooperation Between Subclasses of Ly+ Cells in the Generation of Killer Activity". *J. Exp. Med.* 141:1390, 1975.

48. Stout, R.D., Waksal, S.D., and Herzenberg, L.A., "The Fc Receptor on Thymus Derived Lymphocytes, III. Mixed Lymphocyte Reactivity and Cell-Mediated Lymphocytic Activity of Fc- and Fc+ Lymphocytes". *J. Exp. Med.* 144:54, 1976.

49. Gershon, R.K., "T-Cell Control of Antibody Production" in *Contemporary Topics in Immunobiology*, Cooper, M.D. and Warner, N.L. (Eds.), Plenum Publishing Corporation, New York, Vol. 3, 1-49, 1974.

50. Cautinho, A., and Moller, G., "Thymus-Independent B-Cell Induction and Paralysis". *Adv. Immunol.* 21:113, 1975.

51. Cantor, H., McVay-Boudreau, L., Hugenberg, J., et al., "Immunoregulatory Circuits Among T-cells Sets II. Physiologic Role of Feedback Inhibition *in vivo*: Absence in NZB Mice", *J. Exp. Med.* 147:1116, 1978.

Antigenic Mimicry Exhibited Between BCG and Human Neoplastic and Normal Tissue Extracts†

Peter Maxim[1]
R. Veltri[1,2]

SUMMARY—Reports from various laboratories indicate that microorganisms possess antigens that are also expressed on tumor cells. This sharing of common antigens between widely diverse groups of organisms has been termed antigenic mimicry. Our objective was to determine whether mimicry existed between microorganisms and human lung carcinoma extracts. Antisera were raised in rabbits to several different genera of bacteria. These antisera were tested by Ouchterlony double diffusion and by an agarose adsorption modification of this procedure for cross-reactivity to human serum and tissue extracts. Of all the antisera tested only those to BCG reacted with human tissue extracts. These antisera reacted to 100,000xg soluble extracts of human lung tumors, normal human lung soluble extracts and fetal lung soluble extracts giving two precipitan bands. The major BCG cross-reactive antigen also reacted with human serum and could be adsorbed by serum or Cohn fraction II and III of normal human serum. This antigen was also found to be present in the sera of several different animal species. The minor BCG cross-reactive antigen remained following adsorption with serum, but was present in normal as well as tumor soluble extracts. This antigen, however, could not be detected in extracts of breast, colon or cervical tumors. Supported by NCI contract NO1-CB-43890.

INTRODUCTION

Antigenic mimicry is said to occur when a microorganism and mammalian cell share a common antigenic determinant. There is abundant information in the literature supporting the concept that such sharing does occur and this has been the subject of a review (1). The most commonly cited examples of antigenic determinants shared by microorganisms and mammalian cells include blood group substances (1,2), Forssman antigens (1, 2), and histocompatibility antigens (3, 4).

Microorganism can acquire these heterogenetic antigens by several different means. While many are synthesized under the control of the microbial genome still others can be adsorbed from the environment. The acquisition of new antigenic determinants by microbes and multicellular

---

[1]Department of Surgery, West Virginia University, Morgantown, West Virginia.
[2]Department of Microbiology, West Virginia University, Morgantown, West Virginia.
†Supported by NCI contract N01-CB-43890.

parasites from their environments has been established (1, 5). A final mechanism involves those intracellular parasites that reproduce by budding. For example, influenza virus (2) and members of the Herpes viruses (6) acquire host cell membrane antigens by this process.

The presence of antigens on both a microorganism and host tissue may give rise to immunopathological injury subsequent to the infectious process. A classic example being the cross-reactivity of streptococcal antigens and heart antigens that has been implicated in the pathogenesis of rheumatic fever (7).

While the above situation has obvious deleterious effects, the presence of shared antigens between microbes and tumor cells could contribute to enhance the hoste immune defenses of tumors. Borsos and Rapp (8) demonstrated an antigen present on *Mycobacterium bovis* BCG which was also present in transplantable guinea pig hepatoma line 10 cells but not in line 1 cells. This finding was extended to show cross-reactivity between BCG and cultured human melanoma cells (9). Minden et al. (10) have confirmed the above findings in tissue culture cells and found cross reactive antigens in human tumors. This group was also able to show antibodies to both melanoma and BCG antigens in the sera form melanoma patients and non tumor bearing individuals (11). Similarily, cross-reactions have been shown for several other microorganisms and tumor cells (12, 13).

The value of BCG and other microorganisms as a therapeutic technique (reviewed in 14) in cancer, therefore, may well have part of its value associated with the presence of cross reacting antigens.

The objective of this study was to examine the possibility of antigenic mimicry occuring between selected microorganisms and human lung cancer extracts. The choice of bacterial antigens to be considered was influenced primarily by a report from Ruckdeschel et al. (15) In a retrospective analysis of patients undergoing surgical resection for lung cancer, it was found that the five year survival rate for patients that developed empyema was 50%. Another group of patients that did not develop empyema had a 5 year survival rate of 18%. The organisms isolated from these patients were *Staphylococcus aureus, Escherichia coli, Pseudomonas aeruginosa* and *Candida albicans*. In another study of nonsurgical patients with empyema the same organisms were commonly found as well as *Streptococcus pneumoniae* and *Klebsiella* (16). Antisera to these organisms as well as BCG were raised and tested to determine whether cross reactive antigens could be detected in lung extracts.

MATERIALS AND METHODS

Organisms

The Phipps strain of *Mycobacterium bovis* BCG grown on Proskaur-Beck media with tween-80 (Difco) was obtained from the Trudeau Institute and

86

the National Institute of Health supplied the Pasteur strain. The Eli Lilly Company supplied pneumococcal vaccine prepared from type 14 *Streptococcus pneumoniae* and a second vaccine with twelve capsular polysaccharides included. *Staphylococcus aureus* Cowan I and *Klebsiella pneumoniae* were obtained from culture collections maintained at West Virginia University.

Tissue Processing Protocol

Human tumor tissues, embryonic tissues and normal tissue specimens were obtained through the cooperation of the Departments of Surgery and Pathology at West Virginia University. The tissues were minced, washed, homogenized and separated into soluble and membrane fractions by centrifugation at 100,000xg. The details of this procedure and methods used for various chemical and mechanical extractions of the membrane pellets have been published previously (17).

Serum Sources

Normal human sera were obtained from healthy laboratory personnel and from blood bank donors. Sera from various animal species were supplied by Dr. Robert Burrell, Department of Microbiology, West Virginia University. Cohn fractions (18) of normal human serum were purchased from Pentax Laboratories.

Immunization Protocol

New Zealand white rabbits were obtained from local suppliers and acclimated to conventional facilities for two weeks before use. Ten days before starting active immunization the animals were "primed" by injecting 2.5ml of Freund's incomplete adjuvant at four sites: two i.m. in each thigh and two s.c. in the neck region. The immunization protocol consisted of injections of 1×10^7 organisms or 50ug of the pneumococcal vaccines mixed with 2.0ml of the adjuvant Alhydrogel (Gallard Schlesinger) at two week intervals. The animals received 5 injections before test bleeds were taken. The sera were tested for cross reactivity to normal human serum and normal human lung soluble extract. If reactive, the animals received one booster injection and were exsanguinated one week later. If nonreactive, the animals were boosted and retested for a maximum of 4 more injections. If nonreactive at the end of this time the animals were terminated.

Immunodiffusion

All immunodiffusion assays were performed in 0.75% agarose prepared in 1.0M glycine, 0.85% NaCl, and 0.1% sodium azide, pH 7.1. Immunodiffusion plates were prepared by coating 7.5 x 10 cm glass plates with 20ml of agarose solution. Patterns were cut with wells 7mm in diameter and 6mm apart.

Adsorption analyses were performed by the agarose diffusion method of DeCarvalho (19). Antiserum wells were filled with normal human serum and/or soluble tissue extracts and incubated at 37°C for 2 hours. Thereafter, the antiserum and antigen wells were filled and incubated overnight at 37°C. Precipitation of antibodies to the adsorbent fluid occurred in a zone surrounding the antiserum well.

Immunoelectrophoresis

Immuno-Tec-II kits (Behring Diagnostics) were used with a barbital buffer, ionic strength 0.04, pH-8.6, to perform immunoelectrophoretic analyses. The samples were applied to the wells and electrophoresed at 125 volts for 2 hours. After addition of antisera to the troughs, the plates were incubated overnight at room temperature.

RESULTS

Analysis of Antisera

Antisera raised to the various microorganisms as described in materials and methods were confirmed to have reactivity to the immunogens. They were then tested by immunodiffusion against normal human serum. After adsorption with pooled normal human sera, they were again tested against lung soluble extracts.

The antisera raised to *S. aureus, K. pneumoniae,* and the pneumococcal vaccines had no reactivity against serum or lung soluble extracts. The antisera to BCG, however, did react with normal human serum and tissue extracts giving several bands (Figure 1). Following adsorption with normal human serum, reactivity to normal human lung soluble extracts remained (Figure 2). These reactivities were collectively referred to as serum (S-band) and tissue (T-band) for further studies. (Figure 1 & 2)

A summary of the reactivity of several different antisera is presented in Table 1. Of those antisera that reacted with serum or lung solubles the response was varied. Three antisera to BCG-Phipps reacted with serum giving one or two precipitin bands. Four reacted with lung soluble pools giving from 1 to 4 bands. (Table 1)

Immunoelectrophoretic analysis of an unadsorbed antiserum to BCG is presented in Figure 3. It can be seen that this antiserum gives three precipitin arcs against normal human serum and two against normal lung extract. The cathodally migrating antigen is common to both antigen mixtures. (Figure 3)

Figure 1—CROSS REACTIVITY BETWEEN ANTI-BCG AND NORMAL HUMAN SERUM, NORMAL LUNG SOLUBLE EXTRACT AND LUNG TUMOR SOLUBLE EXTRACT

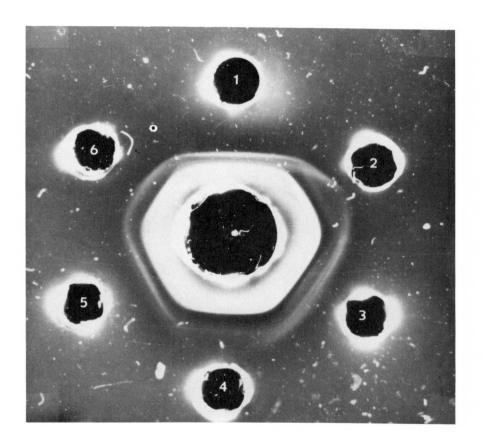

Center well contains unadsorbed anti-BCG. Outer wells 1, 3, 5 contain normal human serum diluted 1:5, 1:10, and 1:20 respectively. Wells 2 and 6 contain normal lung extract and well 4 contains tumor soluble extract.

Figure 2—CROSS REACTIVITY BETWEEN ANTI-BCG ADSORBED WITH NORMAL HUMAN SERUM AND LUNG EXTRACTS

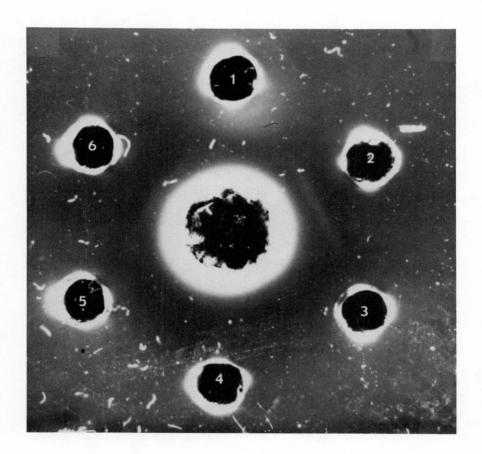

Center wells contain anti-BCG adsorbed with normal human serum. Outer wells are as in Figure 1. A faint precipitin band is present against the normal lung extracts in wells 2 and 6.

Table 1—SUMMARY OF IMMUNIZATION EXPERIMENT

Antiserum	Normal Human Serum		Normal Human Lung	
	Animals Reactive	Number of Bands	Animals Reactive	Number of Bands
Staphylococcus aureus	0/5	—	0/5	—
Klebsiella pneumoniae	0/5	—	0/5	—
Type 14 pneumococcal polysaccharide	0/5	—	0/5	—
Dodecyl pneumococcal vaccine	0/5	—	0/5	—
BCG-Phipps	3/5	1,2,1	4/5	1,2,4,2
BCG-Pasteur	0/3	—	1/3	1

Figure 3—IMMUNOELECTROPHORETIC ANALYSIS OF ANTI-BCG CROSS REACTIVITY

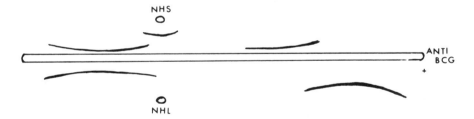

Unadsorbed anti-BCG is in the trough. Normal human serum (NHS) and normal human lung (NHL) soluble extract were placed in the wells.

Analysis of Serum Cross Reactivity

To further characterize the serum component cross-reacting with the anti BCG antisera adsorption studies were performed with Cohn fractions of a normal serum pool. Antiserum wells in diffusion plates were first filled with the specified Cohn fraction (10mg/ml) and later filled with the anti-BCG serum. It can be seen in Table 2 that all Cohn fractions except II-III removed the S-band reactivity but did not affect the reactivity of the antiserum to tissue. Similar results were obtained when the anti-BCG serum was tested unadsorbed against Cohn fractions and normal serum pool. A line of identity formed with all Cohn fractions except II-III.

Table 2—CROSS-REACTIVITY BETWEEN ANTI-BCG AND COHN FRACTIONS OF NORMAL HUMAN SERUM

Cohn Fraction	Adsorption Analysis		Identity Analysis	
	S-Band	T-Band	S-Band	T-Band
I	—	+[a]	+[b]	—
II, III	+	+	—	—
IV	—	+	+	—
V	—	+	+	—
VI	—	+	+	—

[a] + indicates that antiserum still gives either S or T band in immunodiffusion after adsorption with specified Cohn Fraction.
[b] + indicates that line of identity forms between antigen in specified Cohn Fraction and normal human serum.
S-Band denotes the reaction between anti-BCG and normal human serum.
T-Band is that reaction that occurs between anti-BCG adsorbed with normal human serum and soluble tissue extracts.

Because of the cross-reactivity with human serum we also wanted to determine whether the anti-BCG serum cross reacted with sera of other animal species. Table 3 shows that the cross reacting antigenic determinant was present in the serum of a variety of different animal species representing several different phyla.

Reactivity of Antiserum with Tissue Extracts

Table 4 and 5 present the results obtained when the anti BCG serum was tested by immunodiffusion against various tissue extracts. The serum reactivity was present in virtually all extracts as would be expected. Following adsorption of the antiserum with normal human serum, however, the T-band reactivity was demonstrated in all but one of the normal lung soluble extracts. Only 4/19 lung tumor soluble extracts reacted. The membrane extracts of lung tumors were less reactive and 0/2 embryonic lung extracts reacted. When soluble extracts of other tumor types were tested none reacted with the antiserum to give the T-band (Table 5).

Table 3—REACTIVITY OF VARIOUS ANIMAL SERA WITH ANTISERUM TO BCG

Serum Source	S-Band	T-Band
Mouse	+[a]	—
Chicken	+	—
Duck	+	—
Goose	+	—
Opossum	+	—
Bush baby	+	—
Horse	+	—
Sheep	+	—
Rabbit	+	—
Dog	+	—
Hamster	+	—

[a]Line of identity forms between normal human serum and specified animal serum.
S-Band and T-Band are defined in legend to Table 2.

Table 4—REACTION OF ANTISERUM TO BCG WITH HUMAN LUNG EXTRACTS

Lung Tissue Extracts	S-Band	T-Band
Normal Lung Soluble Extracts	7/7[a]	6/7[a]
Lung Tumor Soluble Extracts	17/17	4/19
Lung Tumor 3M KC1 Extracts	9/9	1/9
Lung Tumor Sonicate Extracts	9/10	0/10
Human Embryonic Lung Soluble Extracts	2/2	0/2

[a]Number of extracts giving positive precipitin band/number tested.
S- and T-Band are defined in legend in Table 2.

Table 5—CROSS REACTIVITY BETWEEN ANTI-BCG AND EXTRACTS OF HUMAN TUMORS OTHER THAN LUNG

Tumor Tissue Extract	S-Band	T-Band
Breast Soluble Extracts	5/5[a]	0/5
Colon Soluble Extracts	3/3	0/3
Cervical Soluble Extracts	7/7	0/7

[a]Number of extracts giving precipitin band/number of extracts tested.
S- and T-Band are defined in legend in Table 2.

Recently, we have immunized rabbits with *Corynebacterium parvum* (Burroughs Wellcome) according to the same protocol. Preliminary results are presented in Figure 4 and show that this organism also induces antibodies in rabbits that cross react with normal human serum and normal lung extracts. Experiments are currently in progress to determine whether the cross reactive antigens are similar in both systems.

DISCUSSION

It is well established in the literature that antigenic sharing occurs between microorganisms and mammalian cells (1-4). It is also documented that there are shared antigens between microorganisms and tumor cells (8-13). The presence of common antigens on microorganisms and tumor cells offers one explanation for the therapeutic value of organisms such as BCG in the treatment of certain malignancies.

Ruckdeschel (15) found that the five year survival rate was much greater in a group of lung cancer patients that developed empyema subsequent to surgical resection. We felt that the observation could be associated with shared antigens between the microorganisms most commonly associated with empyema in these patients and lung tumor cells. To investigate the possibility we raised antisera in rabbits to *S. aureus*, *S. pneumoniae*, *polysaccharides* and *Klebsiella* and tested for cross-reactivity with human serum, normal lung extracts and lung tumor extracts. No cross-reactivity could be detected by our immunodiffusion assay procedure between these antisera and human tissue extracts. This was not due to a failure of the immunization protocol as all antisera did have detectable titers to the respective immunogens.

When rabbits are immunized to *Mycobacterium bovis* BCG the antibodies that were produced cross reacted with normal human serum and soluble extracts of normal human lung. When the serum cross-reactivity was

Figure 4—CROSS REACTIVITY BETWEEN
ANTI-*C. PARVUM* AND NORMAL HUMAN SERUM AND
LUNG EXTRACTS

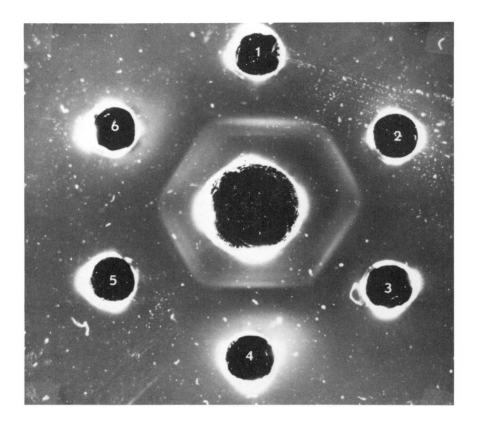

Center well contains unadsorbed anti-*C. parvum*. Outer wells are as in Figure 1.

examined it was found that the cross reactivity was due to at least three antigens present in serum. These antigens were present in all but one of the Cohn fractions (18) of normal human serum and were also uniformly present in a variety of normal and tumor extracts tested. The antisera were also tested against the sera from a variety of different animals. A broad phylogenetic range of serum cross-reactivity was noted that encompassed species ranging from birds to rodents and man.

The distribution of these serum reactive antigens will be further analyzed when they have been separated. The individual occurrence of these proteins in the above mentioned tissue extracts may be more meaningful that the uniform presence of the S-band in all samples tested here.

In addition to the serum cross-reactivity, the antisera after adsorption with normal human serum continued to react with lung soluble extracts. This reaction was termed the T-band but there was evidence that there were several antigens present in both normal and tumor lung extracts. No reactivity was noted with breast, colon or cervical tumor extracts. There appears then to be antigens present in lung tissue that do cross react with antisera to BCG. These cross reactions also will have to be re-analyzed on an individual basis when the different antigens can be separated. Then one considers the difference in reactivity of normal lung extracts (6/7) and lung tumor extracts (4/19) an accurate definition of antigen distribution becomes critical.

The finding of mimicry antigens of BCG which cross react with both human serum components as well as lung-specific associated antigens provide important issues to discuss in terms of immunoregulation as well as pathogenesis of lung-related diseases. The non-specific effects of BCG on the immune response of an animal are well established (20, 21). Both suppressive and stimulatory effects on several immune parameters are noted *in vivo* and *in vitro*. Thus BCG has been shown to induce natural killer cells (22), T suppressor cells (23), macrophage-like suppressor cells (24), cytotoxic T cells (20) and act as a polyclonal B cell mitogen (25-27). Consider also that experimental tuberculosis in rabbits results in the production of autoantibodies to lung-associated antigens (28). Furthermore, the sera of patients with chronic pulmonary diseases including asthma, emphysema, tuberculosis, and even cancer produce such autoantibodies to lung-associated antigens (29). It now becomes apparent that defining the mimicry antigens of BCG may be relevant not only to immunoregulation and adjuvant immunotherapy of cancer but also to our understanding of the pathogenesis of diseases such as tuberculosis. Future experiments will be directed toward resolving the antigen systems and their relevance to these latter questions.

ACKNOWLEDGMENT

The authors would like to thank Ms. Jeanne Boehlecke, Ms. Joanne Wright, Ms. Winnie Larue and Mr. John McKolanis for their assistance.

REFERENCES

1. Springer, G.F., "Blood Group and Forssman Antigenic Determinants Shared Between Microbes and Mammalian Cells". *Prog. Allergy,* 15: 9-77, 1971.
2. Rott, R., Drzeniek, R., Saber, M.S., et al., "Blood Group Substances, Forssman and

Mononucleosis Antigens in Lipid Containing RNA Viruses". *Arch. Ges. Virus forsch.* 19: 273-288, 1966.

3. Mittal, K.K., Terasaki, P., Springer, G.F., et al., "Inhibition of Anti-HLA Alloantisera by Glycoproteins, Polysaccharides, and Lipopolysaccharides From Diverse Sources". *Transpl. Proc.* 5: 499-506, 1973.

4. Rapaport, F.T., "Cross-reactive Antigens, Cancer, and Transplantation". *Transpl. Proc.* 6: 39-44, 1974.

5. Diggs, C.L., "Immunodiffusion Studies of *Plasmodium berghei:* Interactions of an Extract of the Erythrocytic Form With Rabbit Antisera". *Exper. Parasit.* 19: 237-248, 1966.

6. Reed, C.L., Cohen, G.H. and Rapp, F., "Detection of a Virus Specific Antigen on the Surface of Herpes Simplex Virus Transformed Cells". *J. Virol.* 15: 668-673, 1975.

7. Zabriskie, J.B., "Streptococcal Cross-Reactive Antigens in Relation to Rheumatic Fever". *Zbl. Bakt. Hyg. I. Abt. Orig. A.* 214: 339-351, 1970.

8. Borsos, T. and Rapp, H.J., "Antigenic Relationship Between *Mycobacterium bovis* (BCG) and a Guinea Pig Hepatoma". *J. Natl. Cancer Inst.* 51: 1086-1087, 1973.

9. Bucana, C. and Hanna, M.G. Jr., "Immunoelectronmicroscopic Analysis of Surface Antigens Common to *Mycobacterium bovis* (BCG) and Tumor Cells". *J. Natl. Cancer Inst.* 53: 1313-1323, 1974.

10. Minden, P., McClatchy, J.K., Warnberg, M., et al., "Shared Antigens Between *Mycobacterium bovis* (BCG) and Neoplastic Cells". *J. Natl. Cancer Inst.* 53: 1325-1331, 1974.

11. Minden, P., Jarret, C., McClatchy, J.K., et al., "Antibodies to Melanoma Cell and BCG Antigens in Sera From Tumor-free Individuals and From Melanoma Patients". *Nature* 263: 774-777, 1976.

12. Black, M.M., Zachrau, R.E., Shore, B., et al., "Prognostically Favorable Immunogens of Human Breast Cancer Tissue: Antigenic Similarity to Murine Mammary Tumor Virus". *Cancer* 35: 121-128, 1975.

13. Yeh, J., Ahmed, M. and Mayyasi, S.A., "Detection of an Antigen Related to Mason-Pfizer Virus in Malignant Breast Tumors". *Science* 190: 583-584, 1975.

14. Bast, R.C., Jr., Zbar, B., Borsos, T., et al., "BCG and Cancer". *N. Eng. J. Med.* 290: 1413-1420, 1458-1469, 1974.

15. Ruckdeschel, J.C., Codish, S.D., Stranahan, A. et al., "Post-Operative Empyema Improves Survival in Lung Cancer". *N. Eng. J. Med.* 287: 1013-1017, 1972.

16. Bartlett, J.G., Gorbach, S.L., Thadepalli, H., et al., "Bacteriology of Empyema". *Lancet* 1: 338-340, 1974.

17. Veltri, R.W., Mengoli, H.F., Maxim, P.E., et al., "Isolation and Identification of Human Lung Tumor-Associated Antigens". *Can. Res.* 37: 1313-1322, 1977.

18. Cohn, E.J., Strong, L.E., Huges, W.L., et al., "Preparation and Properties of Serum and Plasma Proteins". *J. Am. Chem. Soc.* 68: 459-475, 1946.

19. DeCarvalho, S., "Detection of Neoantigens in the Serum of Patients With Active Neoplastic Diseases by the Absorption-Immunodiffusion Method". *Oncology* 27: 193-234, 1973.

20. Mitchell, M.S., Kirkpatrick, D., Mokyr, M.B., et al., "On the Mode of Action of BCG." *Nature* (New Biol.) 243: 216-217, 1973.

21. Florentin, I., Huchet, R., Burely-Rosset, M., et al., "Studies on the Mechanisms of Action of BCG". *Cancer Immunol. Immunother.* 1: 31-40, 1976.

22. Wolfe, S.A., Tracey, D.E. and Henney, C.S., "The Induction of Natural Killer Cells by BCG". *Nature* 262: 584-586. 1976.

23. Geffard, M., Orback-Arbouys, S., "Enhancement of T Suppressor Activity in Mice by High Doses of BCG." *Cancer Immunol. Immunother.* 1: 41-43, 1976.

24. Klimpel, G.R. and Henney, C.S., "BCG-Induced Suppressor Cells. I. Demonstration of a Macrophage-Like Suppressor Cell That Inhibits Cytotoxic T cell Generation *in vitro*". *J. Immunol.* 120: 563-569, 1978.

25. Sultzer, B.M., "Infection with Bacillus Calmette-Guérin Activates Murine Thymus-Independent (B) Lymphocytes". *J. Immunol.* 120: 254-261, 1978.

26. Nilsson, B.S., Sultzer, B.M. and Bullock, W.W., "Purified Protein Derivative of Tuberculin Induced Immunoglobulin Production in Normal Mouse Spleen Cells". *J. Exp. Med.* 137: 127-139, 1973.

27. Coutinho, A. and Moller, G., "Thymus-Independent B Cell Induction and Paralysis". *Adv. Immunol.* 21: 113-236, 1975.

28. Rheins, M.S. and Burrell, R.G., "Further Studies on Auto-Tissue Substances in Tuberculous Rabbits". *The American Rev. of Respiratory Dis.* 81: 213-217, 1960.

29. Burrell, R.G., Wallace, J.P. and Andrews, C.E., "Lung Antibodies in Patients With Pulmonary Disease". *The American Rev. of Respiratory Dis.* 89: 697-706, 1964.

The Isolation of Tissue and Tumor Antigens

Isidore Faiferman[1]
S. Nerenberg[1]
R. Prasad[1]
N. Biskup[1]
L. Pedersen[1]

SUMMARY—We have developed a general procedure for the isolation of soluble tissue-specific antigens consisting of: 1) fractionation of soluble tissue extracts by preparative polyacrylamide gel electrophoresis, 2) sections of the polyacrylamide gel containing protein bands are mixed with Freund's adjuvant and injected into rabbits, 3) the rabbit antiserum is rendered specific by sequential absorption with polymerized normal human serum and 'other tissue' extracts, 4) antigen antibody complexes (precipitin arcs) of tissue extract and monospecific antiserum, are injected into rabbits, and 5) rabbit antiserum, rendered specific by absorption, is polymerized with glutaraldehyde and used for the purification of tissue-specific antigen by affinity chromatography.

Using these procedures we have isolated and characterized a pancreas-specific antigen and an antigen present in nuclei of liver and kidney (the hepatorenal antigen). The pancreatic antigen has been determined in serum using a radioimmunoassay: The results indicate an increase in levels of pancreatic antigen in sera of alcoholics. Similarly, experiments indicate an increase in levels of hepato-renal antigen in sera of patients with hepatitis or recipients of kidney transplants. The same methodological approach is being used in the purification of pancreatic-carcinoma antigen.

Pathological processes in tissues and organs usually produce tissue damage with a concomitant release of proteins into the circulation. Although many of these proteins are shared by many tissues, others are specific for a given tissue or organ and therefore their detection in the circulation can be used to pinpoint the tissue of their origin; furthermore, quantitation and knowledge of their half-life in the circulation would aid in determining the degree of damage. A variety of normal tissue or organ-specific proteins have now been identified as orginating from the heart (1), liver (2,3), kidney (4), and other tissues of human and animal origin (5,6). Moreover, it has been shown that such tissue-specific antigens can be identified in the circulation in a number of pathological conditions viz, hepatitis, renal disease, and others (7,8,9). Similarly, tumor-associated antigens have been detected by cytotoxicity studies, migration inhibition

---

[1]Department of Pathology, University of Illinois Medical School, Chicago, Illinois.

assays, and by use of specific antisera to these antigens; shedding of tumor antigens has been shown for melanoma, breast, and colon carcinomas (9,10,11). Hopefully, the quantitative determination of circulating tumor antigens will provide a means for detecting tumor growth before it produces clinical manifestations, and thereby allow for earlier and more effective treatment.

The work of our group has been devoted to developing highly reproducible procedures for the isolation of normal tissue and tumor antigens. The established format is as follows: 1) fractionation of soluble tissue extracts by preparative polyacrylamide gel electrophoresis, 2) protein bands located within the polyacrylamide gel are mixed with Freund's complete adjuvant and injected into rabbits, 3) resulting rabbit antisera are rendered specific by sequential absorption with polymerized normal human serum and 'other tissue' extracts, 4) antigen-antibody complexes (precipitin arcs) of tissue extracts and specific antiserum are mixed with Freund's complete adjuvant and injected into a new set of rabbits, 5) rabbit antisera (from step 4) are rendered specific by absorption, and 6) specific antisera are polymerized with glutaraldehyde to form insoluble immunoadsorbents which are used to purify tissue-specific antigens by affinity chromatography. Using these procedures, we have isolated a liver and kidney-specific antigen (Hepato-Renal antigen) and a pancreas-specific antigen.

I. Isolation of Hepato-Renal (HR) Antigen
A. Preparation of antiserum to H-R antigen

Saline extracts of human liver were fractionated by preparative polyacrylamide gel electrophoresis (PAGE). Preparative PAGE was carried out in 35.0x4.5 cm columns of 7.5% acrylamide gels in 0.04 M Tris-glycine buffer, pH 9.3. Five ml liver extracts with a protein concentration of 30 mg/ml were applied to the gels, following which electrophoresis was carried out at 300 V and 100 mA for 18 hours at 4°C. Protein bands were localized by staining a thin, longitudinal slice of the gel with 0.01 M amido black in 0.5% acetic acid. The unstained gels were then divided in 8 sections each of which was crushed, homogenized with Freund's complete adjuvant and injected intradermally into 25-30 sites of the backs of two 3kgm rabbits. To boost the immunogenicity of the antigens, aqueous eluates of the respective sections of the gels were injected intravenously three weeks later and at weekly intervals thereafter. Antisera were collected weekly, absorbed with pooled normal human serum polymerized with glutaraldehyde (12) and tested by double gel diffusion and radial immunodiffusion against normal human serum and extracts of different human tissues. The antiserum obtained by injecting section 4 of the preparative gel (Figure 1) appeared specific for liver and kidney. Additional antiserum specific for liver and kidney was subsequently produced by injecting rabbits with precipitin arcs obtained by immunoelectrophoresis of human liver saline extracts followed by reaction with rabbit antiserum prepared as described above (13).

Figure 1—FRACTIONATION OF HUMAN LIVER SALINE EXTRACTS BY PREPARATIVE POLYACRYLAMIDE GEL ELECTROPHORESIS

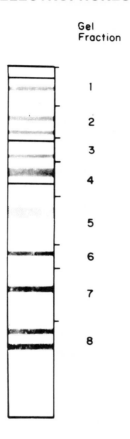

B. Antigen purification.

A two-step procedure was employed for the isolation of human H-R antigen:

1. DEAE-Sephadex. Saline extracts of human liver were dialyzed against 0.01 M Veronal buffer, pH 8.6, then mixed with DEAE-Sephadex (a-50, particle size 40-120, Pharmacia, Uppsala, Sweden) pre-equilibrated with Veronal buffer, in the proportion of 1 ml dialyzate to 2 gm wet gel. The

101

suspension was mixed on a shaker for 1 hour at room temperature, then filtered under vacuum. The filtrate was absorbed again with fresh gel and concentrated under pressure by ultrafiltration in an Amicon filter unit with a UM-10 filter.

2. Affinity chromatography. Rabbit antiserum to human H-R antigen, rendered specific by absorption with polymerized normal human serum, was polymerized with glutaraldehyde at pH 5.5 to form an insoluble immunoadsorbent (IA). The IA was mixed for 30 minutes at room temperature with liver antigen previously absorbed with DEAE-Sephadex; the suspension was then centrifuged for 5 minutes at 3,000 rpm at 4°C. The pellet of IA was washed twice with 0.1 M phosphate-buffered saline (PBS) pH 7.4, then packed in a 22 x 0.7 cm column and washed with PBS until no UV absorbing material was eluted. The antigen was then eluted with 0.1 M glycine-HCl pH 2.5 at a flow rate of 18 ml/hr. Aliquots of 2 ml were collected; those aliquots containing UV absorbing material were taken to pH 7.2-7.4 with 0.4 M Na_2HPO_4 and dialyzed vs. 0.01 M phosphate buffer pH 7.0. The H-R antigen was eluted as a single peak, containing the antigenic activity, as detected by radial immunodiffusion.

C. Characterization of human H-R antigen

Thin layer isoelectric focusing of purified H-R antigen showed a single protein band, with a pH of 7.2-7.4 (14). The molecular weight, determined by SDS-polyacrylamide gel electrophoresis (15) or thin-layer Sephadex Gel filtration (16), was 58,000 and 60,000 daltons respectively (Figure 2). On immunoelectrophoresis in agar, the antigen was localized to the slow gamma globulin region.

D. Properties of the purified antigen

The antigen appeared homogeneous as determined by SDS-analytical polyacrylamide gel electrophoresis and by isoelectric focusing; it contained 19% carbohydrate, as determined by the phenol-sulfuric acid method and was extractable by 0.6 M PCA without loss of antigenic activity. The antigen is relatively thermostable since incubation at 85°C for 1 hour does not affect its antigenic activity. Antigenic activity was preserved following exposure of the antigen to pH's ranging from 2 to 11 and was precipitated by 35-75% saturated ammonium sulfate. The antigen was destroyed by incubation with either trypsin or chymotrypsin; incubation with ribonuclease or deoxyribonuclease had no effect; similarly, incubation of the antigen with neuraminidase followed by exposure to sodium periodate did not affect its antigenic activity, suggesting that the carbohydrate moiety was not part of the antigenic site.

E. Immunogenicity of H-R antiserum

Rabbit antiserum to H-R antigen, rendered specific by absorption, was tested for its reactivity with saline extracts of a variety of human tissues by

102

Figure 2—DETERMINATION OF THE MOLECULAR WEIGHT OF HEPATO-RENAL ANTIGEN BY THIN-LAYER CHROMATOGRAPHY IN SEPHADEX G-100

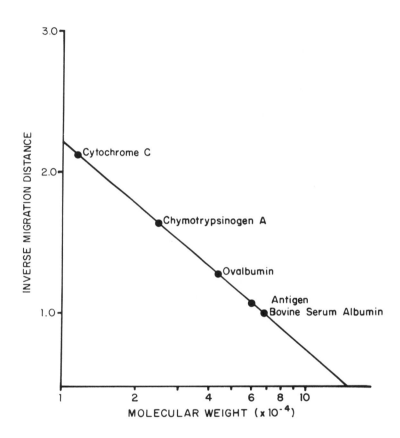

radial immunodiffusion and double immunodiffusion: liver and kidney extracts showed reactivity and complete antigenic identity; no reactivity was detected with extracts of other tissues.

F. Intracellular localization of H-R antigen

Six microns thick cryostat sections of liver and kidney tissues were fixed in ethanol, then incubated with rabbit antiserum to H-R antigen, follwed by incubation with peroxidase conjugated goat anti-rabbit antiserum and substrate (diamminobenzidine tetrahydrochloride: H_2O_2). Under the light microscope, the antigen could be localized in the nucleus but not in the cytoplasm of liver and kidney cells (Figure 3).

103

Figure 3—IMMUNOPEROXIDASE STAINING OF A RAT LIVER SECTION

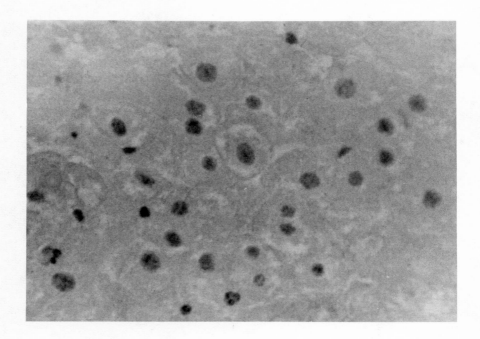

G. Loss of H-R antigen from hepatomas and hypernephromas.

Saline extracts of human hepatomas and hypernephromas and of the rat Morris hepatoma 5123 were tested against rabbit monospecific antiserum by double diffusion or radial-immunodiffusion. No reactivity was detected. Extracts of human and rat liver and kidney tested simultaneously showed a positive reaction. Furthermore, fixed Morris hepatoma cells did not show the characteristic nuclear fluorescence by the indirect immunofluorescent procedure.

II. *Isolation of a Human Pancreatic Antigen (Pan Ag)*
A. Development of antiserum and isolation of the antigen.

A human pancreatic antigen was isolated by procedures similar to those described for the isolation of human hepato-renal antigen.

Saline extracts of human pancreas were fractionated by preparative polyacrylamide gel electrophoresis; sections of the gel containing protein bands were mixed with Freund's adjuvant and injected into rabbits.

Antiserum to one of the sections proved specific for human pancreas extract after absorption with polymerized normal human serum. Additional antiserum specific for pancreas was subsequently developed by injecting rabbits with precipitin arcs. Saline extracts were then fractionated by filtration through a Sephadex G-200 column; eluates containing antigenic activity appeared in the void volume and were futher fractionated by preparative polyacrylamide gel electrophoresis. Four protein bands, detected by staining, were eluted; the antigenic activity, restricted to a single protein band, was further fractionated by affinity chromatography using rabbit monospecific antiserum specific to pancreas, polymerized with glutaraldehyde.

B. Properties of the isolated pancreatic antigen

The molecular weight, determined by filtration through Biogel A-1.5 M and SDS-acrylamide gel electrophoresis, was estimated at 225,000 daltons. The antigen was destroyed by incubation with either trypsin or chymotrypsin and also by extraction with 0.6 N perchloric acid. The antigenic activity was not affected by incubation at 60°C for 1 hour; the antigen precipitated between 30-45% saturation with ammonium sulfate. By means of the indirect immunofluorescence technique, the antigen was located in the cytoplasm of pancreatic acinar cells.

C. Immunogenicity of pancreatic antigen

The antiserum reacted with extracts of fetal and adult pancreas but failed to react with insulin, amylase, lipase, deoxyribonuclease, ribonuclease, chymotrypsin A, elastase, collagenase, leucine aminopeptidase, phospholipase A and B, and γ-Glutamyl transpeptidase. A reaction of complete antigenic identity was obtained with extracts of adult human, fetal human, and adult baboon pancreas.

D. Radioimmunoassay for pancreatic antigen and clinical results

A double-antibody type radioimmunoassay was developed to pancreatic antigen using purified Pan Ag labeled with ^{125}I and rabbit antiserum. The levels of circulating pancreatic antigen were then determined in sera of normal controls, in patients with diseases not affecting the pancreas, in alcoholics, and in patients with clinically diagnosed pancreatitis and compared to amylase levels (Table 1).

The results obtained show high levels of circulating pancreatic antigen in about 40% of alcoholics (patients with acute alcoholic intoxication or patients admitted for detoxification and tested after 2 to 4 weeks of abstinence) and in 100% of patients with clinically diagnosed pancreatitis; levels of amylase were about 4% and 40% respectively.

The procedures described before are now being employed in the isolation of tumor antigens. We have prepared an antiserum that reacts specifically

Table 1—LEVELS OF PANCREATIC ANTIGEN (PAN AG) AND AMYLASE IN SERUM OF PATIENTS WITH:

	Normal Controls	Diagnosed Pancreatitis	Liver Disease	Acute alcoholic Intoxication	Detoxified Alcoholics	Miscellaneous Diseases
Number of Patients	12	15	9	85	29	36
Pan Ag Positive[a]	1/12(8%)	15/15(100%)	1/9(11%)	36/85(42%)	11/29(38%)	2/36(5%)
Range	1.0-7.0	10-52	0.-7.0	0-12.5	0-12	0-20
Amylase positive[b]	0/12(0%)	6/15(40%)	2/9(22%)	3/85(4%)	1/29(3%)	2/36(5%)
Range	66-135	65-915	57-199	49-270	54-218	34-175

[a]Normal levels: 3.0 ± 3.2 (2SD) ng/ml. Values over 6.2 ng/ml are considered positive.
[b]Normal levels: 110 ± 50 U/dl. Values over 160 U/dl are considered positive.

with pancreatic carcinoma extracts (primary and metastatic tumors) in 12 out of 12 cases tested. Thin sections prepared from pancreatic tumors stained with rabbit antiserum following the immunoperoxidase procedure, showed the antigen present in the cytoplasm. The isolation of pancreatic tumor-associated antigen and the development of a radioimmunoassay for its determination is in progress.

REFERENCES

1. Chaturvedi, U.C., Davies, J.W. and Flewett, T.H., "Separation and Characterization of Cardiac Antigen Proteins." *Clin. Exp. Immunol.* 15: 613-622, 1973,
2. Meyer Zum Buschenfelde, K.H. and Miescher, P.A., "Liver Specific Antigens. Purification and Characterization." *Clin. Exp. Immunol.* 10: 89-102, 1972.
3. Sugamura, K. and Smith, J.B., "Purification and Characterization of Human Liver-Specific F-Antigen." *Clin. Exp. Immunol.* 26: 28-34, 1976.
4. Intorp, H.J. and Milgrom, F., "Thermostable Kidney Antigen and Its Excretion Into Urine." *J. Immunol.* 100: 1195-1203, 1968.
5. Shulman, S., "Tissue Specificity and Auto Immunity." Springer Verlag, New York, 1974.
6. Cohen, S.R., McKhann, G.M. and Guarnieri, M., "A Radioimmunoassay for Myelin Basic Protein and Its Use for Quantitative Measurements." *J. Neurochem.* 25: 371-376, 1975.
7. Smith, J.B. and Iverson, G.M., "Occurrence of Liver-Specific Antigen in Adult Human Serum." *Clin. Exp. Immunol.* 13: 209-212, 1973.
8. Rosenmund, A., "Ein Leberspezifisches Antigen in Serum von Leberkranken." *Schweiz med Wschr* 101: 1023-1026, 1971.
9. Poskitt, P.K.F., Poskitt, T.R. and Wallace, J.R., "Release into Culture Medium of Membrane-Associated Tumor-Specific Antigen by B-16 Melanoma Cells." *Proc. Soc. Exp. Biol. Med.* 152: 76-80, 1976.
10. Nordquist, R.E., Anglin, J.H. and Lerner, M.P., "Antibody Redistribution and Shedding From Human Breast Cancer Cells." *Science* 197: 366-367, 1977.
11. David, G.S., Reisfeld, R.A. and Chino, T.H., "Continuous Production of Carcinoembryonic Antigen in Hollow Fiber Cell Culture Units." *J. Nat. Cancer Inst.* 60: 303-306, 1978.
12. Nerenberg, S.T., Prasad, R., Biskup, N. and Pedersen, L., "Insoluble Human Plasma Protein Immunoadsorbents. Large Scale Production and Storage." *Clin. Chem. Acta.* 74: 237-245, 1977.
13. Goudie, R.B., Horne, C.H.W. and Wilkinson, P.C., "A Simple Method for Producing Antibody Specific to a Single Selected Diffusible Antigen." *Lancet* 1224-1226, 1966.
14. Radola, B., "Analytical and Preparative Isoelectric Focusing in Gel-Stabilized Layers." *Ann. N.Y. Acad. Sci.* 209: 127-143, 1973.
15. Weber, K. and Osborn, M.J., "Proteins and Sodium Dodecyl Sulfate. Molecular Weight Determination on Polyacrylamide Gels and Related Procedures." In *The Proteins,* edited by H. Neurath, and R.L. Hill, Academic Press, London and New York, 179-223, 1975.
16. Johansson, B.G. and Rymo, L., "Thin-Layer Gel Filtration." *Acta. Chem. Scand.* 16: 2067-2069, 1962.

Immunization Against Human Tumors: Generation of Killer Lymphocytes *In Vitro* Against Human Tumor Cells Using Soluble Bacterial Extracts

Brahma Sharma[1]

SUMMARY—Human tumor cells and various cell fractions isolated from cultured tumors were tested for their ability to induce cell mediated cytotoxic immunity against allogeneic and autologous human tumors. Tumor cells were either not immunogenic or were immunogenic usually at low concentrations. Following treatment with mitomycin C, cells became capable of immunizing lymphocytes at large concentrations. Sometimes, tumor cells were unable to immunize lymphocytes. These cells, however, became immunogenic when they were mixed with soluble bacterial components or Poly AU. Cell-free extracts of tumors were immunosuppressive. Cells were fractionated thus to isolate fractions with immunizing and suppressive activities. Fractions isolated from malignant melanoma and carcinomas of colon and breast were capable of transforming lymphocytes into effector lymphocytes with cytotoxic activity against specific and histologically different tumor targets but not against normal lymphoblasts. Fractions isolated from kidney tumor were not immunogenic or were weakly immunogenic. R2 fractions sedimented at 10,000-20,000 x g were significantly more immunogenic than R3 fractions sedimented at 100,000 x g and R3 fractions appeared to have more suppressive activity than R1, R2 or cell-free extracts. Poly AU, water soluble bacterial components and Levamisole were able to potentiate the immunization of lymphocytes against tumor cells. Nylon wool non-adherent and SRBC rosetted lymphocytes could become immunized to tumor cells suggesting that precursors of cytotoxic lymphocytes have SRBC receptors.

INTRODUCTION

The use of microorganisms or their products for the treatment of cancer was initiated by the repeated observations that cancer in some patients was regressed following acute bacterial infections. A patient who had four unsuccessful operations to control his neck cancer recovered fully after suffering two facial erysipelas (an acute streptococcal infection) (1). Encouraged by these observations, Coley started a systematic treatment of cancer by the use of mixed bacterial vaccines (Coley Toxin) (2,3). Even though there was no scientific explanation of how or why these vaccines worked or why some patients responded to such therapy while others did not, these findings provided incentive for further research. As a result of

---

[1]Associate Director of Research, Oncology-Hematology Department, The Children's Hospital, Denver, Colorado.

these observations, a variety of microbes or their soluble or insoluble products have been widely used as immunomodulators for immunotherapy and immunoprevention of animals and human tumors.

Our interest in this area started when we found that lymphocytes from some cancer patients and normal persons have depressed ability to become immunized against cells *in vitro* (4). In an attempt to augment their lymphocyte response, we studied the additional effects of certain water soluble cell wall components (peptidoglycan) of some *Mycobacteria*. The results of these findings described in (5) demonstrated that these water soluble cell wall components were able to potentiate the cytotoxicity of tumor sensitized lymphocytes *in vitro*. Since a relationship between microbes and tumors appeared to exist, we decided to examine further the effects of soluble bacterial products directly on lymphocyte population or lymphocytes stimulated with weakly immunogenic tumor cells.

In this paper, we will discuss results of some of these and other recent studies conducted to learn more about the effects and mode of action of soluble cell preparations from some human and animal strains of *Mycobacteria, Staphylococcus aureus,* and *Listeria monocytogenes*. Most of this work has recently been published (6,7). Various studies described here may provide basic information needed for clinical studies and also for an understanding and improvement of microbial immunotherapy.

MATERIALS AND METHODS

Source of Tumor Cells

Tumor cells were obtained from the following human tumor lines: RPMI-7932 (malignant melanoma) originated from pleural effusion, COLO-205 (colon carcinoma) originated from ascites fluid, and COLO-321 (colon carcinoma) originated from liver metastasis. These tumor cultures were provided by Dr. G.E. Moore, Denver General Hospital, Denver, Colorado. HT-29 (colon carcinoma) established from a solid primary tumor was provided by Dr. J. Fogh, Sloan-Kettering Institute for Cancer Research, New York. SH-3 cells that originated from the pleural effusion of a patient with breast carcinoma were obtained from Dr. G. Seman, MD Anderson Hospital, Houston, Texas. SH-3 may be cross-contaminated with HeLa (cervix) as recently reported by Nelson-Rees (8). 805 (breast carcinoma) cells were established by Dr. Plata and 613 (lung carcinoma) cells were obtained from Dr. Takasugi, UCLA. Leukemic blasts obtained from peripheral blood or bone marrow at the time of initial presentation were purified by Ficoll-Hypaque and stored in liquid nitrogen. These cryopreserved leukemia cells were used as tumor targets and PHA-treated or cryopreserved autologous remission lymphocytes were used as normal control targets. Characteristics of tissue cultured human tumor lines are

110

given in References 9-12. All tumor cells were *Mycoplasma* and virus-free, as determined by electron microscopy and culture methods.

Preparation of Killer Lymphocytes

Peripheral blood lymphocytes from normal persons and leukemia patients in remission were isolated and purified over Ficoll-Hypaque according to the method described previously (13). The purified lymphocytes contained less than 5% polymorphonuclear leukocytes and 5-10% monocytes. Lymphocytes (1 x 10⁶) were stimulated with various concentrations of bacterial extracts by mixing in 0.75 ml of minimal essential medium containing 20% heat inactivated human AB plasma in 15 ml plastic tubes (Falcon Plastics Co., Los Angeles, CA). Tubes were incubated for five days at 37°C in 6-7% CO_2 humid atmosphere. At the end of the incubation period, the cultures were harvested by centrifugation. Cells were suspended in 10% heat inactivated AB plasma. Lymphocytes and lymphoblasts were counted with the use of phase-contrast microscopy. Fewer than 1% monocytes were present in stimulated cell population.

Target Cells

The tumor lines were the source of tumor targets and cryopreserved leukemia cells and autologous remission lymphocytes were the source of leukemic and non-leukemic target cells. Lymphoblasts produced by PHA treatment of lymphocytes from normal donors were the source of autologous and allogeneic normal lymphoblasts (6). Approximately 1 x 10⁶ tumor cells or lymphoblasts were suspended in 100 μc Na_2CrO_4 solution in 1 ml tubes which were then incubated for 1 hour at 37°C. The cells were then washed three times with plasma-free medium and suspended in MEM containing 10% heat inactivated AB plasma and counted.

Cell-Mediated Cytotoxicity

The cytotoxic activity of *in vitro* bacterial stimulated lymphocytes was measured by ⁵¹Cr release assay as previously described (13). In brief, ⁵¹Cr labeled target cells (5,000) and stimulated lymphocytes (50,000) were mixed in 0.4 ml microtubes and incubated for three hours. At the end of the incubation period, the tubes were centrifuged at 800 x g for 2 minutes. The supernatants were carefully removed. The percentage of ⁵¹Cr released into supernatants and percentage of ⁵¹Cr remaining in the residue was counted. The percent specific ⁵¹Cr release was calculated by subtracting the ⁵¹Cr released from targets in the presence of unstimulated lymphocytes from the ⁵¹Cr release from targets in the presence of *in vitro* stimulated lymphocytes.

Preparation of Mycobacterial Products

Water soluble mycobacterial cell wall components were prepared according to procedures of Kotani, et al. and Adam, described previously (5). In brief, delipidated cells were homogenized at high pressure and cell envelop thus obtained were treated with Triton X-100 extracted with sodium dodecyl sulfate and subjected to differential centrifugation. Cell walls prepared this way were treated with lysozyme or L-11 enzymes which release water soluble peptidoglycan. In a few cases, mycobacterial extracts were used which were prepared according to procedures described previously (6) and provided by Dr. Minden.

Preparation of Synthetic Double Stranded Complexes of Poly AU

Polyadenylic acid (Poly A), potassium salt, and polyuridylic acid (Poly U), ammonium salt, were purchased from Miles Laboratory, Elkhart. Prior to use, Poly AU complexes were formed by mixing equimolar amount of each polymer and incubating the mixture for 1 hour at 25°C. If Poly AU were formed, these were dialyzed against H_2O overnight. Prior to use, Poly AU complexes were diluted to the appropriate concentrations with medium.

RESULTS AND DISCUSSION

Effect of Soluble Mycobacterial Cell Components on Lymphocyte Immunization

Lymphocytes from some cancer and normal persons are not able to become cytotoxic after sensitization with tumor cells (5). To determine whether mycobacterial cell preparations are capable of reversing this nonresponsiveness, lymphocytes were stimulated by cocultivation with tumor cells with or without soluble mycobacterial components (SMC). The cytotoxic activity of stimulated lymphocytes was then tested against ^{51}Cr labeled tumor target cells. SMC were not only able to potentiate the cytotoxicity of *in vitro* generated killer lymphocytes against tumor cells, but they were also able to induce the generation of cytotoxic lymphocytes when lymphocytes could not be immunized with tumor cells alone (5,14). As shown in Table 1, cocultivation of lymphocytes from donors A, B (cancer patients) and E, F (normal person) with respective stimulating tumor cells could not generate killer lymphocytes. The addition of a small amount of SMC to the mixed cultures, however, induced the generation of killer lymphocytes. In other cases, C & D, the addition of a small amount of SMC potentiated appreciably the elicitation of cytotoxic reactivity of tumor stimulated lymphocytes. Whereas, higher concentrations usually cause a suppressive effect (6,15). Although there is substantial evidence of a direct nonspecific modulating action on immunologically reactive cells, the exact mechanism of action of these immunomodulators is not yet clear. These may potentiate response by directly acting on the responder lymphocyte subpopulation (B, T, K or N) or by modifying the antigenicity of tumor cells. Low concentrations of SMC may augment the response by reversing the tumor induced immunosuppression through potentiation of T helper

112

Table 1—EFFECT OF SOLUBLE BACTERIAL COMPONENTS (SBC) ON *IN VITRO* GENERATION OF KILLER LYMPHOCYTES AGAINST HUMAN TUMOR CELLS

Responding lymphocyte[a]	Immunizing tumor cells or SBC	%Specific ^{51}Cr release $\pm$ SD Immunizing tumor cells and SBC		
		Tumor cells	SBC	Tumor cells + SBC
A (cancer patient)	805 (breast)	2±0.7	1±1.0	11±0.7
B (cancer patient)	ALB[b]	-9±2.0	10±2.5	20±2.0
C (normal)	805	14±0.7	5±1.0	40±0.7
D (normal)	613 (lung)	37±0.7		70±2.1
E (normal)	SH-3 (breast)	-9±2.0	25±2.0	57±2.0
F (normal)	HT-29 (colon)	-1±2.0	17±3.0	30±2.8
F (normal)	COLO-205 (colon)	-6±1.0	-13±2.3	20±4.9

[a]Lymphocytes from cancer patients or normal persons were sensitized with allogeneic or autologous tumor cells, soluble bacterial components (SBC) or tumor cells in the presence of SBC and then cytotoxicity of sensitized lymphocytes was tested against tumor target cells.
[b]Autologous leukemic blasts.

cell function or through abrogation of suppressor cell activity (15), or simply by activating the activity macrophages (16). The stimulation of mainly T lymphocytes may also result in the production of lymphotoxin capable of killing tumor targets (17). All of these possibilities are currently under investigation.

Generation of Killer Lymphocytes Against Nonlymphoid Tumors

Since some microorganisms are able to regress tumors, and cell-mediated cytotoxicity has been implicated in tumor rejection, studies were carried out to see if bacterial antigens could stimulate lymphocytes to become cytotoxic against tumor cells. The experiments recently reported indicate that not only is this possible, but that the cytotoxicity of bacterial sensitized lymphocytes is sometimes greater than the cytotoxicity of lymphocytes sensitized by intact tumor cells (6).

Lymphocytes from normal persons were stimulated with different concentrations of bacterial extracts prepared from BCG, L. Monocytogenes (LM) and S. aureus (SA). The cytotoxic activity of bacterial stimulated lymphocytes was then tested against RPMI-7932, SH-3, HT-29, COLO-321 tumor cells and allogeneic and autologous normal lymphoblasts. The results were compared with the capacity of the same cells to kill normal lymphoblast cells. In only one donor, there was as much as 25% specific ^{51}Cr release from normal lymphoblasts (Table 2). Accordingly, ^{51}Cr release of 25% or more was chosen in this study as the criteria for specific cytotoxicity. BCG-stimulated lymphocytes from 4 of 6 donors were able to cause significant ^{51}Cr release from RPMI-7932 and SH-3 cells. LM-stimulated cells from 4 of 6 donors were cytotoxic to RPMI-7932 and 3 of 6 donors were cytotoxic to SH-3 tumor cells. Lymphocytes from 3 of 5 donors treated with SA became similarly cytotoxic to RPMI-7932 cells, and 2 of 5 were cytotoxic to SH-3 cells. EC-stimulated lymphocytes were usually not significantly cytotoxic to RPMI-7932 and SH-3 cells. Donor G whose *in vitro* bacterial stimulated lymphocytes were highly cytotoxic to tumor cells also exhibited strong positive skin reactions to LM and SA. The results indicate that this donor might have been previously exposed to these bacterial or similar antigens. The effect of various concentrations of BCG, LM, SA and EC is shown in Figure 1. It appears that bacterial extracts are generally most effective in low concentrations (6). The mechanism of action of bacterial antigens in generating killer lymphocytes against tumor target cells is not clear as yet. It is possible that these agents activate natural killer lymphocytes or the generation of killer lymphocytes might be the result of sensitization of lymphocytes to bacterial antigens. Antigenic relationship between mycobacterial fractions and neoplastic cells has been shown (18). Induction of cytotoxicity may also be due to the mitogenic effect of bacterial antigens (19). Although our previously reported findings (6) and recent

114

results obtained with syngeneic hepatocarcinoma (line-10) tumor model (7) indicate that induction of cytotoxicity is not due to mitogenic effect, but the possibility of mitogenic effect can not yet completely be ruled out.

Table 2—IMMUNIZATION OF LYMPHOCYTES *IN VITRO* AGAINST HUMAN TUMOR CELLS USING BACTERIAL EXTRACTS

Donor of lymphocytes[a]	Stimulating bacterial extract	%Specific ^{51}Cr release ± SD from target cells		
		RPMI-7932	SH-3	Normal lymphoblasts
E	BCG	22±6.0	23±1.0	
	LM	30±4.0	40±1.0	
	SA	28±2.0	29±2.0	
F	BCG	48±7.0	30±1.0	7[b]±2.0
	LM	12±1.0	44±3.0	−3[b]±1.0
	SA	53±4.0	26±1.0	4[b]±1.0
G	BCG	62±1.0	46±1.0	21[c]±2.0
	LM	90±1.0	72±1.0	25[c]±1.0
H	LM	54±1.0	9±1.0	
	SA	13±1.0	3±1.0	
I	SA	9±1.0	11±1.0	
J	BCG	70±2.0	33±4.0	−6[b]±2.0
	LM	74±2.0		−7[b]±2.0
K	BCG	25±2.0	50±5.0	10[b]±2.0
	LM		20±2.0	4[b]±1.0
L	BCG	47±1.7	12±1.9	
	LM	21±1.5	9±3.0	
	SA	40±4.8	5±1.0	

[a]Lymphocytes were stimulated with soluble bacterial extracts, and cytotoxic activity of stimulated lymphocytes was then tested against RPMI-7932 (malignant melanoma), SH-3 (breast tumor cells) and normal lymphoblast target cells.
[b]Autologous lymphoblasts.
[c]Allogeneic lymphoblasts.

115

Figure 1—GENERATION OF KILLER LYMPHOCYTES *IN VITRO* AGAINST HUMAN TUMOR WITH BACTERIAL EXTRACTS

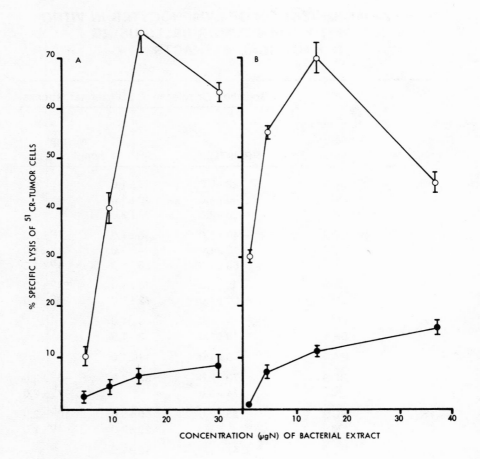

Lymphocytes were stimulated with different concentrations of A, *staphylococcus aureus* extract, B, *Listeria monocytogenes* extract, C, BCG extract, D, *Escherichia coli* extract. Stimulated lymphocytes were tested against target cells: A, ○, melanoma tumor cells, ●, normal lymphoblasts; B, ○, breast tumor cells, ●, normal lymphoblasts; C, ○, melanoma tumor cells, ●, normal lymphoblasts; D, ○, melanoma tumor cells, ●, normal lymphoblasts.

Stimulation of Lymphocytes In Vitro with E. Coli (EC) Extract

Lymphocytes stimulated with EC do not seem to acquire appreciable cytotoxicity against RPMI-7932 and SH-3 cells (6). To test whether EC-stimulated lymphocytes are also not cytotoxic to tumor cells other than RPMI-7932 and SH-3, we exposed lymphocytes to EC and then tested their cytotoxic activity against HT-29. The results show that EC extract rendered lymphocytes cytotoxic significantly more to HT-29 (colon tumor) than to SH-3 (Table 3). To examine whether EC-stimulated cells will be cytotoxic also to cells from another colon tumor line, we stimulated lymphocytes with EC and then their cytotoxic activity against colon tumor line COLO-321 was tested. The results show that cells from this tumor line were also susceptible for lysis by EC-stimulated lymphocytes (Table 3). Whether there is a relationship between *E. coli* and colon tumor cells is remained to be further investigated.

Effect of BCG Antisera on Target Cell Lysis by Bacterial Stimulated Lymphocytes

Tumor specific antibodies have been demonstrated. However, cell-mediated immune reactions rather than tumor antibodies appear to be implicated in rejection or suppression of tumor growth. It is possible that tumor antibodies, especially lymphocyte dependent antibodies, may be involved along with lymphocytes in the rejection of neoplastic cells. To determine whether BCG antibodies will amplify the destruction of tumor target cells by BCG-stimulated lymphocytes, we incubated ^{51}Cr labeled tumor cells with BCG antisera for 30 minutes at 37°C and then lysis of antibody coated and uncoated cells was tested by stimulated lymphocytes. The results show that BCG, $H_{37}Rv$ and LM stimulated lymphocytes were able to lyse the antibody coated targets significantly more than uncoated targets (Table 4). It appears that unstimulated cells were not cytotoxic to either antibody coated or uncoated cells. These results indicate that the antibody dependent cellular cytotoxicity (ADCC) mechanism may be involved. ADCC has been shown to be operative against a variety of tumor cells *in vitro* (20-23).

Generation of Killer Lymphocytes In Vitro Against Autologous Leukemia Cells

Since bacterial antigens were able to stimulate lymphocytes to become cytotoxic to allogeneic human tumor cells but not allogeneic or autologous normal lymphoblasts, we tested whether bacterial antigens are also capable of rendering lymphocytes cytotoxic to syngeneic and autologous tumor cells. When lymphocytes from strain-2 guinea pig were exposed to extracts from BCG, LM or SA, they became cytotoxic to syngeneic line-10 (hepatocarcinoma) tumor cells (7). Similarly, lymphocytes from acute

Table 3—IMMUNIZATION OF LYMPHOCYTES *IN VITRO* AGAINST HUMAN TUMOR CELLS WITH *E. COLI* EXTRACT

Donor of lymphocytes[a]	Stimulating bacterial extract (µgN)	%Specific ^{51}Cr release ± SD from target cells			
		SH-3	HT-29	COLO-321	
E	EC (2.3)	10±1.0	34±5.4		
	(4.6)	15±1.0	40±4.0		
	(18.4)	13±1.0	31±1.8		
	(36.8)	3±2.0	30±4.0		
F	EC (9.2)	21±1.7	49±2.7	52±4.7	
	(18.4)	26±3.6	98±2.2		
	LM (9.2)	36±2.4	34±2.9		

aLymphocytes were stimulated with *E. coli* (EC) or *Listeria monocytogenes* (LM) extracts. The cytotoxic activity of stimulated cells was then tested against SH-3 (breast), HT-29 (colon) and COLO-321 (colon) tumor cells.
bConcentrations of bacterial extracts are given in parentheses.

Table 4—CYTOTOXIC ACTIVITY OF LYMPHOCYTES STIMULATED WITH BACTERIAL EXTRACTS AGAINST BCG ANTIBODIES SENSITIZED AND UNSENSITIZED HT-29

Exp. No.	Donor of lymphocytes[a]	Stimulating tumor cells or bacterial extract	%Specific ^{51}Cr release ± SD from tumor target cells	
			HT-29 or RPMI-7932	HT-29-Ab[b] or RPMI-7932-Ab[c]
1	F	HT-29 (5,000)	3±3.0	5±1.0
		HT-29 (80,000)	13±3.0	64±4.6
		BCG	−1±1.0	−2.9±1.7
		H$_{37}$Rv	25±3.0	37±2.4
			21±4.0	60±2.2
2	F	BCG	58±2.0	74±3.0
		LM	64±3.0	76±2.0

[a]Lymphocytes were stimulated with soluble bacterial extracts. The cytotoxic activity of stimulated lymphocytes was then tested against HT-29 (colon) tumor cells and HT-29 incubated with rabbit antisera to BCG extract.

[b]HT-29 (colon) tumor cells incubated with rabbit antisera to BCG extract for 30 minutes at 37°C, washed twice and used as target cells.

[c]Experiment no. 1 was conducted using HT-29 tumor cells and experiment no. 2 was conducted using RPMI-7932 cells.

lymphoblastic leukemia patients in remission also acquired the ability to kill their leukemia cells but not autologous remission lymphocytes following exposure to bacterial antigens (Table 5) (24). The results indicate that leukemic specific killer lymphocytes are generated following stimulation with bacterial antigens.

Effect of Poly AU on the Generation of Cytotoxic Lymphocytes

Poly AU is known to potentiate *in vivo* and *in vitro* immune responses (25). It has recently been shown to amplify *in vitro* lymphocyte response to a variety of antigens, especially weakly stimulating antigens (26). Lymphocyte response to tumor cells and tumor cell fractions has also been found to be augmented by Poly AU (27). In the present study, we studied the effect of Poly AU on the generation of killer lymphocytes using bacterial extracts. The results show that Poly AU is able to amplify the cytotoxicity of *in vitro* bacterial stimulated lymphocytes in certain cases (Table 6). In some cases, the addition of Poly AU decreased the response of lymphocytes to bacterial antigens. SA-stimulated lymphocytes, although capable of lysing RPMI-7932 cells, were not able to lyse HT-29 cells. Lymphocytes stimulated with SA in the presence of Poly AU were, however, able to kill HT-29 cells. The mode of action of Poly AU potentiating effect has been discussed previously (26). Experiments have been reported which suggest that Poly AU can amplify both B cell as well as T cell activity. The ability of Poly AU to amplify immune responsiveness also appears related to its direct action on macrophage activity (26). It may act directly on cytotoxic precursor cells during the process of development into fully effector cells. This could be achieved through the potentiation of helper T cell functions or through abrogation of suppressor cell activity. These possibilities remain to be investigated.

Nature of Cytotoxic Lymphocytes

Although there is substantial evidence of a direct modulating action of microbial products on immunologic reactive cells, the exact mode of action is not yet established (15). These agents might have a variety of effects under different conditions. The induction of cytotoxic lymphocytes following exposure to these bacterial products suggests that these antigens may have a direct effect on lymphocytes. Are these *in vitro* induced cytotoxic lymphocytes T, B, K or N Cells? To narrow down the cell types involved in cytotoxicity, we first fractionated Ficoll-Hypaque purified cells by nylon wool column techniques. The unfractionated and nylon-wool non-adherent cell populations were then stimulated with BCG, SA and LM extracts and their cytotoxicity was tested against RPMI-7932 or HT-29 cells. The results show that bacterial stimulated nylon-wool non-adherent cells were capable of lysing tumor target cells (Table 7). In most cases, the cytotoxicity of

Table 5—GENERATION OF KILLER LYMPHOCYTES *IN VITRO* AGAINST AUTOLOGOUS LEUKEMIA CELLS USING BACTERIAL EXTRACTS

Remission lymphocytes from ALL donor[a]	Stimulating bacterial extract (µgN)[b]		%Specific ^{51}Cr release ± SD from target cells	
			Autologous	
			Leukemia cells	Remission lymphocytes
M	BCG	(2.3)[b]	32±2.0	4±1.0
		(4.6)	49±3.0	5±1.0
		(9.2)	61±6.0	5±2.0
M	SA	(2.3)	18±2.0	2±1.0
		(4.6)	24±3.0	1±1.0
		(9.2)	3±1.0	1±1.0

[a]Remission lymphocytes were stimulated in 0.75 ml of minimal essential medium (MEM) containing 20% heat inactivated human AB plasma. Cytotoxic activity of stimulated lymphocytes was then tested against autologous leukemic blasts and PHA treated autologous remission lymphocytes. ALL = acute lymphoblastic leukemia.

[b]Concentration in (µgN) of bacterial extracts are given in parentheses.

Table 6—EFFECT OF POLYADENYLIC AND POLYURIDYLIC ACID (PAU) ON GENERATION OF KILLER LYMPHOCYTES *IN VITRO* AGAINST TUMOR CELLS USING BACTERIAL EXTRACT

Effector-stimulator[a]	Concentration of PAU (μg)	%Specific ^{51}Cr release ± SD from tumor targets	
		RPMI-7932	HT-29
F-BCG (2.3 μgN)	0	19±1.0	19±2.0
	41.5	25±1.0	23±0.7
	83.0	33±2.0	20±2.0
	249.0	43±1.0	
F-BCG (18.4 μgN)	0	58±4.0	36±1.0
	41.5	65±2.0	28±4.0
	249.0	69±2.0	44±1.0
F-LM (2.3 μgN)	0	42±4.0	36±1.0
	41.5	52±1.0	41±2.0
	83.0	38±1.0	
	249.0	39±2.0	
F-LM (18.4 μgN)	0	61±4.0	30±2.0
	41.5	45±2.0	31±4.0
	83.0	52±2.0	
F-SA (2.3 μgN)	0	43±4.0	0±2.0
	41.5	31±1.0	22±1.0
	83.0	25±4.0	22±2.0

[a]Lymphocytes were stimulated with different concentrations of BCG, LM (Listeria monocytogenes) and SA (*S. aureus*) with or without the presence of different concentrations of PAU. The cytotoxic activity of stimulated lymphocytes was then tested against RPMI-7932 and HT-29.
[b]Concentrations of soluble bacterial components are given in parentheses.

nylon-wool non-adherent cells was significantly higher than the cytotoxicity of unfractionated cells. The increase in response of non-adherent cells may possibly be due to the removal of nylon-wool adherent suppressor cells. To determine whether T lymphocytes were involved, we tested non-rosette forming and E-rosette forming lymphocytes for their ability to become cytotoxic. Ficoll-Hypaque purified cells were separated into E-rosette and non-rosette forming lymphocytes according to the procedure described in "Materials and Methods". Rosette and non-rosette forming lymphocytes were then stimulated with different concentrations of *S. aureus*, BCG and *L. monocytogenes* extracts. Results shown in Table 8 demonstrate that E-rosette forming lymphocytes were able to become cytotoxic against RPMI-7932 cells following exposure to these bacterial antigens. In some cases, bacterial stimulated non-rosette forming cells also exhibited cytotoxicity but the cytotoxicity exhibited by E-rosette forming lymphocytes was greater than the cytotoxicity of non-rosette forming lymphocytes. Again, the ability of FH lymphocytes increased significantly in several cases following removal of non-rosette forming cells. These results demonstrate that although T lymphocyte populations appeared to have precursor cells which undergo differentiation into fully mature cytotoxic effector cells, non-rosette forming cell populations also seem to contain some responder lymphocytes. Whether this non-rosette forming population is B, N, K, T cells remains to be investigated.

CONCLUSION

Anti-tumor effects of a variety of microorganisms or their products are generally attributed to their nonspecific stimulation of RES-lymphoid system. These immunomodulators may exert their antineoplastic activity through stimulation of macrophages, B, K, N or T cells. The exposure to bacterial antigens (SA, BCG, LM) render lymphocytes highly cytotoxic to allogeneic and autologous human tumors and syngeneic animal tumors *in vitro*. The induction of cytotoxic lymphocytes may be one of the mechanisms by which immunomodulators mediate their anti-tumor activity. E-rosette forming lymphocytes are able to become cytotoxic following exposure to bacterial components, suggesting that T lymphocytes are important effector cells in neoplastic cell destruction. Immunomodulators may also be effective through LDCC mechanism as BCG antibodies are able to potentiate the lysis of tumor cells by BCG stimulated lymphocytes. B cells stimulated by BCG or its products may produce antibodies *in vivo* which may in turn coat (sensitize) tumor cells and make them more susceptible for lysis by K cells. Unstimulated lymphocytes are not able to cause appreciable lysis of coated or uncoated tumor cells, suggesting that stimulated lymphocytes probably are better effectors in causing lysis of antibody sensitized

Table 7—GENERATION OF KILLER LYMPHOCYTES *IN VITRO* AGAINST RPMI-7932 AND HT-29 BY STIMULATION OF FICOLL-HYPAQUE PURIFIED (UNFRACTIONATED) AND NYLON-WOOL NONADHERENT LYMPHOCYTES WITH SOLUBLE BACTERIAL COMPONENTS (SBC)

Donor of lymphocytes[a]	Stimulating SBC	%Specific ^{51}Cr release ± SD from tumor target cells	
		Responder lymphocytes	
		Unfractionated	Nylon-wool nonadherent
L	BCG (2.3 µgN)	7±1.0	47[b]±2.4
	S. aureus (2.3 µgN)	40±4.8	42[b]±2.3
	(9.2 µgN)	18±3.0	27[b]±1.0
	L. monocytogenes (2.3 µgN)	16±1.9	21[b]±1.8
K	BCG (9.2 µgN)	5±4.0	27[c]±1.0
	S. aureus (9.2 µgN)	2±2.0	21[c]±1.0
	L. monocytogenes (9.2 µgN)	10±1.0	28[c]±1.0

[a] Ficoll-Hypaque purified lymphocytes were fractionated on nylon-wool columns. Unfractionated and nylon-wool nonadherent cells were then stimulated with soluble bacterial components. The cytotoxic activity of stimulated lymphocytes was tested against RPMI-7932 or HT-29 tumor cells.
[b] Lysis of RPMI-7932.
[c] Lysis of HT-29.

Table 8—GENERATION OF KILLER LYMPHOCYTES *IN VITRO* AGAINST RPMI-7932 (MALIGNANT MELANOMA) BY STIMULATION OF FICOLL-HYPAQUE PURIFIED LYMPHOCYTES (UNFRACTIONATED) SRBC ROSETTE AND NON-ROSETTE FORMING LYMPHOCYTES WITH SOLUBLE BACTERIAL COMPONENTS (SRBC)

Donor of lymphocytes[a]	Stimulating SBC	%Specific ^{51}Cr release $\pm$ SD from RPMI-7932 target cells	Responder lymphocytes	
		Unfractionated	Non-rosette forming	E-rosette forming
N	S. aureus (2.3 μgN)[b]	9±0.75	15±2.0	18±0.75
	(9.2 μgN)	24±2.0	−15±1.0	17±0.75
	(36.8 μgN)	25±2.0	−2±2.0	26±1.0
	BCG (2.3 μgN)	9±4.0	13±2.0	51±2.0
	(9.2 μgN)	39±1.0	18±1.0	82±1.0
	(36.8 μgN)		36±1.0	77±2.0
	L. monocytogenes (2.3 μgN)	39±1.0	5±1.0	18±1.0
	(9.2 μgn)	29±2.0	39±1.0	35±2.0
	(36.8 μgN)	22±1.0	16±1.0	63±1.0

[a] Ficoll-Hypaque purified lymphocytes (FH) were fractionated into E-rosette forming and non-rosette forming lymphocytes by the procedure described in the text. Unfractionated (FH), E-rosette forming and non-rosette forming lymphocytes were then stimulated with soluble bacterial components and the cytotoxicity was then tested against RPMI-7932 target cells.

[b] The concentrations of SBC are given in parentheses.

tumor targets. Thus, it appears that microbial immunomodulators may mediate their antineoplastic activity by a number of different mechanisms.

Whatever the mode of actions may be in the rejection or suppression of tumor growth or in heightening the resistance, the finding that lymphocytes from some normal persons and cancer patients can be stimulated by bacterial antigens to kill tumor cells suggests that immunization with certain microbial antigens may influence the development of resistance to some cancer, although some genetical and environmental factors may influence the induction of resistance after such immunization. It will be interesting in this respect to see whether there is any relationship between the bacterial and viral vaccination and the development of cancer or if there is any significant difference in the frequency of occurrence of cancer between countries with low sanitation standards and higher standard of living. Interestingly, there are several reports in which difference in leukemia deaths is compared among BCG vaccinated and nonvaccinated children. Leukemia mortality rate for nonvaccinated group appears to be higher as compared to vaccinated children, although some questions are raised to the methods used in these studies.

ACKNOWLEDGMENTS

This investigation was supported by Grant CA 20067-02 awarded by the National Cancer Institute, DHEW and by The Helen S. Fisher Cancer Research Fund of The Children's Hospital.

REFERENCES

1. Bush, W., "Neidderheinische Gesellschaft fur Natur und Heilkunde in Born Aus der Sitzung der Mediz neschen". *Ber., Klin, Wochenschrift* 5:137-139, 1868.
2. Coley, W.B., "Contribution to the Knowledge of Sarcoma". *Amer. Surg.* 14:199-220, 1891.
3. Nauto, H.C., Swift, W.E. and Coley, B., "The Treatment of Malignant Tumors by Bacteria Toxins as Developed by the Late W.B. Coley, Reviewed in the Light of Modern Research". *Cancer Res.* 6:205-216, 1946.
4. Sharma, B. and Terasaki, P.I., "Immunization of Lymphocytes from Cancer Patients". *J. Natl. Cancer Inst.* 52:1925-1926, 1974.
5. Sharma, B., Kohasi, O., Mickey, M.R. and Terasaki, P.I., "Effect of Water-Soluble Adjuvants on *In Vitro* Lymphocyte Immunization". *Cancer Res.* 35:666-669, 1975.
6. Sharma, B., Tubergen, D.G., Minden, P. and Brunda, M.J., "*In vitro* Immunisation Against Human Tumour Cells with Bacterial Extracts". *Nature* 267:845-847, 1977.
7. Sharma, B. and Brunda, M.J., "*In Vitro* Sensitization of Guinea Pig Lymphocytes Against Syngeneic Hepatocarcinoma with Tumor Cells or Bacterial Extracts". *Fed. Proc.* 37:1593, 1978.
8. Nelson-Rees, W.A. and Flandermyer, R.R., "Inter- and Intra-Species Contamination of Human Breast Tumor Cell Lines HBC and BrCa5 and Other Cell Lines". *Science* 195:1343-1344, 1977.
9. Sharma, B., "*In Vitro* Immunization Against Human Tumor Cells with Tumor Cell

Fractions". *Cancer Res.* 37:4660-4668, 1977.

10. Quinn, L.A., Woods, L.K., Merrick, S.B., et al., "Cytogenetic Analysis of 12 human Malignant Melanoma Cell Lines". *J. Natl. Cancer Inst.* 59:301-307, 1977.

11. Fogh, J. and Trempe, G., "New Human Tumor Lines". In *Human Tumor Cell in Vitro.* J. Fogh, (ed.), Plenum Publishing Corp., New York, 115-154, 1975.

12. Semple, T.U., Quinn, L.A., Woods, L.K. and Moore, G.E., "Tumor and Lymphoid Cell Lines from a Patient with Carcinoma of the Colon for a Cytotoxicity Model". *Cancer Res.* 38:1345-1355, 1978.

13. Sharma, B., "*In Vitro* Lymphocyte Immunization to Cultured Human Tumor Cells: Parameters for Generation of Cytotoxic Lymphocytes". *J. Natl. Cancer Inst.* 57:743-748, 1976.

14. Sharma, B., Minden, P. and Brunda, M.J., "Generation of Killer Lymphocytes Against Human Tumor Cells with Tumor Cells and Bacterial Extracts". Submitted for publication.

15. Kedar, E., Nahas, F., Unger, E. and Weiss, D.W., "*In Vitro* Induction of Cell-Mediated Immunity to Murine Leukemia Cells. III. Effect of the MER Fraction of Tubercle Bacilli on the Generation of Anti-Leukemia Cytotoxic Lymphocytes." *J. Natl. Cancer Inst.* 60:1097-1106, 1978.

16. Wagner, H., Feldman, M. and Boyle, W., et al., "Cell-Mediated Immune Response *in Vitro*. III. The Requirement for Macrophages in Cytotoxic Reactions Against Cell-Bound and Subcellular Alloantigens". *J. Exp. Med.* 136:331-343, 1972.

17. Podleski, W.K., "Cytodestructive Mechanisms Provoked by Lymphocytes". *Am. J. Med.* 61:1-8, 1976.

18. Minden, P., McClatchy, J.K., Wainberg, M., et al., "Shared Antigens Between *Mycobacterium bovis* (BCG) and Neoplastic Cells". *J. Natl. Cancer Inst.* 53:1325-1331, 1974.

19. Ben-Efraim, S. and Diamanstein, T., "Mitogenic and Adjuvant Activity of Methanol Extraction Residue of Tubercle Bacilli on Mouse Lymphoid Cells *In Vitro*". *Immunol. Communic.* 4:565-575, 1975.

20. Hellström, K.E. and Hellström, I., "Lymphocyte-Mediated Cytotoxicity and Blocking Serum Activity to Tumor Antigens". *Advan. Immunol.* 18: 209-277, 1974.

21. Cerottini, J.C. and Brunner, K.T., "Cell-Mediated Cytotoxicity, Allograft Rejection and Tumor Immunity". *Advan. Immunol.* 18:67-132, 1974.

22. Baldwin, R.W., "Immunological Aspects of Chemical Carcinogenesis". *Advan. Cancer Res.* 19:1-75, 1973.

23. Herberman, R.B., "Cell-Mediated Immunity to Tumor Cells". *Advan. Cancer Res.* 19:207-263, 1974.

24. Sharma, B. and Odom, L.F., "Generation of Killer Lymphocytes *In Vitro* Against Human Autologous Leukemia Cells Using Soluble Bacterial Extracts". Submitted for publication.

25. Johnson, A.G., Cone, R.E., Friedman, H.M., et al., In, *Biological Effects of Polynucleotides,* edited by R. Beers and W. Braun, Springer-Verlag, New York, 1970.

26. Graziano, K.D., Levy, C.C., Schmukler, M. and Mardine, M.R., Jr., "Parameters for Effective Use of Synthetic Double Stranded Polynucleotides in the Amplification of Immunologically Induced Lymphocyte Triated Thymidine Incorporation". *Cellular Immunol.* 11:47-56, 1974.

27. Sharma, B., "Immunization Against Human Tumors: Generation of Killer Lymphocytes *In Vitro* Against Human Tumor Cells Using Tumor Cells and Cell Fractions". In *Cancer Immunology: Experimental and Clinical,* edited by R.G. Crispen, Science Press, New Jersey (in press).

PANEL DISCUSSION

Chairman: Isaiah J. Fidler

Fidler: The first question, if you don't mind, I would like to ask. The title of this session is Tumor Antigens and I think the first question should deal with tumor antigens. For esoteric value perhaps every speaker ought to comment on "what is a tumor antigen?" but I think we would sit here for two days and nobody would have the answer.

Thank God, I do not occupy myself with isolation and purification of tumor antigens. But, I have been to enough presentations by good friends and when they talk about tumor antigens they are always concerned with the following question: Is it a rejection antigen? Can you demonstrate that what you isolated can protect an animal; that is, either the animal has a tumor, you give the antigen, the tumor goes away; or you give the antigen and you can immunize the animal against that tumor? Do we, in fact, isolate tumor rejection antigens? I was particularly intrigued by Dr. Neal Pellis' findings. Out of the crude extract that he used, and I am glad he called it a CSA or I would have called it CSA, crude soluble extract, he obtains a fraction that enhances and a fraction that causes rejection or regression. Now, if he were not to fractionate these two things and if he were to inject the whole thing, he might get nothing. They might cancel each other and then, by definition, you do not have a tumor antigen. Do you follow me? What he described today is extremely important.

Now, I put forth this question, because I am going to ask Dr. Marchalonis to comment on it first because he has been questioned several times: "Do you have the rejection antigens?" Then anyone on the panel or in the audience can address that point.

John Marchalonis: Well, the simple answer to that, Josh, is I don't know. But, if you will allow me to philosophize, I will try and present a general picture. I feel that at this time we don't know what a tumor associated antigen is. We don't really know their molecular properties except that the three groups seem to have the same molecular weight on SDS from three different tumors. But, we and others have worked on other cell surface components where we do have information. I would like to answer your question by an analogy to other systems, namely, surface immunoglobulins and histocompatibility antigens; then swing back and try to put tumor antigens in that context.

If you would take one molecule, like an immunoglobulin molecule; it has individual determinants, it has allotypic determinants, and it has common determinants. Now, what does this mean? A common determinant, in the case of immunoglobulin, is your class or isotype; i.e., IgM, IgA, kappa or lambda. It's a common antigen and it's an antigen with which you can immunize another species. You can immunize a xenogeneic species and get a strong antibody response. A common determinant is present on all members of a class, and remember, all three determinants are on one molecule. It can be a heavy chain or a light chain. Allotypes are genetically restricted within a species. Different strains would have them. Generally, they are weak antigens and they're not on all molecules of that class.

Now, there is such a thing called an idiotype which is a determinant on the combining site of antibody that is an individual determinant. It induces a very weak response in syngeneic animals. Now, we have three determinants on the same molecule. If we want an antiserum which is potent and isolates all of that surface immunoglobulin, this is what we'd go for. If we are looking at maybe one percent, or less, of our molecules, we would want an anti-idiotype, but the anti-idiotype is a syngeneic antiserum usually and it's very weak compared to the other. We don't know about individual determinants for histocompatibility antigens. There are allotypic determinants. That is why different people, for example, have different histocompatibility types. Again, these are weak determinants and you get your best antiserum in the allogeneic case if you immunize with whole cells. People in the histocompatibility antigen game say that you get terrible antibodies if you immunize with extracts or if you immunize with purified histocompatibility antigen. Now, if you want a good antiserum, which reacts with mouse or human histocompatibility antigen, you inject another species, such as a rabbit. You obtain an antibody which will, in the case of the mouse, for example, immunize a rabbit with a purified H2B molecule. You will get strong antibody which will precipitate all mouse histocompatibility antigens.

What about these unknowns? Well, people seem to be using either syngeneic or xenogeneic immunization. In the case of the xenogeneic immunization, essentially the data I presented today, you get a relatively strong antiserum. You can use a variety of assays and immune absorbents to actually isolate molecules. We've done it, Lloyd Law's group at NCI has done it with two different tumors and Baldwin's group in Nottingham has done it with different tumors. So, we can say from three separate cases, you can immunize xenogeneic species and obtain a strong antiserum to isolate molecules.

Both Law and Baldwin have also looked at syngeneic immunization; again, it's weak. This is the case if you try to do it within the same strain of mice or, certainly, within isogeneic strains. Now, the question would be: can you use this type of isolation using a xeno antiserum, isolate a component and then get something which will protect in the syngeneic situation? The answer is yes. I have not done it; but both Baldwin and Law's group have evidence for it.

They can isolate these antigens from sarcomas and hepatocarcinomas using xenogeneic antiserum or they get apparently the same molecule using syngeneic antiserum which will pick up an individual determinant. Both groups have now been able to protect, in other words, they have been able to immunize with purified antigens.

So, in principle, tumor antigens, whatever cell component they prove to be, are not going to be that different from other surface molecules. If you use a xenogeneic immunization you have a molecule which has a common portion which is shared by all molecules of this type and if you use syngeneic immunization you have some sort of individual specificity. I think the answer will come to the question of whether or not there is a common molecule involved in forming a tumor surface antigen because the antigens that the three groups have isolated seem to look the same on SDS gel, they don't seem to be a virus, and Law's group has certainly eliminated their histocompatibility antigens. So, an interesting comparison would be to obtain antigens from three or four types of tumors and acquire enough structural information to see if they are variants of the same surface molecule. I hope I didn't confuse the issue too much.

Neal Pellis: First, I agree with Dr. Marchalonis' illustration of the hierarchy of cell surface antigen recognition and we have also approached the problem with that in mind. In the syngeneic host one expects a very weak but well directed recognition of the tumor antigen. Whereas, in the xenogeneic host, probably in excess of 90% of the "immunologic effort" is directed toward common features, i.e., taking a mouse crude tumor extract and injecting it into a rabbit. About 90% of the rabbit's effort is directed against mouse tissue antigens and you are asking that rabbit to recognize probably a very, very small region of determinant on the molecule that we call the tumor antigen. So, we have stayed with the syngeneic host and are now making marginally successful attempts at getting antiserum. We don't know whether polymorphism of carcinogen induced tumor antigens relates to the primary sequence of amino acids in that molecule or whether it has to do with various terminal carbohydrates. We feel that our best chances for recognition of that will come in the syngeneic host once we develop an appropriate test for the antibodies.

Our goal is to isolate and characterize that tumor antigen with regard to primary amino acid sequence and possibly the participation of carbohydrate in antigenicity. We chose the model methylcholanthrene induced tumors because if you inject several different sites in a mouse with the same carcinogen, methylcholanthrene happens to be the one in our case, each site will develop a tumor. Analysis of those tumors for their rejection inducing antigens reveals that each tumor that you derive from the singular host will have unique antigens. And induction and protection against one tumor need not necessarily protect the animal against challenge with the other tumor. So, they are highly polymorphic antigens. These tumors do not induce antibodies in syngeneic hosts which can precipitate tumor rejection

131

antigens. We inject crude extracts into rabbits in an attempt to get precipitating antibodies, but this has proven unsuccessful. We have, with partially purified materials, been able to get rabbit antibody to the immunizing fraction; whether this precipitates the immunizing antigen itself, we don't know. We'll have to test the rabbit hetero-antiserum, to see if it precipitates the antigen from the parent and antigenically different tumor cell extracts. If it precipitates both of them, possibly we've detected a common region; if it precipitates only one, then we've potentially detected the unique region of the molecule that confers specificity. That's the problem we face. We do not know whether or not we will detect a specific region with the hetero-antiserum.

Malcolm Mitchell: A very short comment and then a question for Dr. Marchalonis. The different directions in which different extracts of antigen push the immune response is exceedingly interesting. I like the phrase that Dr. Pellis used—a vectorial sum—because Dr. Bennett and I have used the same phrase in describing what the effects of BCG are in the human response. Presumably, the cell surface has within it components that are capable of enhancing or suppressing the immune response by stimulating various parts of it, that is different kinds of cells. I find that an interesting analogy.

Has Dr. Marchalonis, or perhaps, Dr. Pellis, ever tested by serology whether human melanoma antigens are at all related to mouse melanoma? The reason I ask this is because my associates and I studied cell-mediated reactivity of patients with melanoma and found that they did react to mouse B16 melanoma cells. They did not react against mouse neuroblastoma in the same strain, C57 black, and patients who did not have melanoma did not react against the B16. This preliminary evidence suggests a relationship which we can't quite explain in the mouse melanoma. Now the obvious control, which we have not done, is a pigmented melanocyte that is not a melanoma to see whether these patients are reacting to pigment cells or against some kind of a tumor. Is there any serological evidence that there might be some relationship across the species lines?

Marchalonis: Josh, do you want to answer that?

Fidler: About four years ago I wrote a paper which dealt with the cross reactivity among mouse, dog and human melanomas. We had dogs with melanomas and dogs bearing osteogenic sarcoma. You get lymphocytes from both and you do *in vitro* cytotoxicity; it's not chromium now, it's a three day assay. You prelabel DNA with 3H-Thymidine. The dogs bearing melanoma lymphocytes, lyse B16 melanoma, but do not lyse mouse fibrosarcoma. The dog bearing osteogenic sarcoma, the big round cell, against the mouse tumors were the same. Mice immunized against B16 melanoma, lyse dog melanoma but not dog osteogenic sarcoma. Then we obtained some human melanoma, which we called H1, and lo and behold, the mouse B16 lymphocytes also lysed that human tumor. Now it appears you cannot immunize man with mouse melanoma, but you can do the reverse. So then we immunized mice with dog melanomas, dog osteogenic sarcoma, human melanoma, human osteogenic sarcoma, and mouse melanoma, and then challenged the mice. The one that protected the mice was the mouse melanoma. There was absolutely zero protection with the xenogeneic tumor. So there is evidence, but not serological evidence, that it was cellular mediated. In regard to the pigmentation, it doesn't hold because we do have non-pigmented melanomas and they lyse just as well.

Mitchell: No, I meant a normal melanocyte. A non-pigmented melanoma really is the same thing, because you can induce pigment by tyrosinase, so it really had a potential to make pigment.

Fidler: Yes, that's a good point. I guess you are talking about isolated cells.

Mitchell: I meant a normal melanocyte growing on the skin. That would be the best control.

Fidler: I don't think anybody has ever done that to my knowledge.

Mitchell: They are hard to grow.

Fidler: I just wish to point out to the audience that tumor antigen specificity is very exciting but it's about seven light years away. In the meantime, we heard one paper today about the use of MER. If anyone tells me that MER is tumor specific, I will show him about 110 references to the contrary. MER was extremely effective in preventing the emergence of methylcholanthrene induced tumors. The tumors that Dr. Pellis told us he uses to identify and purify tumor antigen. So, we must keep in mind that the host has another system that totally disregards tumor antigens, and that's the macrophage system. We have investigated what the macrophages recognize and by what mechanism the marcophages discriminate between tumors and normal cells. And, I can assure you that the bottom line is not tumor antigens, it's not tumor specific transplantation antigens. It's a common denominator; perhaps, it's something that Dr. Marchalonis outlined. Dr. Kollmorgen, do you want to comment on nonspecific immunization or protection? Then we can go from there to the BCG and lung tissue.

G. Mark Kollmorgen: I have evidence on the lack of specificity with the MER studies that were done. The question that I would like to ask you, though, Josh, is can you derive a specific reaction with the macrophage induced immunological event that may be nonspecific but having components of specificity associated with it?

Fidler: No one seems to be able to find or publish the so-called specific macrophages. I looked into why it is so difficult to find specific macrophages and I think I concluded the following: If you use tumor immunized mice and the immunization does not involve complete Freund's adjuvant, the peritoneal exudate cells from those mice appear to have cytotoxic specificity *in vitro*. If you now take those mice that are the donors of the so-called "smart" macrophages, and you wound them, cut the tail, cut the ear, and let the wound develop, those mice now have nonspecific macrophages, because they respond to the infection. If you use complete Freund's adjuvant in your regimen of immunization, you enlisted nonspecific macrophages; if you use allogeneic tumors, you enlisted nonspecific macrophages. It appears that the only specific macrophages in response to TSTA are in clean mice. Malcolm, you did a lot of work in that area.

Mitchell: I think macrophages show up with a cytophilic antibody which I think is the equivalent of the specific macrophage arming factor that Evans and Alexander say comes from the T cell counterpart. Macrophages can be reasonably specific but the specificity is derived from elsewhere. You can nonspecifically turn on macrophages and they kill whatever is in sight; not normal cells apparently, but certainly embryonic fiberblasts in early passage and discriminate tumor cells. It is uncertain what they discriminate, whether it's mitotic rate or a new antigen. You can turn on macrophages with BCG nonspecifically so that they kill nonspecifically. But, to say that a macrophage is totally nonspecific is erroneous because under certain conditions they can be armed by other sources, an antibody or SMAF.

Kollmorgen: May I comment on the macrophages while we are still discussing them? The serum that we identified did not support blastogenic activity and was sent to Dave Talmage in Colorado. Dr. Talmage is interested in macrophage activating and has defined that among other things they need serum constituent. One of the major constituents seems to be arginine. They look for urea production indicative of arginase being produced in the activation process. The serum that inhibited the mitogen-induced blastogenic activity of the lymphocyte did not support macrophage activation. The serum that gives good blastogenic activity gives very good macrophage activation. Now, his philosophy has been that serum is deficient and not inhibiting. One of the deficiencies that he has found in some of his systems is the fact that arginine is limiting. When he added arginine back into these reactions there was no activation at all. I'm not supposing or suggesting that the factors which inhibit the lymphocyte are necessarily the same factors that inhibit the macrophages. What I am suggesting is that there seems to be paralysis of other lymphoid cells in serum from these animals that have been on the high fat diets.

Unidentified Speaker: I might sound a little philosophical but the tumor cells and embryonal cells don't necessarily attack the macrophages. They behave more like crippled cells. In other words, they have a deficiency when in contact with other cells, like natural killer cells from macrophages. Tumor cells are deficient in some intercellular recognition system which prevents the tumor cells from dying. In other words, the system is the law upside down. The macrophage is not attacking the tumor cells, the tumor

134

cell or the embryo cell is sensitive to interactions with other cells, including the monocytes. This might sound philosophical but I think the problem should be put in a different perspective than it is. Would anyone care to comment?

Fidler: You have a very good point, and as a matter of fact, it occupied a great deal of our attention.

Is the macrophage the active selector or is the tumor cell susceptible? We have evidence that in some systems it's both.

CANCER IMMUNODIAGNOSIS AND VIRAL IMMUNITY

Virus-Specific Nuclear Antigens
of Transformed Cells†

Saul Kit[1]

SUMMARY—Many DNA-containing viruses induce tumors in animals or transform cells in culture. Even the most common human herpesvirus, herpes simplex virus (HSV), has oncogenic potential. HSV causes acute and latent infections, but is also suspected on seroepidemiological grounds of involvement in squamous cell carcinoma of the cervix. In tissue culture, HSV can transform normal hamster, rat, and mouse embryo cells to malignant cells *(morphological transformation)* and it can convert thymidine kinase (TK)-negative human and mouse cell mutants to the TK-positive phenotype *(biochemical transformation).*

Transformed cells and tumor cells induced by DNA-containing viruses often do not contain infectious virus particles. However, viral DNA sequences integrated with cellular DNA can be detected by nucleic acid hybridization procedures. Some of the integrated viral DNA sequences are transcribed and translated to produce virus-specific antigens, which can serve as viral diagnostic markers. Recent research efforts have been concerned with the purification and characterization of these tumor (T) antigens and on the elucidation of their biological functions.

Virus-specific tumor (T) antigens were first detected as complement-fixing or CF antigens present in polyoma virus, SV40, and adenovirus-induced tumors, respectively, that reacted with antibodies derived from hamsters bearing these tumors. Further studies showed that the T antigens were produced in acutely and abortively infected cells prior to the initiation of virus DNA replication, suggesting that the T antigens also functioned in virus replication.

Antigens analogous to the papovavirus and adenovirus T antigens have likewise been visualized by anti-complement immunoflourescence (ACIF) tests in nuclei of lymphoblastoid cells transformed by human and chimpanzee strains of Epstein-Barr virus (EBV), and by the acid-fixed nuclear-binding technique in nuclei of lymphocytes transformed by the EBV-related baboon herpesvirus, *Herpesvirus papio* (HVP). The papovavirus and adenovirus T antigens bind strongly to DNA-cellulose, a useful property for their purification by affinity chromatography.

Reviewed are some of the properties of the papovavirus and adenovirus T antigens and EBV EBNA and a new HSV-related antigen recently detected in nuclei of cells *biochemically* transformed by HSV. The function of the HSV-associated nuclear antigen (HANA) is as yet unknown and there is no

[1]Division of Biochemical Virology, Baylor College of Medicine, Houston, Texas.
†Supported by USPHS Grants Nos. CA-06656-16 and 1-K6-AI-2352-15 from the National Cancer Institute and the National Institute of Allergy and Infectious Diseases.

information regarding its presence or absence in tumor cells morphologically transformed by HSV. However, it has the interesting property of binding to chromosomes.

INTRODUCTION

Many DNA-containing viruses induce tumors in animals or transform cells in culture. Among the viruses with oncogenic potential are papovaviruses isolated from man (JC, BK), monkeys (SV40), and mice (polyoma), adenoviruses isolated from man (Ad12), monkeys (SA7), and chickens (CELO), and herpesviruses isolated from man (EBV), chimpanzees (EBV-Ch), and baboons (HVP) (Table 1). Even the most common human herpesvirus, herpes simplex virus (HSV), has oncogenic potential. HSV causes acute and latent infections, but is also suspected on seroepidemiological grounds of involvement in squamous cell carcinoma of the cervix. In tissue culture, HSV can transform normal hamster, rat, and mouse embryo cells to malignant cells *(morphological transformation)* and it can convert thymidine kinase (TK)-negative human and mouse cell mutants to the TK-positive phenotype *(biochemical transformation)*.

Transformed cells and tumor cells induced by DNA-containing viruses often do not contain infectious virus particles. However, viral DNA sequences integrated with cellular DNA can be detected by nucleic acid hybridization procedures. Some of the integrated viral DNA sequences are transcribed and translated to produce virus-specific antigens, which can serve as viral diagnostic markers. The persistence of virus-specific antigens in transformed cells and tumors suggests that they may have a role in the maintenance of the transformed phenotype. Recent research efforts have been concerned with the purification and characterization of these tumor (T) antigens and on the elucidation of their biological functions. Furthermore, as antisera to the viral-specific tumor antigens became available, it was possible to test tumor samples of unknown etiology to determine whether they expressed viral genetic information.

Virus-specific tumor (T) antigens were first detected as complement-fixing or IF antigens present in polyoma virus, SV40, and adenovirus-induced tumors, respectively, that reacted with antibodies derived from hamsters bearing these tumors (1-7). T antigens have since been found in cells transformed by all known strains of papova- and adenoviruses (8-11) (Table 1). Further studies showed that the T antigens were produced in acutely and abortively infected cells prior to the initiation of virus DNA replication, suggesting that the T antigens also functioned in virus replication.

Antigens analogous to the papovavirus and adenovirus T antigens have likewise been visualized by anti-complement immunofluorescence (ACIF) tests in nuclei of lymphoblastoid cells transformed by human and chim-

Table 1—NUCLEAR ANTIGENS INDUCED BY PAPOVAVIRUSES, ADENOVIRUSES, AND HERPESVIRUSES

Class of virus	Virus species	Antigens	Methods of detection
Papovaviruses	Simian virus 40 (SV40) Polyoma virus Human papovavirus JC Human papovavirus BK	T antigens	Immunofluorescence Complement fixation Immunoperoxidase staining Anti-complement immuno- fluorescence
Adenoviruses	Human subgroup A (Ad 12, 18, 31) Human subgroup B (Ad 3, 7, 11, 14, 16, 21) Human subgroup C (Ad 1, 2, 5, 6) Chicken embryo lethal orphan (CELO) Simian adenovirus 7 (SA7) Bovine Adenovirus type 3	T antigens	Immunofluorescence Complement fixation
Herpesviruses	Human Epstein-Barr virus (EBV)	EBNA	Anticomplement immuno- fluorescence Acid-fixed nuclear binding technique
	Chimpanzee virus related to EBV	Ch-NA	Anticomplement immuno- fluorescence
	Herpesvirus papio (baboon)	HUPNA	Acid-fixed nuclear-binding technique
	HSV-1 and HSV-2	HANA	Peroxidase-antiperoxidase Immunofluorescence

panzee strains of Epstein-Barr virus (EBV), and by the acid-fixed nuclear-binding technique in nuclei of lymphocytes transformed by the EBV-related baboon herpesvirus, *Herpesvirus papio* (HVP) (12-14). The human EBV-associated nuclear antigen was named EBNA and the corresponding chimpanzee and baboon nuclear antigens were called Ch-NA and HUPNA, respectively (Table 1). The papovavirus and adenovirus T antigens bind strongly to DNA-cellulose, a useful property for their purification by affinity chromatography. EBNA is also a DNA-binding protein. In addition, EBNA has been found associated with metaphase chromosomes of EBV tumor cells.

In the discussion that follows, I will briefly review some of the properties of the papovavirus and adenovirus T antigens and EBV EBNA. I will also describe a new HSV-related antigen recently detected in nuclei of cells biochemically transformed by HSV (15). The function of the HSV-associated nuclear antigen (HANA) is as yet unknown and there is no information regarding its presence or absence in tumor cells morphologically transformed by HSV. However, like EBV EBNA, the HSV-related antigen has the interesting property of binding to chromosomes.

SV40 and Polyoma Virus Tumor Antigens

T antigens were initially defined as virus-coded proteins present in virus-induced tumors that the host recognized as foreign. However, as will be apparent from the discussion that follows, certain virus-induced tumor cells may synthesize viral antigens not synthesized by other tumor cells transformed by the same virus. The particular antigens expressed in viral-induced tumors (and transformed cells) depend on the viral DNA sequences integrated in the tumor cells, possibly their chromosomal sites of integration, and also the state of the viral genome in the tumor cells (repressed vs derepressed, whether or not the cells are producing virus DNA or virus particles). A more restrictive definition of T antigens might be those antigens in virus-induced tumors that are the products of the viral genes critical for the initiation and/or maintenance of tumor cell transformation.

The T antigens of SV40 and other papovaviruses are found mainly, but not exclusively, in nuclei of transformed and infected cells. The SV40 T antigens are coded by the "early" region (gene A cistron) of SV40 DNA (16). Another SV40-specific antigen, also coded by the early region of SV40 DNA, is the tumor-specific transplantation antigen (TSTA). It is recognized through tests in which SV40-induced tumor cells are rejected by animals previously immunized with SV40 virus. TSTA is found in the membrane of SV40 transformed cells and will not be considered further in this discussion.

Studies with SV40tsA mutants have shown that gene A function is continuously required to initiate each round of viral DNA replication and transiently required to initiate late viral transcription in productive infection of permissive cells. In infection of restrictive cells, gene A function is necessary to establish the transformed state. SV40tsA mutants overproduce at the restrictive temperature in either productive or transforming infections two immunologically related polypeptides, large-T and small-t, with apparent molecular weights of about 94,000 daltons and 15,000-20,000 daltons (17). Biochemical and electron microscopic studies have shown that T antigen binds preferentially at the origin of SV40 DNA replication (0.67 on the physical map of SV40 DNA, where 0.0 is conventionally designated as the EcoRI restriction endonuclease site) (18). This site is also close to the origin of gene A transcription, which serves to explain the finding that SV40 gene A protein regulates its own synthesis (19, 20). The 94,000 dalton protein of cells transformed by tsA mutants has been partially purified and shown to be more thermolabile than the corresponding protein from wild-type SV40-transformed cells in both immunoreactivity and DNA-binding properties (21, 22).

Large-T and small-t SV40 proteins not only share immunological determinants recognized by antisera from hamsters bearing SV40-induced tumors, but they also yield a common set of methionine-containing tryptic peptides. Furthermore, two polypeptides virtually indistinguishable from large-T and small-t (by electrophoretic mobility and tryptic peptide maps) are synthesized *in vitro* with mRNA from the early region of SV40 DNA (23, 24). One of the tryptic polypeptides of large-T contains a serine phosphate residue.

The early region of SV40 DNA is transcribed counterclockwise to 19S mRNAs. The SV40 DNA physical map coordinates for this transcribed region start at about 0.65 and terminate at about 0.165. This portion of the SV40 genome includes part of Hind restriction endonuclease fragment A and fragments H, I, and B. SV40 mutants temperature-sensitive in gene A function map in Hind fragments H, I, and occasionally B.

To locate the coding sequences for large-T and small-t in SV40 DNA, the production of these proteins was examined after infection of monkey cells with wild-type virus and deletion mutants (17). It was found that a deletion at the distal portion of the early region (0.43-0.325) altered the structure of large-T but not of small-t. In contrast, deletions within the region between map coordinates 0.59-0.55 resulted in alteration or absence of small-t but a normal large-T. Deletions at map positions 0.17 or at 0.68 (outside the early region) had no effect on either large-T or small-t. These findings have been rationalized by a model that proposes the existence of two early mRNAs, one coding for large-T and the other for small-t. Both mRNAs span virtually the entire early region, but the mRNA coding for large-T lacks the nucleotide sequence between map coordinates 0.59-0.54. Small-t is translated from the larger of the two mRNAs, beginning at or near its 5'-end and terminating at a codon at about map coordinate 0.54. Large-T, on the other hand, is translated from the shorter mRNA, beginning at the same initiator codon, but because of the deletion of the terminator codon at 0.54, translation proceeds to a terminator codon at or near map position 0.175.

The early region of polyoma virus corresponds to that of SV40. Two early gene functions, defined by the hr-t and ts-a complementation groups, have been identified in this early region and shown to be essential for neoplastic transformation (25). It appears that the hr-t gene controls the synthesis of polyoma virus small-t while the ts-a gene controls the formation of large-T. When isolated by means of anti-polyoma tumor (T) antisera, the major product of mouse cells productively infected by wild-type polyoma virus is a polypeptide with a molecular weight of about 80,000-90,000, but in addition, immunoprecipitates contain four more polypeptides with apparent molecular weights of 63,000, 56,000, 36,000, and 22,000. The 90,000, 56,000, and 36,000 polypeptides are phosphorylated. As with SV40tsA mutants, polyoma ts-a mutants show altered immune reactivity of large-T, as judged by immunofluorescence, complement fixation, and the disappearance of a 90,000 dalton band on sodium dodecyl sulfate gels. In cells infected by an hr-t mutant carrying a deletion of about 150 base pairs in the early region of polyoma virus DNA, the large-T polypeptide appears to be unchanged. However, all four of the lower molecular weight bands are absent or drastically reduced in the immunoprecipitate from hr-t-infected cells. The findings could be explained by the mRNA "splicing" model described for early SV40 mRNA.

Human papovavirus BK, which was initially isolated from the urine of a renal transplant recipient on immunosuppressive therapy, replicates in human cells and transforms hamster cells. BK virus and SV40 share approximately 20-25% of their base sequences. This base sequence homology is localized mainly in the regions of the virus DNAs transcribed late in infection, but a small degree of sequence homology involving the early gene regions of SV40 and BK virus DNA has also been found (26). The T antigens induced by SV40 or BK virus in virus-infected or transformed cells react quite strongly with serum directed against the heterologous T antigens, but neither of the T antigens cross-reacts with polyoma virus T antisera. The BK virus T antigen immunoprecipitated from extracts of BK virus-transformed hamster and BK virus-infected human cells, respectively, have molecular weights of about 113,000 and 97,000, but, in addition, polypeptides with smaller molecular weights have been detected. Some of the smaller polypeptides may have been derived by protease cleavage of the 97,000 or 113,000 molecular weight polypeptides. Because the SV40 and BK virus T antigens strongly cross-react, and because the viruses share some base sequence homology in the early regions, the peptide compositions of the two papovavirus T antigens have been analyzed (26). Out of a total of 20 SV40-and 21 BK virus-specific methionine labeled tryptic peptides, there were seven pairs of similar peptides on the basis of coelution from ion exchange columns. These coeluting peptides contained about 25 to 30% of the total methionine radioactivity.

Human papovavirus JC is the virus most commonly associated with the rare demyelinating disease, progressive multifocal leukoencephalopathy (PML) (27). A frequent histological finding in old lesions of PML is enlarged astrocytes with bizarre nuclei, that resemble malignant astrocytes in glioblastomas. JC virus is extremely neurooncogenic in newborn Syrian hamsters. Eighty-three per cent of inoculated hamsters develop malignant gliomas within six months. There is considerable cross-reactivity between the T antigens of JC virus, BK virus, and SV40 (3, 10).

SV40, and BK viruses also are capable of inducing brain tumors in hamsters. A high incidence of ependymomas has been found in hamsters inoculated intracerebrally with BK virus and SV40 (28, 29). These observations and the fact that both JC virus and an SV40-variant strain (SV40-PML) have been isolated from the brains of patients with PML have raised a suspicion that some brain tumors in humans may have a viral etiology. Tabuchi and coworkers (30) screened 39 human brain tumors for the presence or absence of SV40-related T antigens by direct and indirect immunoperoxidase methods. Two tumors of ependymal origin (malignant ependymoma and choroid plexus papilloma) revealed markedly positive nuclear staining for T antigens. In view of the high incidence of papovavirus infection in man, further work along these lines would be worthwhile.

Adenovirus Tumor Antigens

Oncogenic human adenoviruses are readily divisible into two chief subgroups: A (types 12, 18, and 31), and B (types 3, 7, 11, 14, 16, and 21), based on similar biological and biochemical properties. Subgroup A viruses are highly oncogenic when inoculated into newborn hamsters, while subgroup B viruses are weakly oncogenic. Adenoviruses of both groups A and B readily transform rodent cells in tissue culture. A third human adenovirus subgroup C (types 1, 2, 5, and 6) fails to induce tumors in animals but does transform rat and hamster cells in tissue culture. These transformed cells develop into tumors when inoculated into animals. Subgroup-specific T antigens are produced in tumor cells, transformed cells, and in cells acutely infected by these human adenoviruses (Table 1) (31). The adenovirus T antigens resemble the papovavirus T antigens in that they are not incorporated into mature virus particles and they are thermosensitive to 5 min. of heating at 56°. In contrast, viral (V) structural antigens are relatively thermostable. However, unlike papovavirus T antigens, which stain the entire nucleus (exclusive of nucleoli), but not the cytoplasm of transformed and infected cells, the adenovirus T antigens are detected as flecks and dots in nuclei of transformed and infected cells and are found in the cytoplasm as well.

Several investigators have reported partial purification of adenovirus 12 (subgroup A) tumor antigens. However, the number and sizes of the adenovirus T antigens reported initially presented a confusing picture. The presence of up to four components was described after rate zonal centrifugation in linear sucrose gradients, but it was uncertain whether they represented different conformational or polymeric forms of a single protein, or were distinctive viral gene products. Gilead and Ginsberg (33), Gilden et al. (31), and Tavitian et al. (34) each identified only one molecular form, but the estimated molecular weights were 20-25,000, 40-50,000, and 150,000, respectively. Hollingshead et al. (35) also described a 20-25,000 molecular weight form of adenovirus 12 T antigen, but in addition, found an 80-90,000 molecular weight species. Potter et al. (36) likewise reported two T antigen species, but with apparent molecular weights of 40-50,000 and 80-90,000, while Tockstein et al. (37) detected the presence of four T antigen species with estimated molecular weights of 22,000, 40,000, 52,000, and 84,000. Hollingshead and coworkers (38) achieved a 160,000-fold purification of the 25,000 molecular weight species, but found that this T antigen yielded three protein bans on vertical gel electrophoresis.

In more recent studies, Biron et al. (39) extracted adenovirus 12 T antigen from Ad12-transformed hamster cells and purified it about 500-fold by chromatography on double-stranded DNA cellulose. A further two-fold purification was achieved by filtering the preparation through a single-stranded DNA cellulose column. The T antigen activity was recovered in the void volume while some contaminating proteins were retarded. The T antigen polypeptides were immunoprecipitated by antibodies from tumor-bearing hamsters and were identified as a major peptide of molecular weight 50,000 and a minor species of molecular weight 11,000.

Van der Vliet and Levine (40) and Gilead et al. (41) purified two single-stranded DNA-binding proteins from adenovirus type 2 and type 5 (subgroup C) infected cells and demonstrated by the use of temperature-sensitive mutants that they were viral-coded and essential for virus DNA replication. The proteins had molecular weights of about 72,000 and 48,000. Comparison of tryptic peptides suggested that the 48,000 component was a degradation product of the 72,000 polypeptide. The polypeptides were early gene products, for they were synthesized soon after infection in the presence of ara-C, an inhibitor of DNA synthesis. The structural gene for the 72,000 dalton polypeptide was mapped in the EcoRI-B fragment of adenovirus 2 DNA (about 0.65 physical map units).

Studies by Gilead et al. (41) and Levinson and Levine (42) with antisera from hamster tumors induced by Ad1-SV40 and Ad2-SV40 hybrid viruses demonstrated that the single-stranded DNA-binding proteins from cells infected with adenovirus 2 and 5 had T antigen specificity. In addition, this antisera reacted with another virus-specific polypeptide having a molecular

146

weight of 58,000.

Recent experiments suggest that the 58,000 MW polypeptide rather than the 72,000 (and 48,000) MW polypeptides is the T antigen with critical functions in adenovirus-transformed cells and tumors. The particular virus polypeptides detected in tumor cells depend on the source of the antisera from tumor-bearing animals and on the viral DNA sequences integrated. Tumors induced by adenovirus particles often contain integrated DNA sequences from most, if not all, of the viral genome. Sera from animals bearing these tumors react with several early adenovirus proteins. In contrast, the smallest adenovirus type 2 and 5 DNA fragment found to contain transforming activity is the HsuI-G fragment (MW 1.7×10^6), which represents the left terminal 7% of the adenovirus genome (43, 44). Cells transformed by the HsuI-G fragment DNA express T antigen activity and they produce tumors in animals. Sera from tumors induced by the left terminal DNA fragment react with the 58,000 MW polypeptide, but not with the 72,000 MW polypeptide (42, 45). Sera of hamsters bearing tumors induced by cells containing the left-hand 14% of the adenovirus 2 genome immunoprecipitate the 58,000 MW polypeptide, but in addition, the sera precipitate another polypeptide of molecular weight 17,000 (45).

The early adenovirus genes carried in the left terminal DNA sequences are common to all adenovirus 2-transformed cell lines. Furthermore, Yano et al. (46) and Shiroki et al. (47) have shown that the left terminal 7.2% of adenovirus 12 DNA contains the transforming genes for this subgroup A adenovirus. They analyzed rat lines that had been transformed by whole adenovirus DNA, EcoRI fragment C (left terminal 16%) or Hind III fragment G (left terminal 7.2%). The transformed cell lines were named WY1, CY1, and GY1, respectively. Three kinds of antisera were used to characterize these transformed lines: (i) broad tumor-bearing hamster sera (TBHS) which contained antibodies to T antigens and other viral antigens, such as single-stranded DNA-binding proteins; (ii) narrow tumor-bearing hamster sera which contained antibody to T antigen but not to other viral antigens; and (iii) tumor-bearing rat sera from animals that has been transplanted with either CY1 or GY1 cells. Complement fixation and immunofluorescence tests with broad TBHS and narrow TBHS showed that the CY1 and GY1 cells contained only T antigen, while WY1 cells contained not only T antigen but also single-stranded DNA-binding proteins. In the case of adenovirus 12-infected cells, the single-stranded DNA-binding proteins had molecular weights of 60,000 and 48,000 (48). The sera from rats with CY1 and GY1 tumors contained antibody only to T antigen while sera from rats bearing tumors induced by the whole adenovirus DNA contained antibodies to T antigen and to single-stranded DNA-binding proteins.

Finally, proteins corresponding to 44,000 to 50,000, and to 15,000 MW polypeptides have been identified as the products of the left-end early genes

(1.3 to 4.0 and 4.9 to 11.1 map units, respectively) of adenovirus 2 DNA. This has been done in two ways. First, Harter and Lewis (49) have shown by two dimensional isoelectric focusing-polyacrylamide gel electrophoresis that the 44,000 to 50,000 and the 15,000 MW polypeptides are among virus-specific proteins synthesized early after lytic infection of human cells by adenovirus 2. Second, Lewis et al. (50) obtained early adenovirus type 2 mRNA that hybridized to the leftmost HpaI adenovirus 2 DNA fragments E and C. They translated this mRNA in a cell-free synthesizing system. The translation products were polypeptides with molecular weights of 44,000-50,000 and 15,000.

What is the function of the adenovirus T antigen in virus replication? A clue to the answer to this question has come from a recent study by Rekosh and coworkers (51). They identified a 55,000 MW protein which is directly attached to 5' ends of each of the adenovirus type 2 DNA strands, probably via covalent linkages. They proposed that the protein functions during the viral DNA replication by facilitating priming of the progeny strands, thus allowing the 5'-ends of the DNA to be replicated. Adenovirus DNA replication begins at or near each of the ends of the adenovirus DNA and proceeds in a 5' to 3' direction by a displacement mechanism with the copying of each complementary strand. The model postulates that during DNA replication, a newly synthesized molecule of the 55,000 dalton terminal protein recognizes a region near the 3'-end of a parental DNA strand and binds strongly but noncovalently to it, remaining on the outside of the phosphodiester chain. The fact that there is an inverted terminal repetition in adenovirus DNA means that the sequence at either 3'-end is identical and thus could function as a binding site. The protein would become attached covalently to the 5' terminal deoxycytidine of the progeny strand either by acting directly as a primer for the DNA polymerase or by a mechanism involving direct recognition of dCTP by the protein either before or after the protein is bound to the DNA. The free 3'-OH on the protein-bound cytidine could then be used to prime DNA synthesis or to allow completion of the 5'-ends of the molecules.

It is noteworthy that purified adenovirus T antigen has about the same molecular weight as the protein which binds to the terminal end of adenovirus DNA (42, 45, 51). It remains to be determined whether the terminal protein and T antigen are the same molecule.

The finding that the adenovirus terminal protein binds at or near the origin of adenovirus DNA replication is of interest by comparison with the SV40 T antigen. The SV40 T antigen binds to the origin of SV40 DNA replication and is essential for initiating SV40 DNA replication.

Epstein-Barr Virus—Associated Nuclear Antigen

Reedman and Klein first described a nuclear antigen present in all

148

producer and nonproducer human lymphoblastoid cell lines containing Epstein-Barr virus (EBV) (12). This antigen was defined using antisera from patients with diseases associated with EBV infection in the anticomplement immunofluorescence assay (ACIF). EBNA is the only EBV-associated antigen present in all EBV genome carrying lymphoid cell lines, and it is also present in biopsies of Burkitt lymphoma tissues. In contrast, other EBV-related antigens [early antigen (EA), membrane antigen (MA), and viral capsid antigen (VCA)] are expressed in some, but not all, Burkitt tumor cells, although expression of EA, MA, and VCA can sometimes be enhanced by chemicals. EBNA is likewise found in the nucleus of the epithelial cells of nasopharyngeal carcinoma, a second human tumor associated with infection by EBV, and in all human cord blood lymphocytes transformed *in vitro* by the B95-8 strain of EBV. In view of the regular presence of EBNA in all cells carrying the EBV genome and the direct relationship between the number of EBV DNA copies and the amount of EBNA per nucleus (52), it appears possible that EBNA may play an important regulatory role in lymphocyte immortalization and/or in keeping the multiple viral genome latent.

EBV-transformed cells contain a soluble complement-fixing antigen which appears to be identical to the antigen detected by the ACIF test. The evidence for this connection between EBNA and the soluble CF antigen is indirect and based on the following facts: (i) there is a good correlation between the anti-EBNA titers and the antibody titers against the soluble CF antigen in a collection of human sera; (ii) partially purified CF antigen specifically absorbs anti-EBNA antibodies from human sera; and (iii) EBNA is chromosomally localized in metaphase while the soluble CF antigen binds to DNA cellulose columns. Also noteworthy is the striking demonstration that purified complement-fixing antigen from EBV-transformed human cells can be bound by methanol/acetic acid-fixed metaphase chromosomes. On addition of this antigen to the fixed metaphase chromosomes, followed by exposure to human sera containing antibodies against EBNA, brilliant positive staining was obtained by ACIF (53).

Sucrose gradient centrifugation and gel filtration experiments have shown that purified EBNA has a molecular weight of 174,000 (53, 54). In neutral buffers containing 0.5-1.0 M NaCl, the antigen dissociates into a form of approximately one-half the original molecular weight with retained complement-fixing activity (98,000). The 174,000 and 98,000 MW forms of EBNA are probably tetrameric and dimeric molecular forms of the antigen. EBNA "monomer" appears to be a polypeptide with a molecular weight of 49,000 (55). EBNA has been purified 85- to 150-fold by Baron and Strominger (55) from nuclear pellets derived from an EBV-transformed B-lymphoblastoid cell line by a five step procedure. This procedure, which took advantage of the heat-stability and the affinity of EBNA for double-stranded DNA, consisted of heating nuclear extracts at 80°C in phosphate buffer, ammonium sulfate precipitation, preparative ultracentrifugation, and affinity chromatography on double-stranded DNA-cellulose. The purified complement-fixing antigen had specific blocking activity in the ACIF assay for EBNA. After SDS-polyacrylamide slab gel electrophoresis of the purified antigen, a prominent polypeptide band with a molecular weight of 49,000 was seen. In addition, there were 5 to 6 minor polypeptide bands ranging in size from 12,000 to 70,000 daltons. The relationship, if any, of the minor polypeptide bands to EBNA has not as yet been determined.

Herpes Simplex Virus-Associated Nuclear Antigen

HSV-related antigens are of interest in relation to investigations on virus latency and on the suspected involvement of HSV in cervical cancer (56-58). In this section, I will describe a new HSV-related intranuclear antigen(s) detected in biochemically transformed human and mouse cells (15). Herpesvirus-specific antigens have previously been detected in the cytoplasm and on the membranes of cells morphologically transformed or biochemically transformed by HSV (59-63). The experiments to be described represent the first demonstration of HSV-related intranuclear antigens in biochemically transformed cells.

Detection of the HSV-related nuclear antigens was accomplished by using the highly sensitive peroxidase-antiperoxidase (PAP) immunological staining technique, and also by immunofluorescence, with rabbit antisera that had high neutralizing titers against HSV-specific deoxypyrimidine kinase and virus infectivity. This antisera had been used in previous immunoadsorbent experiments to detect HSV deoxypyrimidine kinase polypeptides in cells labeled with ^{35}S-methionine (64).

To prepare HSV antigens for rabbit immunization, primary and secondary cultures of rabbit cells were infected for 6 hr with either HSV-1 or HSV-2, cytosol extracts were made, and the extracts were repeatedly inoculated into rabbits. The cytosol extracts were prepared 6 hr post-infection because this is the time of maximal induction of HSV deoxypyrimidine kinase. It was anticipated that the extracts would be enriched in "early" HSV nonstructural proteins, but that they would also contain "late" structural proteins. The virus neutralizing activity of the antisera verifies that antibodies to structural proteins were present. An immunoadsorbent prepared by coupling the antisera to Sepharose 4B bound several ^{35}S-methionine-labeled HSV polypeptides in cytosol extracts of infected cells, showing that the antisera recognized HSV antigens other than HSV deoxypyrimidine kinase polypeptide. The labeled polypeptides were detected by SDS-PAGE analyses of the polypeptides eluted from the anti-HSV-IgG-Sepharose 4B immunoadsorbent (unpublished experiments). To obviate nonspecific antibody staining, immunoglobulin fractions from

150

HSV-1 and HSV-2 antisera and from normal rabbit sera were absorbed with fetal calf serum and with cell packs and sonicates from uninfected mouse and human cells. A point worth emphasizing is that this antisera differed from that used previously by others. Other investigators have generally used human convalescent sera, sera obtained from rabbits immunized with virus, sera derived from rabbits that had been inoculated with HSV-transformed cells, or sera from hamsters bearing HSV-induced rodent tumor cells (59-63).

To obtain biochemically transformed cells, thymidine kinase-negative human HeLa(BU25) or mouse LM(TK⁻) cells were transformed to the thymidine kinase-positive phenotype by infection with UV-irradiated HSV-1 or HSV-2, and selected in hypoxanthine-aminopterin-thymidine (HAT) medium. Biochemical and immunological experiments demonstrated that all biochemically transformed cell lines expressed the type-specific HSV deoxpyrimidine kinase. Clones of human and mouse cells biochemically transformed by HSV-1 (strains KOS and clone 101) are designated HeLa(BU25)/KOS-8-1, HeLa(BU25)/KOS-8-2, LM(TK⁻)/KOS-10, and LM(TK⁻)/HSV-1 clone 7. Human and mouse lines, respectively, biochemically transformed by HSV-2 strain 333 are designated HeLa(BU25)/HSV-2-6 Cl 4 and LM(TK⁻)/HSV-2-8.

Diffuse nuclear staining with relatively little cytoplasmic staining was observed in human and in mouse cells biochemically transformed by HSV-1 (Table 2). The PAP immunological staining method was more sensitive than indirect immunofluorescence for detection of the HSV-related antigens. For example, anti-HSV-1 sera number 46 was diluted 1:60 for PAP immunological staining, but only 1:3 for indirect immunofluorescence tests.

In the case of human and mouse cells biochemically transformed by HSV-2, both nuclei and cytoplasm were stained with anti-HSV-2 serum number 29. Human and mouse cells biochemically transformed by HSV-2 did not cross-react with the anti-HSV-1 sera, nor did human and mouse cells biochemically transformed by HSV-1 cross-react with anti-HSV-2 serum. Uninfected HeLa(BU25) and LM(TK⁻) cells and SV40-transformed cells did not react with either HSV-1 or HSV-2 antisera and none of the cell types reacted immunologically with normal rabbit serum (Table 2).

HSV-related antigens were likewise detected in both the nucleus and cytoplasm of mouse or human cells productively infected for 6 hr with either HSV-1 or HSV-2 (Table 2). As expected, the staining of acutely infected cells was very intense. In contrast to biochemically transformed cells, cells acutely infected by either HSV-1 or HSV-2 reacted in the PAP immunological staining test with either anti-HSV-1 or HSV-2 sera, indicating that the HSV-related type-specific antigens in biochemically transformed cells were a subset of the HSV-antigens synthesized in acutely infected cells.

The nuclear localization of the HSV-related antigens in biochemically

Table 2—REACTIONS[1] OF HSV-1 ANTISERA AND OF HSV-2 ANTISERA WITH ANTIGENS IN BIOCHEMICALLY TRANSFORMED HUMAN [HeLa(BU25)] AND MOUSE [LM(TK⁻)] CELLS, IN SOMATIC CELL HYBRIDS (LH81-11) PREPARED BY FUSING LM(TK⁻) WITH HeLa(BU25)/KOS-8-1 CELLS, AND IN LM(TK⁻) AND HeLa(BU25) CELLS PRODUCTIVELY INFECTED WITH EITHER HSV-1 OR HSV-2

Cells	Immuno-PAP			Immunofluorescence		
	Anti-HSV-1 serum No. 46	Anti-HSV-2 serum No. 29	NRS[2]	Anti-HSV-1 sera No. 46	No. 159	NRS[2]
HeLa(BU25)	-	-	-	-	-	-
LM(TK⁻)	-	-	-	-	-	-
HeLa(BU25) infected for 6 hr with HSV-1 (KOS)	+	+	-	+	+	-
LM(TK⁻) infected for 6 hr with HSV-1 (KOS)	+	+	-	+	+	-
HeLa(BU25)/KOS-8-1	+	-	-	+	+	-
HeLa(BU25)/KOS-8-2	+	-	-	+	+	-
LM(TK⁻)/HSV-1 Clone 7	+	-	-	ND[3]	+	-
LM(TK⁻)/KOS-10	+	-	-	ND[3]	ND[3]	ND[3]
HeLa(BU25) infected for 6 hr with HSV-2 (333)	+	+	-	+	+	-
LM(TK⁻) infected for 6 hr with HSV-2 (333)	+	+	-	+	+	-
HeLa(BU25)/HSV-2-6 Clone 4	-	+	-	-	-	-
LM(TK⁻) HSV-2-8	-	+	-	-	-	-
LH81-11 Clones 11-15	+	ND[3]	ND[3]	ND[3]	ND[3]	ND[3]

[1] + : HSV antigens detected; - : HSV antigens not detected.
[2] NRS : normal rabbit sera.
[3] ND : not done.

transformed cells suggested that they might be DNA-binding proteins. About 16 different virus-determined DNA-binding proteins have been found in mammalian cells lytically infected by HSV-1 and HSV-2 (65-67). Therefore, the possible association of HSV-related antigens with metaphase chromosomes was investigated (68). Table 3 shows that anti-HSV-1 serum number 46 did, in fact, stain metaphase chromosomes of biochemically transformed human and mouse cells, but not chromosomes of uninfected cells. Normal sera did not react with any of the constituents of biochemically transformed cells. Methanol/acetic acid treatment of the biochemically transformed cells, which removes most of the chromatin-bound proteins, eliminated their staining for HSV-related antigens. The PAP immunological staining of biochemically transformed cells was blocked by mixing anti-HSV-1 sera with high salt extracts from cells acutely infected by HSV-1 prior to PAP staining.

Table 3—PAP IMMUNOLOGICAL STAINING OF HSV-1-ASSOCIATED ANTIGENS ON CHROMOSOMES OF CELLS BIOCHEMICALLY TRANSFORMED BY HSV-1

Cell Type	PAP immunological staining[1]	
	Anti-HSV-1 serum Number 46	Normal rabbit serum
Parental cells		
HeLa(BU25) (human)	-	-
LM(TK-) (mouse fibroblast)	-	-
Cells biochemically transformed by HSV-1		
HeLa(BU25)/KOS-8-1	+	-
HeLa(BU25)/KOS-8-2	+	-
LM(TK-)/KOS-10	+	-
LM(TK-)/HSV-1 Clone 7	+	-
LH81-11 Clone 12	+	ND[2]

[1] + : HSV-1 antigens detected; - : HSV-1 antigens not detected.
[2] ND : not done.

The results shown in Tables 2 and 3 indicate that the HSV-related antigens of biochemically transformed cells resemble EBNA in that both the EBV and HSV antigens bind to metaphase chromosomes. We therefore propose that the HSV-associated nuclear antigens be named "HANA".

Ohno et al. (53) demonstrated that EBNA binds *in vitro* to

153

methanol/acetic acid-fixed chromosomes, a further indication of the DNA-binding capacity of EBNA. To learn whether anti-HSV-1 serum number 46 could recognize DNA-binding proteins in the *in vitro* reconstitution test, methanol/acetic acid-fixed chromosomes of biochemically transformed or uninfected cells were treated *in vitro* with high salt extracts from HSV-1-infected cells, followed by exposure to anti-HSV-1 sera and PAP staining. The results showed that antigens in the extracts from the HSV-1-infected cells do bind to methanol/acetic acid-fixed chromosomes. Similarly, using anti-HSV-2 sera, *in vitro* binding of high salt extracts from HSV-2-infected cells to methanol/acetic acid-fixed chromosomes was demonstrated, but there was no staining when soluble extracts from uninfected cells were substituted for those from HSV-infected cells.

The detection of both HSV deoxypyrimidine kinase and HANA in biochemically transformed cells raises the question as to whether the genes determining these two HSV proteins might be closely linked on the HSV genome. The HSV deoxypyrimidine kinase and HANA genes might have been co-integrated in the original transformation event or alternatively, they could have been integrated independently as a result of distinct recombinational events with host DNA. To investigate this question, we have utilized somatic cell hybrids prepared by fusing LM(TK⁻) cells with HeLa(BU25)/KOS-8-1 cells and HAT-ouabain selection. Human-mouse somatic cell hybrids prepared in this way lose most of the human chromosomes, but of necessity retain the human chromosome that carries the integrated HSV deoxypyrimidine kinase gene (69). The somatic cell hybrids isolated after fusing LM(TK⁻) cells with HeLa(BU25)/KOS-8-1 cells are called "LH81" cells. They express HSV-1 TK. Isozyme and karyological analyses of subclones of LH81 cells are in progress. The results at this writing indicate that they contain few human chromosomes. Five out of 5 LH81 subclones tested also express HANA, suggesting that the genes for HSV deoxypyrimidine kinase and HANA may, in fact, be integrated on the same human chromosome.

Five additional comments are appropriate. First, it should be emphasized that although cells morphologically transformed by UV-irradiated HSV form tumors in animals, biochemically transformed cells have not as yet been shown to be oncogenic. However, both morphologically and biochemically transformed cells contain HSV DNA integrated with cellular DNA (69, 70). Second, it should now be possible to purify and characterize HANA from biochemically transformed cells and compare its properties with EBNA. Third, it would be interesting to learn whether HANA is expressed in cells that are transformed by HpaI (8.4 kilobase) and Bam H-I (3.4 kilobase) HSV-1 DNA fragments, which are known to code for HSV-1 deoxypyrimidine kinase (70). A positive result would confirm linkage of HSV deoxypyrimidine kinase and HANA genes on HSV DNA.

154

Fourth, we do not know at this time the biological function of HANA, but its association with chromosomes suggests that it might modify gene expression, as already proposed for EBNA (53). Fifth, a search for HANA appears worthwhile in cells morphologically transformed by HSV, in human cancer, and in spinal ganglia where latent infection by HSV occurs. The detection of HANA has opened up new and promising avenues of investigation, which are currently being pursued.

REFERENCES

1. Black, P.H., Rowe, W.P., Turner, H.C. and Huebner, R.J., "A Specific Complement-Fixing Antigen in SV40 Tumor and Transformed Cells." *Proc. Natl. Acad. Sci.* U.S.A. 50:1148-1156, 1963.
2. Habel, K., "Specific Complement-Fixing Antigens in Polyoma Tumors and Transformed Cells." *Virology* 25: 55-61, 1965.
3. Huebner, R.J., Rowe, W.P., Turner, H.C. and Lane, W.T., "Specific Adeno-Virus Complement-Fixing Antigens in Virus-Free Hamster and Rat Tumors." *Proc. Natl. Acad. Sci.* U.S.A. 50: 379-389, 1963.
4. Kitahara, T., Butel, J.S., Rapp, F. and Melnick, J.L., "Correlation Between Complement-Fixing Cell Antibody and Immunofluorescent Nuclear Antibody in Hamsters Bearing SV40-induced Tumors." *Nature* 205: 717, 1965.
5. Pope, J.H. and Rowe, W.P., "Detection of Specific Antigens in SV40-transformed Cells by Immunofluorescence." *J. Exptl. Med.* 120: 121-128, 1964.
6. Pope, JH. and Rowe, W.P., "Immunofluorescent Studies of Adenovirus 12 Tumors and of Cells Transformed or Infected by Adenoviruses." *J. Exptl. Med.* 120: 577-588, 1964.
7. Rapp, F., Butel, J.S. and Melnick, J.L., "Virus-Induced Intranuclear Antigen in Cells Transformed by Papovavirus SV40." *Proc. Soc. Exptl. Biol. Med.* 116: 1131-1135, 1964.
8. Yoshida, T.O. and Ito, Y., "Immunofluorescent Study on Early Virus-Cell Interaction in Shope Papilloma *in vitro* System." *Proc. Soc. Exptl. Biol. Med.* 128: 587-591, 1968.
9. Beth E., Cikes, M., Schloen, L., et al., "Inter-species, Species-, and Type-Specific T Antigenic Determinants of Human Papovaviruses (JC and BK) and of Simian Virus 40." *Int. J. Cancer* 20: 551-559, 1977.
10. Beth, E., Cikes, M. and Giraldo, G., "Microfluorometric Analyses of Anti-Complement and Indirect Immunofluorescence Tests for Human Papovaviruses (JCV and BKV) T Antigens." *Int. J. Cancer* 21: 1-5, 1978.
11. Anderson, J.P., McCormick, K.J., Stenback, W.A. and Trentin, J.J., "Induction of Hepatomas in Hamsters by an Avian Adenovirus (CELO)." *Proc. Soc. Exptl. Biol. Med.* 137: 421-423, 1971.
12. Reedman, B.M. and Klein, G., "Cellular Localization of an Epstein-Barr Virus (EBV)-Associated Complement-Fixing Antigen in Producer and Non-Producer Lymphoblastoid Cell Lines." *Int. J. Cancer* 11: 499-520, 1973.
13. Gerber, P., Pritchett, R.F. and Kieff, E.D., "Antigens and DNA of a Chimpanzee Agent Related to Epstein-Barr Virus." *J. Virol.* 19: 1090-1099, 1976.
14. Ohno, S., Luka, J., Falk, L. and Klein, G., "Detection of a Nuclear, EBNA-Type Antigen in Apparently EBNA-Negative Herpesvirus Papio (HVP)-Transformed Lymphoid Lines by the Acid-Fixed Nuclear-Binding Technique." *Int. J. Cancer* 20: 941-946, 1977.
15. Kurchak, M., Dubbs, D.R. and Kit, S., "Detection of Herpes Simplex Virus-Related Antigens in the Nuclei and Cytoplasm of Biochemically Transformed Cells with Peroxidase/Antiperoxidase Immunological Staining and Indirect Immunofluorescence." *Int. J. Cancer* 20: 371-380, 1977.

155

16. Tegtmeyer, P., Rundell, K. and Collins, J.K., "Modification of Simian Virus 40 Protein A" *J. Virol.* 21:647-657, 1977.
17. Crawford, L.V., Cole, C.N., Smith, A.E., et al., "Organization and Expression of Early Genes of Simian Virus 40." *Proc. Natl Acad. Sci. U.S.A.* 75: 117-121, 1978.
18. Jessel, D., Landau, T., Hudson, J., et al., "Identification of Regions of the SV40 Genome Which Contain Preferred SV40 T Antigen-Binding Sites." *Cell* 8: 535-545, 1976.
19. Tegtmeyer, P., Schwartz, M., Collins, J.K. and Rundell, K., "Regulation of Tumor Antigen Synthesis by Simian Virus 40 Gene A." *J. Virol.* 16: 168-178, 1975.
20. Alwine, J.C., Reed, S.I. and Stark, G.R., "Characterization of the Auto-regulation of Simian Virus 40 Gene A." *J. Virol.* 24: 22-27, 1977.
21. Tenen, D.G., Baygell, P. and Livingston, D.M., "Thermolabile (T) Tumor Antigen From Cells Transformed by a Temperature-Sensitive Mutant of Simian Virus 40." *Proc. Natl. Acad. Sci. U.S.A.* 72: 4351-4355, 1975.
22. Alwine, J.C., Reed, S.I., Ferguson, J. and Stark, G.R., "Properties of T Antigens Induced by Wild-Type SV40 and tsA Mutants in Lytic Infection." *Cell* 6: 529-533, 1975.
23. Prives, C., Gilboa, E., Revel, M. and Winocour, E., "Cell-Free Translation of Simian Virus 40 Early Messenger RNA Coding for Viral T-Antigen." *Proc. Natl. Acad. Sci. U.S.A.* 74: 457-461, 1977.
24. Greenblatt, J.F., Allet, B., Weil, R. and Ahmad-Zadeh, C., "Synthesis of the Tumor Antigen and the Major Capsid Protein of Simian Virus 40 in a Cell-Free System Derived From *Escherichia coli.*" *J. Mol. Biol.* 108: 361-379, 1976.
25. Schaffhausen, B.S., Silver, J.E. and Benjamin, T.L., "Tumor Antigen(s) in Cells Productively Infected by Wild-Type Polyoma Virus and Mutant NG-18." *Proc. Natl. Acad. Sci. U.S.A.* 75: 79-83, 1978.
26. Simmons, D.T., Takemoto, K.K. and Martin, M.A., "Relationship Between the Methionine Tryptic Peptides of Simian Virus 40 and BK Virus Tumor Antigens." *J. Virol.* 24: 319-325, 1977.
27. Padgett, B.L., Walker, D.L., Zu Rhein, G.M. and Varakis, J.N., "Differential Neurooncogenicity of Strains of JC Virus, a Human Polyoma Virus, in Newborn Syrian Hamsters." *Cancer Res.* 37: 718-720, 1977.
28. Corallini, A., Barbanti-Brodano, G., Bortoloni, W., et al., "High Incidence of Ependymomas Induced by BK Virus, a Human Papovavirus: Brief Communication." *J. Natl. Cancer Inst.* 59: 1561-1564, 1977.
29. Kirschstein, R.L. and Gerber, P., "Ependymomas Produced After Intercerebral Inoculation of SV40 into Newborn Hamsters." *Nature* 195: 299-300, 1962.
30. Tabuchi, K., Kirsch, W.M., Low, M., et al., "Screening of Human Brain Tumors for SV40-Related T Antigen." *Int. J. Cancer* 21: 12-17, 1978.
31. Gilden, R.V., Kern, J., Freeman, A.E., et al., "T and Tumour Antigens of Adenovirus Group C-Infected and Transformed Cells." *Nature* 219: 517-518, 1968.
32. Lewis, A.M., Jr., Wiese, W.H. and Rowe, W.P., "The Presence of Antibodies in Human Serum to Early (T) Adenovirus Antigens." *Proc. Natl. Acad. Sci. U.S.A.* 57: 622-629, 1967.
33. Gilead, Z. and Ginsberg, H.S., "Characterization of the Tumorlike (T) Antigen Induced by Type 12 Andenovirus. II. Physical and Chemical Properties." *J. Virol.* 2: 15-20, 1968.
34. Tavitian, A., Peries, J., Chuat, J. and Boiron, M., "Estimation of the Molecular Weight of Adenovirus 12 Tumor CF Antigen by Rate-Zonal Centrifugation." *Virology* 31: 719-721, 1967.
35. Hollingshead, A.C., Alford, T.C., Oroszlan, S., et al., "Separation and Description of Adenovirus 12-Induced Cellular Antigens Which React With Hamster Tumor Antisera." *Proc. Natl. Acad. Sci. U.S.A.* 59: 385-392, 1968.
36. Potter, C.W., Oxford, J.S. and McLaughlin, B.C., "A Comparison of Adenovirus 12-Induced T and Tumour Antigens by Rate-Zonal Centrifugation." *J. Gen. Virol.* 6: 105-116, 1970.

37. Tockstein, G., Polasa, H., Pina, M. and Green, M., "A Simple Purification Procedure for Adenovirus Type 12 T and Tumor Antigens and Some of Their Properties." *Virology* 36: 377-386, 1968.

38. Hollingshead, A., Bunnag, B., Alford, T. and Cusumano, C., "Purification and Analysis of Adenovirus Group-Specific T. Antigen." *J. Gen. Virol.* 4: 433-435, 1969.

39. Biron K.K., Morrongiello, M.P., Raskova, J. and Raska, K., Jr., "Adenovirus Type 12 Tumor Antigen. I. Separation From DNA Polymerase α and Immunoprecipitation of Tumor-Antigen Polypeptides." *Virology* 85: 464-474, 1978.

40. Van der Vliet, P.C. and Levine, A.J., "DNA-Binding Proteins Specific for Cells Infected by Adenovirus." *Nature New Biology* 246: 170-174, 1973.

41. Gilead, Z., Arens, M.Q., Bhaduri, S., et al., "Tumor Antigen Specificity of a DNA-Binding Protein From Cells Infected with Adenovirus 2. *Nature* 254: 533-536, 1975.

42. Levinson, A. and Levine, A.J., "The Isolation and Identification of Adenovirus Group C Tumor antigens. *Virology* 76: 1-11, 1977.

43. Van der Eb, A.J., Mulder, C., Graham, F.L. and Houweling, A., "Transformation with Specific Fragments of Adenovirus DNAs. I. Isolation of Specific Fragments with Transforming Activity of Adenovirus 2 and 5 DNA." *Gene* 2: 115-132, 1977.

44. Van der Eb, A.J. and Houweling, A., "Transformation with Specific Fragments of Adenovirus DNAs. II. Analysis of the Viral DNA Sequences Present in Cells Transformed with a 7% Fragment of Adenovirus 5 DNA." *Gene* 2: 133-146, 1977.

45. Gilead, Z., Jeng, W.H., Wold, W.S.M., et al., "Immunological Identification of Two Adenovirus 2-Induced Early Proteins Possibly Involved in Cell Transformation." *Nature* (London) 264: 263-266, 1976.

46. Yano, S., Ojima, S., Fujinaga, K., et al., "Transformation of a Rat Cell Line by an Adenovirus Type 12 DNA Fragment." *Virology* 82: 214-220, 1977.

47. Shiroki, K., Handa, H., Shimojo, H., et al., "Establishment and Characterization of Rat Lines Transformed by Restriction Endonuclease Fragments of Adenovirus 12 DNA." *Virology* 82: 462-471, 1977.

48. Rosenwirth, B., Shiroki, K., Levine, A.J. and Shimojo, H., "Isolation and Characertization of Adenovirus Type 12 DNA-Binding Proteins." *Virology* 67: 14-23, 1975.

49. Harter, M.L. and Lewis, J.B., "Adenovirus Type 2 Early Proteins Synthesized *in vitro* and *in vivo*. Identification in Infected Cells of the 38,000- to 50,000-Molecular Weight Proteins encoded by the Left End of the Adenovirus Type 2 Genome." *J. Virol.* 26: 736-749, 1978.

50. Lewis, J.B., Atkins, J.F., Baum, P.R., et al., "Location and Identification of the genes for Adenovirus Type 2 Early Polypeptide." *Cell* 7: 141-151, 1976.

51. Rekosh, D.M.K., Russell, W.C., Bellet, A.J.D. and Robinson, A.J., "Identification of a Protein Linked to the Ends of Adenovirus DNA." *Cell* 11: 283-295, 1977.

52. Ernberg, I., Andersson-Anvret, M., Klein G., et al., "Relationship Between Amount of Epstein-Barr Virus-Determined Nuclear Antigen Per Cell and Number of EBV-DNA Copies Per Cell." *Nature* (London) 266: 269-270, 1977.

53. Ohno, S., Luka, J., Lindahl, T. and Klein, G., "Identification of a Purified Complement-Fixing Antigen as the Epstein-Barr Virus-Determined Nuclear Antigen (EBNA) by its Binding to Metaphase Chromosomes." *Proc. Natl. Acad. Sci. U.S.A.* 74: 1605-1609, 1977.

54. Luka, J., Siegert, W. and Klein, G., "Solubilization of the Epstein-Barr Virus-Determined Nuclear Antigen and its Characterization as a DNA-Binding Protein." *J. Virol.* 22: 1-8, 1977.

55. Baron, D. and Strominger, J.L., "Partial Purification and Properties of the Epstein-Barr Virus-Associated Nuclear Antigen." *J. Biol. Chem.* 253: 2875-2881, 1978.

56. Baringer, J.R., "Herpes Simplex Virus Infection of Nervous Tissue in Animals and Man." *Progress in Med. Virol.* 20: 1-26, 1975.

57. Pacsa, A.S., Kummerlander, L., Pejtsik, B., et al., "Herpes Simplex Virus-Specific Antigens in Exfoliated Cervical Cells From Women With and Without Cervical

Anaplasia." *Cancer Res.* 36: 2130-2132, 1976.

58. Choi, N.W., Shettigara, P.T., Abu-Zeid, H.A.D. and Nelson, N.A., "Herpesvirus Infection and Cervical Anaplasia—a Seroepidemiological Study." *Int. J. Cancer* 19: 167-171, 1977.

59. Duff, R. and Rapp, F., "Oncogenic Transformation of Hamster Embryo Cells After Exposure to Inactivated Herpes Simplex Virus Type 1." *J. Virol.* 12: 209-217, 1973.

60. Reed, C.L., Cohen, G.H. and Rapp, F., "Detection of a Virus-Specific Antigen on the Surface of Herpes Simplex-Transformed cells." *J. Virol.* 15: 668-670, 1975.

61. Li, J.L., Jerkofsky, M.A. and Rapp, F., "Demonstration of Oncogenic Potential of Mammalian Cells Transformed by DNA-Containing Viruses Following Photodynamic Inactivation." *Int. J. Cancer* 15: 190-202, 1975.

62. Gupta, P. and Rapp, F., "Identification of Virion Polypeptides in Hamster Cells Transformed by Herpes Simplex Virus Type 1." *Proc. Natl. Acad. Sci. U.S.A.* 74: 372-374, 1977.

63. Chadha, K.C. and Munyon, W., "Presence of Herpes Simplex Virus-Related Antigens in Transformed L Cells." *J. Virol.* 15: 1475-1486, 1975.

64. Kit, S., Jorgensen, G.N., Dubbs, D.R., et al., "Detection of Herpes Simplex Virus Thymidine Kinase Polypeptides in Cells Labeled with ^{35}S-Methionine." *Intervirology* 9: 162-172, 1978.

65. Purifoy, D.J.M. and Powell, K.L., "DNA-Binding Proteins Induced by Herpes Simplex Virus Type 2 in HEp-2 Cells." *J. Virol.* 19: 717-731, 1976.

66. Powell, K.L. and Purifoy, D.J.M., "DNA-Binding Proteins of Cells Infected by Herpes Simplex Virus Type 1 and Type 2." *Intervirology* 7: 225-239, 1976.

67. Bayliss, G.J., Marsden, H.S. and Hay, J., "Herpes Simplex Virus Proteins: DNA-Binding Proteins in Infected Cells and in the Virus Structure." *Virology* 68: 124-134, 1975.

68. Kit, S., Kurchak, M., Wray, W. and Dubbs, D.R., "Binding to Chromosomes of Herpes Simplex-Related Antigens in Biochemically Transformed Cells." *Proc. Natl. Acad. Sci. U.S.A.* 75: 3288-3291, 1978.

69. Donner, L., Dubbs, D.R. and Kit, S., "Chromosomal Site(s) of Integration of Herpes Simplex Virus Type 2 Thymidine Kinase Gene in Biochemically Transformed Human Cells." *Int. J. Cancer* 20: 256-267, 1977.

70. Pellicer, A., Wigler, M., Axel, R. and Silverstein, S., "The Transfer and Stable Integration of the HSV Thymidine Kinase Gene Into Mouse Cells. *Cell* 14: 133-142, 1978.

Detection of C-Type Virus Immune Molecules in Man During Gestation†

Sandra Panem[1]
T. Neal[1]

SUMMARY–C-type RNA retroviruses have been studied as etiologic agents for some naturally occurring neoplastic and immune complex diseases in several animal models. With increasing evidence that virtually all mammals carry multiple, endogenous C-type viruses, it has been suggested that these viruses have a normal physiologic function, perhaps during development, in addition to their pathogenic roles. We have utilized HEL-12 virus, a retrovirus isolated from human embryonic lung cells, as a probe for identifying C-type viral immune molecules in man. The techniques employed are immunofluorescence, competition radioimmunoassay and electrophoretic analysis of precipitates formed between antiviral sera and extracts of human tissues. Data will be presented suggesting that C-type viral antigen is expressed during normal human gestation. These findings will be evaluated in light of other reports on the occurrence of viral antigen and antiviral antibody in man and their association with disease.

INTRODUCTION, MATERIALS AND METHODS

C-type RNA retroviruses have been studied as etiologic agents for some naturally occurring neoplastic and immune complex diseases in several animal models. With increasing evidence that virtually all mammals carry multiple, endogenous C-type viruses, it has been suggested that these viruses play a role in normal, physiologic functions in addition to their participation in pathogenesis. In this regard, C-type viruses are postulated to participate in differentiation, immune recognition and speciation (1, 2, 3).

C-type viruses may be transmitted vertically (endogenous viruses) or horizontally (exogenous viruses). Furthermore, C-type viruses undergo extensive recombination and recombinants may be formed between endogenous and exogenous viruses. It is possible that endogenous viruses have functions which are distinct from those of exogenous viruses. A currently popular idea is that endogenous viruses may play positive or neutral biologic roles whereas exogenous and/or recombinant viruses may mediate pathogenesis. In assessing the possible role of C-type viruses in man it is of interest to delineate the variety of C-type viruses and their modes of transmission.

[1]Department of Pathology, University of Chicago, Chicago, Illinois.
†Supported by grants from the Elsa U. Pardee Foundation, The National Foundation: March of Dimes, and the American Cancer Society Illinois Division.

159

Although endogenous viruses have been isolated from numerous species, no human endogenous virus has yet been identified. As there is no standard virus to use as a probe for viral expression in human tissue, it has been necessary to rely on antigenic cross-reactivity postulated to occur between known viruses of sub-human primates and those of man. Such cross-reactivity is predicted in analogy to extensive studies of C-type viruses of numerous species which have shown that (i) C-type viruses have evolved with the species; (ii) viruses of closely related species (as determined by the fossil record) are more closely related antigenically than are those of distantly related species; (iii) viruses isolated from related species share conserved antigenic determinants (interspecies antigens) (2, 4). In our attempts to demonstrate C-type viral expression in man, we have looked for antigens and antibodies in human tissues which specificites shared with HEL-12 virus (5-7). HEL-12 virus is a C-type retrovirus isolated from human embryonic lung cells (8). It is unique among the currently available C-type retroviruses of primates in that it derived from a normal human tissue and that it shares antigenic and nucleic acid homology with a group of exogenous primate viruses (SiSV/GALV) and a group of endogenous primate viruses (BaEV/Rd-114) (5-10).

In this communication we will summarize the evidence that C-type viruses are expressed during gestation and that these viral antigens can be found during the pathogenesis of systemic lupus erythematosus (SLE).

RESULTS AND DISCUSSION

C-type viruses have been detected in the placentas and germinal tissues of numerous species including man (11-15). As there is extensive ultrastructural evidence for C-type virus like particles in human placenta we examined normal, term human placenta for viral antigen expression using indirect immunofluorescence and a hyper-immune antiserum raised to HEL-12 virus (7). Our previous results can be summarized as follows: (1) 24 of 24 normal term placentas reacted with anti-HEL-12 virus serum but not preimmune serum; (2) the reaction could be blocked completely by HEL-12 virus; partially by SiSV or BaEV but not by Rous sarcoma virus, Rauscher murine leukemia virus, fetal calf serum, bovine serum albumin, human serum albumin, immunoglobulin and hemoglobin; (3) fluorescence was predominantly associated with cells in contact with fetal circulation; (4) a high-molecular weight glycoprotein rich fraction β-μ could be isolated from placenta and blocked the reaction of anti-viral serum with placenta or virus infected cells; (5) antisera raised to β-μ reacts with virus infected cells but not controls and (6) antisera to SiSV showed a similar immunofluorescence pattern with 2 term placentas.

160

Although anti-HEL-12 virus serum reacts with each term placenta tested, we have not yet found a normal adult tissue which reacts with the serum (i.e., heart, lung, skin, liver, spleen, etc.). To date, the only tissues other than placenta in which we have detected HEL-12 virus like antigen have been those of patients with SLE containing immune deposits (5, 6, 7, 16).

In view of observations that C-type virus-like particles are more easily demonstrated in 1st trimester placenta as compared with term placenta of subhuman primates (17) and reports that pregnant women show variable cell mediated immunity to primate C-type viruses during pregnancy (18, 19), we asked whether HEL-12 virus antigen expression varies during gestation. Table 1 shows the immunofluorescence end-points of immune IgG prepared from rabbit-anti-HEL-12 virus serum with placentas of varying gestational age. Preimmune IgG did not react with any specimen. The reaction of immune IgG and placenta could be blocked by β-μ (Table 2). Previously, the specificity of the anti-viral serum for HEL-12 virus has been demonstrated (5, 6). The fluorescence end-points of 1st trimester placenta were between 1:4-1:8, for 2nd trimester between 1:8-1:16 and for term placenta 1:4. The validity of the measurement of 2 term placentas is supplemented by previous findings with whole anti-viral serum showing that 10 randomly chosen term placentas had a common fluorescence end-point (7). These data, based on a small population are preliminary. Nevertheless, they suggest that antigenicity persists throughout gestation and that the variation in antigen quantity is limited. The four-fold variation in end-point dilutions are confirmed by the amount of β-μ needed to absorb the reaction (Table 2). The suggestion that antigenic variation is limited must be evaluated in view of the fact that anti-HEL-12 IgG detects multiple viral antigens (J.T. Reynolds, unpublished data).

As β-μ blocked the reaction of anti-HEL-12 serum with placenta it was of interest to determine the complexity of β-μ. On SDS-polyacrylamide gel electrophoresis (SDS-PAGE), β-μ is found to contain 3 components of approximate molecular weights 70,000, 35,000 and 15,000 (Figure 1). β-μ is isolated by binding the 70-80,000 molecular weight protein in a placenta eluate to concanavalin A-sepharose. The concanavalin binding protein eluted with alphamethylmannoside is defined as β-μ (7). The molecular sieve and affinity chromatography are performed in PBS at neutral pH. The size heterogeneity of β-μ on SDS-PAGE may be explained (i) by the low molecular weight components being breakdown products of the 70,000 molecular weight component; (ii) by the low molecular weight components being specifically bound in a 70,000 molecular weight structure which is disrupted on SDS-PAGE or (iii) by the low and high molecular weight components being unrelated. These alternatives have yet to be assessed. It is of interest to note that the avian leukosis virus envelope contains a high molecular weight glycoprotein which can be cleaved into two smaller

Table 1—HEL-12 VIRUS RELATED ANTIGEN EXPRESSION DURING GESTATION*

Sample	Immunofluorescence with Immune IgG to HEL-12 Virus			Preimmune IgG
	1:4	1:8	1:16	1:4
1st Trimester Placenta				
# 738	+	–	–	–
# 741	+	+	–	–
# 778	+	+	–	–
# 782	+	–	–	–
# 824	+	–	–	–
# 891	+	+	–	–
2nd Trimester Placenta				
# 911	+	–	–	–
# 970	+	+	+	–
Term Placenta				
# 42	+	–	–	–
# 45	+	–	–	–
2nd Trimester Fetal Tissue				
# 970 Liver	–	–	–	–
Kidney	–	–	–	–
Lung	+	+	–	–

*Tissue was snap frozen in isopentane and 4 mμ sections were obtained with a cryostat. Sections were examined by indirect immunofluorescence. Sera were immunoglobulin G (IgG) prepared by ammonium sulfate fractionation and ion-exchange chromatography from pre-immune and rabbit-anti-HEL-12 virus sera. The IgG's were prepared at 8 mg/ml in phosphate buffered saline (PBS) and diluted just prior to use.
+, positive immunofluorescence
–, no immunofluorescence

components held together by disulfide bonds (20). In that system, the high molecular weight and the disulfide bonded low molecular weight components co-purify from gradient purified virus in the absence of reducing agents.

We previously described HEL-12 virus–related antigens in immune deposits of patients with SLE (5, 6, 16). We were interested to know if the virus antigens found in SLE were the same as those expressed in placenta. Table 3 summarizes results comparing placenta antigen and SLE immune deposits using immunofluorescence and antisera prepared to HEL-12 virus

Table 2—ABSORPTION OF IMMUNOFLUORESCENCE BY β-μ*

Sample	No Absorbent	β-μ Absorbent		
		10 μg	50μg	100μg
1st Trimester Placenta (778)	+	+	+	$-/+$
2nd Trimester Placenta (970)	+	+	+	$-$
Term Placenta (45)	+	+	$-$	$-$

*Immune IgG to HEL-12 virus (1:4) was used in indirect immunofluorescence. For absorption, 0, 10, 50 or 100 μg of β-μ was added to immune IgG for 30 minutes at 25°C and 30 minutes at +4°C prior to reaction with tissue sections.

Figure 1—POLYACRYLAMIDE GEL ANALYSIS OF β-μ

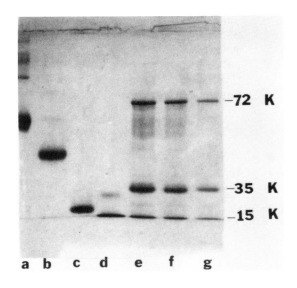

An 8.5% acrylamide-bisacylamide slab gel containing 0.2% SDS was used to analyze β-μ. The stacker gel was 3% and the samples were solubilized with SDS, 2-β-mercaptolethanol and Cleland's reagent. The gel was run in tris-glycine, pH 8.0 at 100 volts. After fixation, proteins were demonstrated by staining with coomassie brilliant blue. (a) Bovine serum albumin, 68,000 molecular weight, (b) ovalbumin, 45,000 molecular weight, (c) chymotrypsin, 25,000 molecular weight, (d) RNase, 13,500 molecular weight, (e)β-μ , 65 μg, (f) β-μ , 32.5 μg, (g) β-μ , 16 μg.

163

and β-μ. The patterns of reactivity were the same for each serum. Both reacted with virus infected cells, placenta and immune deposits in a kidney from a patient with SLE but not with normal kidney, a kidney from a patient with non-SLE immune complex nephropathy, or uninfected control cells. Furthermore, the reaction of either serum for placenta could be blocked by absorption with HEL-12 virus. These data strongly suggest, but do not prove that a similar antigen may be shared by SLE immune complexes and placenta. Whether all viral antigens found in SLE are present in placenta is unknown. We are currently employing competitive radio-immunoassays to address this question more directly.

Table 3—IMMUNOFLUORESCENCE WITH ANTI-SERUM TO β-μ AND HEL-12 VIRUS*

Target	Infecting Virus	Species	Immunofluorescence with Sera to		
			β-μ	HEL-12 Virus	Pre-immune
HEL-12 p.21	HEL-12	Human	+	+	−
A204	Uninfected	Human	−	−	−
NMF	HEL-12	Mink	+	+	−
NMF	Uninfected	Mink	−	−	−
71AP1	SiSV	Marmoset	+	+	−
MFS	Uninfected	Marmoset	−	−	−
BILN	BaEV	Baboon	+	+	−
Human Term Placenta		Human	+	+	−
Normal Kidney		Human	−	−	−
Non-SLE Immune Complex Kidney		Human	−	−	−
SLE Kidney		Human	+	+	−

*Immunofluorescence was performed with human tissues and cells grown in-vitro.
+, positive immunofluorescence
−, no immunofluorescence

In summary, antigen related to HEL-12 virus, SiSV and BaEV is expressed throughtout gestation. The antigen is not normally expressed in adult tissue. An antigen which reacts with antisera prepared to the placenta antigen can be found in immune deposits of patients with SLE. The data are consistent with a hypothesis that a virus which plays a normal role during embryogenesis may be activated during the pathogenesis of SLE. We have yet to determine whether the antigens of the placenta are cross-reactive or identical to those found in SLE.

164

REFERENCES

1. Levy, J.A., "Xenotropic Type C Viruses." *Current Topics in Microbiology and Immunology* 79: 113-213, 1978.
2. Todaro, G., "Evolution and Modes of Transmission of RNA Tumor Viruses." *Am. J. Path.* 81: 590-605, 1975.
3. Moroni, C. and Schumann, G., "Are Endogenous C-Type Viruses Involved in the Immune System?" *Nature* 269: 600-601, 1977.
4. Strand, M. and August, J.T., "Structural Proteins of RNA Tumor Viruses as Probes for Viral Gene Expression." *Cold Spring Harbour Symp. Quant. Biol.* 39: 1109-1116, 1975.
5. Panem, S., Ordóñez, N.G., Katz, A.I., et al., "C-Type Virus Expression in Systemic Lupus Erythematosus." *N. Engl. J. Med.* 295: 470-475, 1976.
6. Panem, S., Ordóñez, N.G., Katz, A.I., et al., "Viral Immune Complexes in Systemic Lupus Erythematosus: Specificity of C-Type Viral Complexes." *Lab. Invest.*, In Press.
7. Sawyer, M.H., Nachlas, N.E., Jr., Panem, S., "C-Type Viral Antigen Expression in Human Placenta." *Nature*, In Press.
8. Panem, S., Prochownik, E.V., Reale, F.R., Kirsten, W.H., "Isolation of Type C Virions from a Normal Human Fibroblast Strain." *Science* 189: 297-299, 1975.
9. Prochownik, E.V. and Kirsten, W.H., "Inhibition of the Reverse Transcriptases of Primate Type C Viruses by 7S Immunoglobulin from Patients with Leukemia." *Nature* 260: 64-67, 1976.
10. Prochownik, E.V. and Kirsten, W.H., "Nucleic Acid Sequences of Primate Type C Viruses in Normal and Neoplastic Human Tissues." *Nature:* 267; 175-177, 1977.
11. Kalter, S.S., Helmke, R.J., Heberling, R.L., et al., "C-Type Particles in Normal Human Placentas." *J. Natl. Cancer Inst.* 50: 1081-1084, 1973.
12. Vernon, M.L., McMahon, J.M., Hackett, J.J., "Additional Evidence of Type C Particles in Human Placentas." *J. Natl. Cancer Inst.* 52: 987-989, 1974.
13. Imamura, M., Phillips, P.E., Mellors, R.C., "The Occurrence and Frequency of Type C Virus-like Particles in Placentas from Patients with Systemic Lupus Erythematosus and from Normal Subjects." *Am. J. Pathol.* 83: 383-394, 1976.
14. Dirksen, E.R. and Levy, J.A., "Virus like Particles in Placentas from Normal Individuals and Patients with Systemic Lupus Erythematosus." *J. Natl. Cancer Inst.* 59: 1187-1192, 1977.
15. Panem, S., "C-Type Virus Expression in Placenta." *Current Topics in Pathology,* In Press.
16. Panem, S., Ordóñez, N.G., Dalton, H. and Soltani, K., "Viral Immune Complexes in Systemic Lupus Erythematosus: C-Type Viral Immune Complex Deposition in Skin." *Arch. Derm.,* In Press.
17. Kalter, S.S., Heberling, R.L., Helmke, R.J., et al., "A Comparative Study on the Presence of C-Type Viral Particles in Placentas from Primates and Other Animals." *Bibl. Haematol.* 40: 391-401, 1975.
18. Hirsch, M.S., Kelly, A.P., Chapin, D.S., Reinhard, K., "Immunity to Antigens Associated with Primate C-Type Oncornaviruses in Pregnant Women." *Science* 199: 1337-1340, 1978.
19. Thiry, L., Sprecher-Goldberger, S., Bossens, M., Neuray, F., "Cell Mediated Immune Response to Simian Oncornavirus Antigens in Pregnant Women." *J. Natl. Cancer Inst.* 60: 527-532, 1978.
20. Leamnson, R.N. and Halpern, M.S., "Subunit Structure of the Glycoprotein Complex of Avian Tumor Virus." *J. Virol.* 18: 956-968, 1976.

Primate Models for Studying Herpesvirus-Induced Malignant and Self-Limiting Lymphoproliferative Diseases

Lawrence A. Falk, Jr.[1,2]

SUMMARY—Lymphotropic herpesviruses, either the B-tropic viruses of man and Old World primates or the T-tropic agents of New World Primates, cause lymphoproliferative diseases in the natural or experimental hosts. These agents are of interest and warrant study because: 1) of the putative role of Epstein-Barr virus in Burkitt's lymphoma and its proven etiologic role in infectious mononucleosis, 2) distinct host immune responses occur during malignant disease, arising spontaneously or induced experimentally as a result of virus infection, 3) of cytogenetic markers which distinguish virus-carrying malignant cells from virus-carrying non-malignant cells, 4) lymphocytes can be transformed *in vitro* by virus and 5) nonhuman primate models have been established for lymphotropic herpesviruses for studying lymphoproliferative diseases.

Herpesvirus papio (HVP), an indigenous virus (B-tropic) of baboons and *Herpesvirus saimiri* (HVS), a T-tropic virus of squirrel monkeys, offer good models for studying virally-induced malignant or self-limiting lymphoproliferative diseases in experimentally-infected marmoset monkeys. HVP infection of adult marmosets of one species caused a fatal lymphoproliferative disease and death (13-22 days PI) whereas infection of newborn marmosets resulted only in a persisting latent infection. Lymphoblastoid cell lines were established and studied from marmosets dying after HVP infection.

HVS causes malignant lymphoma/leukemia in marmoset monkeys but an attenuated strain of HVS (A-HVS) has been derived which fails to induce malignancy. Comparative studies of marmosets infected with either HVS or A-HVS suggest that the initial events are similar but in A-HVS infected animals the acute stage of lymphoproliferation resolves to a persisting, lifelong (>4 years) latent infection. In marmosets infected with A-HVS, humoral and cell-mediated immunologic responses may control the outcome of infection.

INTRODUCTION

A property unique to members of the herpesvirus group is that once the natural host becomes infected, the infection persists for life. The primary infection may result in a transient clinical disease (Figure 1), such as fever

---

[1]Department of Microbiology, Rush-Presbyterian-St. Luke's Medical Center, Chicago, Illinois.
[2]Present Address: Chairman, Division of Microbiology, New England Regional Primate Research Center, Harvard Medical School, Southborough, Massachusetts.

blisters or genital lesions after infection with herpes simplex virus, chicken pox with varicella-zoster virus or infectious mononucleosis after Epstein-Barr virus infection. Primary infection may also result in only a latent infection with subclinical manifestations which is probably what occurs in the majority of primary infections. Throughout life, latent infection may be completely inapparent without clinical disease, recurrent disease at periodical intervals i.e. fever blisters or in the case with certain herpesviruses, it has been suggested that they may be oncogenic in the host.

Figure 1—PRIMARY INFECTION WITH HERPESVIRUSES

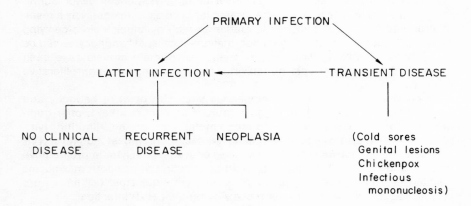

Representative human and primate herpesviruses (Figure 2) are classified on the basis of the tissue in which they exist in a repressed state: neurotropic or lymphotropic. The neurotropic group is exemplified by herpes simplex virus types I and II which are harbored repressed in cells of the trigeminal or sacral ganglion respectively. The lymphotropic viruses are further subdivided into the B- or T-tropic on the basis of the lymphocyte population they infect and transform both *in vivo* and *in vitro*. EBV of man is the best known member of this group but recently viruses have been identified in Old World primates—specifically *Herpesvirus papio* of baboons (1-3), viruses of chimpanzees (4) and orangutans (5). By the fact that gorillas and gibbon apes have antibodies cross reacting with EBV viral capsid antigens makes it reasonable to predict that these primates also have their own B-lymphotropic herpesviruses. All of these viruses possess cross-reacting viral capsid antigens with EBV and partial genome homology with EBV DNA.

Figure 2—REPRESENTATIVE HUMAN AND PRIMATE HERPESVIRUSES

HUMAN-PRIMATE HERPESVIRUSES

NEUROTROPIC	LYMPHOTROPIC	
	T-	B-
HERPES SIMPLEX I & II	HERPESVIRUS SAIMIRI	EPSTEIN—BARR VIRUS
VARICELLA-ZOSTER	HERPESVIRUS ATELES	HERPESVIRUS PAPIO
		CHIMPANZEE-VIRUS
		ORANG-UTAN VIRUS
		(GORILLA, GIBBON)

Two T-lymphotropic herpesviruses have been identified in primates: *Herpesvirus saimiri* (HVS) of squirrel monkeys (6) and *Herpesvirus ateles* of spider monkeys (7,8). There appears to be a distinct division: B-tropic herpesviruses have thus far been identified only in man and Old World primate species and the T-lymphotropic viruses appear restricted to New World primates. One can ask the question whether T-viruses exist in man or Old World primates or if New World monkeys have B-tropic viruses. This of course is a possibility but on the basis of serologic studies we have performed, such viruses must be unrelated to these agents for man and Old World primates lack antibodies reactive against HVS or HVA and New World monkeys lack anti-EBV antibodies.

The etiologic association of EBV with heterophile-positive infectious mononucleosis and the possible cocarcinogenic role of EBV in Burkitt's lymphoma make the lymphotropic herpesviruses of nonhuman primates of interest as laboratory models for investigating the role of EBV in lymphoproliferative diseases of man. In the last decade we have employed the nonhuman primate models for examining the oncogenic potential of lymphotropic herpesviruses and have devoted little attention to utilizing these same virus-host models for investigating herpesvirus latent infections.

Herpesvirus papio of baboons and *Herpesvirus saimiri* of squirrel monkeys are good models for studying both viral induced malignancies or persistent, latent infections because it is possible to study latent infections in the natural hosts, baboons or squirrel monkeys respectively, or induce experimentally malignancies or latent infections in marmoset monkeys *(Saguinus, Callithrix* sp.).

169

Properties of Baboon Lymphoblastoid Cell Lines: Lymphoblastoid cell lines (LCL) were established from splenic or circulating lymphocytes of *Papio hamadryas* or *P. anubis* baboons (Table 1) (1). With exception of one cell line, all cultures contained antigen-reactive cells that reacted with antibodies to EBV viral capsid or early antigens (VCA/EA). A nuclear antigen, similar or analogous to EBV specified nuclear antigen (EBNA) cannot be detected in cells of these cultures by immunofluorescence staining *in situ* with VCA+ human or baboon sera. A nuclear antigen has been detected in cells of some of these cultures by an acid-fixed nuclear binding technique (9).

There was an excellent correlation between lack of detectable EBNA-NA by staining *in situ* and absence of EBNA-NA antibodies in baboon sera. Serum from two separate baboon colonies were tested and 55 of 62 sera had anti-VCA antibodies at titers of 1:4—1:128 but all were negative for anti-EBNA antibodies (8).

Table 1—PROPERTIES OF BABOON LYMPHOBLASTOID CELL LINES CARRYING *HERPESVIRUS PAPIO*

| | Baboon species | |
| | P. hamadryas | P. anubis |
Origin of cell cultures	splenic lymphocytes	circulating lymphocytes
LCL established	3	13
VCA/EA reactive	2/3[1] (2-10%)[2]	11/11 (1-10%)
EBNA-NA reactive	0/3	0/11
EBV-related genomes	3/3 (1-6)[3]	7/7 (12-25)
Rosette formation:		
E	0/3	0/8
EAC	3/3 (15-90%)	4/6 (2-7%)
Ig production:		
IgG	0/3	0/8
IgM	2/3 (21-24%)	8/8 (18-39%)

[1]Number positive/number tested
[2]percent positive cells: 200-300 cells examined in each assay
[3]EBV-related genome equivalents per cell: EBV specific cRNA used in DNA-cRNA filter hybridization tests.

Experimental Studies with Marmoset Monkeys:

Transformation of marmoset lymphocytes: Lymphocytes of cotton-topped *(Saguinus oedipus)* or white-lipped *(S. nigricollis, S. fuscicollis)* marmosets were transformed *in vitro* after cocultivation with X-irradiated HVP-producing baboon lymphoblastoid cells (10). The majority of cotton-topped LCL contained VCA/EA reactive cells (Table 2), but all white-lipped LCL were antigen-negative. EBNA-NA was not detected in any HVP-transformed marmoset LCL.

Table 2—TRANSFORMATION *IN VITRO* OF MARMOSET LYMPHOCYTES WITH *HERPESVIRUS PAPIO*

	Marmoset species	
	S. nigricollis S. fuscicollis	S. oedipus
Transformation	20/32[1]	9/15
VCA-EA reactive cells	0/12	5/9
EBNA-NA reactive cells	0/9	0/9
EBV-related genomes	3/3	2/2

[1]Number positive/number tested

Experimental inoculation of marmosets with HVP: Three of 4 adult cotton-topped marmosets developed generalized lymphoproliferative disease and died 13-22 days postinoculation (PI) with 10^8 HVP-producing baboon lymphoblastoid cells (Table 3) (11). At necropsy, necrotic tumors were present at the inoculation site and in addition pronounced hepatosplenomegaly and generalized lymphadenopathy were found. Lymphoid hyperplasia was the prominent microscopic lesion observed in spleen, lymph nodes, tonsils and thymus. Mild infiltration of lymphoid cells was detected in liver, heart, lung, kidney and adrenal glands.

In contrast to the apparent susceptibility of adult cotton-topped marmosets to HVP infection, experimental inoculation of newborn marmosets with HVP-producing cells resulted in no overt clinical manifestations. In order to assess whether or not such marmosets might respond differently when inoculated as adults, the marmosets described above were re-inoculated with HVP-producing cells about 18 months after their first inoculation. These studies are summarized in Table 4. Each member of 4 twin pairs of marmosets were inoculated with 5-30 x 10^7 13CB-1 cells (*P. hamadryas*), 2-3 days after birth. None of the animals developed a recognizable clinical illness and only 1 of 8 developed measurable anti-HVP antibodies. One member of each twin pair (#1 of each pair) was re-inoculated with 7.5 x 10^8 13CB-1 cells 508-605 days after the first inoculation. Since we had never evaluated the susceptibility of adult common marmosets *(Callithrix jacchus)* to experimental HVP infection, one common marmoset, 76CT-2, without prior 13CB-1 cell inoculation, was inoculated with 7.5 x 10⁸ cells.

Table 3—INOCULATION OF ADULT COTTON-TOPPED OR WHITE-LIPPED MARMOSETS WITH 13CB-1 BABOON LYMPHOBLASTOID CELLS

Marmoset Species	Animal number	Sex	Inoculum dose of	VCA antibodies	Survival PI (days)
Cotton-topped	KZ-1	M	1.3 x 10⁸		17: generalized lympho-proliferative disease
	DF-3	F	"	19[1]	22: " "
	5833	M	5.0 x 10⁸		13: " "
	4472	F	"		>550
White-lipped	5471	M	5.0 x 10⁸	16	>550
	4261	F	"	16	>550

[1]Day PI when VCA antibodies first detected in plasma of marmoset.

As shown by the data presented under "second inoculation" of Table 4, 3 of 4 re-inoculated marmosets and the control marmoset (76CT-2) developed measurable levels of anti-HVP antibodies 10-24 days PI at titers ranging from 1:4-1:32. Only marmoset 76EL-1 had failed to become seropositive.

Additional evidence suggesting HVP infection of these marmosets comes from the ability to establish continuous lymphoblastoid cell lines after cultivation *in vitro* of their circulating lymphocytes. Continuous cell cultures were established from lymphocytes of marmosets 76CT-2, 76EL-1, 76EH-1 and 76DZ-1 at weekly intervals PI. Preliminary characterization of these cultures indicated they possessed a marmoset karyotype, were antigen negative and had surface membrane properties of B-lymphocytes.

HERPESVIRUS SAIMIRI (HVS) AND *HERPESVIRUS ATELES* (HVA)

HVS and HVA are indigenous herpesviruses of squirrel and spider monkeys respectively and experimental infection of susceptible nonhuman primates with HVS or HVA causes lymphoma and/or lymphocytic leukemia (7,8,12,13). In contrast to EBV and HVP which are B-lymphotropic, HVS and HVA are T-lymphotropic and are carried repressed in T-lymphocytes of the experimental or the natural hosts (14). Another distinct and important difference is that HVS/HVA replicate *in vitro* in

Table 4—EXPERIMENTAL INOCULATION OF MARMOSET MONKEYS WITH *HERPESVIRUS PAPIO* CARRYING, BABOON LYMPHOBLASTOID CELLS (13CB-1)

Marmoset Species	Marmoset Number	First Inoculation		Second Inoculation		
		Age	Seroconversion	Inoculated	Days	Seroconversion
C. jacchus	76-DZ-1[a]	2 days	–	Yes[c]	605	+(10 days PI: 1:4)
	76-DZ-2		–	No		
S. oedipus	76-EH-1[a]	2 days	–	Yes[c]	591	+(24 days PI: 1:4)
	76-EH-2		–	No		–
S. nigrifrons	76-EL-1[a]	3 days	–	Yes[c]	586	–
	76-EL-2		–	No		–
	76-FR-1[b]		–	Yes[c]	508	+(10 days PI: 1:32)
	76-FR-2	3 days	1:4	No		+
C. jacchus	76-CT-2		None	Yes[c]	683	+(24 days PI: 1:8)

[a] Inoculated with 5-6.5 x 10^7 13CB-1 cells
[b] Inoculated with 2.9 x 10^8 13CB-1 cells
[c] Inoculated with 7.5 x 10^8 13CB-1 cells

monolayer cell cultures of nonhuman primate origin (vero, owl monkey kidney, etc.). More information has been accumulated on HVS and this presentation will focus on this virus system with particular emphasis on recent studies with an attenuated strain of HVS.

HVS in the Natural Host: HVS was first isolated from primary kidney cell cultures of squirrel monkeys *(Saimiri sciurues)* (6) and subsequently from squirrel monkey lymphocytes after cocultivation with permissive monolayer cells (15). Sero-epidemiology studies performed with several large groups of squirrel monkeys (16) showed that monkeys are born free of infection although they possess maternal antibodies: during the first year of life the majority of animals acquire infection from cage-or troopmates and by two years of age 100% of monkeys have acquired HVS infection as determined by virus isolation and/or serologic studies. Thus far no overt clinical disease has been observed in squirrel monkeys that is associated with latent, HVS infection. Furthermore, colony-born and reared squirrel monkeys, maintained free of HVS infection, have been inoculated with HVS and they failed to develop any clinical manifestations (17, 18). However, infection was confirmed several weeks after inoculation by virus isolation from cocultivated lymphocytes and development of viral specific antibodies. In addition, these monkeys transmitted HVS infection to uninoculated, HVS-negative cagemate monkeys. Once squirrel monkeys acquire HVS infection, they remain latently infected for the remainder of their lives.

HVS in Experimental Hosts: A variety of nonhuman primate species have been evaluated for their susceptibility to HVS infection and these studies have been reviewed and summarized by Deinhardt, et al. (19). Marmoset *(Saguinus* and *Callithrix* sp.) and owl *(Aotus trivirgatus)* monkeys have been employed the most extensively for experimental studies. HVS infection of marmoset monkeys invariably results in fatal disease and in owl monkeys only about 50% of inoculated monkeys develop malignant disease and the remainder develop a persistent, latent infection.

In marmoset monkeys, once HVS infection has been demonstrated by virus rescue or serologic techniques, the infection is ultimately fatal in all monkeys. Previously we conducted a minimal oncogenic dose study, comparing the susceptibility of cotton-topped *vs.* white-lipped marmosets. As few as 2 PFU of HVS caused infection and death of cotton-topped marmosets whereas 20 PFU were required to achieve infection in white-lipped marmosets.

Attenuated Strain of HVS: In collaboration with Dr. Priscilla Schaffer (20), a variant or attenuated strain of HVS (A-HVS) was derived which lacked oncogenic potential. Inoculation of squirrel monkeys or cotton-topped, white-lipped or common marmosets with attenuated HVS resulted in development of a persistent, latent infection: virus could be recovered from cocultivated circulating lymphocytes and antibodies to viral specified

174

early and late antigens were detectable in plasma. Shown in Figure 3 is a longitudinal study of two cotton-topped marmosets inoculated over four years previously with about 600 plaque forming units (PFU) of A-HVS: during the entire observation period it has been possible to rescue virus from these animals and they have maintained relatively constant antibody titers to early and late antigens.

A question of interest was whether or not such animals would be resistant to challenge with oncogenic HVS: two cotton-topped marmosets, latently infected for 142 days and two marmosets without prior exposure to A-HVS were inoculated with about 770 PFU of oncogenic HVS. The control marmosets died 22-23 days PI with malignant disease whereas the two marmosets with A-HVS infection survived 74 and 79 days PI. Therefore A-HVS infection was not completely protective against challenge with oncogenic virus although the survival period was prolonged (20).

Recently we have demonstrated that common marmosets were as susceptible to experimental infection with oncogenic HVS as cotton-topped or white-lipped marmosets (21) and they were studied also for susceptibility to A-HVS infection. All of eight marmosets inoculated with A-HVS developed persistent latent infection and have survived over 2 years PI. Six marmosets were challenged with 100-800 PFU of oncogenic HVS and all of these marmosets have now survived over 12 months postchallenge, whereas two control marmosets without latent A-HVS infection, died 24 and 25 days PI with lymphoma (22).

Presently the fate of oncogenic virus in the challenged marmosets is unknown and we have proposed three possibilities:

1. challenge virus is eliminated immediately by humoral and/or cell mediated immune responses

2. challenge virus infects and transforms target T-lymphocytes which are eventually eliminated or

3. challenge virus infects and transforms target T-lymphocytes which coexist with lymphocytes harboring A-HVS repressed.

Now it is impossible to determine experimentally which of these alternatives is correct because we have not identified differences between A-HVS and oncogenic virus that can be used for distinguishing the two strains *in vitro*. From our previous challenge studies in cotton-topped marmosets it seems likely that oncogenic virus does infect T-lymphocytes, therefore it seems reasonable that the animals are latently infected with both viruses.

The important question which emerges from these studies with A-HVS is how two viruses which are so similar can induce such contrasting disease courses. One feasible hypothesis would be a differential alteration in the cell membranes of virus-infected lymphocytes: T-lymphocytes are target cells for both A-HVS and oncogenic HVS (O-HVS) and infection of T-lymphocytes leads immediately to lymphoproliferation. In marmosets infected

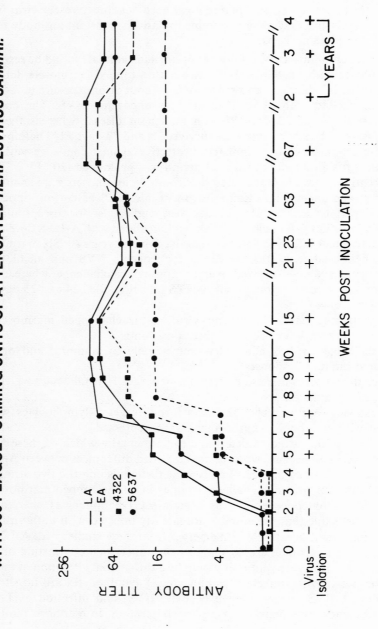

Figure 3—TWO COTTON-TOPPED MARMOSET MONKEYS, 4322 AND 5637, INOCULATED WITH 600 PLAQUE FORMING UNITS OF ATTENUATED *HERPESVIRUS SAIMIRI.*

Blood samples were collected at various intervals postinoculation and used for virus rescue and serologic studies.

176

with O-HVS lymphoproliferation continues unabated until death whereas in A-HVS infected animals, lymphoproliferation is abrogated and resolves to a latent infection. This difference may only be a question of quantitative or qualitative differences in viral induced membrane antigens: on O-HVS infected lymphocytes, neoantigens may be weakly immunogenic or exist not at all therefore there is no humoral or cell-mediated immune response. In contrast, lymphocytes infected with A-HVS may possess neomembrane antigens which are strongly immunogenic and hence stimulate an effective immune response.

DISCUSSION

HVP and HVS are representative of B- and T-lymphotropic herpesviruses which in the natural hosts cause no overt clinical disease but in marmoset monkeys, HVP and HVS induce malignant or persistent, latent infections. The studies with HVP are relevant because of common properties shared with EBV: cross-reacting viral antigens, partial genome homology, transformation of lymphocytes *in vitro* and potential for inducing lymphoproliferative disease. In contrast, HVS/HVA are T-lymphotropic viruses: HVA transforms lymphocytes *in vitro* and both cause lymphoma in marmosets. The isolation of an attenuated strain of HVS, apparently lacking oncogenic potential, adds another approach for studying herpesvirus-induced malignancy/latent infections.

Until recently we have pursued these virus-host models for gaining insight into the oncogenic potential of herpesviruses to further support the assumption that EBV and Herpes simplex virus cause neoplasia in man. While such studies are necessary and important, these models present an excellent opportunity to also study herpesvirus latency in the natural host, baboons and squirrel monkeys, and in an experimental host, marmoset monkeys. In the latter system we have some choice over the outcome of experimental infection: malignancy *vs.* persistent, latent infection. In the area of latent infections with lymphotropic herpesviruses, our information is incomplete. Although we know these viruses are carried in either B- or T-lymphocytes, such lymphocytes have a definite lifespan and therefore there must be some means for perpetuating a given number of cells harboring repressed virus. This could be explained by at least one of two mechanisms: progenitor, hematopoietic stem cells harbor latent viral genomes which are passed to progency cells or the infection is random and cyclic whereby a small percentage of infected lymphocytes are directed to enter the lytic cycle, infectious virus is produced which infects new lymphocytes.

Finally, an area that offers great promise is the use of these viruses for "immunologic engineering" whereby specific antibody producing cells are converted into continuously growing cell cultures after cell transformation with either EBV or HVP. For experimental evaluation *in vivo,* it would be possible to employ either baboons or marmosets with autochthonous or allogeneic lymphocytes. The T-tropism of HVS/HVA provides the potential for conversion of specific, cytotoxic T-lymphocytes to a state of continued proliferation. With the identification and characterization of an attenuated strain of HVS, introduction of T-lymphocytes carrying such a virus will eliminate a fatal HVS-induced disease in the host.

ACKNOWLEDGMENTS

These studies were supported by Research Contract NO1-CP-33219 within the Virus Cancer Program of the National Cancer Institute, US Public Health Service and Research Grant VC-185 from the American Cancer Society.

We thank the Board of Health, City of Chicago, for housing most of our experimental animals.

REFERENCES

1. Falk, L., Deinhardt, F., Nonoyama, M., et al., "Properties of a Baboon Lymphotropic Herpesvirus Related to Epstein-Barr Virus." *Int. J. Cancer* 18:798-807, 1976.
2. Rabin, H., Neubauer, R. H., Hopkins, R. F., et al., "Transforming Activity and Antigenicity of an Epstein-Barr-Like Virus from Lymphoblastoid Cell Lines of Baboons with Lymphoid Disease." *Intervirology* 8:240-249, 1977.
3. Gerber, P., Kalter, S. S., Schidlovsky, G., et al., "Biologic and Antigenic Characteristics of Epstein-Barr Virus-Related Herpesviruses of Chimpanzees and Baboons." *Int. J. Cancer* 20:448-459, 1977.
4. Gerber, P., Pritchett R.F., and Kieff, E. D., "Antigens and DNA of a Chimpanzee Agent Related to Epstein-Barr Virus." *J. Virol.* 19:1090-1099, 1976.
5. Rasheed, S., Rongey, R.W., Bruszweski, J., et al., "Establishment of a Cell Line with Associated Epstein-Barr-Like Virus from a Leukemic Orangutan." *Science* 198:407-409, 1977.
6. Melendez, L. V., Daniel, M. D., Hunt, R. D., and Garcia, F. G., "An Apparently New Herpesvirus from Primary Kidney Cultures of the Squirrel Monkey *(Saimiri sciureus)."* *Lab. Animal Care* 18:374-381, 1968.
7. Melendez, L. V., Hunt, R. D., King, N. W., et al., "A New Lymphoma Virus of Monkeys: *Herpesvirus ateles."* *Nature New Biology* 234:182:184, 1972.
8. Falk, L. A., Nigida, S. M., Deinhardt, F., et al., *"Herpesvirus ateles:* Properties of an Oncogenic Herpesvirus Isolated from Circulating Lymphocytes of Spider Monkeys *(Ateles* sp.)." *Int. J. Cancer* 14:473-482, 1974.
9. Ohno, S., Luka, J., Falk, L., Klein, G., "Detection of a Nuclear, EBNA-Type Antigen in Apparently EBNA-Negative *Herpesvirus papio* (HVP)-Transformed Lymphoid Lines by the Acid-Fixed Nuclear Binding Technique." *Int. J. Cancer* 20:941-946, 1977.
10. Falk, L. A., Henle, G., Henle, W., et al., "Transformation of Lymphocytes by *Herpesvirus papio."* *Int. J. Cancer* 20:219-226, 1977.
11. Deinhardt, F., Falk, L., Wolfe, L. G., et al., "Susceptibility of Marmosets to Epstein-Barr Virus-Like Baboon Herpesviruses." In: *Primates in Medicine,* edited by E. I. Goldsmith and J. Moor-Jankowski, S. Karger, Basel, V. 10, 163-170, 1978.

178

12. Melendez, L. V., Hunt, R. D., Daniel, M. D., et al., "*Herpesvirus saimiri*. II. Experimentally-Induced Malignant Lymphoma in Primates." *Lab. Animal Care* 19:378-386, 1969.

13. Wolfe, L. G., Falk, L. A., and Deinhardt, F., "Oncogenicity of *Herpesvirus saimiri* in Marmoset Monkeys." *J. Nat. Cancer Inst.* 47:1145-1162, 1971.

14. Wright, J., Falk, L. A., Collins, D., Deinhardt, F., "Mononuclear Cell Fraction Carrying *Herpesvirus saimiri* in Persistently Infected Squirrel Monkeys." *J. Nat. Cancer Inst.* 57:959-962, 1976.

15. Falk, L. A., Wolfe, L. G., and Deinhardt, F., "Isolation of *Herpesvirus saimiri* from Blood of Squirrel Monkeys *(Saimiri sciureus)." J. Nat. Cancer Inst.* 48:1499-1505, 1972.

16. Falk, L., Wolfe, L., Deinhardt, F., "Epidemiology of *Herpesvirus saimiri* Infection in Squirrel Monkeys." In: *Medical Primatology, Part III,* Karger, Basel, 151-158, 1972.

17. Falk, L. A., Wolfe, L. G., and Deinhardt, F., "*Herpesvirus saimiri:* Experimental Infection of Squirrel Monkeys *(Saimiri sciureus)." J. Nat. Cancer Inst.* 51:165-170, 1973.

18. Klein, G., Pearson, G., Rabson, A., et al., "Antibody Reactions to *Herpesvirus saimiri* (HVS)-Induced Early and Late Antigens (EA and LA) in HVS-Infected Squirrel, Marmoset and Owl Monkeys." *Int. J. Cancer* 12:270-289, 1973.

19. Deinhardt, F. W., Falk, L. A., Wolfe, L. G., "Simian Herpesviruses and Neoplasia." In: *Advances in Cancer Research,* Academic Press, 19, 167-205, 1974.

20. Schaffer, P. A., Falk, L. A., Deinhardt, F., "Brief Communication: Attenuation of *Herpesvirus saimiri* for Marmosets after Successive Passage in Cell Culture at 39°C." *J. Nat Cancer Inst.* 55:1243-1246, 1975.

21. Wright, J., Falk, L. A., Wolfe, L. G., et al., "Susceptibility of Common Marmosets *(Callithrix jacchus)* to Oncogenic and Attenuated Strains of *Herpesvirus saimiri." J. Nat Cancer Inst.* 59:1475-1478, 1977.

22. Wright, J., Falk, L. A., Wolfe, L. G., and Deinhardt, F., "*Herpesvirus saimiri:* Protective Effect of Attenuated Strain Against Lymphoma Induction." Manuscript in preparation.

Coagulation Changes in Patients With Breast Lesions: A Possible Test for Detecting Cancer

Joseph A. Caprini[1,2]
L. Zuckerman[2]
J. Vagher[2]
J. Mitchell[2]
E. Cohen[2]

SUMMARY—This report summarizes our experience with celite-activated thrombelastrography which has developed over the past seven years to evaluate clotting characteristics in a variety of clinical settings. Patients entering the hospital for breast biopsy were studied preoperatively with clotting tests as well as standard measurements of hemostasis. Previously we reported 99% accuracy with 100% specificity and 97% sensitivity comparing breast biopsy patients to thrombelastographic results. That report only included those not on medication and since that time we have studied an additional group of 129 patients without exclusion because of medication or additional medical complications. The results show 65% specificity and 93% sensitivity.

Ten patients were deleted from this analysis because of known factors which cause either hypercoagulable or hypocoagulable conditions. Therefore, all patients having >380,000 platelets or a diagnosed acute clinical infection were eliminated as false positives, and all patients having <50,000 platelets or a hematocrit of 18% or less were removed as false negatives. Four patients with a negative TEG had demonstrable tumor. In two of these, however, there was no definite evidence of invasion. The test would seem to be very good, indeed, for correctly classifying patients with invasive cancer unless they have markedly deranged clotting systems. From previous work, if patients on certain medications are deleted the figures dramatically improve. We are planning to study drug interactions as they relate to hematologic changes in order to further refine the method of analysis. It is hoped with additional studies that this analytical method will be useful in the diagnosis of invasive cancer and define a high risk group for screening on the basis of the blood results.

INTRODUCTION

Although clinical evidence has shown that patients with cancer are often hypercoagulable (1-18) and that the cancer cells may be stimulating this phenomenon (19), no reproducible coagulation test has been successful in the detection of occult cancer. Progress in this area has been slow partially due to the lack of a uniform definition of the hypercoagulable state and the

---

[1]Department of Surgery, Evanston Hospital, Evanston, Illinois.
[2]Northwestern University Medical School, Chicago, Illinois.

181

lack of coagulation tests with the sensitivity needed for early detection.

These problems are compounded since many of the coagulation factors are involved in biologic feedback systems. One could postulate that a consumptive process may be homeostatically balanced by increased synthesis. Furthermore, most clotting assays do not measure total factor levels in excess of levels needed to form a clot. If consumptive processes only effect the excess factors, then the *in vitro* test would be insensitive to detecting a hypercoagulable condition. Therefore, there remain several hidden parameters that might be useful in defining homeostatic balance and the hypercoagulable state. With this concept in mind, we evaluated the thrombelastograph (TEG) because of its sensitivity in measurement of whole blood clotting kinetics plus the interactions of many clotting factors, including the levels of fibrinogen, platelets and red cells. In an attempt to measure the static reserves of the individual, we compared the clotting formed during whole blood (*in vitro*) coagulation to that of an identical sample with the addition of celite (1% W/V) simultaneously (20). The celite stimulation of the contact activation factor (Factor XII) causes an increase in clotting kinetics and consequently, more utilization of clotting factors in proportion to their reserve levels. Subsequently, we utilized the results of both native and celite activated TEG to provide a functional definition of the accelerated coagulability. This state does not imply 100% incidence of detectable clinical thrombosis but rather altered clotting balance above that seen in normals. This was accomplished by studies on a group of patients with known cancer compared to normal individuals on no medication (21, 22). The analysis was 99% accurate, with 100% specificity and 97% sensitivity. However, we should emphasize that although the data looked promising, patients and normals were carefully selected that were not on any medications or had any known disease at the time of their test. This report deals with a prospective study based on all subjects coming into the hospital for breast biopsy regardless of medications.

MATERIALS

TEG analyses were performed approximately 24 hours prior to the scheduled biopsy on 119 patients. The TEG analysis consisted of a native and celite activated TEG on whole blood samples taken through a 19-gauge butterfly needle utilizing a two-syringe method into a 5 ml plastic syringe (21). In addition, a microhematocrit and phase platelet count were performed on these individuals. Ten of the patients who signed consent forms had either a hypercoagulable or hypocoagulable condition as judged by an acute infection and/or by platelet counts >380,000 or <55,000 and/or a hematocrit of <18%. These patients were removed from the final analysis.

RESULTS

Tissue biopsy results indicated 43% of the 119 cases were malignant and were clinically staged after operation (Table 1). The TEG results (Table 2) show 94% sensitivity, which is the probability that a person having cancer will be correctly classified. It also shows a 74% specificity, which is the probability that a person free from cancer will be classified as a normal. This specificity is lower than the 100% we reported previously which considered a larger group of normal healthy volunteers not receiving medication. The distribution of the result of TEG analysis is shown in Fig. 1.

Table 1—DISTRIBUTION OF PATIENTS HAVING BREAST BIOPSY

PATHOLOGY REPORTS	NUMBER OF SUBJECTS	% OF TOTAL
BENIGN	68	100
BREAST		
CANCER		
STAGE I	8	16
STAGE II	14	27
STAGE III	15	29
STAGE IV	11	22
OTHER		
CANCERS	3*	6
TOTAL CANCERS	51	100%

*Patients had negative breast biopsy, but were found to have cervical cancer.

Table 2—TEG CLASSIFICATION

PATHOLOGY REPORT	NEGATIVE	POSITIVE	TOTAL
BENIGN	50	18	68
MALIGNANT	3	48	51
TOTAL	53	66	119*

$X^2=55.5$ Significance at $P \leq .001$
82% (98/119) of cases classified according to pathology report.
94% (48/51) Sensitivity of test
74% (50/68) Specificity of test
* Patients (5) were excluded from this TEG analysis because of platelet counts of <55,000 or >380,000 and Hct $\leq$18%.

Figure 1—FREQUENCY DISTRIBUTION OF THROMBELASTOGRAPHIC ANALYSES OF 68 SUBJECTS WITH BENIGN BREAST LESIONS AND 51 SUBJECTS WITH VERIFIED BREAST CARCINOMA

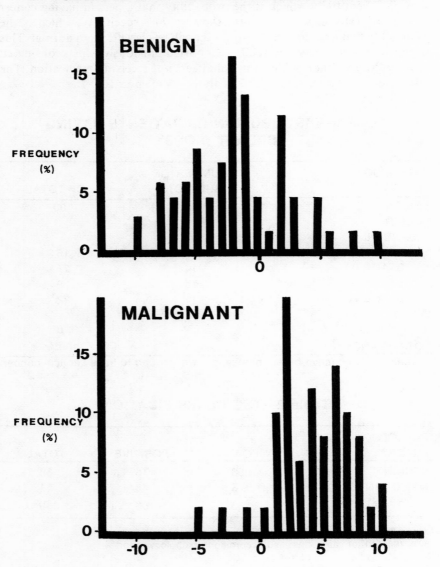

The TEG classification index (abscissa) is + for hypercoagulable and — for normal or hypocoagulable states.

184

Although the distribution for the hypercoagulable group is similar to our previous publication, the benign group is significantly shifted toward the false positives.

DISCUSSION

There is no doubt that the TEG provides sensitive measures of hyper-coagulable states. From this paper we note that there is a significant increase in our population of false positives over a mixed population of normals and breast biopsy negatives without medications. This suggests that among breast biopsy patients there is a higher incidence of hypercoagulability and/or that there are significant drug interactions that must be explained before offering this as a possible screening procedure for cancer. Our experience with a limited number of patients and normals who have been on agents such as birth control pills, aspirin, and thyroid has shown coagulation abnormalities. When these subjects discontinued the drugs their coagulation profile returned to normal.

In the group of 18 false positives, we noted five patients on thyroid medication, one on aspirin, two on steroids and aspirin, two on steroids and two insulin-requiring diabetics. These agents or disease states have been associated with altered coagulability and if dealt with in larger populations may provide a useful weighting index for our classification analysis. We hasten to add that this interference is far from being uniform or predictable in all subjects. Indeed, we have subjects that are correctly classified while on these medications, and even some false negatives could be anticipated. Out of the six remaining false positives, only two had no medications indicated. One other had a positive culture for infection and another was digitalized for heart disease. Although we have not tested our classification index on these disease states, clinical evidence has shown a higher frequency of clotting occurs in these groups. Therefore, our intent is to continue working with this procedure to determine the specific changes related to drugs which interfere with the analysis and to improve the statistics to a point where the test can be used as a screening device.

It is very evident that this coagulation test is not specific for cancer, and that there appears to be a high incidence of false positives (26%) in a population of subjects being hospitalized for a breast biopsy. Although much of this is related to drug interference, we cannot rule out the fact that this is a rather select population of patients. As reported earlier, normal healthy subjects had no false positives. Therefore, the test is successful when applied to analyses of hyper- and hypocoagulation states, which is often linked to a malignant process. The hypocoagulable state usually occurs only after widespread dissemination of the disease state and near fatal conditions are reached. In spite of this, the ease and cost effectiveness of this type of analysis makes this test worthy of further investigations to reduce the number of false positives and achieve wider clinical applicability.

REFERENCES

1. Davis, R.B., Theologides, A., and Kennedy, B.J., "Comparative Studies of Blood Coagulation and Platelet Aggregation in Patients With Cancer and Nonmalignant Diseases." *Ann. Intern. Med.* 71:67, 1969.
2. Kennedy, W.E., "The Association of Carcinoma in the Body and Tail of the Pancreas with Multiple Venous Thrombi." *Surgery* 14:600, 1943.
3. McKay, D.G., Mansell, H., and Hertig, A., "Carcinoma of the Body of the Pancreas with Fibrin Thrombosis and Fibrinogenopenia." *Cancer* 6:862, 1953.
4. Soulier, J.P. and LeBolloch, A.G., "Le Test de Tolerance à l'Heparine *In Vitro:* Test d'Hypocoagulabilité." *Rev. Hematol.* 5:148, 1950.
5. Waterbury, L.S. and Hampton, J.W., "Hypercoagulability With Malignancy." *Angiology* 18:197, 1968.
6. Amundsen, M.A., et al., "Hypercoagulability Associated With Malignant Disease and With the Postoperative State—Evidence for Elevated Levels of Antihemophilic Globulin." *Ann. Intern. Med.* 58:608, 1963.
7. Soong, B. and Miller, S.P., "Coagulation Disorders in Cancer III. Fibrinolysis and Inhibitors." *Clin. Res.* 16:362, 1968. (Abstr.)
8. Davis, R.B., Theologides, A. and Kennedy, B.J., "Observations on the Frequency and Predictability of the Hypercoagulable State in Patients With Cancer." *J. Lab Clin. Med.* 72:870, 1968. (Abstr.)
9. Fumorda, D. and Del Bueono, G., "The Blood Coagulation Pattern in Malignancies." *Prog. Med.* (Napoli), 14:327, 1958.
10. Lewis, J.H., et al., "Studies of Hemostatic Mechanisms in Leukemia and Thrombocytopenia." *Am. J. Clin. Pathol.* 28:433, 1957.
11. Rapaport, S.I., Chapman, C.G. and Ames, S.B., "Coexistent Hypercoagulability and Acute Hypofibrinogenemia in a Patient With Prostatic Cancer." *Am. J. Med.* 27:144, 1959.
12. Kwaan, H.C., Lo, R., and McFadzean, A.J.S., "Antifibrinolytic Activity in Primary Carcinoma of the Liver." *Clin. Sci.* 18:251, 1959.
13. Levy, J. and Conley, C.L., "Thrombocytosis Associated With Malignant Disease." *Arch. Intern. Med.* 114:497, 1964.
14. Rosenthal, M.D., Nuemetz, J., and Wisch, N., "Hemorrhage and Thromboses Associated With Neoplastic Disorders." *J. Chronic Dis.* 16:667, 1963.
15. Greenberg, E., Divertie, M.B., and Woolner, L.B., "Review of Unusual Systemic Manifestations Associated With Carcinoma." *Am. J. Med.* 36:106, 1964.
16. Durham, R.H., "Thrombophlebitis Migrans and Visceral Carcinoma." *Arch. Intern. Med.* 96:380, 1955.
17. Olef, I., "Differential Platelet Count." *Arch. Intern. Med.* 57:1163, 1936.
18. Morrison, M., "Analysis of Blood Picture in 100 Cases of Malignancy." *J. Lab. Med.* 17:1071, 1932.
19. Hall, T.C., (ed.) "Paraneoplastic Syndrome." *Annals of the New York Acad. of Science* 230:1-577, 1974.
20. Caprini, J.A., Zuckerman, L., and Cohen, E., "Thrombelastographic Analysis of Patients With Cancer." *Diagnostica* 30:4-9, 1974.
21. Caprini, J.A., Zuckerman, L., Cohen, E., et al., "The Identification of Accelerated Coagulability." *Thromb. Res.* 9:167-180, 1976.
22. Cohen, E., Caprini, J.A., Zuckerman, L., et al., "Evaluation of Three Methods Used to Identify Accelerated Coagulability." *Thromb. Res.* 10:587-604, 1977.

186

The Proteinuria of Patients With Disseminated Neoplastic Disease+

Daniel Rudman[1,2]
R.K. Chawla[1]
D.W. Nixon[1]
W.R. Vogler[1]
J.W. Keller[1]
R.C. McDonell[3]

SUMMARY—Low-grade proteinuria occurs in most patients with disseminated cancer. Twenty-four hour urine protein (ave ± SD, N =9-17) was <80 mg in normals; 223 ± 154 mg in patients with acute myelocytic leukemia; 177 ± 98 mg in subjects with stage IV Hodgkin's; 215 ± 147, 229 ± 186, 233 ± 163, and 280 ± 240 mg in patients with metastatic cancer of colon, breast, ovary, and pancreas respectively. The novel glycoprotein EDC1 (mol wt 27,000) was previously isolated from the urine of patients with several types of cancer and shown to be a fragment of plasma inter-α-trypsin inhibitor (IATI) (mol wt 170,000). Both EDC1 and IATI are antiproteolytic. By radial immunodiffusion and radioimmunoassay of the 41 recognized plasma proteins and of EDC1, the composition of urine protein has now been analyzed in: (i) five nephrotics ("Glomerular proteinuria"), (ii) four patients with cystinosis and four with hereditary renal tubular acidosis ("tubular proteinuria"), and (iii) 26 proteinuric (200-800 mg/day) patients with the six types of disseminated cancer listed above. In (i), (ii) and (iii) the 41 plasma proteins accounted for 100%, >95%, and 33-60% of the urine protein, respectively, while EDC1 accounted for <1%, <1%, and 40-63% respectively. In normals, (i), (ii) and (iii), plasma EDC1 averaged <1, <1, <1 and 65 µg/ml respectively. Renal clearance of EDC1 in (iii) averaged 3% of creatinine clearance. Postmortem renal histology in three cancer patients with EDC1-proteinuria was normal. Conclusion: most types of cancer cell interact with plasma IATI to generate plasma EDC1 which is rapidly filtered by the glomeruli, with a resultant "overflow" or "prerenal" proteinuria which is unique to disseminated neoplastic disease.

INTRODUCTION

In 1968 we reported that about one half of cancer patients in the last six months of life excrete in the urine 100-1000 mg/day of a mixture of several proteins 10,000 to 60,000 daltons in mol wt (1). Immunodiffusion analysis indicated that most of these substances were immunologically distinct from

[1]Department of Medicine, Emory University School of Medicine, Atlanta, Georgia.
[2]Director, Clinical Research Facility, Emory University Hospital, Atlanta, Georgia.
[3]Department of Pediatrics, Emory University School of Medicine, Atlanta, Georgia.
+Supported by USPHS grants CA12646, CA20997, and RR00039.

the normal plasma proteins. A program was undertaken to isolate and identify these novel components from the urine of patients with advanced cancer. During 1973-1977, five such proteins were isolated (Table 1) (2-5). All proved to be glycoproteins. Quantitative immunochemical methods for measuring them were developed.

Table 1—PROPERTIES OF 5 NOVEL URINARY GLYCOPROTEINS ISOLATED FROM URINE OF PATIENTS WITH DISSEMINATED CANCER

Protein	BJC1	BJC2	JBB5	EDC1	HNC1β
Disease of origin (ref.)	Chronic myelocytic leukemia (2)	Chronic myelocytic leukemia (2)	Metastatic carcinoma of the colon (4)	Acute myelocytic leukemia (3)	Acute monocytic leukemia (5)
Mol wt	29,000	32,000	55,000	27,000	33,000
% Peptide	39	77	77	73	60
% Carbohydrate	61	23	23	27	40

To what extent do these five glycoproteins account for the proteinuria of patients with disseminated cancer? To answer this question, we have analyzed a series of such urines chemically for total protein, and immunochemically for the 41 major plasma proteins and the five novel glycoproteins. For comparative purposes, urines from normal subjects, from patients with nephrotic syndrome ("glomerular proteinuria"), and from patients with cystinosis or hereditary renal tubular acidosis ("tubular proteinuria") were similarly analyzed.

MATERIALS AND METHODS

1. *Subjects.* Twenty-four hour urine samples were collected from 94 subjects (Tables 2 and 3). No patient had pyuria or had taken medication during the preceding five days.

   A. Nine normal individuals excreting <80 mg protein/day.

   B. Five patients with nephrotic syndrome according to the criteria of Berman and Schreiner (6), excreting 6000 to 17,000 mg protein/day. Light microscopy of a needle biopsy of the kidney led to the following diagnoses according to the classification of Ogg (7): renal amyloidosis, 1; membranoproliferative glomerulonephritis, 2; membranous nephropathy, 1; focal proliferative glomerulonephritis, 1; minimal glomerular change, 2.

188

Table 2—PREVALENCE OF PROTEINURIA IN PATIENTS WITH DISSEMINATED CANCER

Diagnosis	Number	mg/24 hr					
		Ave ± SD	0-100	100-200	200-400	400-800	>800
Normal	9	59±17	9				
Acute myelo-cytic leukemia	17	223±154*	4	4	8	1	
Hodgkin's disease (stage IV)	11	177±98*	3	3	5		
Metastatic cancer of colon	12	215±147*	3	3	4	2	
Metastatic cancer of breast	15	229±186†	3	4	6	2	
Metastatic cancer of ovary	11	233±163*	3	1	4	2	
Metastatic cancer of pancreas	14	280±240†	3	2	4	3	1

* Differs from normal with P <.005
† Differs from normal with P <.01

C. Four children with cystinosis, excreting 114 to 700 mg protein/day. Diagnosis was confirmed by examination of bone marrow by polarized light. All patients exhibited renal glycosuria, hyperaminoaciduria and bicarbonate wasting.

D. Four adolescent or adult patients with proteinuria of 210-940 mg/day caused by hereditary renal tubular acidosis. These individuals have been described in an earlier publication (patients III-2, III-4, III-7 and IV-6 in reference 8).

E. Twenty six patients with six types of disseminated cancer (acute myelocytic leukemia; stage IV Hodgkin's; disseminated carcinoma of colon, breast, ovary or pancreas) who were excreting >200 mg protein daily. These patients came under study as follows. During January to December 1975, 80 patients with these types of cancer admitted to Emory University Hospital had 24-hour urinary protein measured (9). As shown in Table 2, and as reported previously (1), 50% (41 patients) were excreting >200 mg protein daily. Fifteen of the 41 had evidence of renal or urologic disease which could have contributed to the proteinuria (stone, 2; chronic urinary tract infection, 10; hypertension and/or diabetes with proteinuria which preceded the diagnosis of cancer, 3); these patients were excluded. The remaining 26 individuals were included in the present study.

Table 3—CLINICAL CHARACTERISTICS OF THE SUBJECTS WHOSE URINE PROTEIN WAS ANALYZED

Diagnosis	Number	Age (yr)	Duration of illness (yr)	Bun (mg/dl)	Creatinine clearance (ml/min/1.73 M²)	Urine Protein (mg/24 hr)	Mol wt >100,000	class of urine proteins by gel-filtration (% of total urine protein)			
								60,000-100,000	40,000-60,000	20,000-40,000	10,000-20,000
Normal	9	31 (23-59)		12 5-15)	110 (93-130)	59 (29-89)	9 (3-8)	56 (41-67)	26 (21-30)	7 (6-	5
Nephrotic syndrome	5	32 (15-50)	2 (0.5-4)	21 (10-60)	50 (15-110)	12000 (6050-1680)	7 (3-10)	71 (50-83)	16 (11-21)	5 (3-7)	1 (0-4)
Cystinosis	4	3.3 (2.5-5.0)	3.3 (2.5-5.0)	25 (12-70)	41 (16-45)	420 (114-700)	4 (1-9)	20 (13-30)	23	28 (18-30)	25 (21-30)
Hereditary renal tubular acidosis	4	19 (14-29)	19 (14-29)	18 (10-40)	73 (43-100)	510 (210-940)	3 (2-6)	20 (11-29)	17 (12-35)	31 (24-40)	29 (20-33)
Acute myelocytic leukemia	7	36 (18-69)	0.3 (0.1-1.2)	12 (6-15)	93 (86-110)	260 (210-290)	2 (1-5)	10 (6-13)	15 (11-21)	59 (41-72)	14 (11-19)
Hodgkin's disease (stage IV)	4	34 (22-49)	4 (2-6)	10 (6-15)	82 (83-105)	240 (210-400)	6 (3-12)	15 (12-18)	24 (19-29)	55 (39-65)	1 (0-2)
Metastatic cancer of colon	4	62 (41-69)	3 (2-5)	11 (7-14)	104 (90-135)	290 (200-420)	4 (2-10)	23 (16-29)	30 (21-39)	49 (40-69)	4 (0-6)
Metastatic cancer of breast	5	55 (43-63)	4 (3-6)	10 (5-14)	98 (82-110)	320 (210-530)	5 (1-6)	14 (9-17)	36 (31-45)	49 (39-64)	3 (0-5)
Metastatic cancer of ovary	3	54 (46-59)	2 (1-4)	12 (6-12)	90 (81-103)	280 (200-340)	3 (2-5)	27 (21-35)	18 (11-22)	52 (41-68)	1 (0-2)
Metastatic cancer of pancreas	3	63 (52-66)	2 (1-5)	10 (7-13)	104 (92-115)	230 (200-310)	4 (1-6)	22 (15-28)	25 (20-32)	43 (30-51)	2 (1-2)

Urine protein was analyzed by gel-filtration and radial immunodiffusion/radioimmunoassay; results of gel-filtration Values represent ave (range).

2. *Urine Collections* were made for 24 hours at 5°C with several drops of 1% sodium azide as preservative; the samples were then stored at −20°C until analysis.

3. *Urine Concentration* was done at 4°C, after clarification by centrifugation (5000 rpm, 10 minutes, 4°C), by ultrafiltration through Visking cellophane dialysis tubes to achieve a protein concentration of 30-100 mg/ml.

4. *Gel-Filtration of Urine.* Typical elutions profiles of 5 ml unconcentrated urine on a 2 x 200 cm column of Sephadex G-75 in 0.1M tris-HCl buffer, pH 7.4 are shown in Fig. 1. The column had been calibrated with purified proteins of known mol wt (1). To quantify the distribution of mol wt classes of urine protein, and to isolate each class for subsequent immunochemical analysis,* 5 ml of each concentrated urine (30-100 mg/ml) was fractionated on the same type of column (3). Effluent was divided into fractions corresponding to mol wt >100,000, 60,000-100,000, 40,000-60,000, 20,000-40,000 and 10,000-20,000. Each of these five fractions was concentrated by ultrafiltration through Visking cellophane dialysis tubes to a protein level of 3 to 50 mg/ml. Total protein content of each fraction was measured by the biuret reaction, with albumin as standard, and contents of 46 individual proteins (41 plasma proteins and the five glycoproteins) were determined immunochemically as described below.

5. *Antisera* to 41 normal plasma proteins and to the five novel glycoproteins are described in Table 4.

6. *Immunochemical Analysis of Urinary Proteins.* The techniques used are indicated in Table 4. For 43 proteins, the analysis was by radial immunodiffusion (10). The reference standards were either homogeneous preparations of the protein antigen or a serum of specified antigen concentration furnished by Behring Diagnostics (Somerville, NJ) as listed in Table 4. For two of the five novel proteins, analysis was by radioimmunoassay (3, 5). Lysozyme was measured by the "lysoplate" method of Osserman and Lawlor (11).

7. *Renal Clearance of EDC1 and Creatinine.* The concentrations of both substances were measured in a urine sample collected from 8 AM to noon and in a plasma obtained at 10 AM (3, 8). In order to estimate plasma EDC1, one ml of plasma was fractionated by gel-filtration on a 1 x 100 cm Sephadex G-200 column at pH 7.0 (3) and EDC1-immunoreactivity in the effluent fraction corresponding to 15,000-35,000 mol wt was measured by radioimmunoassay (3).

---

*The major proportion of each protein generally appears in the effluent fraction corresponding to its mol wt (Table 4), with minor proportions in the two adjacent fractions of higher and lower mol wt. We summed the content of the protein in these three fractions.

Table 4—PROTEINS MEASURED IN THE URINE

Protein	Mol wt	Conc'n in normal plasma (mg/100 ml)
β_2-microglobulin	11,000	.03-.3
lysozyme	17,000	.07-0.2
retinol-binding protein	21,000	3-6
β_2-glycoprotein III	35,000	5-15
β_2-glycoprotein I	40,000	15-30
Zn-α_2-glycoprotein	41,000	2-15
L-chain dimers	44,000	Not reported
α_1-acid glycoprotein	44,100	55-140
α_2-HS glycoprotein	49,000	40-85
prealbumin	50,000	10-40
α,β-glycoprotein	50,000	15-30
Gc-globulin	50,800	20-55
α_1-antitrypsin	54,000	200-400
hemopexin	57,000	50-115
α_1-T glycoprotein	60,000	5-12
albumin	65,000	3500-5500
antithrombin III	65,000	17-30
α_1-antichymotrypsin	68,000	30-60
prothrombin	72,000	5-10
C3 proactivator	80,000	10-40
C1s-component	86,000	2-4
haptoglobin	100,000	100-300
C1s inactivator	104,000	15-35
ceruloplasmin	132,000	15-60
C-reactive protein	140,000	<1.2
IgG	150,000	800-1800
inter-α-trypsin inhibitor	160,000	20-70
IgA	160,000	90-450
IgD	170,000	<100 IU/ml
α-lipoprotein	180,000→350,000	290-770
C3-component	185,000	55-120
IgE	190,000	<800 IU/ml
C4-component	230,000	20-50
fibrinogen	341,000	200-450
α_2-AP glycoprotein	350,000	<0.5
C1q-component	400,000	10-25
α_2-macroglobulin	820,000	150-420
IgM	900,000	60-280
Coagulation-factor VIII	1-2 million	<1
β-lipoprotein	2,400,000	190-740
EDC1	27,000	<0.1
BJC1	29,000	<1

192

HNC1β	33,000	<0.1
BJC2	32,000	<1
JBB5	55,000	<2

All proteins were determined by radial immunodiffusion (ref. 10) except: lysozyme (by enzymatic assay); EDC1 and HNC1β, by radioimmunoassay (ref. 3, 5). All antisera were of rabbit origin except for anti-IgG, from the horse. Standards for the following analyses were the purified protein antigens: β_2-microglobulin, lysozyme, α_1-acid glycoprotein, EDC1, HNC1β, BJC1, BJC2, JBB5. For the remaining assays (all of which were radial immunodiffusion), the standards were sera furnished by Behring Diagnostics. All antisera were from Behring except for the following raised in this lab: anti-β_2-microglobulin, anti-BJC1/BJC2, anti-EDC1, anti-HNC1β, anti-JBB5.

8. *Renal Histology.* Five patients with disseminated cancer died and came to autopsy within one month after the study of the urinary proteins. The light microscopic sections of the kidneys were reviewed.

RESULTS

1. *Gel-Filtration.* Representative elution profiles are shown in Fig. 1. Data are summarized in Table 3. The small amount of protein in normal urine was mostly >60,000 in mol wt. In patients with nephrotic syndrome, 78% of the massive proteinuria was >60,000 daltons. In the cystinosis and hereditary renal tubular acidosis urines, contrastingly, <25% was >60,000 daltons and the major proportions were 10,000-40,000 in size. In the cancer urines, <30% was >60,000; 65% to 85% was recovered in the 20,000-60,000 mol wt range. Except for acute myelocytic leukemia, <4% of the urine protein of cancer patients was of 10,000-20,000 size.

2. *Immunochemical Analyses of Urine Protein (Table 5).*

Normals. Total protein averaged 59 mg/day. Albumin accounted for 40% of the urine protein; other recognized plasma proteins accounted for 25%; none of the novel glycoproteins constituted >1% of the urinary protein.

Nephrotic Syndrome. In these patients, daily urinary protein averaged 12,000 mg, of which 75% was albumin. The remaining 25% was accounted for largely by IgG, transferrin, α_1-acid glycoprotein, α_2-HS glycoprotein and other normal plasma proteins. Each of the five novel glycoproteins constituted <1% of the urinary protein.

Cystinosis and Renal Tubular Acidosis. Sixty to 70% of the 100-900 mg of daily urine protein was accounted for by β_2-microglobulin, lysozyme, retinol-binding protein, L-chain dimers, and other normal plasma proteins in the 10,000-40,000 mol wt range; albumin constituted only about 20%. Each of the five novel glycoproteins constituted <1% of the total.

Cancer Patients. Forty to 70% of the 200-500 mg of daily urine protein was accounted for by the novel glycoproteins EDC1 and HNC1β. The ratio of EDC1 to HNC1β was generally 5-10 to 1. The other 30-60% of urinary

Figure 1—ELUTION PROFILES FROM CHROMATOGRAPHY OF 5 ML UNCONCENTRATED URINE ON 2 X 200 CM COLUMN OF SEPHADEX G-75 AT pH 7.4 (0.1M TRIS-HC1 BUFFER)

Protein content of effluent was monitored by light absorption at 280 nm (vertical axis).

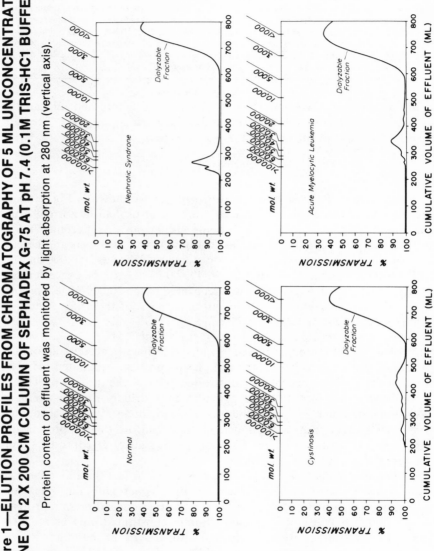

194

protein in the cancer patients was largely a mixture of albumin (ave 15%) and normal plasma proteins <60,000 in mol wt (ave 19%), together with small proportions of the novel glycoproteins JBB5, BJC1 and BJC2, each in a proportion of 1 to 5%. The sum of all immunochemically analyzed proteins in cancer urine was 91-120% of the total urine protein estimated by the biuret method.

3. *Renal Clearances.* Estimations for both EDC1 and creatinine were made in eight patients with disseminated cancer and in four normals (Table 6). The plasma concentration of the glycoprotein averaged 65 μg/ml in the cancer patients compared to <1 μg/ml in normals. Its renal clearance in the former subjects averaged 3% of the clearance of creatinine.

4. *Renal Histology.* Five of the cancer patients (carcinoma of breast, 2; colon, 3) came to autopsy within one month after their urine had been studied. Their daily urinary protein, and its per cent of EDC1, were 250-400 mg and 35-60% respectively. The kidneys were essentially normal on gross and microscopic examination in three of the cases. The other two showed respectively, mild vascular sclerosis and occasional bile plugs in tubules and collecting ducts.

DISCUSSION

The proteinuria of the nephrotic syndrome consisted mostly of albumin (ave 75%), together with smaller proportions of other plasma proteins in the >60,000 mol wt class. Similarly in patients with cystinosis or renal tubular acidosis, essentially all the urine protein could be accounted for by normal plasma proteins; but the principal components were now those proteins in mol wt range 10,000-40,000. These findings are in general agreement with earlier studies of the "glomerular" and "tubular" varieties of proteinuria in patients with intrinsic renal disease (see review by Heinemann, et al (12)).

The proteinuria of cancer differed in composition from that in nephrotic syndrome, cystinosis or hereditary tubular acidosis. It was largely (40-70%) a mixture of the novel low molecular weight glycoproteins EDC1 and HNC1β. Less than 12% of the urine protein was accounted for by the other three novel proteins, BJC1, BJC2, or JBB5, and only 33-60% by normal plasma proteins. EDC1 and HNC1β have the same amino acid composition and differ only in their carbohydrate sidechains (3, 5). They are antigenically related to the larger (mol wt 170,000) normal plasma protein inter-alpha-trypsin inhibitor (IATI) (13). EDC1 and HNC1β may be produced by proteolytic cleavage of IATI, possibly via the enhanced proteolytic capacity of neoplastic cells (14, 15).

The present findings indicate that the five novel proteins in Table 1 largely explain the low-grade proteinuria found in the majority of patients with disseminated cancer (Fig. 1 and Table 2). This proteinuria has a different

Table 5—COMPOSITION OF URINE PROTEIN IN 10 GROUPS OF SUBJECTS

Per cent of total protein in urine

Protein (mol wt)	Normal	Nephrotic syndrome	Cystinosis	Renal tubular acidosis	Acute myelocytic leukemia	Hodgkin's	Ca of colon	Ca of breast	Ca of ovary	Ca of pancreas
	(9)	(5)	(4)	(4)	(7)	(4)	(4)	(5)	(3)	(3)
β_2-microglobulin (11,600)	<1	<1	8±3	5±2	1±0.2	<1	2±1	2±0.6	1±0.2	3±1
Lysozyme (17,000)	<1	<1	14±4	10±2	15±5	<1	1±0.2	<1	2±1	1±0.3
Retinol-binding protein (21,000)	<1	<1	21±5	22±5	2±1	1±0.3	1±0.3	3±1	2±0.5	1±0.2
α_1-acid glycoprotein (44,000)	2±1	5±2	6±2	2±1	4±2	2±1	8±2	6±2	10±3	9±2
α_2-HS glycoprotein (49,000)	1±0.3	4±1	5±2	3±1	1±0.5	<1	1±0.5	2±1	1±0.5	3±1
L-chain dimers ($\kappa + \lambda$) (44,000)	12±2	1±0.3	12±3	14±3	4±2	3±1	3±1	5±2	2±1	1±0.2
Hemopexin (57,000)	<1	1±0.3	5±2	2±1	11±3	<1	<1	2±1	<1	1±0.2
Albumin (68,000)	40±8	75±10	18±5	22±5	14±4	14±3	16±4	11±3	21±5	14±3
Transferrin (88,000)	1±0.3	6±2	2±1	1±0.5	1±0.3	1±0.2	3±1	2±1	2±1	1±0.2
IgG (150,000)	<1	5±2	2±1	1±0.2	<1	1±0.4	<1	2±0.6	1±0.5	<1
26 other plasma proteins†	9±3	18±5	14±3	13±4	7±2	11±2	12±3	8±2	13±4	9±2
BJC1/BJC2 (29,000/32,000)	<1	<1	<1	<1	5±2	5±1	3±1	2±1	5±1	2±1
JBB5 (55,000)	<1	<1	<1	<1	2±1	2±1	6±2	6±2	3±1	5±1
EDC1 (27,000)	<1	<1	<1	<1	54±6	63±7	40±7	40±6	52±5	49±6
HNC1β (33,000)	<1	<1	<1	<1	7±2	8±2	4±2	3±1	7±2	4±1
Unaccounted	39	—*	—*	5	—*	—*	—*	9	—*	1

Values, which represent ave ± SE, are listed only for those proteins which constituted >1% of urine total protein in one or more groups of patient.

† All proteins listed in Table 4 do not appear in this table. None of these 26 proteins averaged >1% of total proteins in normal, renal disease, or neoplastic urine.

* Σ all proteins determined by immunochemical and enzymatic assays was 5 to 20% greater than total protein measured by biuret. The discrepancy is attributed to use of albumin as the standard for biuret method; different proteins do not all have identical color values in the biuret method.

Table 6—RENAL CLEARANCES OF EDC1 AND CREATININE

	Plasma		Urinary excretion per 4 hr		Renal clearance	
	EDC1	Creatinine	EDC1	Creatinine	EDC1	Creatinine
Normal (4)	<1 μg/ml	0.8±0.1 mg/100 ml	<1 mg	280±28 mg	—	146 ml/min±15
Acute myelocytic leukemia (4)	92±9.2 μg/ml	0.9±0.2 mg/100ml	66±12 mg	254±16 mg	3.0±0.4 ml/min	118 ml/min±31
Metastatic cancer of the colon (4)	38±9.1 μg/ml	0.8±0.2 mg/100 ml	39±9 mg	239±31 mg	4.3±0.6 ml/min	124 ml/min±31

Values are ave ± SE.

197

pathogenesis than those which occur in the three types of intrinsic renal disease studied. In the nephrotic syndrome, proteinuria results from glomerular lesions of varying selectivity causing abnormally increased filtration of a mixture of normal plasma proteins >60,000 in size, of which albumin is the main component (12). In cystinosis and hereditary renal tubular acidosis, proteinuria results from a failure of reabsorption by the abnormal tubules of plasma proteins 10,000-40,000 in size, which are constantly being filtered even by normal glomeruli (primarily lysozyme, retinol-binding protein, β_2-microglobulin and light chain dimers) (12). Contrastingly in patients with neoplastic disease, the origin of the pro-teinuria is probably the accumulation of the abnormal protein EDC1 in the plasma with its subsequent prompt filtration through normal glomeruli in amounts which exceed the capacity of normal tubular reabsorption. Sup-porting this view, an accumulation of EDC1 in the plasma of patients with acute myelocytic leukemia and other types of disseminated cancer is known to occur (3) (Table 5); the renal clearance of plasma EDC1 in these patients, 3% that of creatinine, is consistent with the relationship between molecular weight and sieving coefficient for macromolecules across the normal glomerulus (16). A saturation of renal tubular reabsorption by the filtered EDC1 could lead secondarily to excretion of smaller proportions of normal low molecular weight plasma proteins, which constitute 6-27% of the urine protein in cancer patients (Table 5). Thus, we propose that the mechanism for EDC1- and HNC1β-proteinuria is analogous to that for Bence Jones proteinuria in myeloma patients, viz. that it is a "prerenal" or "overflow" proteinuria in contrast to the "glomerular" and "tubular" varieties. Consis-tent with this conclusion is the lack of either glomerular or tubular lesions in three of the five cancer patients with EDC1-proteinuria studied at autopsy.

HNC1β and EDC1 are both antiproteolytic proteins (13, 17). They are probably fragments of the normal plasma antiprotease IATI (13). Reich and coworkers have shown increased proteolytic activity in most tumor cell lines (14, 15), this activity parallels tumorigenicity (18). The regular excretion of two antiproteolytic proteins probably derived from IATI in the urine of patients with advanced cancer is further evidence of a disturbance in the proteolytic activities of cancer cells.

ACKNOWLEDGMENTS

The authors are grateful for the technical assistance of L.J. Hendrickson and the late J. Roler.

REFERENCES

1. Rudman, D., DelRio, A., Akgun, S., et al., "Novel Proteins and Peptides in the Urine of Patients With Advanced Neoplastic Disease." *Am J Med* 46:174-187, 1969.
2. Rudman, D., Chawla, R.K., DelRio, A., et al., "Isolation of a Novel Glycoprotein from the Urine of a Patient With Chronic Myelocytic Leukemia." *J Clin Invest* 53:868-874, 1974.
3. Rudman, D., Chawla, R.K., Hendrickson, L.J., et al., "Isolation of a Novel Glycoprotein (EDC1) from the Urine of a Patient With Acute Myelocytic Leukemia." *Cancer Res* 36:1837-1846, 1976.
4. Chawla, R.K., Heymsfield, S.B., Wadsworth, A.D., et al., "Isolation and Characterization of a Glycoprotein (JBB5) in the Urine of a Patient With Carcinoma of the Colon." *Cancer Res* 37:873-878, 1977.
5. Rudman, D., Chawla, R.K., Nixon, D.W., et al., "Isolation of Novel Glycoprotein HNC1β from the Urine of a Patient With Acute Monocytic Leukemia." *Cancer Res* 1978. In press.
6. Berman, L.B., Schreiner, G.E., "Clinical and Histologic Spectrum of the Nephrotic Syndrome." *Am J Med* 24:249-267, 1958.
7. Ogg, C.S., Cameron, J.S., White, R.H.R., "The C'3 Component of Complement (β_{1c} Globulin) in Patients with Heavy Proteinuria." *Lancet* 2:78-81, 1968.
8. Buckalew, V.M. Jr., Purvis, M.L., Shulman, M.G., "Hereditary Renal Tubular Acidosis. Report of a 64 Member Kindred with Variable Clinical Expression Including Idiopathic Hypercalciuria." *Medicine* 53:229-254, 1974.
9. Savory, J., Pu, P.H., Sunderman, F.W. Jr., "A Biuret Method for Determination of Protein in Normal Urine." *Clin Chem* 14:1160-1171, 1968.
10. Mancini, G., Carbonara, A.O., Heremans, J.F., "Immunochemical Quantitation of Antigens by Single Radial Immunodiffusion." *Int J Immunochem* 2:235-254, 1965.
11. Osserman, R.F., Lawlor, D.R., "Serum and Urinary Lysozyme (Muramidase) in Monocytic and Monomyelocytic Leukemia." *J Exp Med* 124:921-952, 1966.
12. Heinemann, H.O., Maack, T.M., Sherman, R.L., "Proteinuria." *Am J Med* 56:71-82, 1974.
13. Rudman, D., Chawla, R.K., Wadsworth, A.D., et al., "A System of Cancer-Related Urinary Glycoproteins: Biochemical Properties and Clinical Applications." *Tr Am Assoc Phys* 1978. In press.
14. Ossowski, L., Quigley, J.P., Reich, E., "Fibrinolysis Associated With Oncogenic Transformation." *J Biol Chem* 248:4312-4320, 1974.
15. Unkeless, J., Dano, K., Kellerman, G.M., et al., "Fibrinolysis Associated With Oncogenic Transformation: Partial Purification and Characterization of the Cell Factor, a Plasminogen Activator." *J Biol Chem* 249:4295-4305, 1975.
16. Hulme, B., Hardwicke, J., "Human Glomerular Permeability to Macromolecules in Health and Disease." *Clin Sci* 34:515-529, 1968.
17. Chawla, R.K., Wadsworth, A.D., Rudman, D., "Antitryptic Property of Cancer-Related Glycoprotein EDC1." *Cancer Res* 38:452-457, 1978.
18. Christman, J.K., Acs, G., Silagi, S., et al., "Plasminogen Activators: Biochemical Characterization and Correlation With Tumorigenicity, Proteases and Biological Control." In *Cold Spring Harbor Laboratories,* Edited by E. Reich, D.B. Rivkin, E. Shaw, Cold Spring Harbor Laboratories, Cold Spring, NY, 827-839, 1975.

Bacterial Tumor Isolates

Lewis Affronti,[1]
Y. Charoenvit[1]

SUMMARY—Pleomorphic, refractile, motile bacterial forms have been isolated in several laboratories from both human and animal malignant tumors. Well-controlled experiments in mice have suggested that there may be an etiological or augmenting association between these bacteria and the neoplasm. Using sophisticated immunological procedures, Cohen and Strampp (1976) have confirmed the provocative earlier reports of the Livingstons (1974) that certain bacteria isolated from urine of cancer patients produced a human chorionic gonadotropin-like substance (hCG) when cultivated in vitro. More recently, Acevado et al (1978) reported on the presence of choriogonadotropin-like protein in bacteria isolated from cancer patients using immunohistochemical techniques. Our laboratory has been studying and attempting to characterize bacterial tumor isolates for some time. We have not only succeeded in substantiating these earlier reports by isolating a gram-negative bacillus that repeatedly produces an hCG-like substance from the tissue of colon carcinomas but, moreover, we have demonstrated a filterable bacterial tumor isolate (a Staphylococcus epidermidis-like organism) originally obtained from a breast adenocarcinoma that also produces an immunological-ly active substance similar to hCG. Since both hCG and hCG-like substances have been associated with various tumors, neoplastic cells, and tumor-related bacteria, we believe that a systematic and thorough study of their presence, the agents that produce them, and their possible interrelationships in colon cancer should shed new light and meaning on the underlying mechanisms of tumor development.

A number of laboratories, including our own, have demonstrated that some bacterial isolates of human and animal neoplastic origin have several unusual properties. For example, pleomorphic, refractile, and filterable forms have been repeatedly isolated from both human and animal malignant tissues and from the blood of tumor bearing hosts (1). None of these bacteria reported have been identified with assurance, because of their remarkable pleomorphism, although they may culturally and fermentatively resemble a variety of common bacteria. Thus, their various growth phases have been said to resemble viruses, diphtheroids, micrococci, bacilli, and fungi. Moreover, a possible etiologic or augmenting association between the bacterial isolates and the neoplasms from which the organisms have been derived has been described. Thus, the pioneering work of Virginia Liv-

[1]Department of Microbiology, George Washington University Medical Center, Washington, D.C.

ingston and Eleanore Alexander-Jackson (2) in 1970 even favored a new taxon within the order *Actinomycetales* for these unique organisms and they proposed the name *Progenitor cryptocides* for their intermittently acid-fast, filterable bacterium which they had isolated from human cancer patients.

A critical point involving these studies of bacterial tumor isolates is whether neoplastic change can be induced by injecting the suspected organisms into suitable hosts. A number of workers have shown that tumors can indeed be produced by animal inoculation of pure cultures of these bacterial forms, some of which were derived from human cancers (3). Thus, the well-controlled study of Diller (4) indicated that several isolates when injected into ICR albino mice doubled the incidence of tumors. Moreover, she was able to recover the organism with the same characteristics as the one injected from tumors arising in the injected mice, thus fulfilling Koch's postulates. In addition, mention should be made of the recent work of Seibert (5) who showed a delay in tumor development in C3H female mice. In this work she utilized a heat killed vaccine prepared from a bacterial isolate from a tumor which occurs spontaneously in these mice. Regrettably little attention has been paid to such observations and most cancer investigators tended either to regard these associations as fortuitous or to consider them to be a reflection of a marked propensity of neoplastic tissue to support microbial growth.

The possibility that a relationship may exist between these "cancer associated" bacteria and the tumors from which they were isolated has prompted us to pursue a directed study of these organisms. As we hope will become evident during the course of this report, the relationship between the tumor bacterial isolates and known bacterial strains is certainly unclear and if only for this reason alone, we believe that these bacterial forms should be thoroughly studied. Therefore, recognizing that a need existed to study these bacterial isolates in a systematic way, our laboratory undertook investigations which were designed to characterize and compare these isolates.

Among the interesting features of these unusual organisms which have been isolated from human and animal malignant tumors so frequently and by many different laboratories are their remarkable pleomorphism, their intermittent property of acid-fastness, their unique ability to pass through bacterial filters at certain stages of their growth cycle and indeed the most unusual and recently confirmed observation—the presence of an hCG-like protein in their cell wall or membrane.

The obvious pleomorphism which these organisms demonstrate suggested the importance of studies in this area. A series of experiments was therefore designed to study this property. For this phase of our study, we concentrated on an isolate from a human breast adenocarcinoma with the cultural characteristics as summarized in Table 1. The organism is a gram-positive coccus, negative for coagulase, hemolysis production, and mannitol fermentation. The colonial characteristics of this strain on Trypticase Soy Agar (TSA) showed an abundant growth having smooth white, or at times rather opaque colonies that appeared in 24 hrs at 37°C.

Table 1—CULTURAL CHARACTERISTICS OF BACTERIAL ISOLATE FROM A HUMAN BREAST CARCINOMA

Morphology	gram+ cocci in groups
Coagulase	—
Hemolysis	—
Pigment on TSA or Blood Agar	—
Growth on MacConkeys	—
Mannitol-Salt Agar	purple color
Liquify Gelatin	—

Since growth of this organiam was found to be abundant on either Trypticase Soy Agar or in Trypticase Soy Broth, this medium was therefore chosen for study of its growth characteristics. Because a number of earlier investigators reported that these isolates were at times filterable, growth curves and their relationships to filterability were studied.

Curves were made by plotting Klett density readings, using a 660 nm filter, against days of growth. At the period of least density, which, as can be noted from Figure 1, is between day 4 and day 8, filterable forms can be most often recovered by filtering original cultures through either millipore or Seitz filters. It should be mentioned that the growth curve pattern for each strain studied appeared to be characteristic for the strain regardless of the original concentration of bacteria or when it was grown. Twenty-one such filtrations through 0.22 μ millipore filters yielded organisms from the clear filtrate whose morphology was similar to that of the organisms in the original broth culture. The reproducible and characteristic growth curve pattern of these filterable forms can serve as a helpful method of showing also that a culture regrown from its filtrate has, in fact, originated from that strain and is not a contaminant.

Figure 1—GROWTH CURVE OF BACTERIAL ISOLATE 5100

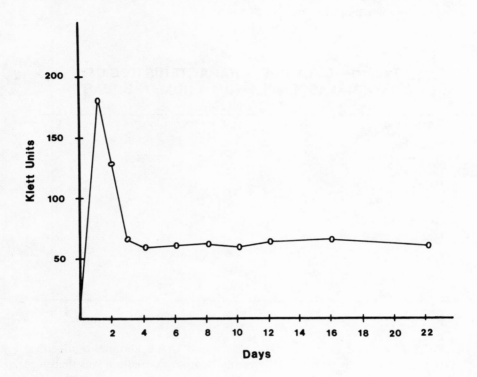

Repeated Scanning electron microscopic (SEM) studies of trypticase soy broth cultures have shown that the cells have a hardy appearance (Figure 2) and this observation is in agreement with transmission electron microscopic studies of other workers (6) who have recently demonstrated by that technique that the organisms possess a rather thick cell wall.

SEM studies of broth cultures over the extent of their growth curve, also confirm the pleomorphic nature of these forms. Great variation in shapes and sizes especially during the extended growth period could be noted (see Figure 3). There was more uniformity in cell size in 24-hour cultures than in later cultures. Larger sized cells were predominant by 2 days incubation and persisting up to 8 days, after which there was a decrease and degeneration of cells. This closely paralled the early rise and rapid decrease in the growth curve experiments.

Figure 2—SCANNING ELECTRON MICROGRAPH OF *STAPHYLOCOCCUS EPIDERMIDIS*-LIKE ISOLATE (5100) FROM A HUMAN BREAST ADENOCARCINOMA

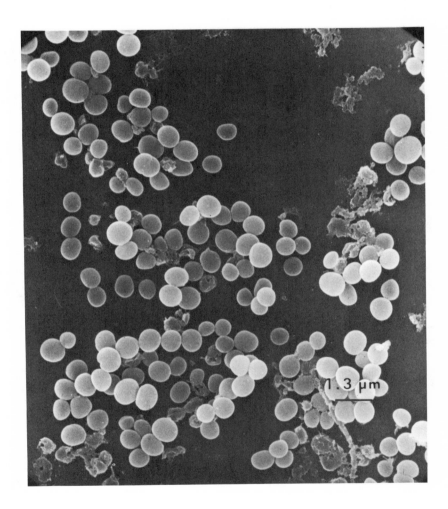

At six days there is minimal degeneration; the cells appear healthy and well formed.

205

Figure 3—SCANNING ELECTRON MICROGRAPH
EPIDERMIDIS-LIKE ISOLATE (5100) AFTER OF *S.* EXTENDED GROWTH

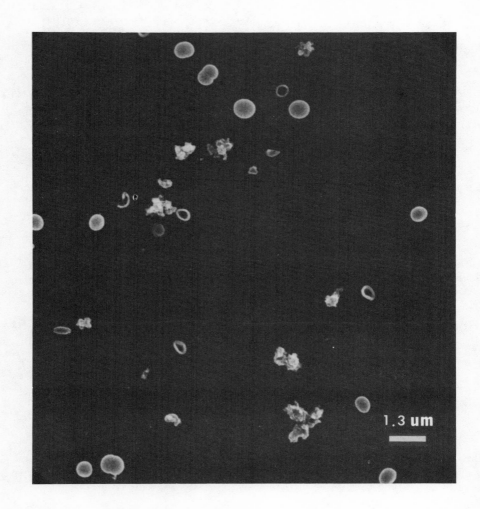

1.3 um

An interesting feature of these cells when viewed under high magnification (30,000 to 40,000) is the presence of a small bud or protuberance which appears to pinch off or separate from the parent cell (Figure 4). The panel on the left is a 3 day old culture showing the presence of a small bud. By 6 days, as shown in the panel on the right, these small forms have separated. These forms range in size from 0.16 to 0.31 μ - and are of sufficient diameter size to pass through filters used in these studies.

Figure 4—SCANNING ELECTRON MICROGRAPH OF WHAT APPEARS TO BE "BUDDING" FORMS OF THE S. EPIDERMIDIS-LIKE ISOLATE (5100)

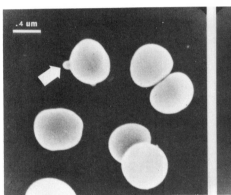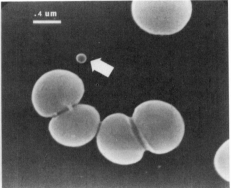

Presence of small forms (arrows) are characteristic of the cultures. The left panel is a 3 day old culture showing the presence of a small bud. By day 6, right panel, these forms have separated. These forms range in size from 0.16 to 0.31 μ and are of sufficient diameter size to pass through the filters used in these studies.

Although the filterable forms could regrow to the original morphology and the growth curves of the filterable form and the strain from which it was derived were very similar, a polyacrylamide gel electrophoresis (PAGE) profile to further characterize these 2 forms, revealed striking differences. In this study, 4-stage polyacrylamide gel columns were prepared using 3.5, 4.5, 7.0 and 12% acrylamide solutions. Samples prepared from ammonium sulfate precipitated culture filtrate material of the experimental and control strains were electrophoresed at 5 milliamps per gel using a standard tris-glycine buffer and bromphenol tracking dye. Upon completion, the gels were stained with Coomassie Blue for 1 hr., destained with 20% TCA and preserved in 7% acetic acid. Based on equivalent amounts of protein sample, it can be seen in Figure 5 that these organisms differ markedly in protein

Figure 5—POLYACRYLAMIDE GEL ELECTROPHORESIS (PAGE) PROFILES OF PROTEIN PREPARATIONS FROM TWO *S. EPIDERMIDIS*-LIKE ORGANISMS COMPARED WITH A CONTROL *S. EPIDERMIDIS* STRAIN

PAGE

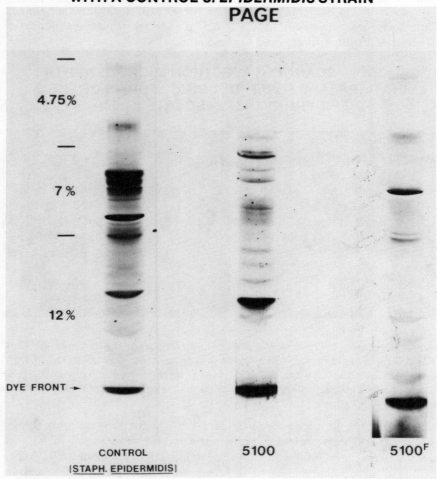

Three hundred fifty micrograms of protein from each sample were applied to four-stage PAGE columns. The three organisms appear to be closely related and yet, each has a unique electrophoretic profile. The tumor isolate (5100) is missing two major components from the 7% gel segment that are present in both the control *S. epidermidis* strain and the filtered form (5100F). In addition the uppermost band in the *S. epidermidis* is less concentrated than in the other two organisms. The *S. epidermidis* also has more highly concentrated components in the 12% gel.

208

composition both among themselves and when compared with *Staphylococcus epidermidis,* an organism which was introduced in these experiments as a control strain, since these tumor isolates in some cases resemble staphylococci morphology. It should be pointed out, however, that the tumor isolates, although cocci in morphology, were coagulase negative, did not give hemolysis on blood agar and neither produced pigment nor fermented mannitol—characteristics which distinguish them from *Staph. aureus.* They also neither grew on MacConkey's medium or liquified gelatin. It is of interest that it has been reported that these unusual forms can produce a purple color when grown on mannitol salt culture plates whereas known strains of *Staph. aureus* and *Staph. epidermidis* produce yellow and orange colors respectively on this same medium (1). Consequently, it appears that these tumor isolates are not closely related to either *Staph. aureus* or *Staph. epidermidis,* two forms that are commonly associated with humans.

It was mentioned at the beginning of this report that one of the most interesting characteristics of these organisms besides their pleomorphism, filterability, and ability to double the incidence of tumors in susceptible animals, is the unique finding that a chorionic gonadotropin-like protein is present in their cell wall or membrane. In 1974, Livingston and her associates (7) reported on the production of an hCG-like protein by organisms which had been isolated from cancer tissue and body fluids of patients with malignant neoplasms. In 1976, obtaining 2 of Livingston's cultures, Cohen and Strampp (8) of Princeton Laboratories, Inc., confirmed the production of an hCG-like glycoprotein by the radioimmunoassay (RIA) using specific antibody to the B subunit of the trophoblastic hormone and by 2 other assays: radioreceptor analysis and testosterone stimulating assay. It was of interest that the bacteria reported by Cohen and Strampp received from Dr. Livingston were gram positive cocci. These investigators further described in their reports that they isolated gram-negative bacteria from the urine of a patient with terminal carcinoma of the colon which also produced an hCG-like material.

Working independently, we in our laboratory described and reported at the ASM and Federation Meetings in 1977 that the bacterial tumor isolates which we had been studying were also capable of producing hCG-like proteins (9,10). This property is regarded as a useful marker in characterizing these unique microbial isolates. In our investigations, hCG-containing acetone precipitates of the culture filtrate from the various tumor isolates under study were prepared according to the method of the Livingstons (7).

Immunodiffusion studies were conducted to determine whether these acetone precipitated culture filtrate products prepared from a number of different colon tumor isolates contain components antigenically related to those of pure hCG. Figure 6 shows the immunodiffusion patterns of hCG-containing acetone precipitates from 5 colon tumor isolates and rabbit anti-hCG antiserum (Cappel Laboratories, Inc.). HCG, serving as the known antigen in this system, is included for comparison. It can be noted that all five products show bands of partial or full identity with the hCG Ag against hCG Ab indicating that the test materials contain components antigenically related to components of hCG. It should be further pointed out here that these immunodiffusion bands can be removed by absorption of specific hCG antiserum (Cappel) by both commerically available highly purified hCG, as would be expected in this system, *and* the hCG-containing acetone precipitated bacterial product, thus demonstrating the specificity of the reaction.

Figure 6—IMMUNODIFFUSION PATTERNS OF COLON TUMOR *ESCHERICHIA COLI*-LIKE ISOLATES AGAINST RABBIT ANTI-hCG ANTISERUM

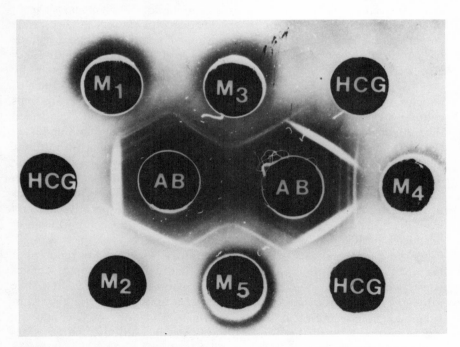

HCG=Human Chorionic Gonadotropin Antigen. AB=Rabbit Anti-human Chorionic Gonadotropin.

M_1-M_5=Cell extracts from *E. coli*-like bacilli isolated from five different colon carcinomas. All five extracts from colon bacterial isolates show bands of partial and/or full identity with hCG antigen against hCG antibody.

Further substantiation for the presence of hCG in our tumor isolates have been recently obtained by the use of immunohistochemical techniques. Utilizing 2 of our organisms—one a gram-positive coccus obtained from an adenocarcinoma of the breast and the other a gram-negative rod isolated from a patient with carcinoma of the colon, Dr. Acevado of the Wm. Singer Memorial Institute of Pittsburgh, confirmed the presence of the chorionic gonadotropin protein in these 2 bacterial forms by the application of the indirect fluorescein-labeled and peroxidase-labeled antibody techniques (6). In these double Ab studies, specific rabbit antiserum to the B subunits of hCG as well as specific rabbit antiserum to total hCG were used as the first Ab. After a suitable reaction period, fluorescein-labeled goat anti-rabbit antiserum or the peroxidase-labeled goat anti-rabbit antiserum were utilized as the second Ab. Controls on the reagents were included in addition to cell controls, which were proven chorionic gonadotropin producing cells. At the same time, proven non-chorionic gonadotropin producing cells, served as "negative controls." All the controls which have been mentioned were performed every time cell tests were done and every time new reagents were received. Figure 7 shows the indirect immunoperoxidase anti-peroxidase reaction of a coccus from a breast tumor with antiserum to hCG as first antibody. Figure 8 shows the same organism with the immunofluorescent technic. Note the intensity of the reaction. Figure 9 shows the hCG-producing rod from a colon tumor using the immunofluorescence reaction with antiserum to total hCG. Figure 10 is the same organism showing the indirect peroxidase-antiperoxidase reaction. Note the intensity of the reaction localized in the cell wall.

The immunohistochemical localization technique therefore leaves little doubt of the presence of the hCG-like protein in these bacterial isolates from a human breast carcinoma and from tumors from patients with colon cancers. These isolates indeed appear to be representative of a group of similar microorganisms which have been described and reported by a number of previous investigators. However, these findings have no doubt raised more questions than they have answered. For example, is the ability of these bacteria to produce hCG a result of *in vivo* genetic exchange between human and bacterial cells? Is there a cause and effect relationship between hCG producing bacteria and the pathogenesis and growth of a tumor; and what role does increased hCG levels—locally, systemically, and/or both play in tumor development? Could detection of elevated levels of hCG be useful in the diagnosis of certain tumors? Answers to these questions must obviously await additional work. The demonstration recently by Richert and Ryan (11) of the *de novo* bacterial biosynthesis of a glycoprotein so similar to the human chorionic gonadotropin that it shares not only antigenic sites but also membrane receptor binding sites offers additional proof that a hormone-like substance can be produced by certain

Figure 7—INDIRECT IMMUNOPEROXIDASE ANTI-PEROXIDASE REACTION OF A *S. EPIDERMIDIS*-LIKE ISOLATE (5100) FROM A BREAST TUMOR WITH ANTISERUM TO HCG AS FIRST ANTIBODY

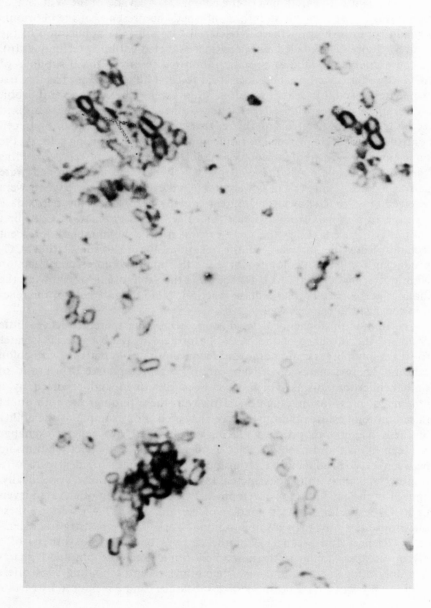

Figure 8—REACTION OF A *S. EPIDERMIDIS*-LIKE ISOLATE (5100) FROM A BREAST TUMOR WITH ANTISERUM TO HCG AS FIRST ANTIBODY WITH THE IMMUNOFLUORESCENT TECHNIQUE

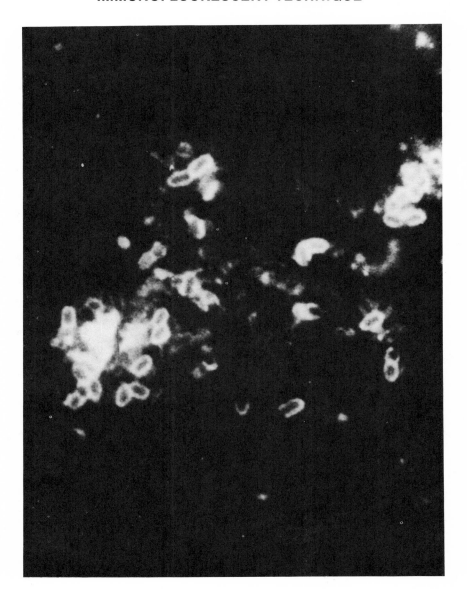

**Figure 9—AN HCG-PRODUCING *E. COLI*-LIKE BACILLUS
FROM A COLON TUMOR USING THE
IMMUNOFLUORESCENCE REACTION WITH
ANTISERUM TO TOTAL HCG**

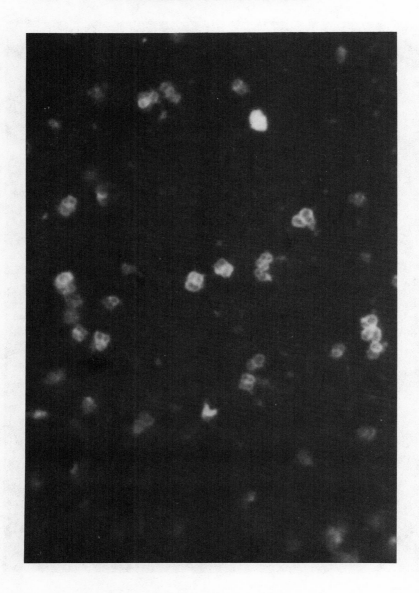

**Figure 10—AN HCG-PRODUCING *E. COLI*-LIKE
BACILLUS FROM A COLON TUMOR SHOWING THE
INDIRECT PEROXIDASE-ANTI-PEROXIDASE REACTION.
INTENSE REACTION IS LOCALIZED IN THE CELL WALL**

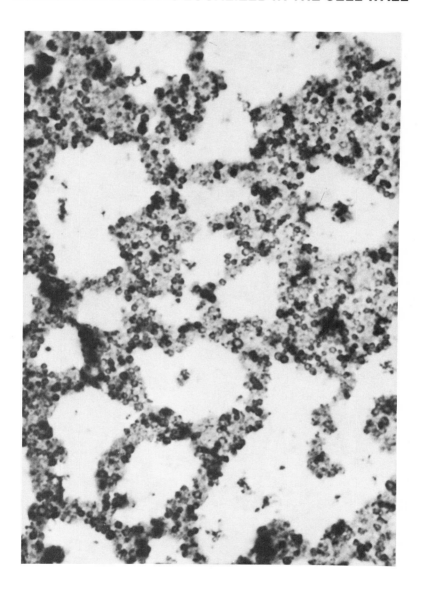

215

bacteria and has significant biological implications. It is clear that these observations warrant serious consideration in that they can provide a new and meaningful approach to the study of cancer. It is also apparent that the impact of such an approach would have provocative implications for biology in general.

REFERENCES

1. Seibert, F.B., Feldman, F., Davis, R.L. and Richmond, I., "Morphological, Biological, Immunological Studies on Isolates from Tumors and Leukemic Bloods." *Ann. N.Y. Acad. Sci.* 174:690-728, 1970.

2. Wuerthele-Caspe Livingston, V. and Alexander-Jackson, E., "A Specific Type of Organism Cultured from Malignancy: Bacteriology and Proposed Classification." *Ann. N.Y. Acad. Sci.* 174:636-654, 1970.

3. Clark, G.A., "Successful Culturing of Glover's Cancer Organism and Development of Metastasing Tumor in Animals Produced by Cultures from Human Malignancy." *Proc. Cong. of Microbiol.* Rome, Italy, 1953.

4. Diller, I., "Tumor Incidence in (CR) Albino and C57/B 16 JNIw Male Mice Injected with Organisms Cultured from Mouse Malignant Tissue," *Growth* 38:507-517, 1974.

5. Seibert, F.B. and Davis, R.L., "Delay in Tumor Development Induced with a Bacterial Vaccine." *J. Reticuloendothel. Soc.* 21:279-282, 1977.

6. Acevado, H., Lifkin, M., Pouchet, G. and Pardo, M., "Immunohistochemical Localization of a Chorionogonadotropic-like Protein in Bacterial Isolated from Cancer Patients." *Cancer* 41:1217-1239, 1978.

7. Wuerthele-Caspe Livingston, V. and Livingston, A.M., "Some Cultural, Immunological and Bacteriological Properties of *Progenetor cryptocides.*" *Trans. N.Y. Acad. Sci.* 36:569-582, 1974.

8. Cohen, H. and Strampp, A., "Bacterial Synthesis of a Substance Similar to Human Chorionicgonadotropin." *Proc. Soc. Expt. Biol. and Med.* 152:408-410, 1976.

9. Affronti, L.F., Chu, Y.M., Grow, L. and Brumbaugh, R., "Production of a Human Gonadotropin-like Substance by Bacterial Tumor Isolates". *Abst. Ann. Meeting Am. Soc. Micro.,* p. 84, New Orleans, 1977.

10. Affronti, L.F., Grow, L., Brumbaugh, R. and Chu, Y.M., "Further Characterization of a Bacterial Tumor Isolate: Production of a Human Chorionicgonadotropin-like Substance." *Federation Proc.* 36, 1977.

11. Richert, N.D. and Ryan, R.J., "Specific Gonadotropin Binding to *Pseudomonas Maltophilia.*" *Proc. Natl. Acad. Sci.* 74:878-882, 1977.

Detection of Colorectal Tumor Associated Antigens by Leukocyte Adherence Inhibition Assay

Albert T. Ichiki[1]
Y. Quirin[1]
S. Krauss[1]
I. Collmann[1]

SUMMARY—The leukocyte adherence inhibition (LAI) assay, now being tested in many laboratories, is finding increasing acceptability as a method to assess anti-tumor immunity. The assay is based on the fact that peripheral blood leukocytes (PBL) from cancer patients are sensitive to a tumor associated antigen (TAA). When the specific TAA is present, PBL will not adhere to a glass surface. In our study, we employed the tube LAI assay to ascertain if the LAI assay could assess anti-tumor immunity in colorectal cancer patients. The colorectal tumor associated antigen (CTAA) was prepared by 3 M KCl extraction of tumor specimens. Non-specific antigens employed included similarly prepared extracts of normal colon tissues and specimens of malignant melanoma. Our sequential LAI results paralleled the changes which occurred in the clinical status of the patients, i.e., an increased nonadherence index (NAI) in patients with a favorable prognosis and in patients who responded to therapy, and a decreased NAI in patients with progressive disease.

We also found that the LAI assay can be adapted as an immunochemical method to determine the properties of the CTAA. An antiserum prepared against CTAA abrogated CTAA activity with PBL from colorectal cancer patients, but did not affect the melanoma associated antigen activity with PBL from melanoma patients. By determining the capacity of other specific antisera to abrogate the CTAA activity, we observed cross reactivity between CTAA and T antigen as well as carcinoembryonic antigen.

Based on these results, we conclude that the LAI assay could be an important method for assessing anti-tumor immunity in colorectal cancer patients and for characterizing the CTAA.

INTRODUCTION

The leukocyte adherence inhibition (LAI) assay was described by Halliday and Miller (1) as a simple test to determine cell-mediated tumor immunity. Under the conditions of the assay, leukocytes adhere to glass; however, leukocytes from tumor-bearing mice do not adhere to the glass surface when the specific soluble tumor extract is present. Maluish and

[1]University of Tennessee Memorial Research Center, Knoxville, Tennessee.

219

Halliday (2) extended the LAI studies by utilizing peripheral blood leukocytes (PBL) from a variety of human cancer patients, and demonstrated organ specificity of the test. In the studies of Halliday and his colleagues the hemacytometer has been employed as the surface for leukocyte adherence. Recently, the assay method was modified to be performed in a glass test tube (3,4), or in microtiter plates (5,6). At the May 1978 International Workshop on the LAI Assay, the hemacytometer method was demonstrated by Drs. W.J. Halliday and A.E. Maluish and the tube method by Dr. D.M.P. Thomson (4). Their demonstrations confirmed the organ specificity of these two assay methods.

As a direct result of our interest in assessing anti-tumor immunity in colorectal cancer patients (7,8), we have developed the capability to perform the tube LAI assay as an adjunct test. The LAI assay has become an integral part of our study. Our purpose was two-fold: First, to perform sequential LAI studies with peripheral blood leukocytes from colorectal cancer patients with a 3 M KCl extract of tumor materials as a means of determining whether the LAI assay did, indeed, reflect the clinical status of the patient; secondly, to ascertain some of the properties of the colorectal tumor associated antigen.

MATERIALS AND METHODS

Subjects

After their informed consent had been obtained, 41 patients with adenocarcinoma of the colon or rectum were included in this study. The diagnosis was confirmed by histologic examination of the surgically resected tumor. The control group was composed of 9 normal subjects, 5 patients with chronic nonmalignant diseases, and 19 patients with unrelated malignant diseases.

Leukocyte Adherence Inhibition Assay

Approximately 20 ml of heparinized blood, drawn from each patient or control, was allowed to settle at 37° C for 1 hour. The leukocyte-rich plasma was drawn off and centrifuged at 200 x g for 5 minutes at 4° C. The cell pellet was suspended in Boyle's solution to lyse the contaminating erythrocytes. The leukocytes were washed twice with Medium 199 and adjusted to a final concentration of 1×10^7 cells/ml.

The tube LAI method of Grosser and Thomson (4) was employed. Briefly, the method is as follows: 0.1 ml antigen extract (2 mg/ml) was added to 0.1 ml leukocyte suspension and made up in 20 ml glass test tubes to a final volume of 0.5 ml with Medium 199. The tubes were laid horizontally with the cell suspension covering 3/4 of the tube side and incubated for 2 hours at 37° C in a humidified 5% CO_2 atmosphere. The tubes were then placed upright and the contents mixed with a Pasteur pipette. The cell suspension was recounted in a hemacytometer and the number of nonadherent cells/ml determined. Each sample was tested in quadruplicate and the tubes were number coded for blind testing. The formula for calculating the nonadherence index (NAI) was as follows:

$$NAI = \frac{A - B}{B} \times 100$$

A = %nonadherence in the presence of the specific antigen
B = %nonadherence in the presence of the nonspecific antigen

An NAI value of 30 or greater was considered to be a positive inhibition of leukocyte adherence.

Preparation of Tumor Extracts

Colorectal tumors, melanoma specimens, and normal colon tissues were received shortly after surgery. The tissue was minced with scissors and homogenized for 20 seconds in a Tissuemizer (Tekmar Company, Cincinnati, OH). After the homogenate was passed through a 60 mesh screen, the cells were extracted with 3 M KCl according to a method of McCoy, et al. (9) and described by Ichiki, et al. (8). The protein concentration of the tumor extract was adjusted to a final concentration of 2 mg/ml. Aliquots were stored at −20° C and later thawed at room temperature for assaying.

Molecular Sieving of the Tumor Extract

Colorectal tumor extracts were pooled and fractionated on a Sephadex G-200 column 2.5 x 100 cm. Approximately 40 mg of the protein were applied to the column which was eluted with phosphate-buffered saline, 0.01 M PO_4 − 0.15 M NaCl, pH 7.2, at a flow rate of 20 ml/hour. The eluted protein was collected in 5 ml fractions which were pooled into five groups, concentrated, and tested in the LAI assay for tumor antigen activity.

Abrogation of LAI Reactivity With Antisera Against the Tumor Extract

Antisera prepared against the colorectal tumor associated antigen (CTAA), was assayed by its capacity to abrogate CTAA activity in the LAI assay (Quirin and Ichiki, paper in press). Contaminating carcinoembryonic antigen (CEA) and serum proteins, especially albumin, were removed from the tumor extract by adsorption with immobilized antibodies. The nonabsorbed materials were used to immunize rabbits.

Before the LAI assay was performed, the anti-CTAA activity was determined by preincubating the tumor extract with the antiserum. The abrogation of the CTAA activity was interpreted to be due to the anti-CTAA antibodies.

RESULTS

The results of the LAI assay with PBL from normal subjects, patients with chronic nonmalignant diseases, nonrelated malignant diseases, and colorectal cancer are summarized in Figure 1. The NAI values were calculated with normal colon extract and with the melanoma extract as the nonspecific antigens. Patients with chronic nonmalignant diseases included those with ileitis, polymyositis, and chronic ulcerative colitis. In the latter case, the patient had a positive NAI value when calculated with both

Figure 1—NONADHERENCE INDEX (NAI) FOR ALL PATIENTS TESTED

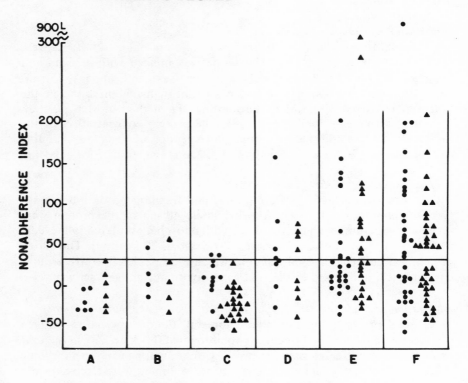

A. control subjects, B. patients with chronic nonmalignant diseases, C. patients with unrelated malignant diseases, D. colorectal cancer patients staged Duke's A and B, E. colorectal cancer patients staged Duke's C, and F. colorectal cancer patients with metastatic disease. ▲ = NAI calculated with the melanoma extract as the nonspecific antigen and ● = NAI calculated with the normal colon tissue extract as the nonspecific antigen.

222

nonspecific antigens. Patients with unrelated malignant diseases included those with Hodgkin's disease, malignant melanoma, and mycosis fungoides. Colorectal cancer patients were grouped by the staging of the tumor according to the Duke's classification. As a result of this grouping, wide distribution of NAI values was obtained.

Our test included 19 colorectal cancer patients who had at least 3 LAI determinations. The results (Table 1) group the patients according to their clinical evaluation and by whether the trend in the NAI values observed was upward or downward. Decreasing NAI values were observed in 6 of 9 patients with progressing disease, while an increasing NAI was observed in 8 of 10 patients with no evidence of recurring disease.

Table 1—TRENDS OF THE RESULTS OF THE SEQUENTIAL LEUKOCYTE ADHERENCE INHIBITION ASSAY DETERMINATIONS

	Increasing NAI	Decreasing NAI
Colorectal Cancer Patients		
Patients with progressing disease	3 of 9*	6 of 9
Patients with no evidence of disease	8 of 10	2 of 10

*8 of 9 patients died

Figure 2 outlines the results of the LAI studies on patient NC, a 65-year-old-female who was found to have recurring disease 15 months after resection of the sigmoid colon. A 5 x 2 x 4 cm tumor mass, found on the anterior abdominal wall, had metastatic spread to the liver. The patient received 3 courses of combined chemotherapy consisting of 5-fluorouracil (5-FU), 1 gm/m²/24 hours by I.V. drip for 4 days every 4 weeks, and mitomycin C, 20 mg/m² by I.V. once every 8 weeks. An increased NAI was determined in April 1977, when the patient was observed to respond to the chemotherapy. When progressive tumor growth was detected in August, the NAI value decreased. The LAI values thus reflected the clinical course of the patient, showing an increased NAI when there was response to therapy and a decreased NAI when the disease progressed.

A pooled preparation of 3 M KCl extracts of colorectal tumor materials was subjected to gel filtration on a Sephadex G-200 column in order to determine the relative molecular weight of the CTAA. The elution profile is illustrated in Figure 3. The fractions were pooled into 5 groups and concentrated either by lyophilization or ultrafiltration. The CTAA was detected by determining which fraction could inhibit leukocyte adherence

Figure 2—THE NAI VALUES FOR THE PATIENT NC, A 65-YEAR-OLD WOMAN, WITH RECURRING DISEASE

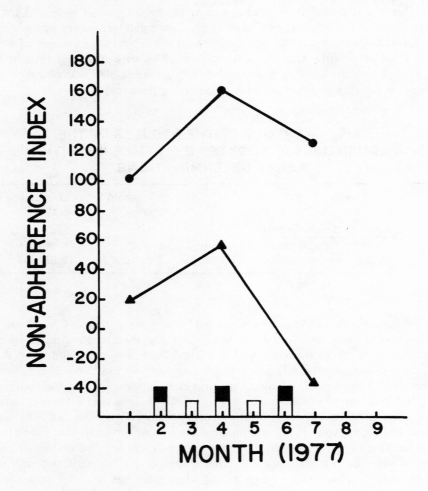

▲ = NAI calculated with the melanoma extract as the nonspecific antigen and ● = NAI calculated with the normal colon tissue extract as the nonspecific antigen. The patient received 5-FU chemotherapy, the unshaded boxes, and Mitomycin C chemotherapy, the shaded boxes.

224

with PBL from 2 colorectal cancer patients (Figure 4). The CTAA activity appears to be located in the first two fractions. The CTAA was predominantly in Fraction 1 for Patient AJ and Fraction 2 for patient SP. As indicated by the elution profile with purified proteins, the minimal molecular weight of the CTAA would be greater than 50,000 daltons.

Figure 3—THE SEPHADEX G-200 FRACTIONATION OF A 3 M KCl POOLED COLON TUMOR EXTRACT

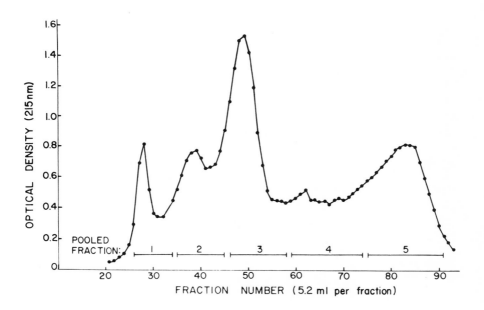

The proteins were eluted with PBS, and approximately 5.2 ml fractions were collected.

Antiserum prepared against the CTAA inhibited the reactivity of the CTAA in the LAI assay when PBL from a colorectal cancer patient was tested (Figure 5). On the other hand, the reactivity of normal colon extract was not affected after it had been preincubated with the anti-CTAA antiserum in the LAI assay. Nor did anti-CTAA affect the CTAA and NCE reactivity with PBL from a patient with malignant melanoma.

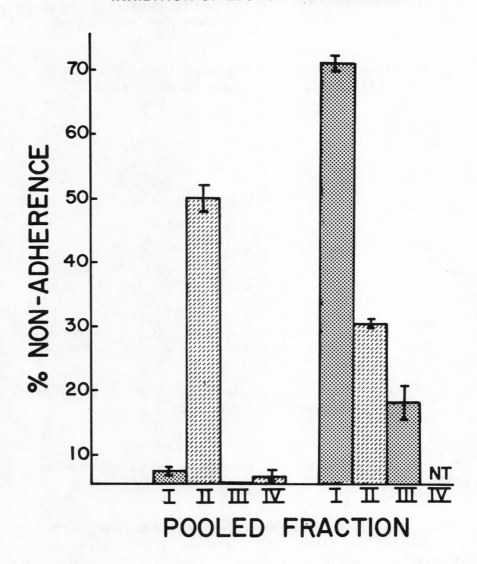

Figure 4—THE LOCATION OF CTAA ACTIVITY IN THE SEPHADEX G-200 FRACTION POOLS BY THE INHIBITION OF LEUKOCYTE ADHERENCE

Peripheral blood leukocytes from patient AJ on the right and patient SP on the left.

Figure 5—THE CAPACITY OF ANTI-CTAA ANTISERUM TO ABROGATE THE CTAA ACTIVITY BY THE LAI ASSAY

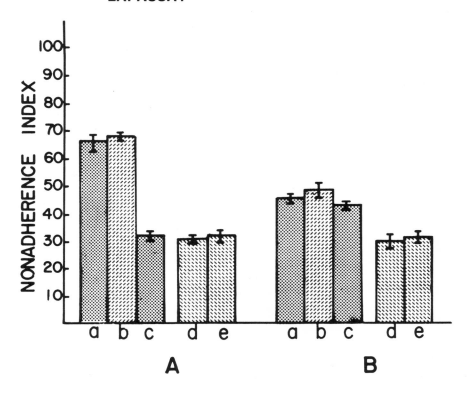

The nonadherence index with PBL from a colorectal cancer patient (A) and a normal subject (B) are compared. The test materials include: a. tumor extract control, b. tumor extract + normal rabbit serum, c. tumor extract + anti-CTAA antiserum, d. normal colon extract, e. normal colon extract + anti-CTAA antiserum.

DISCUSSION

According to our observations of the LAI assay, PBL from colorectal cancer patients are more sensitive to 3 M KCl extracts of colorectal tumors than are PBL from normal subjects or from patients with chronic nonmalignant diseases and nonrelated malignant diseases. Unfortunately, some positive LAI results (>30) were observed with PBL from the control groups and negative LAI results (<30) were observed with PBL from some colorectal cancer patients. Our results to date do not suggest that the LAI

227

assay could be of diagnostic value as has been suggested by Halliday, et al. (10). However, the LAI assay could be useful for monitoring anti-tumor immunity in individual patients because the results do reflect the clinical course of the patient. An increased NAI has been observed in patients with no evidence of disease or in those who have responded to therapy. On the other hand, a decreased NAI was seen in patients with progressive disease. Similar results from a modified tube LAI assay method were reported by Vetto, et al. (11) with melanoma and neuroblastoma patients.

We have taken two approaches in our preliminary studies to characterize the CTAA. The first was to determine the approximate molecular weight of the CTAA. Maximal CTAA activity was observed in fraction 1 which included the macromolecules included in the void volume to approximately a molecular weight of 150,000 daltons as well as in fraction 2 which included proteins with a minimum molecular weight of 50,000 daltons. These observations strongly suggest that more than one colorectal tumor associated antigen is involved in the LAI assay. One would be in the same molecular weight range as CEA, even though CEA is apparently not involved in the LAI assay for colorectal cancer patients (12). Therefore, we have found it necessary to determine the antigenic properties of the CTAA.

The 3 M KCl extract of the colorectal tumors used to immunize rabbits was depleted of CEA and serum proteins, especially albumin, with immobilized antibodies. The resulting antiserum did not form precipitin lines with either CEA or serum proteins (Quirin and Ichiki, paper in press). This antiserum abrogated the CTAA activity when tested with PBL from colorectal cancer patients but did not affect the reactivity of the tumor extract with PBL from patients with malignant melanoma. Ichiki and Quirin (12) have reported that antisera prepared against human thymocytes abrogated the CTAA in the LAI assay with PBL from colorectal cancer patients thus suggesting that the CTAA and T cell antigen share antigenic determinants. On the other hand, antisera prepared against CEA abrogated the CTAA reactivity to some degree but statistically the results were not different from that of the control samples. This finding appears to indicate CEA and CTAA do share some antigenic cross reactivity even though CEA is not involved in the LAI assay.

The LAI assay is a fast, simple, and sensitive method for the detection of CTAA. It also appears to assess anti-tumor immunity via its capability to reflect the clinical course of the patient. It is possible that CTAA may not be a single macromolecule and that the minimal molecular weight for the CTAA would be greater than 50,000 daltons. To a lesser degree, the antigenic determinants on the CTAA critical for the reactivity in the LAI assay cross reacts with the T cell antigen and CEA.

228

ACKNOWLEDGMENT

This study was supported in part with funds from the Physicians Medical Educational and Research Foundation and Biomedical Research Support Funds.

We gratefully acknowledge the technical assistance of Kathy Wenzel and John MacGuire.

REFERENCES

1. Halliday, W.J. and Miller, S., "Leukocyte Adherence Inhibition: A Simple Test for Cell-Mediated Tumour Immunity and Serum Blocking Factors." *Int. J. Cancer* 9:477-483, 1972.

2. Maluish, A.E. and Halliday, W.J., "Cell-Mediated Immunity and Specific Serum Factors in Human Cancer: The Leukocyte Adherence Inhibition Test." *J. Natl. Cancer Inst.* 52:1415-1420, 1974.

3. Holan, V., Hasek, M., Bubenik, J., and Chutna, J., "Antigen-Mediated Macrophage Adherence Inhibition." *Cell. Immunol.* 13:107-116, 1974.

4. Grosser, N. and Thomson, D.M.P., "Cell-Mediated Antitumor Immunity in Breast Cancer Patients Evaluated by Antigen-Induced Leukocyte Adherence Inhibition in Test Tubes." *Cancer Res.* 35:2571-2579, 1975.

5. Holt, P.G., Roberts, L.M., Fimmel, P.J., and Keast, D., "The L.A.I. Microtest: A Rapid and Sensitive Procedure for the Demonstration of Cell-Mediated Immunity *in vitro.*" *J. Immunol. Methods* 8:277-288, 1975.

6. Leveson, S.H., Howell, J.H., Holyoke, E.D., and Goldrosen, M.H., "Leukocyte Adherence Inhibition: An Automated Microassay Demonstrating Specific Antigen Recognition and Blocking Activity in Two Murine Tumor Systems." *J. Immunol. Methods* 17:153-162, 1977.

7. Ichiki, A.T., Collmann, I.R., Sonoda, T., et al., "Inhibition of Rosette Formation by Antithymocyte Globulin. An Indicator for T-Cell Competence in Colorectal Cancer Patients." *Cancer Immunol. Immunother.* 3:119-124, 1977.

8. Ichiki, A.T., Collmann, I.R., Wenzel, K.L., et al., "Immunologic Studies of Colonic Cancer: Evaluation of Immunocompetence." *South. Med. J.* 71:271-276, 1978.

9. McCoy, J.L., Jerome, L.F., Dean, J.H., et al., "Inhibition of Leukocyte Migration by Tumor-Associated Antigens in Soluble Extracts of Human Breast Carcinoma." *J. Natl. Cancer Inst.* 53:11-17, 1974.

10. Halliday, W.J., Maluish, A.E., Stephenson, P.M., and Davis, N.C., "An Evaluation of Leukocyte Adherence Inhibition in the Immunodiagnosis of Colorectal Cancer." *Cancer Res.* 37:1962-1971, 1977.

11. Vetto, R.M., Berger, D.R., Vandenbark, A.A., and Finke, P.E., "Changes in Tumor Immunity During Therapy Determined by Leukocyte Adherence Inhibition and Dermal Testing." *Cancer* 41:1034-1039, 1978.

12. Ichiki, A.T. and Quirin, Y.P., "Evidence for the Immunological Cross Reactivity of a Colorectal Tumor-Associated Antigen, Carcinoembryonic Antigen, and the T Antigen." Abstract 1797. *Federation Proc.* 37:1596, 1978.

230

PANEL DISCUSSION

Chairman: Saul Kit

Malcolm Mitchell: Dr. Panem, one of the problems with the immunofluorescent technique in general is its specificity. Have you tried other adsorptions? Specifically, since the virus was isolated from embryonic lung tissue, have you adsorbed with embryonic lung to see if this is truly a viral reactivity that you are identifying or whether it is an anti-embryonic lung? Did you adsorb with other viruses? Also, I suppose more difficult to do, have you made antiserum to placenta tissue and then adsorbed it with viral protein? In other words, did you do the reciprocal?

Sandra Panem: We did show that the reaction of antiserum raised to B-M, which is a human placenta antigen, can be blocked with adsorption with viral protein. The reaction of the anti-HEL-12 serum could be blocked by HEL-12 virus, but not unrelated C-type viruses such as Rous sarcoma virus, Rous murine leukemia virus or Rickard feline leukemia virus. What I didn't present, because of time, is that the specificity of all the serum we utilized has been checked by doing the appropriate immunoprecipitations with labeled virus, and then analysis of the products of immuniprecipitation by electrophoresis. By these criteria, we can show that the determinants, which are in the sera, are viral proteins. That should answer the question whether there were amino acid sequences which were detected as the antigenic determinants which were either similar or different from other materials. Now you asked the question: Is it a normal lung antigen, such as a tissue specific antigen? Is it a viral antigen? Those are two different questions which may have the same answer. Perhaps these viruses have normal roles. An antigen which may be coded by a sequence and finds its way into a viral genome may, in fact, be a legitimate antigen which plays the role of a tissue specific antigen. There are a number of cases in which this has been considered. This is not a unique idea and Dr. Kennel might wish to comment on similar findings in the murine system. There are a number of antigens which are known to be viral, by the criteria that I just asked myself to generate in the future, which do appear to act as differentiation antigens. The system where this is best known is the G9 antigen in mice which seems to act as a thymocyte differentiation antigen. There has been some interesting data generated out of the Scripps Institute which suggests that murine C-type viral envelope proteins can act as differentiation antigens in a number of tissues. So, I think that those are questions which we would like to look at and intend to look at and they may have the same answer.

Saul Kit: Your experiments, however, do rule out the more trivial explanation that the envelope protein was incorporated into the viral particle accidently.

Panem: Yes.

231

Kit: That is in terms of your host cells and the various simian and other virus cells.

Panem: Yes. However, I think all of the points are well taken and deserve being addressed.

Stephen Kennel: What is the status of the human virus that is reported from Kaplan's lab at Stanford?

Panem: I really don't know, so I can't tell you. What I do know is that there is a suggestion in a number of cell lines derived from patients with Hodgkin's disease which express reverse transcriptase which I understand have antigenic specificity similar to primate C-type viruses. What has been done with the virion isolates from any or all of a number of lines, I'm really not aware.

Kennel: One other thing, the fluorescence that you showed is fairly evenly distributed around the cell. Do you interpret that as antigen being present on the surface of budding virus or is it possibly just present on the cell, so-called normal cell membrane?

Panem: There have been extensive EM surveys of these tissues and the cells. It's a curiosity that the cells with whom the antigen is associated are cells in which it is very difficult to demonstrate budding virion forms. I think the pattern of fluorescence is consistent with the antigen being adsorbed onto the surface of the cell, as in the fetal circulation. In addition, it is consistent with the possibility that those cells are actually synthesizing the antigen. I don't think that we can distinguish it at this point and that is part of the reason that we want to address the question of where the antigen is made. The only thing that I would comment on in that regard is that the general virus cell interaction in primates, both subhuman as well as human, appears to be a non-productive virus interaction. So, whether one finds antigen in the absence of particles is open to discussion.

George Mathé: Dr. Caprini, is it too early to predict with your data the metastatic evolution of the disease according to hypercoagulability?

Joseph Caprini: With the present state of the art, this can be done. It would require more funds to study the population. For example, patients who have stage II breast cancer and no evidence of metastasis at the time of operation. We feel that by utilizing this analysis in concert with specific analysis of fibrinolytic complement and kind of systems as a package, that we definitely would be able to predict gross metastatic problems. We have done studies in rabbits where we have injected either saline or V2 carcinoma cells intraperitoneally. We found that in those animals with just a local irritation from the saline, the analyses of their coagulability returned eventually to normal after several weeks, whereas in those animals where the tumor caught hold and metastasis developed, the analyses continued to show a progressive alteration in the direction of the positive reactions. Those animals that were injected with tumor that didn't take returned to

232

normal. So, I think it does have some possibilities in that regard. It always has to be interpreted in light of the clinical situation. We picked the breast biopsy group since we would have an answer in 24 hours. You must remember that just because a patient has a negative breast biopsy doesn't mean that she is free of cancer or that she cannot subsequently get cancer. It is ironic, but one of my good friends had a positive test for three years and later developed an invasive carcinoma of the breast, despite earlier biopsies that were negative. So, we don't know exactly where we stand. We need more time and we need to analyze more patients.

Unidentified Speaker: In your patients with early breast cancer did their results return to normal after they had surgery?

Caprini: We haven't studied a large group of these individuals. In those we did study, there is a high incidence of eventually returning to normal. The changes which occur postoperatively reach their zenith at the 7th to 10th day and then the test results come back to normal by about one month postoperatively.

Olusola Alaba: Is there any indication as to which stage in the clotting cascade is defective, say factor IX or X or whatever?

Caprini: That is a very interesting and timely question. Prior to 1971 this was subject to a wide degree of speculation, but the work of Oscar Ratinoff linked the clotting fibrinolytic and immunologic systems together through Hageman factor, factor XII, the contact activation factor. His work was based on experiments that were done 50 to 70 years earlier. There is a definite evidence now from our laboratory and others that a broad multi-system activation occurs as a result of the neoplastic process which broadly stimulates these systems and is mediated through Hageman factor. Factor XII not only can trigger clotting, but can trigger the fibrinolytic network which then can directly trigger complement and kinin activation. There is now a number of postulates ranging from infection around the tumor, necrosis as a result of the tumor, neoendothelialization of tumor blood vessels, and direct tumor toxins secreted under certain cases. All of these substances and processes are known to trigger contact activation, which then, according to this theory and school of thought, triggers this multi-system activation.

Alaba: Then will the assay for Hageman factor increase the sensitivity of your tests?

Caprini: So far, experience in both burn patients and in neonatal patients who are on the respirator gives us very definite evidence that Hageman Factor is not the right place to look because it is rapidly inactivated, but rather at the sequential activation products down the line. Specifically, plasminogen, C3, C4, and the five minute kinin. But, in burn patients we can tell in 7 days with over 93% accuracy whether they are going to live or die depending on the status of these systems. In a small group of patients that were premature and on the respirator, we had 100% accuracy in predicting eventual demise based on activation of their clotting and immunologic system. So, we think this test has great promise and has been greatly overlooked.

Robert Kerry: What is the cost to carry out this test? Secondly, on what other types of cancer have you administered this test and have your impressions been similar?

Caprini: Yes, the test can be done for $5 to $10. It must be remembered that these tests have been done for years in Europe. We have worked with a center in Paris and a center in Romania, as well as Memorial in this country, and there is work being done. The data has to be analyzed and studied very carefully. You go ten steps forward and nine back, but there is something there that merits further investigation. Now, we have studied a broad range of patients with cancer and our first two publications were taking those patients with a brand new histologic diagnosis of cancer and it doesn't seem to make much difference as long as they are invasive cancers, as to the stimulation of these changes. We see a little more stimulation with pancreas, lung, and colon, but we have also seen a lot of stimulation with advanced breast cancers. It is of interest that the three mistakes in our analysis, in the 48 out of 51 group, were the three that were incorrect. One of those patients had borderline invasion and the other two patients had very early invasion of the tumor so they were very nearly stage 0 or stage 1/2 or stage 1 tumors. This definitely seems to be related, in some cases, to tumor size.

Kerry: That is for colon and lung did you say?

Caprini: Yes, indeed.

Kit: Dr. Rudman, where does the IATI, itself, originate?

Daniel Rudman: IATI has received very little attention in the past. It has been an obscure plasma protein and is one of the seven known anti-proteinases.

Unlike alpha antitripsin, which has received a lot of attention, there has been virtually no work done on IATI. We presume that like other plasma proteins except for the immunoglobulins, that IATI is made in the liver. What its life span in the blood is, what its turnover time is, where it's degraded, and what are the physiological targets of its anti-proteolytic function are totally unknown.

Unidentified Speaker: In your opinion, is there any value in following 24 hour urines if you can't be as specific on following the progress of patients with advanced cancer?

Rudman: There are two kimds of clinical application that come to mind. One would be for a patient who comes into the hospital without a clear diagnosis. Metastatic cancer is one possibility in differential diagnosis of ascites of unknown origin, or pleural effusion of unknown origin or lymphadenopathy of unknown origin, and the test which I described costing about 1¢ and interpreted in 24 hours, can have a real value in working up the patient in whom metastatic cancer needs to be excluded. In addition, you would probably want radioimmuno assays of 24 hour urines and monitor the plasma level of the glycoprotein. Another application would be in the patient who has known disseminated cancer and is going to be treated with chemotherapy. In this situation a prompt reduction in the urinary excretion and the disappearance of the proteinurea occurs in the patient who is going to have a favorable response to the chemotherapeutic program. There has been a tendency in a number of the patients for the change in the proteinurea to precede by several days or a week the clinical improvement. This is especially useful in patients with solid tumors who may be a month or two in chemotherapy before you are sure they are in remission. Monitoring the urinary excretion or the plasma level may be of assistance in planning a chemotherapeutic program and after the patient has gone into a remission as an early chemical indicator that relapse is approaching.

Melvin Klegerman: Dr. Affronti, you say that you get specific reaction with antibeta sub unit. Has anybody looked at the antialpha sub unit, or anti LH?

Lewis Affronti: Yes, there has been some work done with the alpha subunit. The beta subunit is more specific of hCG than the other polypeptide of the molecule which is the alpha subunit.

Klegerman: Yes, I was wondering if it was the entire hCG or if it was specifically the beta subunit that this bacterium was putting out?

Affronti: I think that Dr. Acevedo, who is our biochemist, can address your question.

Hernan Acevedo: The material isolated from the microbes has biological activity. The fact that it has biological activity means that we have a complete molecule similar to the complete molecule of human choriogonadotropin. By the biological test used, the end that is utilized which is characteristic in endocrinology, like the effect on the production of testosterone by the isolatic ledig cell, the production of progesterone by the granulosa cells, the increase in the uterine weight, and so on . . ., requires not only the presence of the two subunits but also the presence of the oligosaccharides. The alpha subunit and the beta subunit by themselves do not have biological activity. Moreover, the behavior of the material in Con A Sephadex columns as shown by Strampp indicated the presence of oligosaccharide chains as well as sialic acid that is characteristic of the terminal carbohydrate.

John Marchalonis: I wish to ask a question with respect to the specificity of the antisera used to detect the hCG. Is the reaction directed against the glycoseal moieties or is it directed against the polypeptide chain?

Affronti: I believe it is directed against the polypeptide chain; but perhaps

235

Dr. Acevedo whould want to address that question?

Acevedo: We have utilized antiserum to the beta subunit which was given to us by Dr. Vernon Stevens from Ohio State University. This antiserum is also utilized by the World Health Organization. We have utilized antiserum to the beta subunit from NIH that is highly specific according to them. We have utilized antiserum to the thirty-two terminal carbonyl that is highly specific only for the choriogonadotropin and that accounts for the difference between the LH and the choriogonadotropin irrespective of where the antiserum is obtained and the results in cancer cells we have studied are positive. Now it is known that when antiserums are prepared against sialorglyco proteins some antigenic determinants can be formed in the animal, especially, against sialic acid. Now, the antiserums used react also with dessilated glycoprotein; so we cannot say, from the point of view of utilizing the antiserum, whether the sialic acid is present or not. We, as well as investigators from NIH, demonstrated that the material from the cancer cells as well as the material from the bacteria does contain sialic acid because, and I repeat again, the biological activity, in this case the dessilated protein, is lost because of a lack of resistance through the liver and because of the maintenance of the biological activity.

Kit: With respect to the oncogenicity what was the sex of the mice that were used? What kind of tumors were formed? Is the choriogonadotropin itself, oncogenic in mice?

Affronti: Referring to the work that Dr. Beck has reported, there is some evidence that the hCG itself can make a cell somewhat immunosuppressive, that is, it inhibits the blastogenesis. I think that one of Dr. Beck's proposals is that you have an immunologically inert cell that hCG has an apparent effect on.

Acevedo: I don't want to get involved in a taxonomy discussion. I want only to mention that it is well known in microbiology that when you have aerobic bacteria, they can be adaptive anaerobic, like *Staph epidermidis, E. coli,* and so on. We have never known of a case of a totally anaerobic bacteria being converted into aerobic bacteria. I suppose microbiologists who are here would agree with me. In our systematic study of the production of this material in the microbes as well as in the cancer cell, we encountered an American type Culture Collection, neotype, . . . the only one that is available of a very strange bacteria that is totally anaerobic. It is named *Ubacterium lentum* and is a very small bacteria. This bacteria was isolated in 1938 from a rectal tumor. We did an immune electron microscopy of *Ubacterium lentum* showing the immunoperoxidase complex of the level of the inner and outer membranes.

Mitchell: Dr. Ichiki, would you discuss the biological basis for the LAI test? What are you detecting when you do the test?

Albert Ichiki: There is considerable controversy as to the difference

236

between the tube LAI and the hemacytometer methods. The people who use the hemacytometer method have demonstrated that there is a lymphokine involved. It's an assay mediated by a lymphokine when the lymphocytes are incubated with the tumor antigen. In their studies, they say that T cells are involved. There is not very much data on the tube LAI, but it appears that monocytes armed with specific cytophilic antibodies are involved and that is the basis for the cells not being able to adhere to the glass.

Unidentified Speaker: Have you tried isolated CEA instead of KCI abstracts?

Ichiki: Yes, we have used isolated CEA and there is no activity involved. CEA has no effect on the assay.

Robert Epstein: Briefly, what are the adherent cells you use, leukocytes? What kind of leukocytes? Separate lymphocytes from granulocytes and monocytes? What cells adhere? What cells come off?

Ichiki: It is a mixture that we start with and it's a mixture that results. So, you really can't say that there is a specific population of leukocytes.

Kit: Are there additional comments by any of the speakers? I would like to make one comment and possibly direct a question. There has been some suggestion that hCG was acting as an immunosuppressant. I think this has been looked at by a large number of people and by a variety of assays and no one has really shown this to be consistently true. Ron Pattillo from the Medical College of Wisconsin published a study two years ago showing that most of the hCG suppressive activity was related to contaminants found in hCG and when these were dialyzed out there was no suppressive activity. There is another study that I can think of relating to hCG in viral tumor production and this was found to be related to progesterone rather than hCG.

Acevedo: It is unfortunate that the term immunosuppressive continues to be used with respect to hCG. You have pointed out that current research work on hCG shows that it does not have systemic immunosuppressive activity. Now, Pattillo recognizes that we do not know the activity of hCG when it is at a high concentration in the cell membrane. So, it is a matter of concentration. We already talked about the possibility of the physical influence of hCG in relation to the high electronegative charges. That would change completely the picture and we better talk about how a cell can be rendered immunologically inert.

Kit: I suppose it would be remiss of me if I didn't make at least one comment. There were some implications with respect to the oncogenicity of these bacterial forms. I think that anyone who has worked with cellular tissue culture or viral preparations knows that they can be contaminated with microplasma. I can't help raising the question with respect to this particular organism whether, for example, it has reverse transcriptase activity. I would hate to think that this is the Rous sarcoma agent.

CELLULAR AND HUMORAL IMMUNITY

On the Role of Tumor Antigen in the Escape of Tumors from Immunological Destruction

Ingegard Hellström[1]
K.E. Hellström[2]

SUMMARY—Evidence is discussed which indicates that tumor antigen can facilitate the growth of immunogenic tumors *in vivo* and that a mechanism involving radiosensitive T cells plays an important role in this facilitation.

Neoplasms which possess strong tumor specific transplantation antigens (TSTA), for example mouse sarcomas induced by a large dose of 3-methylcholanthrene (MCA), can often grow when transplanted to syngeneic recipients immunized against the respective TSTA, as long as a relatively large number of tumor cells is used for challenge (generally more than 10^5). They generally grow progressively *in vivo,* in spite of the fact that lymphocytes which are cytotoxic to their cells *in vitro* can be demonstrated in regional and distal lymph nodes, in spleens and peripheral blood, and often also within the tumor tissue itself. Furthermore, lymphoid cells from mice with small immunogeneic tumors can often prevent the outgrowth of admixed cells from the respective tumors, when assessed by "Winn type" neutralization tests. Obviously then, there must be some mechanisms preventing the destruction of the growing tumor in the face of an immune response to its TSTA (1).

We postulated about ten years ago that circulating "specific blocking factors" (SBF) provide such a mechanism (2). This was based on the finding that sera from animals with growing tumors can "block" (inhibit, suppress) the *in vitro* killing of plated tumor cells by lymphocytes from syngeneic donors immune to their TSTA. Later work showed that tumor antigens, alone or complexed with antibody, is a common SBF (3, 4). A third SBF, a protein with a molecular weight of approximately 56,000 daltons, and with the ability to bind to tumor cells having the appropriate TSTA, has also been identified. We have speculated that this SBF is similar to T cell derived immunosuppressive molecules in non-tumor systems, and that it is formed by host T lymphocytes in response to specific tumor antigens and/or complexes (5).

[1]Division of Tumor Immunology, Fred Hutchinson Cancer Research and Department of Mirobiology/Immunology, University of Washington, Seattle, Washington.
[2]Division of Tumor Immunology, Fred Hutchinson Cancer Research Center and Department of Pathology, University of Washington, Seattle, Washington.

241

Tumor preparations containing TSTA have been shown to block cell-mediated anti-tumor reactivity *in vitro,* as assayed by standard micro-cytotoxicity techniques, involving about 36 hours' incubation of target cells in the presence of immune lymphocytes (4). Such preparations have also been shown to facilitate ("enhance") tumor growth in animals which have not been previously immunized against the TSTA of the respective neo-plams, as well as in specifically immune ones (6-9). The enhancing effect of the tumor antigen preparations is most apparent, if the antigen is mixed with the challenge tumor inoculum instead of being, for example, given subcutaneously on one side of the back with the tumor challenge on the other (9). Thus, the local milieu in the area of the inoculated tumor cells appears to be crucial as to whether a tumor will grow or be rejected. This may explain "concomitant tumor immunity" (10), the observation that animals with even relatively large tumors are often able to reject a second transplant from the same tumor when given at a different site: since the concentration of TSTA is higher locally then systemically, it may be sufficient for a local turn-off of the immune response but not for a systemic one. However, a variety of other mechanisms may be also contributory to the progressive growth of an established tumor in the face of an immune response to its antigens (1).

Tumor antigen can block the development and/or the expression of an effective tumor immunity in several different ways. Most simply, a large number of cells having the appropriate TSTA can competitively inhibit cell-mediated destruction of (a smaller number of) cells having the same TSTA by "tying up" a large proportion of the effector cells. Likewise, TSTA can absorb out anti-tumor antibodies. Both these mechanisms have been demonstrated *in vitro* (11).

Tumor antigen may also have a more indirect effect: it may, alone or complexed with antibody, modify the immune response by activating suppressor cells (12). The suppressor cells will, in their turn, prevent the development of an effective immune response, perhaps by suppressing the differentiation of killer lymphocytes and also by suppressing the formation of humoral anti-tumor antibodies. They may do this by a mechanism based on cell-to-cell interaction and/or by producing soluble mediators like the 56,000 daltons protein discussed above.

There is evidence that the tumor enhancing effect obtained by giving material containing TSTA at the proper time and location is sensitive to whole body irradiation of the animals with 400 rads, as are many suppressor cell-mediated mechanisms in non-tumor systems. Adoptively transferred T lymphocytes can restore the ability of the irradiated hosts to enhance tumor growth in the presence of TSTA (9). Based on this evidence, and on the observation that T killer cell activity, as assessed by Winn assays, is relatively radioresistant (J. Kant *et al.,* unpublished observations), experi-

242

ments were recently done which showed that whole body irradiation (400 rads) of mice with small MCA-induced sarcomas can lead to tumor inhibition (and even to complete regression of some sarcomas). The effect of radiation was abolished if T cells were given to the irradiated mice (13). Similar observations have been made by giving cyclophosphamide (100 mg/kg body weight) rather than whole body irradiation to tumor-bearing mice, except that the drug has a much stronger direct effect on tumor cells than does 400 rads.

The most likely explanation of the suppressor cell effect, in view of work on suppressor cells done in other systems (14), is that it interferes with the ability of T memory, or T prekiller, lymphocytes to differentiate into full-fledged T killer cells. Most likely, the activated killer cells themselves are not sensitive to T cell suppression. They can, however, be blocked in at least two different ways: by the presence of sufficient numbers of tumor cells having the appropriate TSTA and tying up all the killer cells via a competitive inhibition mechanism, and by the presence of antibodies in sufficient concentrations to mask all the TSTA at the tumor cell surface (11). Conceivably, antibodies to the idiotypic determinants of the killer cells may also abrogate their reactivity, and they may even destroy the killer cells in the presence of complement (15).

We have not studied whether, *in vivo,* the suppressor cells present in tumor-bearing mice suppress immunity to the TSTA of the given tumor specifically or whether, they once activated, nonspecifically suppress reactivity to a variety of antigens including those of the given tumor. We have, however, recently done *in vitro* experiments in collaboration with H.J. Garriques and J.D. Tamerius, which may have some bearing on this point.

These experiments show that spleen cells from BALB/c mice with tumors (approximately 10 mm in diameter) can suppress the development of cytotoxic cells *in vitro,* if they are added at the initiation of a 5 day MLC culture, in which BALB/c spleen cells are primarily sensitized against alloantigens of (irradiated) C57BL spleen cells. However, for suppression to occur, heavily irradiated cells (15,000 rads *in vitro*) from the respective tumor (MCA sarcoma 1425) also had to be added to the MLC system (together with the cells to be sensitized and the spleen cells from mice bearing the 1425 sarcoma). Enrichment of tumor-bearers' spleen cell populations for T cells by passage through nylon wool columns led to the best suppression. We tentatively conclude from this, that spleen (T?) cells from tumor-bearing mice, after further contact with cells containing TSTA, can suppress a third-party immune response. To what extent this mechanism plays a role *in vivo* needs to be studied. One should also study whether the system used can be of value when looking for suppressor cell activity in human cancer patients.

The findings described suggest that it may become possible, with respect to certain immunogenic tumors, to manipulate the immune system in favor of the host. This may be done by removing tumor antigens and complexes in antigen excess, which interfere with the development of an effective immune response and/or its expression, for example by giving high titered antibodies with specificity for the given antigens and creating complexes in antibody excess. A therapeutic effect might be also obtained by giving drugs (or radiation) in such a way that suppressor cells are inhibited more than are the various effector cells.

As more knowledge evolves concerning immune regulation of tumor growth, it should be possible to develop methods with high degree of selectivity for cells having the given TSTA, perhaps by manipulating clones of the specific suppressor cells (and/or their humoral products, if any). One must realize, however, that a variety of different factors are likely to influence the growth of immunogenic tumors *in vivo,* including the release of various nonspecifically acting, immunosuppressive molecules from tumor cells and the modulation of certain TSTA upon contact with humoral antibodies (1). Thus, abolition of suppressor cell-mediated mechanisms may not be sufficient to combat tumor growth.

To what extent mechanisms studied with (highly immunogenic) MCA sarcomas in mice play a role in regulating the growth of tumors in man, needs very much to be studied.

ACKNOWLEDGMENTS

The work of the authors has been supported by grants CA 19148 and CA 19149 from the National Institutes of Health and by grant IM-431 from the American Cancer Society.

REFERENCES

1. Hellström, K.E., and Hellström, I., "Lymphocyte Mediated Cytotoxicity and Blocking Serum Activity to Tumor Antigens". *Adv. in Immunol.* 18:209-277, 1974.
2. Hellström, I., Hellström, K.E., Evans, C.A., et al., "Serum Mediated Protection of Neoplastic Cells from Inhibition by Lymphoyctes Immune to Their Tumor Specific Antigens". *Proc. Natl. Acad. Sci.* 62:362-369, 1969.
3. Sjögren, H.O., Hellström, I., Bansal, S.C., and Hellström, K.E., "Suggestive Evidence That the "Blocking Antibodies" of Tumor-Bearing Individuals may be Antigen-Antibody Complexes". *Proc. Natl. Acad. Sci. U.S.A.* 68:1372-1375, 1971.
4. Baldwin, R.W., and Price, M.R., "Tumor Antigens and Tumor-Host Relationships". *Ann. Rev. Med.* 27:151-163, 1976.
5. Hellström, K.E., Hellström, I., and Nepom, J.T., "Specific Blocking Factors—Are They Important?" *Biochimica et Biophysica Acta.* 473:121-148, 1977.
6. Vaage, J., "Specific and Desensitization of Resistance Against a Syngeneic Methylcholan-threne-Induced Sarcoma in C3HF Mice". *Cancer Res.* 32:193-199, 1972.
7. Thomson, D.M.P., Steele, K., and Alexander, P., "The Presence of Tumor-Specific Membrane Antigen in the Serum of Rats with Chemically Induced Sarcomata". *Brit. J. Cancer* 27:27-34, 1973.
8. Paranjpe, M.S., Boone, C.W., and Takeichi, N., "Specific Paralysis of the Antitumor Cellular Immune Response Produced by Growing Tumors Studied with a Radioisotope Footpad Assay". *Ann. N.Y. Acad. Sci.* 276:254-259, 1976.
9. Hellström, K.E., and Hellström, I., "Evidence That Tumor Antigens Enhance Tumor Growth *in vivo* by Interacting with a Radiosensitive (Suppressor?) Cell Population". *Proc. Natl. Acad. Sci. USA*, 75:436-440, 1978.
10. Gerhson, R.K., Carter, R.L., and Kondo, K., "On Concomitant Immunity in Tumor-Bearing Hamsters". *Nature* 213:674-676, 1967.
11. Hellström, K.E., and Brown, J.P., "Tumor Antigens". In: *"The Antigens"*, Edited by M. Sela, Acadmic Press, N.Y. (In Press).
12. Greene, M.I., Martin, E.D., Pierres, M., and Benacerraf, B., "Reduction of Syngeneic Tumor Growth by an Anti-IJ Alloantiserum". *Proc. Natl. Acad. Sci.* 74:5118-5121, 1977.
13. Hellström, I., Hellström, K.E., Kant, J.A., and Tamerius, J.D., "Regression and Inhibition of Sarcoma Growth by Interference with a Radiosensitive T Cell Population". *J. Exp. Med.* 148:799-804, 1978.
14. Klimpel, G.R., and Henney, C.S., "A Comparison of the Effects of T and Macrophage-like Suppressor Cells on Memory Cell Differentiation *in vitro*". *J. of Immunol.* 21:749-754, 1978.
15. Binz, H., and Wigzell, H., "Induction of Specific Immune Unresponsiveness with Purified Mixed Leukocyte Culture-Activated T Lymphoblasts as Auto-immunogen. III. Proof for the Existence of Autoanti-idiotypic Killer T Cells and Transfer of Suppression to Normal Syngeneic Recipients by T or B Lymphocytes". *J. Exp. Med.* 147:63-76, 1978.

Host Defense Mechanisms in Cancer and Their Modification by Immunotherapy†

Evan M. Hersh[1], Y. Patt[1], J. Gutterman[1], S. Murphy[1],
G. Mavligit[1], S. Richman[1], J. Maroun[1], E. Lotzova[1],
K. Dicke[1], A. Zander[1]

SUMMARY—The status of immunocompetence and immunodeficiency in cancer patients is reviewed. The effects of immunotherapy with active non-specific immunotherapeutic agents such as BCG, C. parvum and MER and the effect of immunorestorative immunotherapy such as thymosin is reviewed. The conventional approach to evaluation of these immunotherapeutic agents includes delayed type hypersensitivity skin testing and measurement of T and B cells. Reactivity in these systems changes relatively slowly with immunotherapy and in addition is relatively insensitive. Newer assays of cell mediated cytotoxicity including measurement of natural killer cells and antibody dependent cell mediated cytotoxicity may be more sensitive and more relevant to the use of some of these agents. Boosting of both of these reactivities by C. parvum MER and interferon are illustrated in this paper. In addition, there is a need for the development of immunotherapy to better define the underlying immunologic functions and defects which are the target for immunotherapeutic agents. In this report we describe the presence of a radiosensitive, thymic hormone sensitive suppressor cell for the lymphocyte blastogenic response to PHA and Con-A found in the peripheral blood of patients with various types of malignancy who manifest immunodeficiency. This suppressor cell activity was shown when the PHA and Con-A responses of normal lymphocytes was depressed by coculture with patients lymphocytes. The suppressor cell was radiosensitive in virtually all the cases and sensitive to thymic hormones, thymosin and THF in approximately 30% of the cases. This was manifested by abrogation of its activity when these hormones were added in vitro. The effects of immunotherapy on the cell and an attempt to eliminate it with immunotherapy are an important current objective of immunotherapy.

INTRODUCTION

The current status of human cancer immunotherapy is that it appears to have a significant but modest effect in prolongation of remission duration and survival among patients with limited disease and in patients with no evident disease after conventional therapy (1). Clinically significant beneficial effects of immunotherapy have been observed in lung cancer, colon

[1]Section of Immunology, Department of Developmental Therapeutics, University of Texas System Cancer Center, M.D. Anderson Hospital and Tumor Institute, Houston, Texas.
†Supported by Grants CA 05831, CA 14984 and Contract NO1 CB 33888 from the National Cancer Institute.

247

cancer, breast cancer, leukemia, lymphoma and malignant melanoma (1). Immunotherapy with BCG, C. parvum and MER, active specific immunization with tumor cells or tumor antigens and immunorestoration with thymic hormones or Levamisole have shown these types of and degrees of effect (1). Unfortunately, the effects have not been long lasting and in most circumstances there is little evidence of this time for a major increase in long-term survivorship or rate of cure.

There seems to be an excellent rationale for the development of immunotherapy in human cancer. Some of the immunological characteristics of human cancer are given in table 1. The ultimate foundation for the development of immunotherapy is the presence on the tumor cell surface, of tumor associated antigens (2). These are recognized as foreign by specific or nonspecific host defense mechanisms and the host can mount an immune or non-immune response against these cells (2). However, this response and the recognition of the tumor as foreign to the host is often impaired because of the immunodeficiency of cancer (3). Progressive immunodeficiency has been observed in almost all types of progressive malignant disease. Its etiology is complex and is related in part to a deficiency in host defense cells, to the development of suppressor cells, to the production and release by the tumor of a variety of immunosuppressive factors and to the immunosuppressive effect of the conventional modalities of treatment (3). Most important is the immunocompetence prognosis relationship. Immunocompetent patients have a relatively good prognosis while immunoincompetent patients have a relatively poor prognosis (3). This has been observed at every stage of malignant disease and in most histologic types or malignancy.

Table 1—IMMUNOLOGICAL BASIS OF IMMUNOTHERAPY

Tumor Antigens and Tumor Immunity
Immunodeficiency in Cancer
Immunosuppressive Serum Factors
Deficiency of Host Defense Cells
Increase in Suppressor Cells
Immunosuppressive Effects of Therapy
Immunocompetence and Prognosis Relationship

There are several current important limitations to the development of immunotherapy for human cancer. These include the production by the tumor of factors which can profoundly inhibit a variety of antitumor host defense mechanisms (4). Also, these include our limited understanding of the mechanisms of host control or failure of host control of tumor growth, our limited understanding of the mechanism of action of some of the immunotherapeutic agents and our lack of appropriate and adequate methods for rapid quantitation and monitoring of the biological effects and toxicities of immunotherapeutic agents.

Recently, attention of tumor immunologists has been refocused on cell mediated cytotoxicity and several assays have been developed which can be utilized to measure T-cell (5), K-cell (6), NK-cell (7) and monocyte (8) mediated cytotoxicity to a variety of target cells. Furthermore, there has been a great increase in our recognition and understanding of suppressor cell mechanisms and these are beginning to appear to be important in the progression of malignancy (9). In this paper we will outline some of the conventional and newer approaches to monitoring and evaluation of immunotherapy. We will indicate that monitoring of natural killer or NK-cell activity and antibody dependent cell-mediated cytotoxicity (ADCC) may be useful methods to study active nonspecific immunotherapy, to monitor it and to guide its clinical use. Furthermore, we will present data on a radiosensitive, thymic hormone sensitive, suppressor cell population in the peripheral blood of immunodeficient cancer patients, which may play a role in the immunodeficiency and progression of malignant disease. This cell may be a target for immunotherapy and its study may be useful in monitoring immunotherapy.

MATERIALS AND METHODS

Recall antigen delayed type hypersensitivity, to dermathophytin, candida, varidase, mumps and PPD was measured using antigens and methods as previously described (10). Antigens were injected in 0.1 ml amounts intradermally in the forearm. Induration was measured at 24 and 48 hours and the average diameter was recorded in millimeters. Peripheral blood T lymphocytes were measured by the fixed slide method (11). Lymphocyte blastogenic responses to PHA, and CON-A were measured ultilizing the previously described microculture system (12). Peripheral blood lymphocytes, separated from defibernated blood by Hypaque-Ficoll density solution centrifugation, were cultured in microwells of Falcon micro test plates at a concentration of 1.5×10^5 cells per well in 0.2 ml of complete media containing RPMI 1640 and 20% pooled normal human AB serum. Cultures were either unstimulated or stimulated with PHA and CON-A. Cultures were harvested at 48 or 72 hours with the MASH II automatic sample harvester. During the last 8 hours of the culture period each culture was incubated with 1 microCurie of tritiated thymidine (SA 1.9 Ci/mM). Thymidine incorporation into DNA was measured by liquid scintillation counting.

For measurement of suppressor cell activity and its modification by irradiation of patient cells or by incubation of lymphocyte cultures with thymic hormones, the schema shown in Table 2 was utilized. Normal lymphocytes were cultured alone at 1.5×10^5 cells per well or with an equal number of allogeneic normal cells or allogeneic patient cells. Patient cells were also cultured alone. In some cultures either patient or normal cells were irradiated with 4,000-6,000 r. When thymic hormones were added their concentration were as follows: Thymosin—100 micrograms per ml and THF—20 micrograms per ml.

Table 2—SUPPRESSOR CELL ASSAY-EFFECT OF PATIENT CELLS ON BLASTOGENIC RESPONSE* OF NORMAL CELLS IN CO-CULTURE

EXPERIMENTAL	INDIVIDUAL CONTROLS	CO-CULTURE CONTROLS
N_1,**	N_1 (Thy, THF)	
P	P (Thy, THF)	
N_1+P		N_1+N_2
N_1+P(XRT)	P(XRT)	N_1+N_2(XRT)
N_1+P(Thy)		N_1+N_2(Thy)
N_1+P(THF)		N_1+N_2(THF)

*PHA, Con-A, MLD
**N=normal; P=patient

The NK cell assay was conducted by incubating 5×10^5 patient lymphocytes with 1×10^4 Chromium^{51} labelled CEM, T lymphoblastoid cell lines cells, in 10×75 mm tubes for 4 hours in 0.2 ml of serum free median at 37°C. After 4 hours supernatants were harvested from cultures which had been incubated with and without effector cells. Total releasable Chromium was determined by a 10 times freezing and thawing. Radioactivity released was counted in a Gamma counter, the percent specific lysis was calculated by the following formula.

$$\frac{\% \text{ specific}}{\text{lysis}} = \frac{\text{cpm experimental—spontaneous release}}{\text{cpm total release—spontaneous release}} \times 100$$

The ADCC Assay

This assay is conducted according to the method of Poplack, et al. (6). Human hyperimmune antiserum to type A and B human red blood cells

(HRBC) is obtained from Dade Company and rabbit antibody to chicken RBC (CRBC) is obtained following three weekly IV injections of 7 x 10^8 CRBC. Both sera are heat inactivated at 56° for 30 minutes, aliquoted in 0.5 cc aliquots and stored at $-80°C$. Type A and type B HRBC and CRBC are obtained weekly and stored in Alsever's solution at 4°C. They are labelled fresh just before the test by incubating 10^9 cells with 100 μCi of Cr^{51} in 0.2 ml for 30 minutes at 37°C and are subsequently washed three times in 100 volumes of media. Mononuclear leukocytes are collected from peripheral blood as described above. Target cells are adjusted to concentrations of 10^6, 3 x 10^6, 10^7, 3 x 10^7, and 10^8 per ml. Effector cells are at a concentration of 10^6 per ml. Then 0.1 ml of effector cells, 0.1 ml of target cells and 0.1 ml of a 1:10 dilution of anti-A or anti-B or a 1:1200 dilution of anti-CRBC were mixed in 12 x 75 ml plastic culture tubes. The experimental and control tubes are incubated 20 hours at 37°. After incubation tubes are centrifuged at 2,000 RPM for 10 minutes and 0.6 ml of the supernatants is counted in a gamma counter. Chromium release is calculated by dividing the CPM in the supernatant by the CPM in the pellet x 100. The final increment of chromium release is obtained by subtracting spontaneous chromium release from the mean chromium release in experimental tubes. All reactions are conducted in triplicates. The maximum percent chromium release is calculated from the data at the red cell concentration at which the maximum number of red blood cells is lysed.

RESULTS

Table 3 shows the delayed hypersensitivity response to recall antigen dermatophytin among patients who received DTIC + BCG for stage IIIB, IVA or IVB malignant melanoma compared to patients who received no therapy for stage IIIB disease. Patients with stage IIIB and IVA disease were treated after being rendered free of disease by surgery. The cumulative percent conversion from negative to positive was calculated. It can be seen that there was a significant cumulative increase in delayed hypersensitivity responses to dermatophytin in the patients with stage III disease who received BCG, compared to the untreated controls. This was not observed in patients with stage IV disease. The change was gradual, took several months to become apparent and was significantly different than the control.

Table 4 indicates that we have made similar observations in the patients receiving IV C. parvum. This table shows data on patients with various advanced solid tumors who were anergic to our battery of recall antigens outlined above. These patients were entered into our phase I trial of intravenous or subcutaneous C. parvum given weekly at increasing doses in successive cases. Chemotherapy was not given simultaneously. For analysis patients were divided into those who receive less than or greater than 5

Table 3—EFFECT OF BCG ON DELAYED HYPERSENSITIVITY TO DERMATOPHYTIN IN PATIENTS WITH STAGE III-IVB MELANOMA ON CHEMOIMMUNOTHERAPY WITH DTIC+BCG

			CUMULATIVE CONVERSION AFTER START OF THERAPY		
Stage	Therapy	n	Percent Conversion After Months Rx		
			1	3	6
III	None	16	0	0	19
III	DTIC+BCG	39	43	58*	62*
IVA	DTIC+BCG	25	32	33	33
IVB	DTIC+BCG	83	13	15	15

*Significant, P<.05

mg/m^2. It can be seen that patients who received greater than 5 mg/m^2 intravenously had significant boosting of delayed hypersensitivity in that they converted from the anergic to the reactive state. This change was significant for the >5 mg/m^2 group of patients but there were individual patients who received a high dose of C. parvum IV who failed to convert while others who received a low dose of C. parvum did convert. Therefore, this measurement is useful for evaluating groups of patients but not for evaluating the effects of individual patients. Similar changes in patients receiving BCG or C. parvum have been observed for lymphocyte blastogenesis and the number of T cells in the peripheral blood but will not be illustrated here.

For the immunorestorative agents such as the thymic hormones or Levamisole we have assays which can directly measure effects of the immunotherapeutic agents on the appropriate target cells or tissues. Results of Thymosin immunotherapy from our phase I trial are illustrated in Table 5. All patients studied had advanced disseminated solid tumors and were not on other therapy. Patients with peripheral blood T cell levels less than 50% showed significant boosting by in vivo administration of Thymosin while patients with levels greater than 50% did not show a significant change after therapy.

Recently we have focused on assays of cell mediated cytotoxicity to target cells in patients receiving immunotherapy. The NK cell assay (7) which measures an antibody independent non-T, non-B killer cell and the ADCC assay (13) which measures K cells when chicken erythrocytes are used as targets and effector monocytes when human erythrocytes are used as targets, were studied before and after about one week after the start of therapy receiving IV C. parvum, IV MER, and interferon immunotherapy. Preliminary data on the effects of immunotherapy on NK cell activity is shown in Table 6. It is clear that the various modalities of immunotherapy studied, appeared to boost NK cell activity.

252

Table 4—EFFECT OF C. PARVUM ON ESTABLISHED DELAYED HYPERSENSITIVITY TO RECALL SKIN TEST ANTIGENS

DOSE OF C. PARVUM mg/m²	TIME OF SKIN TEST READING	NUMBER (%) OF ANERGIC PATIENTS CONVERTING TO REACTIVE ON INDICATED TYPE OF THERAPY			
		SUBCUTANEOUS		INTRAVENOUS	
<5	24h	2/17 (11.8)	P = .36	3/19 (15.8)	P = .03
≥5		0/7 (0)	P = .02	8/19 (42.1)	
TOTAL		2/24 (8.3)	P = .03	11/38 (28.9)	
<5	48h	1/17 (5.9)	P = .30	2/19 (10.5)	P = .04
≥5		2/7 (28.6)	P = .15	7/19 (36.8)	
TOTAL		3/24 (12.5)	P = .14	9/38 (23.6)	

Table 5—EFFECT OF THYMOSIN THERAPY ON NUMBERS OF CIRCULATING E-ROSETTE-FORMING T LYMPHOCYTES

PRE-THERAPY E-ROSETTES (%)			POST THERAPY (%)	P
GROUP	N	MEAN		
<50%	20	34±4	46±3	<.001
≥50%	11	63±3	57±4	N.S.

Table 6—NATURAL KILLER CELLS IN CANCER AND THE EFFECTS OF IMMUNOTHERAPY

SUBJECT	n	THERAPY	PERCENT SPECIFIC LYSIS PRE-THERAPY	POST-THERAPY
normal	49	—	30	—
patient	25	—	24	—
patient	1	C. parvum	7	20
"	1	"	9	30
"	1	"	10	33
"	1	"	15	64
"	1	"	16	21
"	1	"	18	62
"	1	"	59	59
"	1	IV MER	22.3	30.4
"	1	"	11.5	24.1
"	1	Interferon	25	50

The effects of IV C. parvum and IV MER on ADCC to human erythrocyte targets is shown in Figure 1 and to human and chicken erythrocyte targets in one case is shown in Figure 2. Daily intravenous C. parvum caused a progressive increase in ADCC activity in the majority of patients particularly those at the lower end of the pretreatment activity spectrum. In patients receiving IV MER a single dose boosted reactivity on day 4 which appeared to return to baseline by day 7 and which was reboosted by a second dose on day 8. Detailed studies on one patient receiving IV MER showed a striking effect on ADCC to both targets and is

254

Figure 1

Effect of Immunotherapy on ADCC

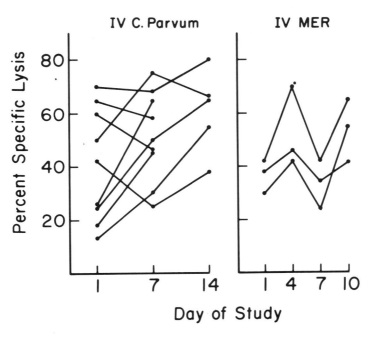

ADCC to HRBC in patients receiving IV C. parvum daily for 14 days at 2 mg/m²/day with studies on days 1 (pre-therapy), 7 and 14 (left hand figure) and in patients receiving IV MER weekly at 1 mg/m² with studies on day 1 (pre-therapy), day 4, day 7 (pre-dose 2) and 10.

detailed in Figure 2. Frozen liquid nitrogen and fresh normal cell control data did not change at most of the points studied. More extensive studies and more closely spaced observations will be necessary to completely clarify the utility of this assay in evaluating active non-specific immunotherapy.

One of the areas of increasing immunological interest in the human immune response in general and in cancer immunology specifically relates to the presence and role of suppressor cells in cancer growth and progression. We have recently detected a radiosensitive, thymic hormone-sensitive suppressor cell for PHA and CON-A induced lymphocyte blastogenic responses in immunodeficient patients with various malignancies. These cells are detected as described above in methods. A typical

255

case is shown in Figure 3. The patient was immunodeficient in terms of having a very poor PHA response. The PHA response of normal lymphocytes was depressed by co-culturing with patients lymphocytes and this depression by patient lymphocytes in co-culture was abrogated by treatment of the patients lymphocytes with 4,000-6,000 r irradiation or by addition to the cultures of 100 micorgrams/ml of Thymosin or thymic humoral factor.

Figure 2—ADCC TO HRBC AND CRBC IN A PATIENT RECEIVING IV MER 1 mg/m² WEEKLY

Effect of Immunotherapy on ADCC

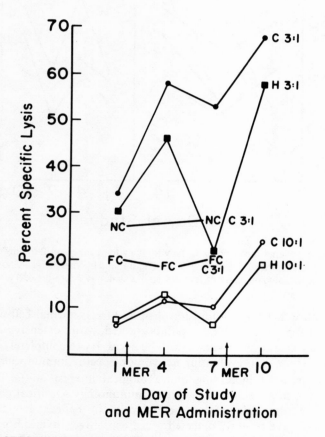

C3:1 is CRBC target, 3:1 target; effector cell ratio; C10:1 is same but 10:1 T:E ratio; h3:1 is HRBC target, 3:L T:E ratio; H10:1 is same but 10:L T:E ratio. NC is a fresh normal cell control. FC is a liquid nitrogen frozen cell control.

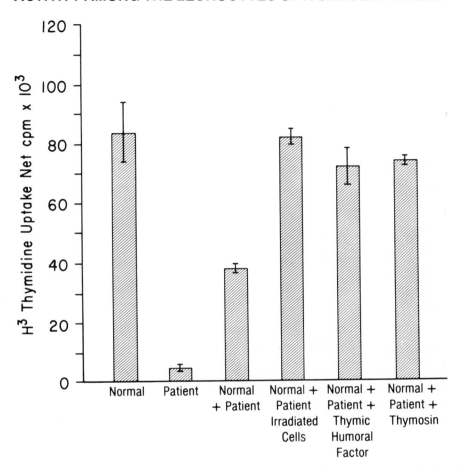

**Figure 3—EXAMPLE OF SUPPRESSOR CELL
ACTIVITY AMONG THE LEUKOCYTES OF A CANCER PATIENT**

Cultures contained 1.5 × 10⁵ normal or patient cells alone or 1.5 × 10⁵ normal plus 1.5 × 10⁵ patient cells. From left to right, bars indicate PHA response of cells from a normal patient, normal plus patient, normal plus patient (irradiated with 4000r), normal plus patient plus Thymic humoral factor and normal plus patient plus Thymosin.

Table 7 summarizes the patient data and the incidence of suppressor cells. We have studied 35 patients, and 60-70% appear to have a suppressor cell for lymphocyte blastogenesis. There was no particular pattern of suppressor cell activity in the various histological type disease. Table 8 summarizes the data in terms of the median values for the blastogenic response of normal lymphocytes, patient lymphocytes and the various co-cultures.

Table 7—SUPPRESSOR CELL IN PATIENTS WITH VARIOUS MALIGNANCIES

Type of Malignancy	Number of Cases	Suppressor Cell[1] Detected by Blastogenic Respose to	
		PHA	CON-A
Lung Cancer	21	12 (57)[2]	13 (62)
Small Cell	2	2	2
Squamous	6	5 (83)	5 (83)
Adenocarcinoma and Large Cell	13	5 (38)	6 (46)
Leukemia	7	3 (43)	5 (71)
Other	7	6 (86)	7 (100)
Sarcoma	2	1	2
Testicular	2	2	2
Lymphoma	2	2	2
Melanoma	1	1	1
TOTAL	35	21 (60)	25 (71)

1. Defined as a 3 fold or greater reduction of normal blastogenesis in co-culture with patient cells.
2. Number and percent of patients in category.

Table 8—SUPPRESSOR CELL ACTIVITY IN HUMAN CANCER MEDIAN H³ THYMIDINE INCORPORATION IN VARIOUS CULTURES

Mitogen	Cell and Additives in Cultures					
	Normal (N)	Patient (P)	N+P	N+P (Irr)	N+P Thymosin	N+P THF
PHA	84	13	9	32	23	22
CON-A	35	6	3	24	6	6

Data in media cpm/1.5 x 10⁵ cells x 10³

Table 9 shows the relationship of the radiosensitive suppressor cell to immunodeficiency and prior chemotherapy. There was a significant trend for the suppressor cell to be more common in patients with immunodeficiency as detected by the PHA and CON-A measurements. There was no significant relationship to the presence or absence of prior chemotherapy although there was a trend towards suppressor cells being more common in

Table 9—RELATIONSHIP OF RADIOSENSITIVE SUPPRESSOR CELL TO IMMUNODEFICIENCY AND PRIOR CHEMOTHERAPY

Category	Radiosensitive Suppressor Cell[1] Detected by Blastogenic Response to	
	PHA	CON-A
Immunodeficient[2]	17/23 (74) [3,4]	21/22 (95)[5]
Immunocompetent	4/11 (36)	4/10 (40)
Prior Chemotherapy	12/19 (63)	16/18 (89)
No Prior Chemotherapy	9/15 (60)	8/14 (57)

1. Defined as 3 fold decrease in normal response by co-culture with patient cells and 2 fold increase compared to co-culture by pre-irradiation of patient cells.
2. Defined as <35,000 cpm PHA response and <12,000 cpm CON-A response.
3. Number with suppressor cell/total in category (percent).
4. $P > .05 < .10$ by x^2 test.
5. $P < .01$ by x^2 test.

patients who had prior chemotherapy as detected by the CON-A measurement. However, this latter was not significant. A relationship to the stage of disease could not be investigated since all of the 35 patients in the current study had disseminated or metastatic disease.

Tables 10 and 11 compare the effects of in vitro radiation, Thymosin or THF in co-cultures of normal patient lymphocytes or normal plus normal allogeneic lymphocytes on the blastogenic response to PHA and CON-A. It can be seen that irradiation boosted PHA and CON-A responses significantly more in normal plus patient cultures than in normal plus normal cultures compared to the appropriate untreated cultures. In the PHA cultures, Thymosin also significantly boosted the group when added to normal plus patient cultures compared to normal plus normal cultures. The groups were not significantly different for THF measured either by PHA or CON-A response. However, individual cases did show significant boosting as indicated and the trend for the overall group was in the same direction, favoring greater boosting of normal plus patient co-cultures compared to normal plus normal cultures.

DISCUSSION

The two major obstacles for a rational development of immunotherapy are our limited understanding of anti-tumor host defense and its failure in

Table 10—SUMMARY OF DATA ON SUPPRESSOR CELL OF PHA RESPONSE

Parameter of PHA Response	Type of Culture and Number and Percent of Subjects in Parameter Category					
	Normal (N)	Patient (P)	N+P	N+P (Irr)	N+P+ Thymosin	N+P+ THF
<35,000 cpm[A]	0/35 (0)[B]	21/35 (60)	23/35(66)	7/34(21)	12/25(48)	13/26(50)
≥3X[C] lower than N	—	23/66	25(71)	7(21)	13(52)	16(62)
≥4X lower than N	—	21(60)	23(66)	4(12)	7(28)	11(42)
↑≥2X in co-culture by Rx	—	—	—	27(79)	12(48)	12(46)
↑≥3X in co-culture by Rx	—	—	—	19(55)	11(44)	11(42)
↑≥4X in co-culture by Rx	—	—	—	13(38)	8(32)	6(23)

A. Lower limit of Normal Range.
B. Number and (Percent) of patients in category showing indicated comparative characteristic.
C. A 2X difference is significant at the .05 level, a 3X difference at the .01 level and a 4X difference at the .001 level.

Table 11—SUMMARY OF DATA ON SUPPRESSOR CELL OF CON-A RESPONSE

Parameter of CON-A Response	Type of Culture and Number and Percent of Subjects in Parameter Category					
	Normal (N)	Patient (P)	N+P	N+P (Irr)	N+P+ Thymosin	N+P+ THF
<12,000 CPM[A]	1/33(3)[B]	23/33(70)	26/33(79)	6/33(18)	12/22(54)	14/22(63)
≥3X[C] lower than N	—	23(70)	25(76)	3(9)	12(54)	16(72)
≥4X lower than N	—	19(58)	22(67)	3(9)	9(41)	13(59)
↑≥2X in co-culture by Rx	—	—	—	26(79)	7(32)	8(36)
↑≥3X in co-culture by Rx	—	—	—	17(52)	6(27)	5(23)
↑≥4X in co-culture by Rx	—	—	—	14(42)	3(14)	4(18)

A. Lower limit of Normal Range.
B. Number and (Percent) of patients in category showing indicated comparative characteristic.
C. A 2X difference is significant at the .05 level, a 3X difference at the .01 level and a 4X difference at the .001 level.

cancer patients and our poor ability to monitor the immunological and other host-defense modifying effects of immunotherapeutic agents. In this paper we have reviewed some of the conventional approaches to monitoring the activation of host defense mechanisms by immunotherapeutic agents and attempted to point out some of their deficiencies. Optimally one would require a relevant assay which would focus on the function of the host defense cells which actually attack and kill tumor cells and would focus on effector cell, tumor target cell interaction. Unfortunately because of lack of reasonable amounts of accessible tumor in most cases, as well as the potential for the tumor to change immunologically with time, it is impractical in most patients with malignant disease receiving immunotherapy to serally monitor effector cell-tumor cell interaction.

However, the discovery and definition of the NK cell (7) and ADCC (6) functions as well as other assays for the cytotoxicity of peripheral blood effector cells (monocytes, T lymphocytes, B lymphocytes) to various malignant and benign target cells, offer a series of assays which can be evaluated for their relevance to anti-cancer host defense and immunotherapy. The NK cell and the ADCC assays as well as other cytotoxicity assays offer the advantage of results being available within 8-24 hours. Therefore, they could conceivably be utilized to both monitor and modify the dose and schedule of immunotherapy. The preliminary results illustrated in this paper suggest that they may be useful for monitoring active non-specific immunotherapy with microbial adjuvants and perhaps also other agents such as interferon.

In both assays, changes induced by immunotherapy appear within a few days after the administration of the agent. Therefore the tests could be used for dose modification. In the second half of this paper we have illustrated that immunodeficient as well as some nonimmunodeficient cancer patients have circulating radiosensitive and at times thymic hormone-sensitive suppressor cells, for the lymphocyte blastogenic response to PHA and CON-A. The spectrum of histological types of cancer in which these cells are found, the relationship of these cells to the stage of disease, their relationship to prognosis, to response to therapy, and the nature of the cells in terms of whether they are T, B, or null lymphocytes or monocytes are yet to be determined. We also do not know whether these cells are responsible for the deficiency of the lymphocyte blastogenic response to PHA and CON-A. Other investigators using a variety of human and animal systems in cancer have found that suppressor T cells (13), suppressor B cells (14) and suppressor monocytes (15) may all play a role in the immunodeficiency of cancer. Histamine receptor positive lymphocytes (16) and prostaglandin E2 secreting monocytes (17) are of particular interest since they may be subject to pharmacological manipulation with agents such as cymetidine (18) and indomethacin (19). Whether the suppressor cells would be responsive to the

262

conventional modalities of immunotherapy such as active non-specific immunotherapy with C. parvum, BCG or MER and their relationship to chemotherapy also need to be investigated. Both chemotherapy and immunotherapy can either induce (20) or abolish (21) the presence of suppressor cells in experimental systems.

ACKNOWLEDGMENTS

The authors wish to acknowledge the provision of thymosin by Dr. Allen Goldstein and the Hoffman La Roche Company and of THF by Dr. Nathan Trainin. The authors also wish to acknowledge the capable technical assistance of Marty Marshall, Charles Gschwind, Marvette Washington, Ruth Goldman and John Morgan.

REFERENCES

1. Hersh, E.M., Mavligit, G.M., Gutterman, J.U., and Richman, S.P., "Immunotherapy of Human Cancer." In: *Cancer, A Comprehensive Treatise,* F.F. Becker (ed.), Plenum Press (New York), 1977.

2. Mavligit, G.M., Hersh, E.M., and McBride, C.M., "Lymphocyte Blastogenesis Induced by Authchthonous Human Solid Tumor Cells: Relationship of Stage of Disease and Serum Factors." *Cancer* 34:1712-1721, 1974.

3. Hersh, E.M., Mavligit, G.M., and Gutterman, J.U., "Immunodeficiency in Cancer and the Importance of Immune Evaluation of Cancer Patient." *Med. Clin. N. Amer.* 60:623-636, 1976.

4. DeLustro, F., and Argyris, B.F., "Mechanism of Mastocytoma-Mediated Suppression of Lymphocyte Reactivity." *The J. of Immunol.* 117:2073-2080, 1976.

5. Shohat, B., and Jashua, H., "Assessment of the Functional Activity of Human Lymphocytes in Malignant Disease by the Local Graft-Versus-Host Reaction in Rats and the T Rosette-Forming Cell Test." *Clin. Exp. Immunol.* 24:534-537, 1976.

6. Poplack, D.G., et al., "Monocyte-Mediated Antibody-Dependent Cellular Cytotoxicity: A Clinical Test of Monocyte Function." *Blood* 48:809, 1976.

7. Takasugi, M., et al., "Decline of Natural Nonselective Cell-Mediated Cytotoxicity in Patients with Tumor Regression." *Cancer Res.* 37:413, 1977.

8. Holden, H.T., Haskill, J.S., Kirchner, H., et al., "Two Functionally Distinct Anti-Tumor Effector Cells Isolated from Primary Murine Sarcoma Virus-Induced Tumors." *Jnl. Immunol.* 117:440-446, 1976.

9. Berlinger, N.T., Lopez, C., Lipkin, M., et al., "Defective Recognitive Immunity in Family Aggregates of Colon Carcinoma." *The J. of Clin. Investigation* 59:761-769, 1977.

10. Hersh, E.M., et al., "Serial Studies of Immunocompetence of Patients Undergoing Chemotherapy for Acute Leukemia," *J. Clin. Invest.* 54:401, 1974.

11. Schafer, L.A., et al., "Permanent Slide Preparations of T-Lymphocyte-Sheep Red Blood Cell Rosettes." *J. Immunol. Meth.* 8:241, 1975.

12. Lewinski, U.H., et al., "Interaction Between Repeated Skin Testing with Recall Antigens and Temporal Fluctuations of *in vitro* Lymphocytes Blastogenesis in Cancer Patients." *Clin. Immunol. Immunopath.* 7:77, 1977.

13. Basten, A., Loblay, R., Pirtchard-Briscoe, H., "T Cell Dependent Suppression of the Immune Response." *Progress in Immunology III,* Elsevier-North Holland Press, Holland, 359-368, 1977.

14. Rollinghoff, M., Starzinski-Powitz, A., Pfizenmaier, K., et al., "Cyclophosphamide-Sensitive T Lymphocytes Suppress the *in vivo* Generation of Antigen Specific Cytotoxic T Lymphocytes." *J. Exptl. Med.* 145:455, 1977.

15. Paglieroni, T. and Mackenzie, M.R., "Studies on the Pathogenesis of an Immune Defect in Multiple Myeloma." *J. Clin. Invest.* 59:1120, 1977.

16. Plaut, M., Lichtenstein, L.M., Gillespie, E., et al., "Studies on the Mechanism of Lymphocyte-Mediated Cytolysis. IV. Specificity of the Histamine Receptor on Effector T Cells." *J. Immunol.* 111:389, 1973.

17. Goodwin J.S., Bankhurst, A.D., and Messner, P.J., "Suppression of Human T-Cell Mitogenesis by Prostaglandin. Existence of a Prostaglandin-Producing Suppressor Cell." *Exptl. Med.* 146:1719, 1977.

18. Schechter, B., and Feldman, M., "Enhancing Lympthocytes in Spleens of Tumor-Bearing Mice: Affinity Chromatography on Insolubilized Histamine." *Int. J. Cancer* 20:239, 1977.

19. Goodwin, J.S., Messner, R.P., Bankhurst, A.D., et al., "Prostaglandin-Producing Suppressor Cells in Hodgkin's Disease." *New England J. Med.* 297:963, 1977.

20. Geffard, M., and Orbach-Arbouys, S., "Enhancement of T Suppressor Activity in Mice by High Doses of BCG." *Cancer Immunol. Immunothera.* 1:41, 1976.

21. Neta, R., Winkelstein, A., Salvin, S.B., et al., "The Effect of Cyclophosphamide on Suppressor Cells in Guinea Pigs." *Cellular Immunol.* 33:402, 1977.

The Relationship of Tumor Induced Cellular Immunity and Cellular Suppression in Tumor Bearing Animals†

Ronald Ferguson,[1]
J. Schmidtke,[1]
R. Simmons[1]

SUMMARY—Thymocytes (TC), spleen cells (SC) and lymph node cells (LNC) from syngeneic EL4 lymphoma bearing C57BL/6 hosts were tested for their capacity to suppress or augment the tumor specific syngeneic cytotoxicity generated by normal C57BL/6 spleen cells against the syngeneic EL4 tumor *in vitro*. After 5 days of EL4 tumor growth TC and SC were capable of suppressing by 50% the *in vitro* generated anti-tumor cytotoxicity. By day 10 suppression by TC and SC was 90%. The suppression was nonspecific in that such cells suppressed the development of immunity *in vitro* to allogeneic antigens. Simultaneously, the LNC of the same tumor bearing animals progressively augmented the amount of cytotoxicity generated in the test cultures against the EL4 tumor. By day 10 (when spleen and thymus suppressed) tumor bearing LNC augmented the generation of test cytotoxicity by over 250%. Thus, the EL4 syngeneic tumor appears to concurrently induce effective tumor destroying immunity in one part of the immune apparatus while preferentially stimulating suppressor activity in thymus and spleen. The net effect of such an immunologic balance may be that effective tumor immunity is inhibited from developing by the dominating influence of suppressor cells in thymus and spleen. Such tumor induced suppression was sensitive to *in vitro* irradiation or mitomycin C treatment and was abrogated *in vivo* by a single dose of 100mg/kg cyclophosphamide given to 10 day tumor bearing animals.

Most autochthonous or transplantable syngeneic tumor systems in experimental animals have demonstrable tumor associated antigens on their cells surfaces which are capable of invoking, within a tumor bearing host, a cellular immune response. A specific cell mediated anti-tumor response is detectable early in the course of tumor bearing, but with increasing time of tumor bearing and tumor load this specific response wanes and the host is overcome by a generalized state of immunounresponsiveness. A variety of explanations for these phenomena, and data to support them, have been generated in recent years (1). These can generally be divided into two categories. The first is the soluble immunodepressive factor which can be tumor specific or non-specific in nature and has been demonstrated to be

[1]Departments of Surgery and Microbiology, The University of Minnesota, Minneapolis, Minnesota.
†Supported by grants CA 21539, AM 13083, CA 11605, AI 14012 from the National Institutes of Health, and grants IM 137 and IR 143 from the American Cancer Society.

265

mediated by immune complexes (2), small molecular weight proteins (3), more peptide fragments (4), and nonspecific alpha globulin (5). A second category involves cell mediated immunosuppression. Much attention has recently been directed toward the possible role of suppressor cells in tumor induced immune suppression and to the possibility of the existence of tumor specific as well as nonspecific suppressor cells that may affect general immunocompetence. Because of the dynamic nature of changing levels of immune responsiveness induced by increasing tumor burden, and the demonstrable nature of a positive cellular immune response directed towards the tumor early in the course of tumor bearing, it was of interest to us to ask several questions about the relationship between these two opposing immunologic phenomena. Are cellular suppressive mechanisms operative in tumor bearing animals? What is the temporal relationship between cytotoxic and suppressive potential in various lymphoid organs of tumor bearing animals? Is there coexistence of suppression and immunity and is this compartmentalized within the lymphoid system? These are all questions we sought to answer in defining the nature of a specific cell mediated immune response directed against the tumor as well as specific and nonspecific cell mediated suppressor effects.

To this end we sought to evaluate the cytotoxic as well as the suppressor potential of various lymphoid compartments over increasing time of tumor bearing in a murine tumor model. The model system was the EL4 lymphoma syngeneic to C57BL6 mice. At varying days after tumor bearing the thymus, regional and distant lymph nodes, and spleen cells were harvested from tumor bearing animals and placed in culture and their cytotoxic and suppressor potentials assayed as described below (Table 1).

Table 1—PROTOCOL FOR EVALUATION OF CYTOTOXIC AND SUPPRESSOR POTENTIAL OF VARIOUS LYMPHOID COMPARTMENTS WITH INCREASING TIME OF TUMOR BEARING

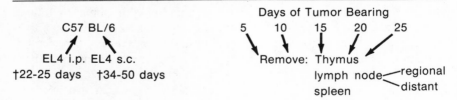

Test: 1) Cytotoxic potential.
Responsiveness to EL4 *in vitro* i.e. MTLC cytotoxicity generation.
Test: 2) Suppressive potential.
Ability to suppress (or augment) normal C57 BL/6 spleen from responding to EL4 *in vitro* i.e. MTLC cytotoxicity generation.

266

MATERIALS AND METHODS

The tumor system utilized throughout was the EL4 lymphoma resident in C57BL6 mice. Murine stocks were obtained from Charles Rivers Laboratories and represented 6 to 12 weeks old female C57BL6 mice. The characteristics of the EL4 tumor showed that as few as 10^2 cells injected intraperitoneally into C57BL6 mice were 100% lethal within 25 to 30 days. When injected subcutaneously the tumors showed progressive growth and ultimate death of the animals within 34 to 48 days. The tumor was not lethal for allogeneic hosts and large inocula were promptly rejected in BALB/C mice.

Sensitization Cultures

The standard assay cultures for suppression and for cytotoxic potential used throughout was a mixed tumor lymphocyte culture (MTLC), where normal C57BL6 spleen cells were placed in culture with irradiated EL4 tumor cells, proliferated and within 5 days developed assayable tumor specific cytotoxicity. 4×10^6 normal C57BL6 spleen cells were placed in culture with 5×10^5 irradiated (5,000 rads) EL4 tumor cells. The cultures were contained in 16 mm. plastic tissue culture dishes in 2 cc. volume of Eagles MEM, supplemented with 10% fetal calf serum, nonessential amino acids and 2-mercaptoethanol (5×10^{-5}M). The cultures were harvested at the end of 5 days and cytotoxicity assayed.

Cytotoxicity Assay

Target cells for assay of syngeneic induced cytotoxicity in MTLC was obtained by chromium labelling of target cells of either EL4 origin or concanavalin A (Con A), or LPS blasts of normal C57LB6 spleen cells. All targets were labelled with chromium 51 by incubating 10^7 cells in a 1 ml. volume with 0.2 microcuries of chromium 51 isotope. Target cells were washed and recounted and the viability was determined. 5×10^4 viable chromium labelled target cells were then placed in a volume of 100 microliters in v bottom microtiter wells and to this was added an appropriate number of *in vitro* generated effector cells from MTLC to reach the desired effector target cell ratio. This was generally an 8 to 1 or 4 to 1 ratio. After 4 hours of incubation at 37°C the plates were spun at 500 rpm for 10 minutes and 0.1 ml of supernatant was removed and counted in a well type gamma counter. Percent cytotoxicity was expressed as

$$\frac{\text{Experimental cpm} - \text{spontaneous cpm}}{\text{total cpm} - \text{spontaneous cpm}}$$

Assay of Cytotoxic Potentials

To assay for cytotoxic potential, lymph node or spleen cells from tumor bearing animals, at varying intervals after tumor innoculation, were harvested and placed in culture with irradiated EL4 tumor cells. As control cultures normal C57BL6 spleen cells, responding to the EL4 were utilized. Cytotoxicity generated was assayed at the end of 5 days as described previously and the cytotoxic potential of the tumor bearing animal was compared to the normal spleen or lymph node response. This was expressed as percent of control.

Assay of suppressive potential and the ability of spleen, regional or distant lymph node, and thymus of tumor bearing animals to suppress normally responsive C57BL6 spleen cells from responding to the EL4 tumor in MTLC was utilized. In each case cell mixing controls using normal lymphoid cells of the same origin as the tumor bearing lymphoid organs being assayed were used. The suppressor potential ws expressed as percent suppression of the cytotoxic response generated in MTLC in the presence of normal as opposed to tumor bearing lymphoid tissue. The ratios in the test mixed lymphocyte culture were 8 responding normal C57BL6 spleen cells to one stimulator irradiated EL4 tumor cell to 4 test lymphoid cells.

RESULTS

Mixed Tumor Lymphocyte Culture Generation of Tumor Specific Cytotoxic Cells

Throughout, the assay for cytotoxic and suppressor potential utilized a MTLC. Table 2 demonstrates that cytotoxicity was generated against EL4 targets when EL4 stimulator cells were mixed with normal syngeneic C57BL6 responder spleen cells. Under these circumstances, however, an allogeneic target (BALB/C, LSTRA) was not killed and there was no cytotoxicity of normal C57BL6 spleen or thymus nor of T or B cell blasts of C57BL6 origin. There was no auto stimulation as C57BL6 spleen cells did not respond to x-irradiated C57BL6 spleen. In the allogeneic circumstance however, the EL4 tumor stimulated allogeneic BALB/C responder cells to give excellent killing of the EL4 target as well as C57BL6 spleen, thymus, or T or B cell blasts of C57BL6 origin. Thus these spleen, thymus, and T and B blasts of C57BL6 spleen were able to be killed. The EL4 tumor cells however, stimulated C57BL6 spleen cells to kill only the EL4. Thus it was apparent that killing of EL4 targets by syngeneic cells was specific for the system in which EL4 was utilized to stimulate the syngeneic spleen cells. In addition, an excellent cytotoxicity at the relatively low effector target ratio of 8 to 1 was generated in this syngeneic, mixed tumor lymphocyte system.

Demonstration of Cellular Suppression in Spleen and Thymus of Tumor Bearing Mice

In order to determine the presence of cells capable of suppression in

268

Table 2—IN VITRO GENERATION OF TUMOR SPECIFIC CYTOTOXIC CELLS IN MIXED TUMOR LYMPHOCYTE CULTURES

		% Cytotoxicity of Targets at 8:1 Effector: Target Ratio					
		TARGET CELL TYPE					
Cell Combination							
Responder+	Stimulator*	EL4	LSTRA	C57 Spleen	C57 Thymus	C57 Con A Blasts	C57 LPS Blasts
C57BL/6	EL4 Tumor	36	-2	-5	-5	-1	-3
C57BL/6	C57BL/6 Spleen	-1	1	0	1	-1	-1
C57BL/6	BALB/C Spleen	1	53	-3	-2	-1	0
BALB/C	EL4 Tumor	84	-5	44	41	50	53

+ 4 x 10⁶ normal spleen cells

* 5 x 10⁵ EL4 tumor cells irradiated with 2000 rads.

269

tumor bearing animals, the above described mixed tumor lymphocyte culture was utilized as a test assay system. To this culture, spleen or thymus from tumor bearing animals, during various days of tumor bearing, were added in the attempt to define the ability of such cells to suppress normally responsive C57BL6 spleen cells from responding to the irradiated EL4 in MTLC and generating tumor specific cytotoxicity. Tables 3 and 4 demonstrate the ability of spleen and thymus from tumor bearing animals to

Table 3—SPLENIC SUPPRESSION OF TUMOR BEARING ANIMALS (TBA)

Day 10 ascites EL4 bearing mouse

Test MTLC*		C57 BL/6 cells added	% cytotoxicity at 8:L/T ratio		% suppression
Responder	Stimulator		EL4	LSTRA	
C57 BL/6 spleen + EL4$_x$ **		———	37	3	—
C57 BL/6 spleen + EL4$_x$	normal spleen	31	3	—
C57 BL/6 spleen + EL4$_x$	TBA spleen	1	-2	97

* MTLC (mixed tumor lymphocyte culture) responder: stimulator: suppressor ratio of 8:1:4.
** x= 2000 rads *in vitro*.

Table 4—THYMIC SUPPRESSION OF TUMOR BEARING ANIMALS (TBA)

Test MTLC*		C57 BL/6 cells added	% cytotoxicity at 8:1 L/T ratio		% suppression
Responder	Stimulator		EL4	LSTRA	
C57 BL/6 spleen + EL4$_x$ **		—	48	-1	—
C57 BL/6 spleen + EL4$_x$	normal thymus	41	0	—
C57 BL/6 spleen + EL4$_x$	TBA thymus	5	0	88

*MTLC (mixed tumor lymphocyte culture) responder: stimulator: suppressor ratio of 8:1:4.
**x = 2000 rads *in vitro*.

270

suppress the generation of C57BL6 anti EL4 cytotoxicity generated in MTLC. In each case, significant amounts of suppression were present at a relatively short time after inoculation of tumor. Figure 1 demonstrates the kinetic pattern of appearance of suppressor potential by splenocytes of tumor bearing animals. Figure 1 shows that three days after inoculation of the ascitic form of the EL4 no suppression was demonstrable. However, by day 5 greater than 50% suppression was apparent and by day 10 suppression was near 100 percent. Spleen cells from 10 day tumor bearing animals were able to totally inhibit normally responsive C57BL6 cells from responding to the EL4 *in vitro*. Similar kinetic patterns of suppressor cells were present when tumor bearing thymus was analyzed. Figure 2 demonstrates that by day 8 tumor bearing thymocytes were capable of strong suppression and this suppression was maintained over time. It thus was apparent that, in at least this tumor system, suppressor cells were induced in both the spleen and the thymus.

Figure 1—KINETIC APPEARANCE OF SUPPRESSOR POTENTIAL IN SPLEEN CELLS FROM ANIMALS BEARING INCREASING TUMOR BURDEN

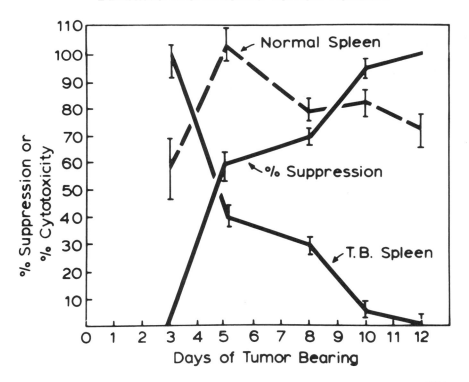

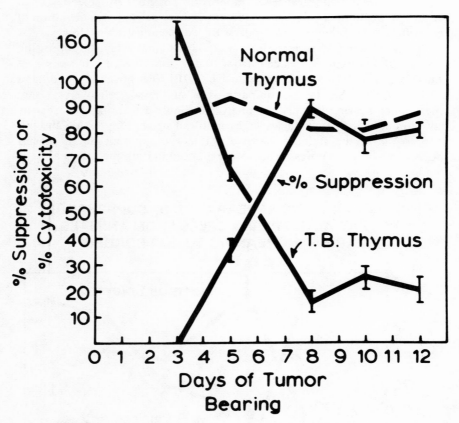

Figure 2—KINETIC APPEARANCE OF SUPPRESSOR POTENTIAL IN THYMOCYTES OF ANIMALS BEARING INCREASING TUMOR BURDEN

Cytotoxic Potential of Spleen and Regional and Distant Lymph Nodes of Subcutaneous Bearing EL4 Animals

The kinetic appearance of responsiveness to EL4 tumor *in vitro* in MTLC was assessed in spleen and regional and distant lymph nodes in animals bearing subcutaneous EL4 tumors. 5×10^5 EL4 tumor cells were injected subcutaneously in the right flank and at various intervals the draining regional lymph nodes as well as distant lymph nodes and spleens were harvested and their ability to respond to the x-irradiated EL4 tumors in MTLC were assessed. This was compared to the response of normal spleen or lymph nodes to respond to the EL4. The results are expressed as percent of control the normal nontumor bearing lymphoid cell responsiveness. These data are shown in Figure 3. Within the first week following

272

inoculation of the tumors, the tumors became palpable in the flank and the spleen and draining regional lymph nodes showed marked augmentation of cytotoxicity generation *in vitro* when compared to normal lymphoid cells. By two weeks of tumor bearing, the regional lymph nodes had increased their enhanced cytotoxic capability. The spleen and distant lymph nodes, however, were showing a decrease in cytotoxic potential while the regional lymph nodes continued to show augmented cytotoxicity. The spleen and distant lymph node showed a markedly depressed ability to respond to irradiated EL4 in culture by 18 days following tumor inoculation. By three weeks of tumor bearing, the spleen and both regional and distant lymph nodes were totally incapable of responding in mixed tumor lymphocyte

Figure 3—CYTOTOXIC POTENTIAL OF CELLS FROM SPLEEN, REGIONAL AND DISTANT LYMPH NODES FROM ANIMALS BEARING SUBCUTANEOUS EL4 TUMORS

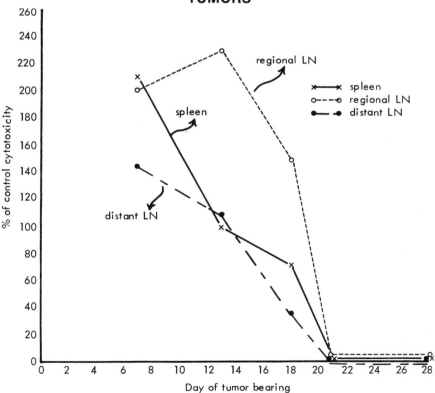

Control cytotoxicity determined by MTLC anti-EL4 response of normal analogous lymphoid tissue.

cultures to the EL4. Thus, there was an apparent enhanced cytotoxic potential in the regional draining lymph nodes of tumor bearing animals concomitant with a rather marked depression of cytotoxic potential in the spleen and the distant lymph nodes of the same animals.

An attempt was then made to correlate the appearance of suppressor capability with this decreased responsiveness in subcutaneous bearing EL4 animals. Again, the assay system was the MTLC with normal C57BL6 spleen cells responding to irradiated EL4 tumor cells and generating cytotoxicity. To a test MTLC were added either thymus, spleen, distant or regional draining lymph node cells of animals bearing subcutaneous EL4 tumors at various times following tumor inoculation. Figure 4 again demonstrates that there was a high degree of augmentation of cytotoxicity generated in test cultures when draining regional lymph nodes from tumor bearing animals were assayed at days 7 through 18 following tumor inoculation. This however, was not the case with thymus, spleen, or distant lymph nodes although they have little effect within the first two weeks

Figure 4—AUGMENTING OR SUPPRESSIVE POTENTIAL OF CELLS FROM VARIOUS LYMPHOID ORGANS FROM ANIMALS WITH SUBCUTANEOUS TUMORS PERFORMED OVER TIME OF INCREASING TUMOR BURDEN

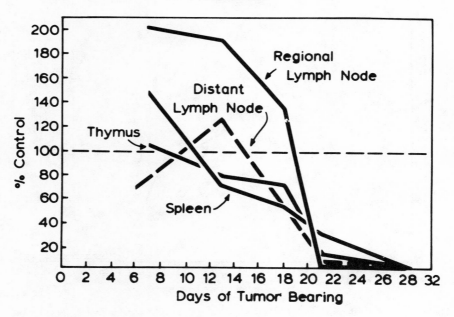

274

following tumor inoculation. By day 18, the spleen, thymus, and distant lymph nodes were capable of suppression by approximately 50% the amount of cytotoxicity generated against irradiated EL4 tumor cells by normal spleen cells. This occurred at the same time that there was an augmented response of regional lymph nodes suggesting the concomitant existence of suppression and immunity within the same tumor bearing animal and that there was some compartmentalization of each function. This however, had totally disappeared by day 21 when it was found that all lymphoid cells, regardless of origin, were capable of suppressing normally responsive spleen cells from generating cytotoxicity *in vitro* against the EL4 tumor. This overwhelming suppressive response occurred fully 10 days prior to the death of the animals.

Specificity of Cellular Suppression Present in Tumor Bearing Animals

We felt it was of some importance to test for the specificity of the cellular suppression in tumor bearing animals especially in light of previous work where the suggestion of both tumor specific (6) as well as nonspecific suppression (7) has been found in tumor bearing hosts. Specificity under these circumstances was defined as being tumor specific if only the response to the EL4 tumor was suppressed and other responses were not. To evaluate this, an allogeneic cell mediated cytotoxicity generation culture similar to the MTLC was utilized only instead of a syngeneic irradiated tumor cell as a stimulator cell in the test culture, an allogeneic irradiated spleen cell, in this case BALB/C, was utilized. The allogeneic target was the LSTRA tumor and the conditions of allogeneic CMC generation cultures were identical to the MTLC with the exception of the presence of an allogeneic stimulator cell. Table 5 demonstrates that ability of spleen, thymus and lymph node cells from ascites bearing EL4 animals to inhibit allogeneic cytotoxicity generated by normal C57BL6 spleen cells directed against allogeneic BALB/C targets. Thymus, spleen, or lymph node cells from 11 day ascites bearing EL4 animals were added to a test allogeneic CMC generation culture containing C57BL6 responder spleen cells and irradiated BALB/C stimulator cells. As cell mixing controls, normal thymus, normal spleen, or normal lymph node cells were also added. It can be seen that the thymus cells and spleen cells from tumor bearing animals markedly suppressed this allogeneic response, thus demonstrating the suppression present in the thymus and spleen was not tumor specific but indeed was capable of inhibiting an allogeneic response. It is interesting to note that the lymph node cells of the same tumor bearing animals were not suppressive. This is consistent with the previous data demonstrating that the appearance of suppression in regional lymph nodes occurs later in the course of tumor bearing than in the spleen or thymus.

275

Table 5—ABILITY OF SPLEEN, THYMUS AND LYMPH NODE FROM ASCITES BEARING EL4 ANIMALS TO INHIBIT ALLOGENEIC CYTOTOXICITY GENERATION BY NORMAL C57 BL/6 SPLEEN CELLS

Test allogeneic CMC generation culture		C57 BL6 cells added	% cytotoxicity at 8:1 L/T ratio		% suppression
Responder	Stimulator		EL4	LSTRA	
C57 BL/6	+ BALB/c	—	3	39	—
C57 BL/6	+ BALB/c	TBA* thymus	0	-1	100
C57 BL/6	+ BALB/c	normal thymus	3	36	—
C57 BL/6	+ BALB/c	TBA spleen	-1	-4	100
C57 BL/6	+ BALB/c	normal spleen	4	51	—
C57 BL/6	+ BALB/c	TBA lymph nodes**	4	49	0
C57 BL/6	+ BALB/c	normal lymph nodes	2	50	—

* TBA (tumor bearing animal) = cells from 11 day ascites EL4 bearing animals.
**Lymph node = non-mesenteric lymph nodes.

DISCUSSION

These data were gathered in an attempt to define a changing cell mediated immunoregulatory balance in a tumor bearing host. Cytotoxic and suppressor potentials of cells from various lymphoid organs of tumor bearing animals were determined over time after tumor inoculation in an attempt to define the relationship and balance between positive antitumor and negative generalized cell mediated immune mechanisms. The assay system used was the generation, in a mixed tumor-lymphocyte culture, of tumor-specific cytotoxic cells. The data demonstrate an early augmented cytotoxic response to tumor cells which is restricted to stimulation by tumor cells (i.e. allogeneic cytotoxicity is not augmented) and is compartmentalized to the draining regional lymph nodes. Eventually, concomitant with the development of immunity, is the appearance, in other lymphoid organs (spleen and thymus), of cells capable of suppressing the response, to tumor, of normally responsive lymphocytes. Ultimately, suppression overtakes all lymphoid tissue within the tumor bearing host and becomes the overwhelming and predominant immunologic mode with complete loss of ability to mount an *in vitro* antitumor response where, with less tumor burden, one had been present previously.

Implicit in the above described data is the concept that, at least in this transplantable tumor system, the tumor itself stimulates both a positive, tumor specific destructive immune response as well as a generalized, negative immunosuppressive cell mediated response. If immune manipulations are to be effective in immunotherapy, either in the experimental model or in man, direct attempts to stimulate a host's immune apparatus, either with active specific or nonspecific active immunostimulation, one must have a immunostimulatable environment. Immunotherapy is designed to modulate the host's immunologic environment which favors tumor growth. One must therefore, prior to any active immunotherapeutic maneuver, remove or assess the presence of any suppressive mode present in a tumor bearing animal before being able to stimulate the antitumor immune system of that animal. Therefore, attempts should be made to shift any possible negative immunoregulatory balances that exist in a tumor bearing host prior to immunotherapeutic stimulation. Perhaps approaches in the future which can be directed at different functional properties of lymphoid subpopulations will prove more promising than past attempts.

REFERENCES

1. Kamo, I., Friedman, H., "Immunosuppression and the Role of Suppressive Factors in Cancer." *Advances in Cancer Research* 25:271, 1977.
2. Hellström, K., and Hellström, I., "Lymphocyte-mediated Cytotoxicity and Blocking Serum Activity to Tumor Antigens." *Advances in Immunology* 18:209, 1974.

3. Nimberg, R.B., Glasgow, A., Menzoion, J., et al., "Isolation of an Immunosuppressive Peptide Fraction from the Serum of Cancer Patients." *Cancer Research* 35:1489, 1975.
4. Holmberg, B., "The Effect on Cell Multiplication *in vitro* on a Dialysable Polypeptide Derived from Tumor Fluids." *Eur. J. Cancer* 4:271, 1968.
5. Cooperband, S., Bondevik, H., Schmid, K., and Mannik, J., "Transformation of Human Lymphocytes: Inhibition by Homologous Alpha Globulin." *Science* 159:1243, 1968.
6. Fujimoto, S., Green, M.I., and Sebon, A.H., "Regulation of the Immune Response to Tumor Antigens. II. The Nature of Immunosuppressor Cells in Tumor-Bearing Hosts." *J. Immunol.* 116:800, 1976.
7. Pope, B., Whitney, R., and Levy, J., "Two Distinct Populations of Suppressor Cells in the Spleens of Mice Bearing Methylcholanthrene-Induced Tumors." *J. Immunol.* 120:2033, 1978.

Properties of Antigens and Adjuvants Which Stimulate Cell Mediated Immunity+

Robert Hunter[1]
F. Strickland[1]

SUMMARY—We are developing procedures for selectively stimulating cell mediated immunity and suppressing the growth of malignant tumors. In our basic model, bovine serum albumin (BSA) is chemically conjugated with a variety of organic moieties. Antigens which can stimulate strong sustained delayed type hypersensitivity (DTH) specific for BSA without stimulating detectable antibody formation have been developed. All of the preparations which stimulate DTH in guinea pigs consist of BSA conjugated with large hydrophobic groups. They are surface active agents with a strong affinity for cell membranes and an unusual ability to localize in the paracortical area of lymph nodes draining the site of injection into animals.

The chemical conjugation procedures developed with BSA have been applied to a membrane antigen preparation from an SV40-induced fibrosarcoma in the hamster. Lipid (dodecanoic acid) conjugation changed this antigen from one which could enhance tumor growth to one which could suppress it. In a number of assays, including microcytotoxicity, blast transformation of lymphoid cells, immunofluorescence, and histology, lipid conjugation of the tumor membrane antigens increased their ability to stimulate cell mediated immunity and decreased their ability to stimulate tumor specific antibody and serum blocking factors.

We are further exploring methods for eliciting cell mediated immunity by varying the adjuvants for these antigens. The detergent-like glycolipid fraction P3 (trehalose dimycolate) isolated from the tubercule bacillus has been shown to be a very effective adjuvant for DTH to protein antigens. We found that certain synthetic detergents (Pluronic polyols) when emulsified with oil and BSA in saline could also act as adjuvants for DTH, as measured by footpad swelling and histology. We are currently determining the physical chemical properties of the antigen-adjuvant complexes required to initiate cell mediated immune responses.

The ability to selectively stimulate cell mediated immunity against important antigens such as those on cancer cells is the goal of our project and is obviously not an accomplished fact. Nevertheless, events of the past few years have made this a realistic goal which we can expect to approach much more closely in the next few years. Tubercle bacilli have long been used as a model of antigens which selectively stimulate delayed type

[1]Department of Pathology, University of Chicago, Chicago, Illinois.
+Supported by USPHS Grants CA14364 and RCDA CA 00032.

279

hypersensivity. One way of stating the basic scientific problem of these studies is to ask why tubercle bacilli stimulate delayed type hypersensivity against tuberculin, while tuberculin itself stimulates only antibody. This question has been studied by many investigators who have taken tubercle bacilli apart and have tried to isolate the active components, then the active molecules of those components, and finally the active sites on the molecules. This approach has been quite successful. Dr. Ribi and his colleagues at the N.I.H. have isolated a simple glycolipid, trehalose dimycolate or P3, which is a very powerful adjuvant (1). In addition, Dr. Chedid and his colleagues in Paris have isolated a small very active molecular component of cell walls, muramyldepeptide (2). When given in the proper vehicles, these two components have many of the adjuvant functions of the intact tubercule bacillus.

Our approach to this problem has been quite different. Instead of looking for the active molecular components of protein adjuvants, we started with the hypothesis that many of the immunologic properties of molecules may not be due to any active site, determinant or receptor, but are due to the physical chemical properties of the entire molecule and vehicle in which it is administered. We were looking for totally nonspecific factors which were able to control both the intensity and the direction specific immune responses. A search for nonspecific factors capable of controlling specific reactions may be unorthodox for immunology, but there is ample precedent for this type of approach in the pharmacology literature. Even though the particular action of a drug is determined by its active sites, the intensity and duration of the action are largely determined by nonspecific factors such as charged hydrophobicity (3). These factors determine how a drug is distributed in body fluids, much of its interaction with cell membranes, and its rate of transport and elimination and a search for them could bring immunology closer to a mainstream of biologic thought.

The basic model for these studies was developed by Dr. John Coon in our laboratory (4). He found that the covalent attachment of relatively large numbers of fatty acids to bovine serum albumin (BSA) depressed and occasionally abolished the ability of the material to stimulate antibody and enhanced its ability to stimulate delayed type hypersensivity in the guinea pig. Subsequent studies with BSA conjugated with a wide variety of materials has suggested that the critical property of the conjugates which stimulate delayed type hypersensivity is that the protein is conjugated with a sufficient quantity of large hydrophobic materials (5,6). In the most active preparations, the protein has been made into a surface active agent which is able to form micelles. These lipid conjugated antigens are localized in the paracortical area of lymph nodes in a pattern quite different from that of the native proteins.

In a related series of experiments, some of the properties of adjuvants which increased the intensity of delayed type hypersensitivity stimulated by lipid conjugated proteins have been studied. A BCG cell wall emulsion prepared by Dr. Ribi was found to be particularly effective (7). This emulsion consists of minute droplets of oil to which BCG cell walls have been attached. This emulsion was found to be an effective antigen if and only if the cell walls were attached to the oil droplets and remained so after injection into the animal. This type of emulsion has served as a model for further studies.

Since the chemically modified proteins which stimulated delayed type hypersensitivity were surface active agents and adjuvants such as trehalose dimycolate, endotoxin and dimethyl dioctadecyl ammonium bromide, DDA, were also surface active agents, a series of experiments were designed in an effort to determine if materials could behave as adjuvants because of their surface active properties and independently of any active sites which they might possess. The pluronic polyol detergents manufactured by BASF Wyandotte, Wyandotte, Michigan were selected for these studies because a wide range of compounds can be obtained which are composed of simple identical subunits. Pluronic polyols consist of a hydrophobic core of polyoxypropylene and two hydrophilic ends of polyoxyethelene, Figure 1.

Figure 1—THE POLYOXYETHYLENE HYDROPHILIC AND POLYOXYPROPYLENE HYDROPHOBIC POLYMERS

STRUCTURE OF PLURONIC POLYOL DETERGENTS

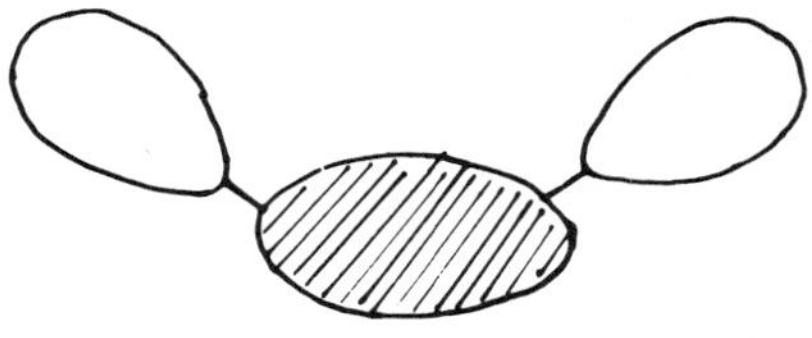

HYDROPHIL - hydrophob - HYDROPHIL

$$HO(CH_2CH_2O)_M (\overset{CH_3}{CHCH_2O})_N (CH_2CH_2O)_M H$$

They have been combined in various configurations and proportions to produce a series of over thirty detergents which vary greatly in their physical, chemical and biologic properties.

By varying the molecular weight of the hydrophobic and hydrophilic portions, a series of detergents have been produced which span almost the entire range of activities of available non-ionic detergents. The detergents were prepared as oil in water emulsions with ^{125}I labeled BSA or lipid conjugated BSA. Fifty microliters of the detergent was homogenized with 100 microliters of oil and 1 milligram of ^{125}I labeled antigen. After thorough mixing, the preparation was homogenized in 2cc of phosphate buffer saline (PBS) containing 0.2% tween 80. The emulsion was then injected into the rear foot pads of random bred CF1 mice, 0.05 ml per foot. Table 1 shows

Table 1—PHYSICAL AND BIOLOGIC PROPERTIES OF SELECTED PLURONIC POLYOLS

Emulsion	Interfacial Tension dynes/cm	Mouse LD_{50}	Emulsion Stability 7 Days	Retention in Foot 10 days	Antibody Day 20	Cell Mediated S.I. Day 20
F108 DRAKEOL L-BSA	14.3	5 gm/kg	0%	0%	0	1
P103 DRAKEOL L-BSA	8.5	1.4gm/kg	0%	0.6%	0	1
L101 DRAKEOL L-BSA	3.5	140mg/kg	48%	53%	1/40	7.5
L101 EICOSANE L-BSA	3.5	140mg/kg	60%	34%	1/20	44
L101 DRAKEOL BSA	3.5	140mg/kg	41%	99%	1/160	1.8
L101 EICOSANE BSA	3.5	140mg/kg	51%	39%	1/160	3.6

The detergents F108, P103, and L101 were prepared in emulsions with BSA or L-BSA and a hydrocarbon as described in the text. The ability of the detergents to reduce interfacial tension between oil and water and their intravenous L.D. 50 were supplied by the manufacturer. Emulsion stability is expressed as the precent of the protein retained by the oil droplets after 7 days at 37°C and as the percent of the injected dose retained near the site of injection in the foot at 10 days. Antibody is expressed as a hemagglutination titer at 20 days after a single foot pad injection. The red cells were coated with BSA. Cell mediated immunity after similar immunization is expressed as the stimulation index (S.I.) of the incorporation of ^{H} 3-thymidine by cells cultured with BSA divided by the unstimulated control values.

some of the results of experiments using these preparations. Three detergents are shown on this table. All have identical polyoxypropylene hydrophobic cores of molecular weight approximately 3250. L101, P103 and F108 have polyoxyethylene hydrophilic groups of 10%, 30% and 80% respectively. These three materials differ greatly in their biologic and physical properties. L101 was very much more toxic to mice following intravenous injection. It was able to retain 48% of the ^{125}I labeled L-BSA in the emulsion at 7 days *in vitro* and it caused 53% retention in the foot following injection into the foot pad. Finally, L101 acted as an effective adjuvant for the production of both antibody and cell-mediated immunity. The other two detergents, P103 and F108, had none of these activities.

Drakeol is mineral oil, USP. It consists of hydrocarbons with an average chain length of about 15. When this was replaced by eicosane, a hydrocarbon of chain length 20, the emulsion produced was more stable *in vitro* but less was retained in the foot. It produced less antibody, but a markedly increased cell mediated immune reaction. If BSA was substituted for lipid conjugated BSA in these emulsions, results were generally similar except that the antibody titer was higher in the cell mediated response lower than that found with L-BSA. In addition, the combination of L101, Drakeol and BSA consistently caused retention of nearly the entire injected dose in the foot.

In the course of these experiments, it was found that relatively minor changes in the vehicle or detergent adjuvant have profound effects on the immune response produced. Four examples of this are shown in Table 2. The small increment in size is accompanied by large differences in physical chemical and biologic properties. The hydrophillipophil balance, HLB, of L121 is 0.5 compared with 1.0 for L101. In addition, a 0.01% solution reduces the interfacial tension between oil and water to 8.2 dynes/cm compared to 3.5 dynes/cm for L101. Finally, the inclusion of L121 in antigen emulsions generally promoted the production of more antibody and

Table 2—EXAMPLES OF THE ABILITY OF DETERGENTS AND VEHICLES TO INFLUENCE THE TYPE OF IMMUNE RESPONSE

Immunogen Preparation[a]	Type of Immune Response[b]
Drakeol L121 BSA	IgG$_1$ antibody
Eicosane L121 BSA	IgG$_2$ antibody
Eicosane L101 L-BSA	Delayed hypersensitivity
Drakeol L131 L-BSA—4 days	Sinus histiocytosis
Eicosane L101 L-BSA—10 days	

[a] All preparations were given as emulsion in single doses as described in the text.
[b] The class of antibody was determined 20 days after immunization by radio-immunoelectrophoresis using ^{125}I-BSA and class specific antisera.

less cell mediated immunity than L101. The combination of L121, Drakeol and BSA regularly produced high antibody titer which was almost exclusively of the IgG 1 subclass as measured by radioimmunoelectrophoresis using subclass specific antibody. L121 is physically similar to L101 except that it is 10% larger. If the Drakeol was replaced by eicosane in these emulsions the animals also produced a high titer of antibody but the majority of this antibody was of the IgG 2 subclass with only a small amount of IgG 1 antibody. Of the preparations evaluated to date, the highest intensity of delayed hypersensitivity was produced by emulsions containing L101, eicosane and L-BSA. The amount of antibody produced by these emulsions was greatly reduced by conjugation of BSA with fatty acids moieties.

Sinus histiocytosis is a histologic pattern of proliferation in lymph nodes which is frequently found in association with malignant tumors. It is associated with a good prognosis. Sinus histiocytosis is characterized by dialated sinuses which are filled with a synctial mass of macrophages or histiocytes and cords which are enlarged and filled with small lymphocytes. It has been quite difficult to find suitable animal models of this histologic change. The two emulsions shown produced an extreme hypertrophy and sinus histiocytosis of popliteal lymph nodes of a portion of the mice injected, Fig. 2.

DISCUSSION

Some of the pluronic polyols are very effective adjuvants and others have no detectable adjuvant activity. Since all of the members of this series are composed of identical subunits, it is difficult to postulate that the huge differences in biologic activity are due to the presence of any specific receptors or determinants on one molecule that are not present in the others. All of the polyol detergents are made with the same chemical reactions in the same equipment. They are highly purified, homogeneous compounds. This makes it unlikely that the differences between them in biologic activity are due to contaminants. It is possible that there are conformational determinants on these molecules, but they have to be composed entirely of polyoxyethylene and polyoxypropylene. It seems much more likely that the differences in biologic activity are, in fact, due to differences in surface active properties. Part of this activity is undoubtedly due to their ability to promote the retention of protein antigen on the oil droplets and to form depots within tissue. However, it is difficult to explain all their biologic activities on this basis. Their abilities to influence the type as well as the intensity of the immune responses seem to require a more complex explanation. Based on available evidence, it is reasonable to postulate that there are at least three components to the adjuvant activity of these detergents. The first is to promote retention of the antigen within the oil

284

**Figure 2—PHOTOMICROGRAPH OF A SECTION OF A
MOUSE POPLITEAL LYMPH NODE REMOVED 10 DAYS
AFTER INJECTION OF EICOSANE-LBSA-L101.**

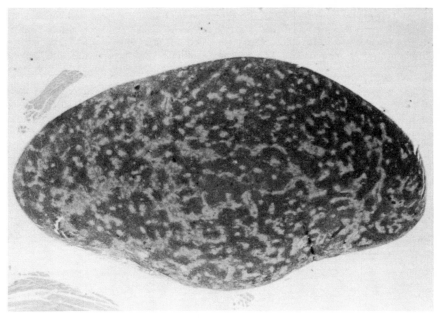

It is massively enlarged and shows the typical changes of sinus-histiocytosis, Hematox-lyn + eosin, 15 x magnification.

droplets and to form a depot within the animals tissue. The second is to have a direct stimulating effect on certain cells of the lymphoid system. This may be simply a manifestation of toxic or irritating properties or it may be more selective. Finally, the particular members of the pluronic polyol series which form effective adjuvants markedly reduce the interfacial tension between oil and water. This property would promote the contact between oil droplets and cell surfaces of many types.

Relatively minor changes in immunizing vehicles and detergent adjuvants are able to produce marked qualitative as well as quantitative changes in immune responses. In studying factors which control the production of various types of immune responses, most immunologists have searched for specific receptors or determinants of various kinds. The present work suggests that nonspecific physical chemical properties such as charge, hydrophobicity, solubility and surface activity may also be very important in determining both the type and intensity of the responses produced. Further study of these factors is likely to produce more effective means of controlling immune responses.

REFERENCES

1. Ribi, E., Toubiana, R., Strain, M.S., et al., "Further Studies on the Structural Requirements of Agents for Immunotherapy of the Guinea Pig Line-10 Tumor." *Cancer Immunol. Immunother.* 3:171-177, 1978.
2. Chedid, L. and Audibert, F., "Recent Advances in the Use of the Synthetic Immunoadjuvants Muramyl Dipeptide and Analogues." In *Microbiology-1977,* edited by David Schlessinger. Amer. Soc. for Microbiol., Washington, D.C., p. 388, 1977.
3. Hansch, C., "A Computerized Approach to Quantitative Biochemical Structure-Activity Relationships." In *Biological Correlations—The Hansch Approach,* edited by Robert F. Gould, Amer. Chem. Soc., Washington, D.C., 1972.
4. Coon, J. and Hunter, R.L., "Selective Induction of Delayed Type Hypersensitivity by a Lipid Conjugated Protein Antigen Which Is Localized in Thymus Dependent Lymphoid Tissue." *J. Immunol.* 110:183-190, 1973.
5. Dailey, M.O. and Hunter, R.L., "Induction of Cell Mediated Immunity to Chemically Modified Antigens in Guinea Pigs. I. Characterization of the Immune Response to Lipid Conjugated Protein Antigens." *J. Immunol.* 118:957-962, 1977.
6. Coon, J. and Hunter, R., "Properties of Conjugated Protein Immogens Which Selectively Stimulate Delayed Type Hypersensitivity." *J. Immunol.* 114:1518-1522, 1975.
7. Champlin, R. and Hunter, R., "Studies on the Composition of Adjuvants Which Selectively Enhance Delayed-Type Hypersensitivity to Lipid Conjugated Protein Antigens." *J. Immunol.* 114:76-80, 1975.

Passive Transfer of Tumor Immunity *In Vivo* Using Cytotoxic Cells Generated *In Vitro*†

Irwin D. Bernstein[1]
O. Alaba[1]
P. Wright[1]

SUMMARY—Although current evidence indicates that prevention of tumor growth is mediated by immune lymphoid cells, an understanding of the mechanism(s) by which immune cells eliminate tumor *in vivo* has not been achieved. We have studied immune cell populations which have been enriched for effector activity following *in vitro* culture in the presence of tumor antigens. Rat lymphoid cells stimulated in an *in vitro* secondary immune response to a Gross virus-induced (C58NT)D syngeneic lymphoma proliferate and differentiate into cytotoxic cells *in vitro*. These cells demonstrate a marked increase in their ability to confer anti-tumor protection *in vivo*. Our studies indicate that *in vitro* sensitized cells inhibit tumor growth by two mechanisms—one involving a direct presumably cytotoxic effect of immune lymphoid cells on tumor target cells, and a second indirect effect mediated by an interaction with a nonimmune, radiosensitive, bone marrow derived host cell. Additional studies have shown these cell-mediated reactions against (C58NT)D to represent at least in part, a response to murine leukemia virus.

Resistance to growth of an inoculum of antigenic tumor cells can be mediated by lymphoid cells *in vivo* or *in vitro* (1-3). Nevertheless, the adoptive transfer of immune cells has not proven in most cases to be effective in causing regression of established neoplastic disease, nor has the mechanism(s) by which immune cells, upon transfer to naive recipients, prevent growth of a tumor inoculum been clarified. We have taken an approach in which lymphoid cells are sensitized *in vitro* against tumor antigen to allow for generation of highly active cells lytic for tumor *in vitro* and which can mediate tumor growth prevention *in vivo*. This approach will hopefully prove effective for the immunotherapy of neoplasia and also may allow a better understanding of the cell-mediated suppression of tumor growth. We have established a rat tumor model system in which spleen cells obtained from rats previously primed to syngeneic virus-induced lymphoma cells can be reactivated *in vitro* so that they generate the capacity to kill tumor cells *in vitro*.

[1]Divisions of Pediatric Oncology and Tumor Immunology, Fred Hutchinson Cancer Research Center, and Departments of Pediatrics, Medicine, and Microbiology, University of Washington, Seattle, Washington.

†Supported by National Cancer Institute, DHEW, grants CA19170 and CA17481.

In the studies presented here, we will (1) briefly describe a model system in which cells activated *in vitro* to tumor antigen can mediate tumor growth prevention *in vivo;* (2) review evidence that these cells eliminate tumor *in vivo* directly and also indirectly by cooperating with host nonimmune bone marrow cells; and (3) present recent studies suggesting antigens of the murine leukemia virus (MuLV) to be associated with the antitumor response *in vivo* and *in vitro*.

The model system used by us is diagrammed in Figure 1. A syngeneic Gross virus-induced transplantable lymphoma in Wistar Furth rats was used (4). When 10^7 lymphoma cells, designated (C58NT)D, are injected subcutaneously into adult males, the tumor grows, reaches maximal size at day 10-12, and then regresses completely by day 20. Herberman and coworkers (5) have shown that lymphoid cells obtained from rats when the tumor is present are cytotoxic for tumor cells in a short-term, direct, chromium release assay, but following regression of tumor, the cytotoxic effect is no longer detectable even though the animal will completely inhibit the growth of a second dose of 10^7 (C58NT)D cells. Reappearance of significant cytotoxic activity within the spleen is not associated with this secondary tumor challenge (5). In order to generate cytotoxic effector cells, we sensitized immune spleen cells obtained following tumor regression at 4-6 weeks in an *in vitro* secondary immune response by co-cultivation with tumor antigen. Co-cultivation of 2.5×10^6 responding spleen cells cultured with 8×10^4 (C58NT)D cells for five days was shown to be optimal (6). Resultant cells were tested for cytotoxic activity using a standard four hour ^{51}Cr release assay. *In vitro* sensitized cells were also tested for *in vivo* activity by injecting the immune lymphoid cells systemically via the intracardiac route followed by a subcutaneous challenge with viable tumor cells with the (C58NT)D cells or 10^7 cells of a variant line designated (C58NT)D-F which will grow progressively and kill non-immune animals.

In initial studies, W/Fu rats previously immunized with syngeneic lymphoma (C58NT)D cells were observed to retain the capacity to generate significant proliferative and cytotoxic activity upon re-exposure to tumor antigens *in vitro* (6, 7). Spleen cells from W/Fu rats obtained 4-6 weeks after immunization with (C58NT)D lymphoma cells lacked cytotoxicity against ^{51}Cr labelled tumor cells *in vitro*. When these same cells were cultivated *in vitro* in the presence of mitomycin C-treated (C58NT)D cells, however, they proliferated and differentiated into cells specifically cytotoxic for the tumor targets.

We found systemic inoculation of as many as 15×10^7 immune spleen cells from rats primed 4-6 weeks earlier with (C58NT)D cells or even 7.5×10^7 spleen cells from animals following rechallenge *in vivo* with living tumor cells 5, 7, or 10 days previously, did not effectively confer antitumor protection on nonimmune recipients against challenge with 10^6 (C58NT)D cells (8). On

288

Figure 1—DIAGRAMMATIC REPRESENTATION OF MODEL SYSTEM USED TO ACTIVATE LYMPHOCYTES *IN VITRO* WHICH CAN LYSE TUMOR TARGETS *IN VITRO* AND CAN MEDIATE TUMOR GROWTH PREVENTION *IN VIVO*

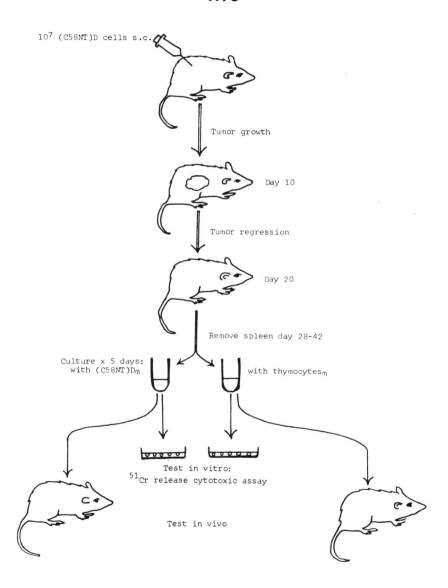

10^7 (C58NT)D cells s.c.

Tumor growth

Day 10

Tumor regression

Day 20

Remove spleen day 28-42

Culture x 5 days: with (C58NT)D$_m$ with thymocytes$_m$

Test in vitro: ^{51}Cr release cytotoxic assay

Test in vivo

289

the other hand, as few as 50 million *in vitro* sensitized cells given to nonimmune recipients could confer complete protection against an otherwise lethal inoculum of 10^7 cells of a variant subline, (C58NT)D-F (8). Thus, *in vitro* sensitized cells will protect animals against a lethal inoculum of tumor cells. This effect was also specific, since the growth of a control polyoma virus-induced tumor was not affected by the restimulated effector cells. This ability to generate antitumor effector activity *in vitro* and measure these effects *in vivo* and *in vitro* was then used to explore the mechanism by which effector cells eliminate tumor *in vivo*.

Mechanism of Tumor Growth Prevention In Vivo. Little is presently known concerning the mechanism by which immune T-cells mediate tumor cell elimination *in vivo*. Although *in vitro* tests show that lymphocytes are necessary and sufficient to kill tumor cells, it is not known whether cytotoxic cell populations eliminate tumor directly *in vivo* or do it, at least in part, by other indirect mechanisms. We therefore asked whether cytotoxic cell populations generated *in vitro* require a host contribution to eliminate tumor *in vivo*, and more specifically whether they eliminate tumor, at least in part, by interacting with host nonimmune radiosensitive cells (9). The design of these experiments is presented in Figure 2. Recipient animals were

Figure 2—DIAGRAMMATIC REPRESENTATION OF EXPERIMENTAL DESIGN TO TEST COOPERATION BETWEEN PASSIVE TRANSFERRED SENSITIZED LYMPHOCYTES AND NONIMMUNE HOST CELLS IN THE IMMUNE SUPPRESSION OF TUMOR GROWTH

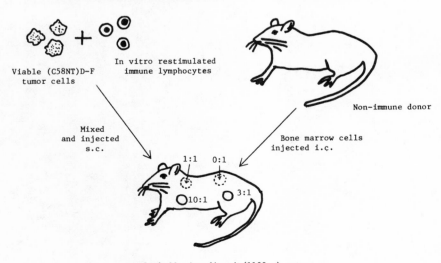

Viable (C58NT)D-F
tumor cells

In vitro restimulated
immune lymphocytes

Non-immune donor

Mixed
and injected
s.c.

Bone marrow cells
injected i.c.

1:1   0:1

10:1   3:1

Lethally irradiated (1100 r) rats

290

heavily irradiated following which some of the animals were reconstituted with 2×10^8 nonimmune cells, including either bone marrow, spleen, lymph node, thymus, or peritoneal exudate cells. These animals were then inoculated intradermally with tumor cells alone or tumor cells admixed with sensitized cells. The results of one such experiment (Figure 3) show that when 10^7 sensitized cells were mixed with the tumor cells and injected intradermally, some inhibition of tumor growth as compared to growth of tumor alone was seen in nonreconstituted rats. However, in rats reconstituted with bone marrow cells, a synergistic effect between sensitized lymphocytes and nonimmune bone marrow was observed. Reconstitution with other cell types was essentially ineffective although peritoneal exudate cells from either immune or non-immune donors contributed to decreased tumor cell growth in the presence or absence of sensitized lymphocytes. This activity possibly could be ascribed to a natural killer (NK) population since it does not represent a cell specifically recruited by immune lymphocytes at the local tumor site as the effect of PE was seen in the presence or absence of sensitized lymphocytes.

In other experiments, we have observed a quantitative relationship between the number of bone marrow cells administered and tumor growth inhibition (9). Similarly, T-cell depleted bone marrow (obtained from thymectomized thoracic duct drained rats) was able to reconstitute lethally irradiated thymectomized recipients suggesting the cooperating cell(s) not to be a T-cell (9).

These data therefore show that nonimmune bone marrow cells, although not required for tumor growth suppression, interact synergistically with immune lymphocytes; they suggest that *in vitro* sensitized cells may inhibit tumor growth *in vivo* by at least two independent mechanisms: a direct, presumably cytotoxic effect on tumor target cells and by indirect recruitment of a nonimmune, radiosensitive, bone marrow derived host cell. The relative importance of host cell recruitment in tumor cell elimination remains to be determined. It may depend on the sensitivity of the tumor to lytic effects of cytotoxic cells as compared to recruited host cells. It also may depend on the magnitude of the cytotoxic response and of the locally recruited host cell component. Thus, results differing from ours have been obtained in studies of allograft rejection. Lubaroff, using a paradigm similar to that used in the experiments described above, has shown that reconstitution of thymectomized, irradiated rats with bone marrow cells did not increase the rate of allograft rejection due to T-cells. His observation, which differs from ours, is likely a consequence of the relatively strong, specific cytotoxic response and a weak or nonexistent effect of recruited nonimmune inflammatory cells in the allograft response. Additionally, a relatively greater susceptibility of tumor to nonspecific inflammatory cells as compared to normal allogeneic cells may also account for the differences.

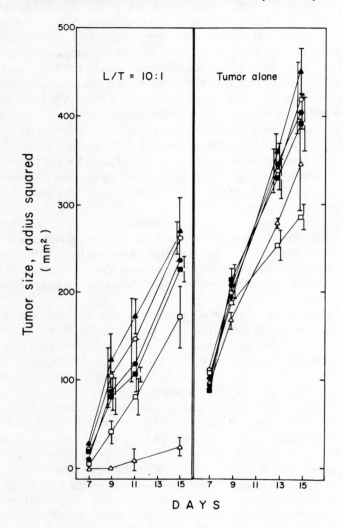

Figure 3—COOPERATION BETWEEN NONIMMUNE BONE MARROW AND SENSITIZED LYMPHOCYTES IN SUPPRESSING THE GROWTH OF (C58NT)D

Rats previously irradiated with 1100 R of total body irradiation were reconstituted with 2×10^8 bone marrow (△—△); peritoneal exudate cells (□—□); thymus (■—■) lymph node (●—●); spleen (○—○) cells or were not reconstituted (▲—▲). Growth of 10^6 (C58NT)D-F tumors alone or with 10^7 (C58NT)D immune lymphocytes mixed specifically restimulated *in* vitro over a 5 day period injected s.c. was determined. Results calculated as average radius of tumor squared (mm²) ± standard error on day of maximal tumor growth.

Association of MuLV Antigen and Cell-Mediated Anti-Tumor Responses. We have recently initiated studies in collaboration with Dr. Robert Nowinski to further define the specificity of the CMI response in our studies. This approach was appealing since there is a strong cytotoxic response and an associated murine leukemia virus of AKR mouse origin (AKR MuLV) is readily available. Earlier studies by Shellam, et al. (10) and Bruce, et al. (11) showed AKR MuLV to stimulate the generation of cytotoxic cells in the *in vitro* secondary response to Gross lymphoma cells.

In our own studies, we first confirmed that AKR MuLV could specifically initiate the *in vitro* differentiation of killer cells from their primed pre-cursors. As few as 0.25 ug/ml concentration disrupted AKR MuLV could stimulate the secondary activation of anti-(C58NT)D killer cells *in vitro*. The effect was specific since cells from rats primed with (C58NT)D, upon culture with virus, became cytotoxic for ^{51}Cr labelled (C58NT)D cells and not allogeneic (BN) Kirsten virus-induced lymphoma cells; on the other hand, cells from W/Fu rats primed to BN alloantigen, upon *in vitro* exposure to the mitomycin inactivated BN lymphoma cells became highly cytotoxic for the allogeneic target (Table 1). However, while confirming the known ability of unlabelled (C58NT)D targets to competitively inhibit (Table 2), we have been consistently unable to competitively inhibit with virus in the ^{51}Cr release assay. Although there have been reports of inhibition of cytotoxicity by p30 (11), the results of our studies suggest to us that the viral antigens are associated with the secondary cytotoxic response,

Table 1—SPECIFICITY OF CYTOTOXIC ACTIVITY GENERATED IN SECONDARY *IN VITRO* RESPONSE TO AKR-MuLV AND BN RAT ALLOANTIGENS

W/Fu responding spleen cells from rats primed with*	Stimulating antigen†	% specific cytotoxicity**	
		(C58NT)D targets	BN targets
(C58NT)D	AKR-MuLV	32.1	-0.3
	BN lymphoma cells	3.5	4.1
BN rat spleen cells	AKR-MuLV	-4.4	0.7
	BN lymphoma cells	-1.0	33.0

*Rats were primed with BN skin grafts or 10^7 (C58NT)D cells 4-6 weeks earlier.
†2.5 x 10^6 responding cells were stimulated with AKR-MuLV at a concentration of 1 ug/ml or 8 x 10^5 mitomycin inactivated BN rat spleen cells.
**Cells were tested for cytotoxic activity at a 30:1 attacker to target cell ratio. Target cells were ^{51}Cr labelled (C58NT)D cells or BN Kirsten virus-induced lymphoma cells. % cytotoxicity calculated as percentage of cytotoxicity of tumor cell cultures—percentage of cytotoxicity of control thymocytes and percentage of cytotoxicity $= S\text{-}S_o/S_m S_o$ where S =supernatant counts after lysis, S_o =supernatant counts from target cells incubated in presence of excess unlabelled target cells at end of assay; and S_m =supernatant counts in three times freeze-thawed tubes, i.e., 100% lysis.

Table 2—INHIBITION OF ANTI-(C58NT)D KILLER CELLS BY LYMPHOMA CELLS BUT NOT AKR-MuLV

Concentration of inhibitor (Ratio of unlabelled inhibitor cells: target cells)†		% specific cytotoxicity*
5×10^5 (C58NT)D cells	20:1	-6.9
5×10^4 (C58NT)D cells	1.1	12.8
200 ug AKR MuLV	——	24.2
50 ug AKR MuLV	——	21.8
——	——	23.8

2.5×10^6 responding spleen cells from rats primed with 10^7 (C58NT)D cells were cultured with AKR-MuLV at 0.25 ug/ml for five days at 37°C in 5% CO_2 in air. Resultant cells were tested for cytotoxic activity against ^{51}Cr labelled (C58NT)D targets.

†Unlabelled tumor cells or virus was added to the reactants as inhibitors in the cytotoxic assay. Effector cells were added at a 30:1 attacker target cell ratio.

*% specific cytotoxicity calculated as in Table 1.

but since they do not effectively compete with the cytotoxic targets, the virus probably represents only a portion or an unmodified form of the antigen.

We next tested whether noninfectious virus could initiate the generation of specific cytotoxic cell precursors. Rats were primed with either 10^7 viable tumor cells, which express viral antigen on the surface, or 40 ug of 10X freeze-thawed noninfectious virus in complete Freund's adjuvant; the rats were then studied for anti-tumor responses *in vitro* and *in vivo*. Table 3 shows that when spleen cells obtained from these rats were activated *in vitro*, both spleen cell preparations proliferated following *in vitro* exposure either to virus or to mitomycin C-inactivated (C58NT)D cells as measured by incorporation of ^3H-thymidine. However, only the cells from the rats primed with tumor could differentiate into lytic cells detectable with the ^{51}Cr release assay. These results suggest that noninfectious cell-free virus initiate a T-helper response, as shown by the proliferative response, but no cytotoxic response. Consistent with this suggestion was our finding that serum from these rats primed with noninfectious virus contain specific anti-viral antibodies directed against gp70 and p30 (Bernstein, I.D., and Nowinski, R., Manuscript in preparation). On the other hand, only cell-bound virus, i.e., tumor cells, stimulated a cytotoxic response.

We also tested the *in vivo* activity of these restimulated spleen cells. 3×10^6 spleen cells obtained following restimulation with mitomycin inactivated tumor cells were mixed with an equal number of (C58NT)D tumor cells and injected subcutaneously into normal recipients; an equal number of tumor cells was injected into the contralateral flank as a control. Both immune cell populations inhibited tumor growth (Table 4). These results demonstrate that noncytotoxic immune cells from rats primed with cell-free virus are

294

Table 3—CELL-MEDIATED REACTIVITY TO TUMOR CELLS AND TUMOR VIRUS

Responding spleen cells from rats primed with:	Stimulating antigen†	Blastogenic response (S/C)* (cpm incorporated ³H-thymidine)	% cytotoxity**
inactivated virus	virus	15.7	-0.1
	NTD	13.9	-0.2
(C58NT)D cells	virus	9.4	48.0
	NTD	16.2	98.0
	——	——	——

Cells obtained from rats primed with 40 ug inactivated AKR-MuLV in complete Freund's adjuvant or with 10^7 (C58NT)D cells were cultivated *in vitro* in the presence of virus or tumor antigen and evaluated for proliferative and cytotoxic activity.

†2.5 x 10^6 responding cells were cultivated with 8 x 10^4 mitomycin inactivated (C58NT)D cells or 1.0 ug/ml AKR MuLV for five days at 37°C in 5% CO_2.

$$*S/C = \frac{\text{cpm incorporated in stimulated cultures}}{\text{cpm incorporated in unstimulated cultures}}$$

**% cytotoxicity calculated as in Table 1. Effector cells tested against ^{51}Cr labelled (C58NT)D cells at a 10:1 attacker to target cell ratio.

Table 4—INHIBITION OF TUMOR GROWTH DUE TO IMMUNE CELLS

Immune cell donor primed with†	Growth of 3 x 10^6 (C58NT)D cells mixed with 3 x 10^6 immune cells*	Growth of 3 x 10^6 (C58NT)D cells alone
virus	0	43.8 ± 30.8
(C58NT)D	0	35.4 ± 10.1

Comparison of *in vitro* restimulated immune cells from donors primed with 10^7 (C58NT)D cells or 40 ug disrupted AKR-MuLV in complete Freund's adjuvant.

†2.5 x 10^6 responding cells were cultivated *in vitro* with 8 x 10^4 mitomycin inactivated (C58NT)D cells for five days at 37°C in 5% CO_2 in air.

*Presented as average radius of tumor squared (mm²) ± standard error on day of maximal tumor growth in unirradiated recipients day 9.

effective *in vivo*. However, their mechanism of action remains to be defined. They may eliminate tumor by a delayed hypersensitivity mechanism which would explain our earlier observation of synergy between sensitized cell and nonimmune bone marrow, since the latter contains cells responsible for the

295

cellular infiltrate at delayed inflammatory reactions. Alternatively, antibody producing cells or cytotoxic immune cells may be induced in the host by these cells. Further studies are in progress to discriminate between these alternatives.

In summary, our studies have shown that lymphoid cells restimulated *in vitro* are effective in eliminating tumor cells both *in vitro* and *in vivo*. They act *in vivo* by a direct, presumably cytotoxic, effect and also indirectly by cooperating with host nonimmune bone marrow cells. The latter mechanisms may represent at least in part, noncytotoxic cells responding to viral antigen; the cytotoxic response to tumor is also directed against viral antigen, but probably in a modified form or in association with other cell surface components.

REFERENCES

1. Klein, G., Sjögren, H.O., Klein, E., and Hellström, K.E., "Demonstration of Resistance Against Methylcholanthrene-Induced Sarcomas in the Primary Autochthonous Host." *Cancer Res.* 20:1561-1572, 1960.
2. Fefer, A., In: *Handbook of Experimental Pharmacology,* Edited by Sartorelli, A.C., and Johns, D.G., vol. 38(1):529.
3. Alexander, P., "Immunotherapy of Cancer. Experience with Primary Sarcoma in the Rat. *Progr. Exp. Tumor Res.* 10:22-71, 1968.
4. Geering, G., Old, L.J., and Boyse, E.A., "Antigens of Leukemias Induced by Naturally Occurring Murine Leukemia Virus: Their Relation to the Antigen of Gross Virus and Other Murine Leukemia Viruses." *J. Exp. Med.* 124:753-772, 1966.
5. Herberman, R.B., and Oren, M.E., "Immune Response to Gross Virus-Induced Lymphoma. I. Kinetics of Cytotoxic Antibody Response." *J. Natl. Cancer Inst.* 46:391-396, 1971.
6. Bernstein, I.D., Wright, P.W., and Cohen, E., "Generation of Cytotoxic Lymphocytes *In Vitro:* Response of Immune Rat Spleen Cells to a Syngeneic Gross Virus-Induced Lymphoma in Mixed Lymphocyte-Tumor Culture." *J. Immunol.* 116:1367-1372, 1976.
7. Bernstein, I.D., Cohen, E.F., and Wright, P.W., "Relationship of Cellular Proliferation and the Generation of Cytotoxic Cells in an *In Vitro* Secondary Immune Response to Syngeneic Rat Lymphoma Cells." *J. Immunol.* 118:1090-1094, 1977.
8. Bernstein, I.D., "Passive Transfer of Systemic Tumor Immunity with Cells Generated *In Vitro* by a Secondary Immune Response to a Syngeneic Rat Gross Virus-Induced Lymphoma." *J. Immunol.* 118:122-128, 1977.
9. Alaba, O., and Bernstein, I.D., "Tumor Growth Suppression *In Vivo:* Cooperation Between Immune Lymphoid Cells Sensitized *In Vitro* and Nonimmune Bone Marrow Cells." *J. Immunol.* 120:1941-1946, 1978.
10. Shellam, G.R., Knight, R.A., Mitchison, N.A., et al., "The Specificity of Effector T Cells Activated by Tumours Induced by Murine Oncornaviruses." *Transplant. Rev.* 29:249-276, 1976.
11. Bruce, J., Mitchison, N.A., and Shellam, G.R., "Studies on a Gross Virus-Induced Lymphoma in the Rat. III. Optimization, Specificity, and Applications of the *In Vitro* Immune Response." *Int. J. Cancer* 17:342-350, 1976.

297

Immunology and Immunotherapy of the Canine Venereal Tumor+

Robert B. Epstein[1]
B. T. Bennett[1]
W. E. Beschorner[1]
A. D. Hess[1]
S. Sarpel[1]
A. Zander[1]

SUMMARY—The canine venereal tumor (CVT) is an unique neoplasm, cellularly transmitted in an outbred mammalian species. Under natural or experimental challenge, initial tumor growth is regularly seen. Approximately 40% of dogs die from local disease, 40% ultimately reject the tumor, and 20% develop metastatic dissemination. The present studies were directed at determining: 1) whether the tumor carries histocompatibility antigens detected by serologic or cell mediated testing, 2) whether the natural history of the tumor correlates with immunologic assays, 3) definition of tumor growth and rejection mechanisms, and 4) the use of the system to assay immunotherapeutic maneuvers. Initial studies revealed that tumor cells contained constant surface antigens detectable by DLA typing sera and that such cells strongly stimulated lymphocytes of prospective recipients in mixed lymphocyte tumor cell culture (MLTC). Progressive growth was associated with specific suppression of MLTC, and rejection with a return of activity. Blocking of inhibition of tumor colony growth in vitro and MLTC was mediated by IgG_{2a} immunoglobulin of progressor dog serum. Attempts to intervene immunotherapeutically in progressive tumor growth were carried out: 1) with serum from regressor animals, 2) lymphocytes from regressor animals, 3) intralesional BCG, and 4) plasmapheresis. Intralesional BCG produced clear systemic immunotherapeutic responses while plasmapheresis was effective in some dogs. Serotherapy and lymphocyte transfer were ineffective. This unique tumor system might provide a model for further studies of immune mechanisms of tumor growth and rejection in a large randomly bred species.

INTRODUCTION

The transmissible venereal tumor of canines (TVT) is a unique neoplasm occurring in an outbred mammalian species. The tumor is consistantly transmitted during intercourse and results in lesions of the genitalia in both

[1]VA West Side Medical Center and Departments of Pathology and Medicine, University of Illinois at the Medical Center, Chicago, Illinois.
+Supported by MRIS funds of the Veterans Administration West Side Medical Center and the American Cancer Society, Illinois Division.

sexes (1). The natural history of the TVT is variable, both as it occurs endemically in the canine population and under experimental conditions. Tumor growth is regularly seen following challenge. Subsequent events include a period of logarithmic growth, followed by (a) complete regression (b) indolent local disease (c) metastatic dissemination (2,3). Of critical importance, indicating the immunogenicity of these tumors, is resistance to rechallenge following regression (3).

Our laboratory has been engaged in a number of studies during the past few years directed at the following questions:

1. What factors account for the ready cellular transplantation of this neoplasm?
2. Can immunogenicity of the TVT be assessed and correlated with the variable clinical course?
3. What immunologic maneuvers alter the course of established tumors?

MATERIALS AND METHODS

Tumor Transplantation. Tumors were regularly produced in random dogs by the subcutaneous injection of 3×10^8 tumor cells per site. Palpable nodular lesions appeared between 7 and 14 days (3). At approximately weekly intervals caliper measurements of the tumors were performed in 3 perpendicular directions and the volume in mm^3 calculated as,

$$V = \frac{\pi}{6} \times \left[\frac{D_1 + D_2 + D_3 - 9}{3} \right]^3$$

(4).

All animals were routinely examined for the presence of local invasive growth or metastasis. Regression was considered to be complete when no palpable tumor could be detected.

Cytotoxicity, Testing. Canine lymphocyte and tumor cell typing were performed by a modification of the two stage microcytotoxicity technique (5). A panel of 40-60 canine alloantisera recognizing DLA specificities at both the A and B loci were used (6). In addition, sera from dogs following tumor regression were tested against random dog lymphocytes and evaluated for DLA specificity by international exchange (6).

Mixed Lymphocyte Tumor Cell Culture (MLTC) (7). Mononuclear cells were isolated from defibriginated blood on a Ficoll-Hypaque gradient. Culture medium consisted of RPMI-1640, supplemented with 100 $\mu g/ml$ streptomycin, 100 units/ml penicillin, 1% glutamine and 20% heat-inactivated pooled normal dog or autologous sera, depending on the experiment. Tumor cells were harvested from freshly excised tumors by mechanical dispersion and were irradiated with 2000 rads by a single ^{60}Co source. Two X 10^5 responder lympocytes and stimulating tumor cells were cultured in microtiter plates and incubated for 5 days at 37°C in 5% CO_2. Cultures were harvested following 16 hours of incubation with 2 μCi ^{3}H-thymidine (sp. act. 2 Ci/mmole). The blastogenic response was expressed as counts per minute of isotope incorporation, or stimulating indices as the ratio of the mixed response to the sum of control values (7).

Cloning of Tumor Cells. Tumor cells were cultured in soft agar as previously described (8). The cells were washed 3 times in a basic media containing TC-199, supplemented with sodium pyruvate, L-asparagine, and DEAE-dextran. The washed cells were combined with media in 0.3% agar so as to yield a final plating concentration of 1-4 $\times$ 10^4 cells per ml. One ml volumes were plated in 35-mm Petri dishes to which 0.1 ml of pooled normal dog sera (NDS) was added to serve as a feeder layer for cell growth. Following 48-72 hrs of incubation colonies of 20 or more tumor cells were enumerated with an inverted phase microscope. Results were expressed as average counts for duplicate plates. The effect of sera from dogs with progressively growing tumors or dogs following regression was evaluated by substituting the relevant sera for normal dog sera in the culture (8).

Immunochemical Techniques. Sera from dogs with progressing or regressing tumors were fractionated by G-200 Sephadex filtration and immunoabsorption with rabbit antiserum specific for canine IgG$_{2a}$ (9). Fractions were characterized by immunoelectrophoresis, radial immunodiffusion and disc gel electrophoresis. Protein eluates from serially removed tumors were fractionated by preparative polyacrylamide electrophoresis. Using ultrafiltration and SDS electrophoresis of tumor associated IgG at low pH, identification of antigen complexed to antibody was attempted.

Immunotherapeutic Evaluations. A series of experiments were performed to explore possible antitumor immunologic maneuvers in altering the course of established TVT lesions.
1. Serotherapy was attempted in 3 dogs. Each dogs received 1 ml/kg of antisera obtained from regressor dogs. The antisera was cytotoxic in vitro to tumor cells at a 1:16 titer and was administered IV on 4 consecutive days. Control animals received sera from normal dogs.
2. For studies of adoptive immunotherapy 5 pairs of histocompatible littermates were challenged with tumor. On days 14 and 15 of tumor growth one member of each pair received 2.5 x 10^9 lymphocytes IV obtained by leukapheresis of a regressor animal. The other member received the same dose of similarly obtained lymphocytes from a normal dog.

3. Intralesional BCG administration was carried out in one of two lesions in 6 dogs (10). One to 4×10^7 viable organisms were injected on days 14, 21, and 28 of tumor growth. Control lesions were injected with saline. Experimental dogs were paired with DLA identical littermates with growing tumors not treated with BCG but injected with saline. Tumors were followed for 100 days.
4. Plasmapheresis of 5 tumor bearing dogs was carried out using discontinuous flow centrifugation. Approximately 2 blood volumes of plasma were removed on each of 4 days over a one week period. The subsequent growth of tumors were compared to DLA identical littermates that were not plasmapheresed.

RESULTS

Course of Experimentally Transplanted TVT. The course of tumors transplanted into 52 random dogs is summarized in table 1. All dogs developed clinically palpable tumors usually within the first two weeks following transplantation. The natural history of tumor growth could be divided into three general categories. In 28 dogs spontaneous regression occurred within 6 months (rapid regressor animals). Tumors persisted in 24 animals beyond 6 months (persister animals.) Most of these dogs were ultimately sacrificed with locally infiltrating disease. Four dogs developed distant metastatic disease. These findings are consistent with the reported natural history of the TVT and the similar course seen in experiments involving cells obtained from dogs with tumors originating in geographically widely separated areas (3).

Table 1—COURSE OF TVT IN RANDOM DOGS

Total number of dogs challenged	52
Regression within 180 days	28
Persistence beyond 180 days	24
Local indolent disease	20
Metastatic dissemination	4

Serologic and Lymphocyte Stimulating Determinants on TVT Cells. Table 2 shows the results of cytotoxic typing with a panel of canine DLA alloantisera of two tumor cell lines and indicates the presence of serologically defined antigens on these cells. Further studies indicated reactivity with a group of unclassified antisera as well. Sera following tumor rejection were also found to type normal dog lymphocytes and were highly associated

Table 2— CYTOTOXICITY TESTING OF TVT CELLS OB-TAINED FROM TWO TUMOR LINES (CTVT AND MTVT)

DLA GROUP 1st SERIES	NOL OF SERA TESTED	CTVT	MTVT
1	2	—	—
2	1	—	—
3	8	+	+
7	3	—	—
8	3	± (*)	±
9	4	—	—
10	6	+	+
2nd SERIES			
4	6	—	—
5	5	—	—
6	6	—	—
11	2	—	—
12	2	—	—
13	2	—	—
UNCLASSIFIED SERA NO.			
110		+	+
113		+	+
7849		—	—
553		+	+
1645		+	+
1679		+	+
1700		—	+
2039		+	+
2075		±	+
2037		+	+
14005		—	—
C21		+	+
D0298		—	±
C16		+	+

(*) Indicates weak reaction with 2 of 3 antisera.
(±) Indicates doubtful reaction.

when analyzed for independence (3,6). Additional family studies related clinical course (regression or persistence) with DLA haplotype segregation patterns in sibships (11).

When mixed lymphocyte tumor cell cultures were carried out, vigorous stimulation was observed of dog lymphocytes prior to challenge and following regression. A significant decrease in responsiveness was noted in dogs during the period of active growth. These results are shown in Fig. 1.

Figure 1—LYMPHOCTYES OF NORMAL, TUMOR-BEARING AND REGRESSOR ANIMALS WERE TESTED IN MLTC INCUBATED IN NORMAL DOG SERA.

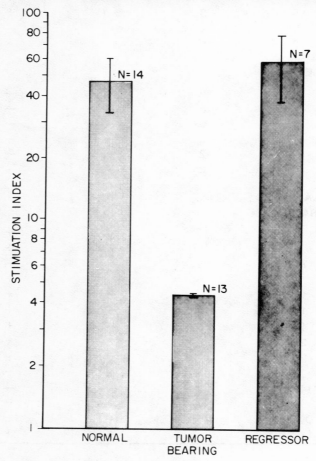

Tumor-bearing animals were tested in the proliferative phase of tumor growth (21-28 days). Results are expressed as the mean S.I. ± S.E.

304

Thus strong evidence exists for the presence of serologically detectable DLA determinants and the lymphocyte stimulating capability of TVT cells.

Serum Factors Modulating the Immunologic Response to the TVT. Initial studies indicated that the mixed lymphocyte tumor cell response was significantly depressed in tumor bearing animals and that animals with the greatest degree of depression tended to develop metastatic disease (7). Fig. 2 illustrates the effect of carrying out the cultures in serum of dogs with progressive tumors as compared to normal dog serum. It is clear that progressor serum markedly suppresses the MLTC. Additional studies using the cloning of tumor cells in soft agar revealed that tumor colony growth was inhibited by the presence of sera from regressor animals but that this inhibition could be blocked by incubating the tumor cells in serum from dogs with growing tumor. Attempts to identify the above serum blocking factors have been carried out by Beschorner, et al (9). Both serum inhibitory (regressor dogs) and blocking activity (progressor dogs) was isolated in the IgG$_{2a}$ subclass of canine immunoglobulin. Table 3 illustrates these activities in whole serum and the IgG$_{2a}$ subclass from regressor and progressor dogs. Eluates of tumor biopsies taken during the course of growth and regression were analyzed for blocking and inhibitory activity. Fig. 3 illustrates the reciprocal relation between inhibition and blocking in this study and shows the correlation of declining blocking activity and rising inhibitory activity as the tumor begins to regress.

Table 3—INHIBITORY AND BLOCKING ACTIVITY OF SERUM AND IgG

Experiment	Dog	Clinical Course	TCFUa*			
			Inhibitory		Blocking	
			Whole	IgG†	Whole	IgG†
1	NDS	—	29	28	0	4
	1666, 1680	Regression	10	6	9	5
	5154	Log Growth	31	28	30	37
2	NDS	—	52	50	4	4
	1048	Regression	6	14	2	2
	5301	Log Growth	50	51	24	40
3	NDS	—	28	ND	0	ND
	5301	Regression	0	4	4	5
	5540	Log Growth	23	15	25	23

*   TCFUa=tumor colony forming units in agar.

†   IgG$_{2a}$ purified by immunoabsorption.

Figure 2—MLTC ASSAYS OF TUMOR BEARING ANIMALS WERE CARRIED OUT USING NORMAL DOG AND AUTOLOGOUS PROGRESSOR SERA.

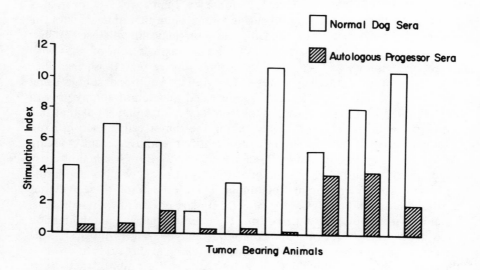

Results are expressed as the stimulating index.

Immunotherapy of the TVT. Because of the immunogenicity of the TVT an attempt was made to survey the effects of immunologic manipulation of the system in dogs with established local tumors. Initial studies consisted of infusions of TVT antisera from regressor dogs at a dose of 1 ml/kg on 4 consecutive days. Tumor growth was followed in 3 dogs and compared to controls given normal dog serum. No differences in subsequent tumor growth were noted. Passive lymphocyte transfer were carried out in 5 pairs of DLA identical littermates. Each member of the pair received 2.5×10^9 lymphocytes IV on two consecutive days, either from normal dogs, or dogs following tumor regression. Again no significant tumor response was observed. As shown in Fig. 4 a clear local and systemic effect of intralesional BCG was obtained when one of two lesions was injected on days 14, 21 and 28 following tumor challenge. In this study 6 DLA identical pairs were used. Each member of a pair was challenged with tumor cells on the right and left flanks. On day 14 when all sites were positive, one of the lesions on experimental dogs was injected with 10^7 viable BCG organisms. The contralateral lesion was injected with saline as were the lesions of the control member of the pair. Fig. 4 shows the growth curves of tumors in control and

306

BCG treated animals. All BCG animals demonstrated regression of injected and noninjected lesions by day 60 while controls had persistent tumors beyond 100 days. On rechallenge BCG treated dogs failed to develop tumors. Serial MLTC assays (Fig. 5) demonstrated a significant increase in activity in the BCG treated group. Thus in this tumor system intralesional BCG was highly effective in producing accelerated rejection of the tumor.

Figure 3—CORRELATION OF TUMOR GROWTH IN DOG # 5540 WITH BLOCKING AND INHIBITORY ACTIVITY OF PURIFIED IgG FROM TUMOR ELUATES

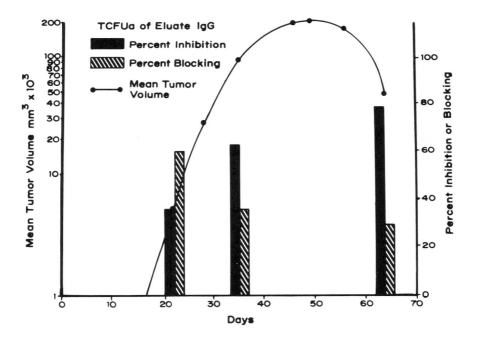

Tumors were biopsied on days 22, 35 and 64. Blocking and inhibition are indicated as percentages of the activity of normal dog serum.

Current interest in plasmapheresis as a possible therapeutic measure to remove putative blocking factors described in human tumors lead us to examine plasmapheresis effects in the TVT (12). Fig. 6 illustrates the course of tumor growth in 5 dogs that underwent plasmapheresis of 2 plasma

307

Figure 4—COURSE OF MEASURED TUMOR GROWTH IN ML (INJECTED PLUS NONINJECTED LESIONS) IN BCG TREATED AND CONTROL DOGS

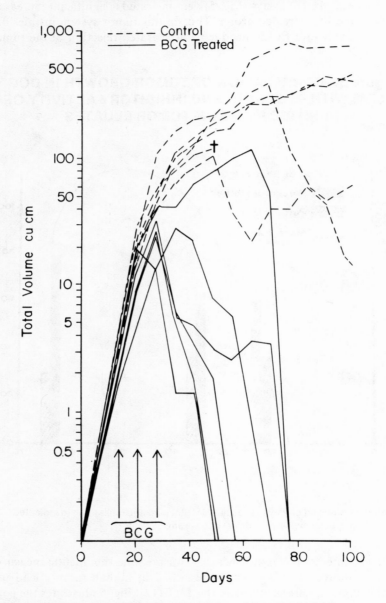

BCG was injected on days 14, 21, 28. +, death from intercurrent infection.

Figure 5—STIMULATION INDEX ± S.E. AS MEASURED IN CONTROL AND BCG TREATED ANIMALS

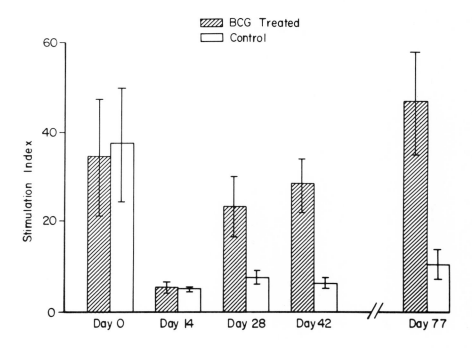

volumes per day for 4 days during the early period of tumor growth. When compared to non plasmapheresed DLA identical littermates the average tumor sizes showed no significant difference. Of interest however, was the wide variation between individual experimental animals when compared to controls suggesting that enhancing or therapeutic effects may be achieved by this technique. Further studies are underway to quantitate removal of blocking factors by plasmapheresis and assess duration and amount removed as a possible guide to therapy.

DISCUSSION

The unique features of the TVT are of interest to both the transplantation biologist and the tumor immunologist. With respect to transplantation, the tumor represents a relatively prolonged survival of a homograft among randomly bred, unmodified hosts. As a tumor it illustrates an impressive ability to escape potent immunologic defenses thought to be more subtly

309

Figure 6—COURSE OF TUMOR GROWTH FOLLOWING PLASMAPHERESIS

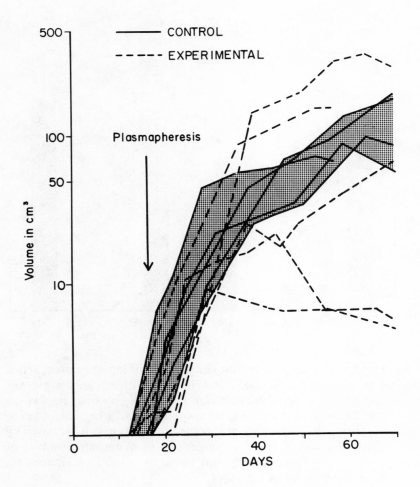

Shaded area represents range of control dogs.

active in other naturally occurring neoplasms.

The present studies confirm that the tumor survival is not due to the absence of DLA antigens. Such antigens were clearly demonstrated by serologic and MLTC testing (3,7). The natural history of the tumor however does appear to relate to histocompatibility as evidenced by family studies (8). Whether associated tumor specific antigens linked to, or independent of DLA can be identified remains to be determined.

It seems likely from studies to date that serum factors significantly modulate the course of the TVT. Suppressive effects of serum from tumor bearings dogs on MLTC responses are consistent with current concepts of blocking effects of serum in other models and in man (13,14). In the TVT such blocking effects were demonstrated in the IgG$_{2a}$ subclass of canine immunoglobulin. In contrast to other systems antigen-antibody complexes were not identified.

The characteristics of the TVT provide a large animal model in which immunotherapeutic maneuvers can be examined against established neoplasms under controlled conditions. It would seem unlikely that regimes unable to promote regression in this immunogenic setting would be of value in tumors of low inherent antigenicity. On the other hand, programs optimal for obviating protective mechanisms in this tumor may assist in evaluating immunotherapeutic protocols proposed for treating established tumors in outbred mammals.

Because of the uniqueness of the TVT, analogies to the human tumor problem can be easily discounted. However, the system does offer a rather clear large animal model for investigating immunologic mechanisms involved in long term homograft tumor survival or rejection in the unmodified host.

REFERENCES

1. Smith, G. B. and Washbourn, J. W., "Infective Venereal Tumours in Dogs." *J. Pathol. Bacteriol.* 5:99, 1898.
2. Rust, J. H., "Transmissible Lymphosarcoma in the Dog." *J. Am. Vet. Med. Assoc.* 114:10, 1949.
3. Epstein, R. B. and Bennett, B. T., "Histocompatibility Typing and Course of Canine Venereal Tumors Transplanted into Unmodified Random Dogs." *Cancer Research* 34:788, 1974.
4. Cohen, D., "The Biological Behaviour of the Transmissible Venereal Tumor in Immunosuppressed Dogs." *European J. Cancer* 9:253, 1973.
5. Terasaki, P. I. and McClelland, J. D., "Microdroplet Assay of Human Serum Cytoxins." *Nature* 206:998, 1964.
6. Vriesendorp, H. M., Westbroek, D. L., D'Amaro, J., et al., "Joint Report of 1st International Workshop on Canine Immunogenetics." *Tissue Antigens* 3:145, 1973.
7. Hess, A., Cunningham, B., Bennett, B. T., and Epstein, R. B., "In Vitro Correlates of the In Vivo Course of the Canine Transmissible Venereal Tumor Studied by Mixed Lymphocyte-tumor Cultures." *Transplantation Proceedings* 7:507, 1975.
8. Bennett, B. T., Debelak-Fehir, M. M. and Epstein, R. B., "Tumor Blocking and Inhibitory Serum Factors in the Clinical Course of Canine Venereal Tumor." *Cancer Research* 35:2942, 1975.
9. Beschorner, W. E., Hess, A. D., Nerenberg, S. T., Epstein, R. B., "Characterization of Serum Blocking and Inhibition of Canine Venereal Tumors". *Proc. of Amer. Assoc. for Can. Res.* 18:187, 1977.
10. Hess, A.D., Catchatourian, R., Zander, A., Epstein, R. B., "Intralesional Bacillus Calmette-Guerin, Immunotherapy of Canine Venereal Tumors." *Cancer Research* 37:3990, 1977.
11. Bennett, B. T., Taylor, Y., and Epstein, R. B., "Segregation of the Clinical Course of Transmissible Venereal Tumor with DL-A Haplotypes in Canine Families." *Transplantation Proceedings* 7:503, 1975.
12. Israel, L., Edelstein, R., Mannoni, P., et al., "Plasmapheresis in Patients with Disseminated Cancer: Clinical Results and Correlation with Changes in Serum Protein." *Cancer* 40:3146, 1977.
13. Hellström, K. E., Hellström, I. and Nepom, J. T., "Specific Blocking Factors—Are They Important?" *Biochimica et Biophysica Acta* 473: 121, 1977.
14. Hellström, K. E. and Hellström, I., "Lymphocyte-mediated Cytotoxicity and Blocking Serum Activity to Tumor Antigens." *Adv. Immunol.* 18:209, 1974.

Immunization Against Human Tumors: Generation of Killer Lymphocytes Against Human Tumor Cells Using Tumor Cells and Cell Fractions

Brahma Sharma[1]

SUMMARY—This study was designed to determine whether soluble bacterial components of *Mycobacteria, Listeria monocytogenes, Staphylococcus aureus, E. coli,* etc. are capable of inducing antitumor immunity *in vitro.* Soluble cell wall components isolated from *Mycobacterium smegmatis* and human mixed mycobacteria strains were able to potentiate immunization of lymphocytes with human tumor cells. Soluble bacterial extracts prepared from whole bacterial cells were able to sensitize lymphocytes (normal and cancer patients) which were highly cytotoxic to allogeneic and autologous tumor cells, but not to allogeneic and autologous lymphoblasts. *E.* coli (EC) extract stimulated lymphocytes from normal donors did not develop significant cytotoxicity against malignant melanoma and breast tumor cells. EC-stimulated lymphocytes from one donor, however, developed cytotoxicity against colon tumor cells. These bacterial components were effective in low concentrations. Not all of the donor's lymphocytes were able to become immunized with bacterial antigens. One donor whose *in vitro* bacterial sensitized lymphocytes were highly cytotoxic to tumor cells also exhibited strong positive skin reactions. The lysis of tumor cells by bacterial sensitized lymphocytes was augmented if tumor targets were coated with antibodies specific for bacterial extracts used. Poly AU was able to potentiate the bacterial induced cytotoxicity against tumor cells. Nylon wool nonadherent and SRBC rosetted lymphocytes became killer lymphocytes following exposure to bacterial antigens suggesting that precursors of cytotoxic lymphocytes have receptors for SRBC.

INTRODUCTION

Immune resistance against syngeneic and autochthonous tumors can be induced by immunization with tumor associated antigens in experimental animals (1-5). Cell-mediated cytotoxic immune reactions are generally considered to be the main factors in suppression of tumor growth and tumor rejection (5-9). Although, cell types responsible for tumor regression are yet to be established, thymus-derived (t) lymphocytes have been generally accepted as major cell types which are responsible for cell-mediated immune reactions against tumors (8). Macrophages, B and K cells seem to be involved as well.

---

[1]Associate Director of Research, Oncology-Hematology Department, Children's Hospital, Denver, Colorado.

The passive transfer of serum from immunized resistant animals to an unimmunized animal does not seem to provide protection against tumors (3-7), but tumor specific antibodies (lymphocyte dependent antibodies) may be capable of destroying tumor target cells through antibody dependent cellular cytotoxic immune mechanisms(10-14).

Since it is not possible to conduct such studies using transplantation techniques in man, except perhaps bone marrow transplantation in genetically identical siblings with leukemia, we have devised an *in vitro* test system in which immunization with cell or cell fractions can induce lymphocyte mediated cytotoxic immunity against allogeneic and autologous human tumors or syngeneic animal tumors (15-19). This *in vitro* immunization system has provided us with the means to study: 1) lymphocyte tumor cell interactions and generation of killer lymphocytes, 2) factors which augment or suppress such interactions and the induction of killer lymphocytes, 3) parameters for immunization against tumor cells, 4) effects of immunomodulators (microbial products, Poly AU, levamisole) on weakly immunogenic or nonimmunogenic tumor cells or cell fractions, and 5) mechanism of actions of immunomodulators. We will discuss here some recent studies from our laboratory on immunization against human tumor cells with tumor cells or cell fractions and the effect of immunomodulators on immunization to tumor cells with weekly immunogenic or nonimmunogenic tumor cell preparations. The results of these studies may provide information which may be useful for designing immunotherapy for the treatment and control of human cancer.

MATERIALS AND METHODS

Source of Tumor Cells. Tumor cells were obtained from the following human tumor lines: RPMI-7932 (malignant melanoma) originated from pleural effusion, COLO-38 (malignant melanoma) originated from primary lesion, COLO-53 (malignant melanoma) originated from a metastatic solid tumor lesion, COLO-205, COLO-321 (colon carcinoma) and COLO-293 (kidney carcinoma). COLO-59 is a normal lymphoid line autochthonous to COLO-53. All of these malignant and nonmalignant cultured cells were provided by Dr. G.E. Moore, Denver General Hospital, Denver, Colorado. HT-29 (colon tumor) established from a solid primary tumor was provided by Dr. J. Fogh, Sloan-Kettering Institute for Cancer Research, New York, and SH-3 cells that originated from the pleural effusion of a patient with breast carcinoma were obtained from Dr. G. Seman, M.D., Anderson Hospital, Houston, Texas. SH-3 may be cross-contaminated with HeLa (cervix) as recently reported by Dr. Nelson-Rees. Leukemic blasts obtained from peripheral blood or bone marrow at the time of initial presentation were purified by Ficoll-Hypaque and stored in liquid nitrogen. These

314

cryopreserved leukemia cells were the source of sensitizing and target tumor cells for autologous remission lymphocytes following stimulation *in vitro*. Characteristics of some of the tissue cultured tumor lines are given in (17, 20, 21). All tumor cells were *Mycoplasma* and virus-free, as determined by electron microscopy and culture methods.

Isolation of Tumor Cell Fractions. Tumor cell fractions were isolated as described previously (17). Cells maintained in MEM containing 10% heat inactivated calf serum or human AB plasma were harvested by gently scraping the monolayers and then passing cells through 22-guage needles. The cells were washed three times with plasma-free medium and suspended in either plasma-free medium or Tris buffer containing 0.25 M sucrose (pH 7.4) at a concentration of 12 x 10^6 cells/ml. The cells in single cell suspension were then disrupted by freezing (-80) and thawing, and various fractions were obtained from cell-free extracts (lysate) by differential centrifugations. The fractions were suspended in equal volumes of medium or Tris buffer (22). Residue and supernatant obtained after centrifugation of cell-free extracts at 2,000 x g for 2 minutes were denoted as R1 and S1, respectively. Residue and supernatant obtained after centrifugation of S1 at 10,000 x g were designated R2 and S2, respectively. Residue and supernatant obtained after centrifugation at 20,000 x g were denoted as R3 and S3, respectively and R4 and S4 were the residue and supernatant obtained after 100,000 x g centrifugation of S3 for 90 minutes. Fractions R1 contained few cells which were not completely lysed and some nuclei, R2 and R3 appeared to contain a few intact nuclei and broken nuclear material, granular cytoplasmic material, and plasma membrane; and R4 seemed to have plasma membranes.

Preparation of Killer Lymphocytes. Peripheral blood lymphoctyes were isolated and purified over Ficoll-Hypaque according to the method described previously (16). Nylon wool adherent and nonadherent cells were separated by nylon wool column by the procedure described by Trizio and Cudkowicz (23). Lymphocytes forming rosettes with sheep RBC were separated by the modification of the method described by West, et al (24). The purified lymphocytes were sensitized with various tumor cell fractions as described before (17). In brief, responding lymphocytes (1 x 10^6) and various concentrations of sensitizing tumor cells or cell fractions were mixed in 15 ml polypropylene tubes in a total volume of 0.75 ml. The tubes were incubated for 5 days at 37° in 6-7% CO_2 humid atmosphere. At the end of the incubation period, the cultures were harvested and cells were suspended in MEM containing 10% heat inactivated AB plasma. Lymphocytes and lymphoblasts were counted with the use of phase contrast microscopy.

Cell-Mediated Cytotoxicity. Cultured nonlymphoid tumors and cryopreserved leukemia cells were the source of tumor target cells. Lymphoid lines autochthonous to tumor lines were the source of normal lymphoblast cells. PHA-treated normal lymphocytes were the source of autologous and allogeneic normal lymphoblasts.

The cytotoxicity of *in vitro* stimulated lymphocytes was measured by 3-hour ^{51}Cr release assay as described previously (16, 17). In brief, ^{51}Cr labeled target cells (5,000) were mixed in 0.4 ml microtubes and incubated for 3 hours. At the end of the incubation period, the tubes were centrifuged at 800 x g for 2 minutes. The supernatants were carefully removed. The percentage of ^{51}Cr released into supernatants and percentage of ^{51}Cr remaining in the residue was counted. The percent specific ^{51}Cr release was calculated by subtracting the ^{51}Cr released from targets in the presence of unstimulated lymphocytes from the ^{51}Cr released from targets in the presence of *in vitro* stimulated lymphocytes.

Preparation of Mycobacteria Products. Water soluble mycobacterial cell wall components were prepared according to procedures of Kotani, et al. and Adam as described previously (25-27). In brief, delipidated cells were homogenized at high pressure and cell envelopes thus obtained were treated with Triton X-100, extracted with sodium dodecyl sulfate and subjected to differential centrifugation. Cell walls prepared this way were treated with lysozyme or L-11 enzymes which release water soluble peptidoglycan. In a few cases, mycobacterial extracts were used which were prepared according to procedures described previously (28) and provided by Dr. P. Minden.

Preparation of Synthetic Double Stranded Complexes of Poly AU. Polyadenylic acid (Poly A), potassium salt, and polyuridylic acid (poly U), ammonium salt, were purchased from Miles Laboratory, Elkhart, Indiana. Prior to use, Poly AU complexes were formed by mixing equimolar amounts of each polymer and incubating the mixture for 1 hour at 25°C. After 1 hour, a sample was taken and kept in a cold room and absorbency at UV was read. Poly AU thus formed was dialyzed against H_2O overnight. Prior to use, Poly AU complexes were diluted to the appropriate concentrations with medium.

Preparation of Levamisole. Levamisole was a gift from Janssen R & D, Inc., New Brunswick, New Jersey. It was reconstituted with medium to a concentration of 15 $\mu g/\mu l$ and stored at -20°C.

RESULTS AND DISCUSSION

Immunization with Tumor Cells. To determine whether tumor cells can sensitize lymphocytes, we mixed lymphocytes with various concentrations

316

of malignant melanoma cells (RPMI-7932) and incubated for 5 days. The cytotoxic activity of lymphocytes was then tested on day 6 against ^{51}Cr RPMI-7932 cells. The results given in Figure 1 show that lymphocytes (1 x 10^6) sensitized with 1 x 10^4 tumor cells acquired maximum cytotoxicity and further increase in the concentration of sensitizing tumor cells followed with a decrease in sensitization and induction of cytotoxicity. Following treatment with mitomycin C, tumor cells were, however, able to immunize lymphocytes at concentrations which were not immunogenic as untreated (Figure 1). Similarly, lymphocytes from a second donor were immunized with various concentrations of SH-3 tumor cells. The results shown in Figure 2 demonstrate that untreated tumor cells were unable to immunize lymphocytes but following treatment with mitomycin C, an increase in concentration of the same sensitizing cells followed with an increase in sensitization and lysis of tumor target cells reaching a maximum at 1.6 x 10^5 tumor cells. Next, we tested whether remission lymphocytes from acute lymphoblastic leukemia patients can be immunized against their own leukemia cells. The results shown in Figure 3 suggest that even mitomycin treated stimulating leukemia cells were able to generate killer lymphocytes usually at a low concentration. The peak response was noted at 2 x 10^4 stimulating leukemia cells. No immunization appears to occur at 1:1 lymphocyte:leukemia cell ratio.

These findings indicate that lack of immunization of lymphocytes is probably not due to lack of antigenicity of stimulating tumor cells, but probably due to suppressive effect of tumor cells. It appears that untreated tumor cells synthesize and release some immunosuppressive factor which inhibits sensitization and generation of cytotoxic lymphocytes. The treatment of tumor cells with mitomycin C presumably blocks the synthesis of the suppressive factor and thus the tumor cells became able to immunize lymphocytes even at higher concentrations following treatment with mitomycin C. Better chemotherapeutic treatment of breast cancer with chemotherapy, including mitomycin C, may be related to this *in vitro* observation.

Immunosuppressive Effect of Tumor Cell-Free Extract. To test whether tumor cells have some suppressive factor, we sensitized lymphocytes from donors I and J with SH-3 cells, with or without the presence of SH-3 cell-free extracts. The results given in Table 1 show that lymphocytes sensitized with SH-3 without the presence of cell-free extract have more cytotoxicity than lymphocytes sensitized with SH-3 in the presence of cell-free extracts. The results thus indicate that SH-3 tumor cells possess some factor(s) which inhibit the immunization of lymphocytes with tumor cells. These *in vitro* findings appear to relate with *in vivo* observations that the larger the tumor mass, the lower is the animal's immune response (29, 30).

317

Figure 1—IMMUNIZATION OF LYMPHOCYTES *IN VITRO* AGAINST MALIGNANT MELANOMA CELLS WITH MITOMYCIN C TREATED AND UNTREATED TUMOR CELLS

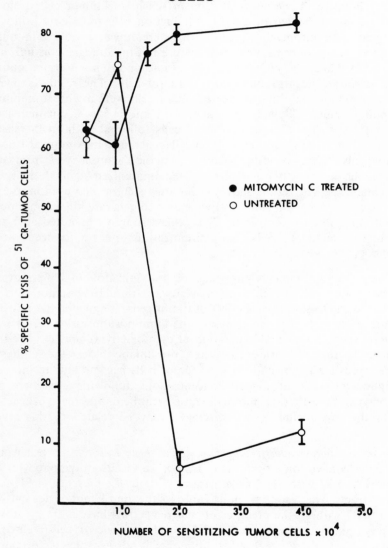

Lymphocytes (1 x 10⁶) were sensitized with different concentrations of melanoma tumor cells and on day 6, the cytotoxic activity of sensitized cells was tested against specific tumor target cells.

318

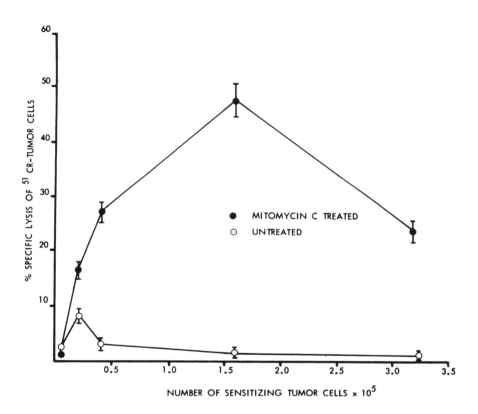

**Figure 2—IMMUNIZATION OF LYMPHOCYTES *IN VITRO*
AGAINST BREAST TUMOR CELLS WITH MITOMYCIN C
TREATED AND UNTREATED TUMOR CELLS**

Lymphocytes (1 x 10⁶) were sensitized with different concentrations of breast tumor cells and on day 6, the cytotoxic activity of sensitized cells was tested against specific tumor target cells.

Fractionation of Tumor Cells. To further characterize suppressive factor and isolate fractions with ability to immunize and suppress, we lysed tumor cells by freezing and thawing, and then isolated fractions from cell-free lysate by differential centrifugation (22). Various cell fractions so obtained were then tested for their ability to immunize or suppress the induction of cell mediated cytotoxic immunity. The ability of cell fractions isolated from

319

Figure 3—IMMUNIZATION OF LYMPHOCYTES FROM ACUTE LYMPHOBLASTIC LEUKEMIA PATIENT IN REMISSION AGAINST HIS LEUKEMIA CELLS WITH MITOMYCIN C TREATED AUTOLOGOUS LEUKEMIC BLASTS

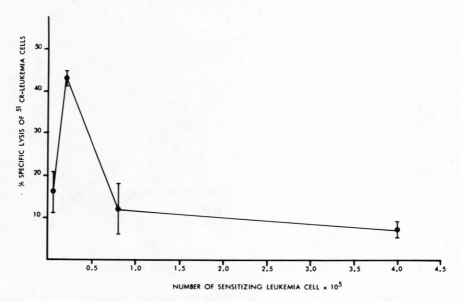

Lymphocytes (1×10^6) were sensitized with different concentrations of leukemic blasts and on day 6, the cytotoxic activity of sensitized cells was tested against specific tumor target cells.

Table 1—EFFECT OF TUMOR CELL-FREE EXTRACT ON *IN VITRO* IMMUNIZATION OF LYMPHOCYTES TO HUMAN TUMOR CELLS

Effector-stimulating tumor cells[a]	%Specific ^{51}Cr release $\pm$ SD	
	Without cell-free extract	With cell-free extract
I-SH-3 (breast)	36±1.0	12±1.0
I-SH-3	30±0.7	23±1.0
J-SH-3 (breast)	52±3.0	18±1.0
J-SH-3 (breast)	39±2.0	7±1.0

[a] Lymphocytes were sensitized with tumor cells with or without the presence of tumor cell-free extract prepared by freezing and thawing single cell suspension of SH-3 tumor. The cytotoxic activity of sensitized lymphocytes was tested against ^{51}Cr-SH-3 target cells.

320

tumor lines RPMI-7932, HT-29, SH-3 and COLO-293 to immunize was determined by measuring their ability to transform lymphocytes from normal persons into cytotoxic effector lymphocytes. Cell fractions sedimented at 2,000 x g, 10,000-20,000 x g and 100,000 x g were able to immunize lymphocytes to various degrees against tumor target cells (Tables 2-5). Cell fractions isolated from COLO-293 were unable to sensitize at all or only weakly (Table 6). R2 fractions appeared to be more sensitizing than R3 or R4 fractions. Although lymphocytes sensitized with cell fractions isolated from RPMI-7932 were able to lyse specific RPMI-7932 target cells, they were also cytotoxic to cells from allogeneic melanoma cells (COLO-38) (Table 2). The lysis of RPMI-7932 was, however, higher than the lysis of COLO-38. For determination of whether immune cells are also equally cytotoxic to cells from other tumor lines, the cytotoxic activity of RPMI-7932 sensitized lymphocytes was tested against HT-29 (colon) and COLO-293 (kidney) tumor cells. Again, lysis of RPMI-7932 target cells was higher than lysis of nonspecific target cells (Tables 3 and 4). Next, we tested the cytotoxic activity of lymphocytes sensitized with cell fractions isolated from HT-29. Results shown in Table 5 demonstrate that HT-29 cell fractions sensitized lymphocytes were markedly cytotoxic to HT-29 but they were also cytotoxic to RPMI-7932. In 3 of 8 cases, the lysis of HT-29

Table 2—CYTOTOXIC ACTIVITY OF LYMPHOCYTES SENSITIZED BY RPMI-7932 (MALIGNANT MELANOMA) CELLS OR CELL FRACTIONS

Effector-stimulating cell or cell fraction[a]	Source of cell or cell fraction	%Specific ^{51}Cr release ± sd	
		RPMI-7932	COLO-38[b]
K-RPMI-7932-cells (80,000)	RPMI-7932 (melanoma)	45±1.0	4±2.0
K-RPMI-7932-R1 (5 µl)		68±2.0	27±1.0
K-RPMI-7932-R1 (10 µl)		−19±2.0	−16±1.0
K-RPMI-7932-R2 (5 µl)		51±1.0	35±2.0
K-RPMI-7932-R2 (10 µl)		73±2.0	21±1.0
K-RPMI-7932-R3 (5 µl)		−5±1.0	−18±1.0
K-RPMI-7932 R3 (10 µl)		26±1.0	8±4.0
K-RPMI-7932-R4 (5 µl)		10±1.0	2±2.0
K-RPMI-7932-R4 (10 µl)		31±2.0	6±1.0

[a] Lymphocytes were sensitized with RPMI-7932 cells or cell fractions and then cytotoxic activity of sensitized lymphocytes was tested against RPMI-7932 and COLO-38 tumor cells. Numbers in parenthesis: concentrations of stimulating cell or cell fraction. Tumor cell fractions sedimented at 2,000 x g, 10,000 x g, 20,000 x g and 100,000 x g are denoted by R1, R2, R3 and R4, respectively.
[b] Malignant melanoma.

Table 3—CYTOTOXIC ACTIVITY OF LYMPHOCYTES SENSITIZED BY RPMI-7932 (MALIGNANT MELANOMA) CELLS OR CELL FRACTIONS

Effector-stimulating cell or cell fraction[a]	Source of Cell or cell fraction	%Specific ^{51}Cr release $\pm$ SD RPMI-7932	HT-29[b]
K-RPMI-7932-cells	RPMI-7932 (melanoma)	52±6.0	1±1.0
K-RPMI-7932-R1		68±2.0	20±1.0
K-RPMI-7932-R2		73±2.0	24±4.0
K-RPMI-7932-R3		26±1.0	−14±2.0
K-RPMI-7931-R4		31±1.0	−14±2.0
L-RPMI-7932-R1		60±1.0	15±2.0
L-RPMI-7932-R2		15±0.7	7±1.0
L-RPMI-7932-R3		20±1.0	5±2.0
L-RPMI-7932-R4		5±0.7	−2±2.0
M-RPMI-7932-R1		51±1.0	11±4.0
M-RPMI-7932-R2		86±2.0	7±1.0
M-RPMI-7932-R3		9±0.7	12±4.0

[a] Lymphocytes were sensitized with RPMI-7932 cells or cell fraction and then cytotoxic activity of sensitized lymphocytes was tested against RPMI-7932 and HT-29 tumor cells. Tumor cell fractions sedimented at 2,000 x g, 10,000 x g, 20,000 x g and 100,000 x g are denoted by R1, R2, R3 and R4 respectively.
[b] Colon carcinoma.

Table 4—CYTOTOXIC ACTIVITY OF LYMPHOCYTES SENSITIZED BY RPMI-7932 (MALIGNANT MELANOMA) CELL FRACTION

Effector-stimulating cell fraction[a]	Source of cell fraction	%Specific ^{51}Cr release RPMI-7932	COLO-293[b]
M-RPMI-7932-R1 (5 μl)	RPMI-7932 (melanoma)	51±2.0	2±2.0
M-RPMI-7932-R1 (10 μl)		12±1.0	1±1.0
M-RPMI-7932-R2 (5 μl)		86±2.0	28±4.0
M-RPMI-7932-R2 (10 μl)		29±1.0	16±1.5
M-RPMI-7932-R3 (5 μl)		−3±1.0	0±2.0
M-RPMI-7932-R3 (10 μl)		9±1.0	6±1.0

[a] Lymphocytes were sensitized with RPMI-7932 cell fraction and then cytotoxic activity of sensitized lymphocytes was tested against RPMI-7932 and COLO-293. R1, R2, R3 and R4 are cell fractions sedimented at 2,000 x g, 10,000 x g, 20,000 x g and 100,000 x g.
[b] Carcinoma of kidney.

322

was higher than lysis of RPMI-7932. In other cases, however, the lysis of RPMI-7932 was about as much as the lysis of HT-29. It is possible that this donor was previously exposed to some antigens related to RPMI-7932 and sensitization with HT-29, which cross react with RPMI-7932, may have also activated RPMI-7932 memory cells. Cell fractions isolated from COLO-293 (kidney carcinoma) were not able to stimulate lymphocytes from three normal persons into cytotoxic lymphocytes in most of the cases (Table 6). The explanation for the inability of COLO-293 cells to stimulate lymphocytes is not yet clear. It is possible that this particular population of cells is not immunogenic (heterogeneity and modulation of tumor population are well known) or they produce more suppressive factor than other lines tested. This remains to be investigated.

The specificity of *in vitro* sensitized lymphocytes was also tested by the comparison of cytotoxic activity against tumor cells and normal lymphoid lines both established from the same patient. As shown in Table 7, sensitized lymphocytes while cytotoxic to tumor cells (SH-3 and COLO-53) were not cytotoxic to lymphoid line COLO-59 which is autochthonous to COLO-53.

Table 5—CYTOTOXIC ACTIVITY OF LYMPHOCYTES SENSITIZED BY HT-29 (COLON) TUMOR CELLS OR CELL FRACTION

Effector-stimulating cell or cell fraction[a]	Source of cell or cell fraction	%Specific ^{51}Cr release $\pm$ SD	
		HT-29	RPMI-7932[b]
F-HT-29-cells (5,000)	HT-29 (colon)	28±1.0	2±2.0
F-HT-29-cells (20,000)		18±5.0	15±1.0
F-HT-29-cells (320,000)		39±1.0	47±2.0
F-HT-29-R1 (5 μl)		17±2.0	−5±4.0
F-HT-29-R1 (10 μl)		23±0.7	
F-HT-29-R2 (5 μl)		61±2.0	60±2.0
F-HT-29-R2 (10 μl)		36±2.0	35±4.0
F-HT-29-R3 (10 μl)		53±1.0	50±2.0
F-HT-29-R4 (5 μl)		47±2.0	31±1.0

[a] Lymphocytes were sensitized with HT-29 tumor cells or cell fractions and then cytotoxic activity of sensitized lymphocytes was tested against HT-29 and RPMI-7932 tumor cells. R1, R2, R3 and R4 are cell fractions sedimented at 2,000 x g, 10,000 x g, 20,000 x g and 100,000 x g.
[b] Malignant melanoma.

Table 6—IMMUNIZATION OF LYMPHOCYTES *IN VITRO* WITH COLO-293 (KIDNEY) TUMOR CELL FRACTION

Experiment	Effector-stimulating cell fraction[a]	Source of fractions and tumor targets	%Specific ^{51}Cr release ± SD COLO-293	HT-29[b]
1	E-COLO-293-cells	COLO-293	7±1.0	5±2.0
	E-COLO-293-S1		8±1.0	4±4.0
	E-COLO-293-R1		6±1.0	0±2.0
	E-COLO-293-R2		8±2.0	9±2.0
	E-COLO-293-R3		2±6.0	0±2.0
	E-COLO-293-R4		8±1.0	2±1.0
2	N-COLO-293-cells	COLO-293	6±2.0	5±1.0
	N-COLO-293-S1		11±2.0	22±1.0
	N-COLO-293-R1		4±0.5	11±2.0
	N-COLO-293-R2		5±4.0	2.5±2.0
	N-COLO-293-R3		9±2.0	1 7±2.0
	N-COLO-293-R4		19±1.0	0±8.0
3	O-COLO-293-cells		−11±4.0	
	O-COLO-293-S1		−9±4.0	
	O-COLO-293-R1		−12±1.0	
	O-COLO-293-R2		−5±1.0	
	O-COLO-293-R3		−15±1.0	
	O-COLO-293-R4		−18±2.0	

[a] Lymphocytes were sensitized with COLO-293 cells or cell fractions and then cytotoxic activity of sensitized lymphocytes was tested against COLO-293 and HT-29 tumor target cells. R1, R2, R3 and R4 are cell fractions sedimented at 2,000 x g, 10,000 x g, 20,000 x g and 100,000 x g.
[b] Colon tumor cells.

The cytotoxicity of effector cells induced by cell fractions was also determined against normal lymphocytes that have been transformed by PHA. Although lymphocytes sensitized with cell fractions lysed specific tumor target cells, there was usually no killing of PHA induced normal lymphoblast cells (Figure 4). These findings suggest that cytotoxic effector cells are not generated against normal histocompatibility antigens. Since lymphocytes sensitized by tumor cell fractions of one histologic type also cross react with tumor cells of different histologic type suggest that sensitization is caused by some common tumor associated antigenic determinants present in tumor cells of various histologic type. In fact, there are many reports which demonstrate the existence of common tumor associated antigens (15, 31-33). Irie, et al (31) recently reported that an

Table 7—SPECIFICITY OF CYTOTOXIC ACTIVITY OF LYMPHOCYTES SENSITIZED BY SH-3 TUMOR CELLS OR CELL FRACTIONS

Effector-immunizing cell or cell fraction	Source of cell or cell fraction[a]	%51Cr release Target alone	%51Cr release Target + unsensitized lymphocytes	%Specific 51Cr release ± SD Targets SH-3	COLO 53	COLO 59	COLO 38
E-SH-3-cells	SH-3 (breast)	10±0.5	10±0.5	50±1.0[b]	43±1.5[b]	−3.0±1.0	34±1.0[b,d]
E-SH-3-cells				25±1.5[b]	18±0.5[b]	−6±4.0	18±1.0[b]
E-SH-3-S1				14±0.5[b]	14±1.0[c]	−12±0.5	11±0.5[b]
E-SH-3-R1				13±0.5[b]	2±1.0	−13±1.0	9±1.0[c,e]
E-SH-3-R2				20±1.0[b]	9±1.0[c]	−18±1.0	10±1.0[c]
F-SH-3-cells	SH-3			14±1.0[b]	9±0.5	−16±1.0	
F-SH-3-R2				10±0.5[b]	5±1.0	−21±0.5	

[a] Lymphocytes were sensitized with SH-3 tumor cells or fractions and then cytotoxic activity of sensitized cells was tested against SH-3, COLO 53, COLO 59, and COLO 38. COLO 53 (tumor line) and COLO 59 (lymphoid line) were established from the same patient.
[b] P value for the test comparing 51Cr release from specific target by sensitized and unsensitized lymphocytes, $P \leq 0.01$.
[c] P value for the test comparing 51Cr release from specific target by sensitized and unsensitized lymphocytes, $0.01 < P \leq 0.05$.
[d] P value for the test comparing 51Cr release from specific and nonspecific targets, $P \leq 0.01$.
[e] P value for the test comparing 51Cr release from specific and nonspecific targets, $0.01 < P \leq 0.05$.

antigen present on a melanoma tumor line was also found on a variety of different histologic types of biopsied and cultured cancer cells. This antigen, however, was not present on biopsied normal tissue. The existence of human tumor associated antigens was further demonstrated by our recent finding that lymphocytes sensitized with autologous leukemic blasts were cytotoxic to autologous leukemic blasts but not to autologous remission lymphocytes (18).

Figure 4—CYTOTOXIC ACTIVITY OF LYMPHOCYTES SENSITIZED WITH VARIOUS TUMOR CELL FRACTIONS AGAINST TUMOR AND NORMAL LYMPHOBLAST TARGET CELLS

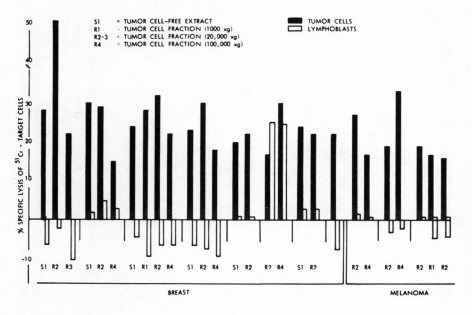

Lymphocytes (1 x 10⁶) were sensitized with tumor cell fractions and on day 6, the cytotoxic activity of sensitized lymphocytes was tested against tumor cells and normal lymphoblasts.

Suppressive Activity in Tumor Cell Fractions. Earlier, we discussed that tumor cell-free extracts appeared to have some suppressive factors (Table 1). In an attempt to separate immunizing and suppressive activities, we fractionated tumor cell-free extracts by differential centrifugations as described earlier in the text. Various cell fractions so obtained were tested

326

for their ability to immunize lymphocytes. The results given in Figure 5 show that the same concentrations of R2 and R3 fractions were more immunizing than R4 fractions. R2 + R3 fractions induced maximum cytotoxicity with 10 μl whereas R4 fractions produced maximal response with 5 μl. R2 + R3 fractions at a concentration of 30-40 μl were quite sensitizing whereas R4 fractions produced little or no sensitization at this concentration. These results indicate that either R4 fractions have components which are not immunizing as good as R2 + R3 fractions or lack some components needed for optimal immunization, e.g. nuclear material, or R4 fractions have more suppressive factors as compared to R2 + R3 fractions. To test these possibilities, we sensitized lymphocytes with or without the presence of R1, R2 + R3, and R4 fractions. The results show that R1, R2 + R3, or R4 fractions were able to suppress the generation of cytotoxic lymphocytes (Table 8). The R4 fractions, however, appeared to have more suppressive activity than R1 or R2 + R3 fractions.

Figure 5—IMMUNIZATION OF LYMPHOCYTES WITH VARIOUS TUMOR CELL FRACTIONS

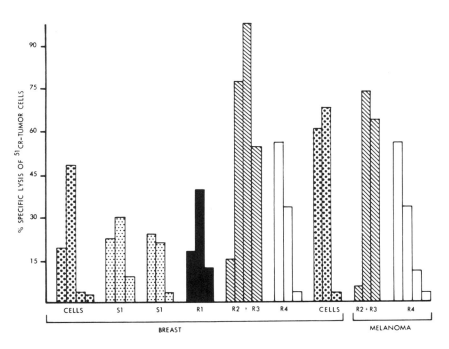

Lymphocytes (1 x 10⁶) were sensitized with different concentrations (5, 10, 20 and 40 μl) of tumor cell fractions and on day 6, the cytotoxicity of sensitized lymphocytes was tested against specific tumor target cells.

327

Table 8—EFFECT OF TUMOR CELL FRACTIONS ON *IN VITRO* IMMUNIZATION OF LYMPHOCYTES AGAINST TUMOR CELLS

Effector-sensitizing[a]	Cell fraction	%Specific ^{51}Cr release $\pm$ SD	
		Without cell fraction	With cell fraction
J-SH-3 (breast)	SH-3-R1	52±3.0	11±2.0
J-SH-3	SH-3-R2 + R3	52±3.0	9±1.0
J-SH-3	SH-3-R4	52±3.0	1±0.7
J-SH-3 (breast)	SH-3-R1	39±2.0	17±1.0
J-SH-3	SH-3-R2 + R3	39±2.0	8±1.0
J-SH-3	SH-3-R4	39±2.0	1±0.7
K-SH-3 (breast)	SH-3-R4	40±1.0	−2±1.0

[a]Lymphocytes were sensitized with SH-3 tumor cells with or without the presence of various SH-3 cell fractions isolated by differential centrifugation. The cytotoxic activity of sensitized lymphocytes was then tested against ^{51}Cr-SH-3 target cells.

Immunization of Lymphocytes With Tumor Cells and Mycobacterial Cell Components. Earlier, we discussed that sometimes lymphocytes could not be immunized with tumor cells (34, 35). So, we decided to test the effect of certain additional mycobacterial components on the generation of killer lymphocytes (35). Lymphocytes were immunized with tumor cells with or without the presence of these agents. The results shown in Table 9 indicate that lymphocytes from cancer patients (A and B) and normal donors (E, F and G) which could not be sensitized with tumor cells and kill specific tumor targets were able to do so when sensitizing tumor cells were mixed with these mycobacterial products. In other cases, the addition of soluble mycobacterial components to mixed lymphocytes (C or D) tumor cell cultures potentiated the immunization of lymphocytes against breast and lung tumor cells (35). Our recent findings as well as of others have demonstrated thay mycobacterial components appeared to have a variety of effects on the induction of immunity (14, 18, 36, 37). The low level of these products were able to: 1) increase the immunization of lymphocytes against tumor cells, and 2) stimulate lymphocytes to become cytotoxic to tumor cells. Large amounts, however, had marked suppressive effects *in vivo* and *in vitro*. The mechanism of action of these immunomodulator (or adjuvants) is not yet established. These may act directly on tumor cells by increasing their immunogenicity or on immunoreactive lymphoid population. They may potentiate lymphocyte tumor cell interactions and generation of killer lymphocytes by inhibiting the tumor induced immunosuppressive mechanism which operate, perhaps, via the induction of suppressor cell population. All of these possible mechanisms of action are currently under investigation. Recently, it has been reported that low level of methanol extract residue of certain mycobacteria could abrogate the induction of nonspecific suppressor cells arising in spleen cell cultures (37).

Table 9—EFFECT OF MYCOBACTERIAL CELL COMPONENTS (MCC) ON *IN VITRO* GENERATION OF KILLER LYMPHOCYTES AGAINST HUMAN TUMOR CELLS

| Responding lymphocyte[a] | Immunizing tumor cells or SBC | %Specific ^{51}Cr release $\pm$ SD Immunizing tumor cells and MCC | | |
		Tumor cells	MCC	Tumor cells + MCC
A (cancer patient)	805 (breast)	2±0.7	1±1.0	11±0.7
B (cancer patient)	ALB[b]	−9±2.0	10±2.5	20±2.0
C (normal)	805	14±0.7	5±1.0	40±0.7
D (normal)	613 (lung)	37±0.7		70±2.1
D (normal)		37±0.7		27±0.7
E (normal)	SH-3 (breast)	−9±2.0	25±2.0	57±2.0
F (normal)	HT-29 (colon)	−1±2.0	17±3.0	30±2.8
F	COLO-205 (colon)	−6±1.0	−13±2.3	20±4.9

[a] Lymphocytes from cancer patients or normal persons were sensitized with allogeneic or autologous tumor cells, soluble bacterial components (SBC), or tumor cells in the presence of MCC and then cytotoxicity of sensitized lymphocytes was tested against tumor target cells.

[b] Autologous leukemic blasts.

Immunization of Lymphocytes With Tumor Cells and Poly AU. Double stranded complexes of polyadenylic and polyuridylic acid (PAU) have been shown to amplify *in vitro* lymphocytes response against a variety of antigens, especially to antigens which cause weak responses (38). We examined, therefore, whether PAU will also potentiate the sensitization of lymphocytes with tumor cells. Lymphocytes from donor G, H and J were sensitized with SH-3 or RPMI-7932 cells or RPMI-7932 cell fractions with or without the presence of PAU. The results shown in Tables 10 and 11 demonstrate that the addition of PAU has the following effects: 1) certain concentrations of tumor cells which were not sensitizing became able to sensitize and generate killer lymphocytes in the presence of PAU, 2) potentiation of immunization of lymphocytes with tumor cells in eight cases, 3) inhibition, in a few cases, in the induction of cytotoxicity, and 4) immunization with R3 and R4 but not with R2 fractions was potentiated by PAU. The understanding of the mechanisms of action of PAU will clarify its variable effects. Our previous findings indicated that amplification produced by water soluble adjuvants from *Mycobacteria* appeared to be similar to the enhancing effect of PAU (35). Various studies reported have suggested that ability of PAU to amplify immune responsiveness appear to be related to its direct effect on T, B and macrophage cell activity. Whether PAU alter the immunogenicity of tumor cells or play a role in tumor induced immunosuppressive mechanism remains to be investigated.

Table 10—EFFECT OF POLYADENYLIC ACID AND POLYURIDYLIC ACID (PAU) ON *IN VITRO* GENERATION OF KILLER LYMPHOCYTES AGAINST HUMAN TUMOR CELLS

Effector-stimulating tumor cells[a]	Concentration of tumor cells	%Specific ^{51}Cr release $\pm$ SD			
		Without PAU	With PAU		
			41.5 μg	83 μg	249 μg
G-SH-3	5 x 10^3	6± 1.0	7±1.0	0±1.0	2±1.0
	2 x 10^4	−3± 1.0	8±2.0	17±2.0	21±4.0
	8 x 10^4	34± 1.0	24±1.0	49±6.0	32±2.0
	3.2 x 10^5	41± 1.0	9±1.0	5±8.0	33±9.0
G-RPMI-7932	5 x 10^3	−7± 2.0	0±1.0	11±1.0	20±2.0
	2 x 10^4	10± 1.0	22±2.0	17±1.0	10±1.0
	8 x 10^4	−17± 1.0	20±4.0	56±2.0	34±4.0
H-SH-3	5 x 10^3	3± 0.7	9±4.0	1±1.0	2±1.0
	2 x 10^4	20± 1.0		15±6.0	30±1.0
	4 x 10^4	31± 2.0	34±4.0	36±2.0	42±2.0
	8 x 10^4	35± 1.0	37±1.0	36±2.0	52±1.0
	3.2 x 10^4	37± 1.0	51±5.0	40±1.0	74±2.0
H-RPMI-7932	2 x 10^4	48± 4.0	60±1.0	69±4.0	62±4.0
	2 x 10^4	52± 4.0	74±2.0	60±2.0	
	8 x 10^4	53±15.0		62±2.0	25±8.0

[a]Lymphocytes were sensitized with different concentrations of tumor cells in the presence and absence of polyadenylic acid and polyuridylic acid and then cytotoxic activity of sensitized lymphocytes was tested against ^{51}Cr tumor target cells.

330

Table 11—EFFECT OF POLYADENYLIC ACID AND POLYURIDYLIC ACID (PAU) ON GENERATION OF KILLER LYMPHOCYTES *IN VITRO* AGAINST MALIGNANT MELANOMA (RPMI-7932) CELLS USING TUMOR CELL FRACTIONS

Responding lymphocytes[a]	Immunizing cell fraction	%Specific ^{51}Cr release ± SD	
		Without PAU	With PAU
J	RPMI-7932-R2	25±4.0	27±2.0
	RPMI-7932-R3	13±2.0	19±0.7
	RPMI-7932-R4	10±0.5	20±1.0

[a] Lymphocytes were sensitized with RPMI-7932 cell fractions with or without the presence of PAU (41.5 μg) and then cytotoxicity of sensitized lymphocytes was tested against RPMI-7932 cells.

Effect of Levamisole on Generation of Killer Lymphocytes. Levamisole has been shown to potentiate T-cell mediated immunity (39-41). It has been used as immunotherapeutic agent for the suppression or regression of tumor growth (42). We tested here whether Levamisole will potentiate the immunization of lymphocytes with tumor cell fractions. Preliminary results given in Table 12 show that it did not have any immunopotentiating effect when R1 fraction was used, however, when R2 fractions were used, lysis of tumor target cells was increased 2-4-fold depending on the concentration of Levamisole used. At slightly higher (450 μg) concentrations there was an inhibiting effect of Levamisole on the induction of lymphocyte mediated cytotoxicity.

Table 12—EFFECT OF LEVAMISOLE ON GENERATION OF KILLER LYMPHOCYTES *IN VITRO* AGAINST HT-29 (COLON) TUMOR CELLS USING HT-29 CELL FRACTION

Effector-stimulating cell fraction[a]	%Specific ^{51}Cr release ± SD	
	Without Levamisole	With Levamisole (μg)
K-HT-29-R1	11±6.0	3.5±2.0 (150)
		6.0±4.0 (300)
K-HT-29-R2	9±1.8	23±4.0 (150)
		37±6.0 (300)
		−1±4.8 (450)

[a] Lymphocytes were sensitized with HT-29 cell fractions with or without the presence of Levamisole and then cytotoxic activity of sensitized lymphocytes was tested against HT-29 target cells. The concentrations (μg) of Levamisole are given in parentheses.

Nature of Responder Lymphocytes. Preliminary experiments to study the nature of cells which are stimulated by tumor cells were done by fractionating Ficoll-Hypaque purified lymphocytes on nylon wool columns. Nylon wool nonadherent and unfractionated lymphocytes were then stimulated with tumor cells. Results are given in Table 13. Lymphocytes from donor F following stimulation with COLO-205, a newly established colon tumor line, were not able to lyse COLO-205 target cells. However, after removal of nylon wool adherent cells, lymphocytes could be immunized against COLO-205. This experiment indicates that unfractionated cell population had some cells which prevented the stimulation of responder lymphocytes to COLO-205. Similarly, the cytotoxicity of HT-29 cell fractions stimulated nonadherent lymphocytes was significantly higher than the cytotoxicity of stimulated unfractionated lymphocytes. In one experiment, however, unfractionated lymphocyte response to SH-3 was reduced significantly after removal of nylon wool adherent cells. Although these preliminary experiments indicate that nylon wool nonadherent cell population has the responder lymphocytes, more experiments are needed to establish the characterization of responder lymphocytes.

Table 13—GENERATION OF KILLER LYMPHOCYTES *IN VITRO* AGAINST TUMOR CELLS BY STIMULATION OF FICOLL-HYPAQUE PURIFIED (UNFRACTIONATED) AND NYLON-WOOL COLUMN FRACTIONATED LYMPHOCYTES WITH TUMOR CELLS AND CELL FRACTIONS

Donor of lymphocytes[a]	Stimulating tumor cells cell fractions and tumor target cells	%Specific ^{51}Cr release ± SD from target cells Responder lymphocytes	
		Unfractionated	Nylon wool non-adherent
F	COLO-205 (colon)	−6±0.5	14±0.5
		−12±2.0	14±2.0
		−17±2.0	9±2.0
G	SH-3 (breast)	30±5.0	10±1.0
P	SH-3 (breast)	31±3.6	45±20.0
	HT-29-R3 (colon)	5±1.0	23±2.0
	HT-29-R4 (colon)	9±1.0	26±2.0

[a] Ficoll-Hypaque purified lymphocytes were fractionated by nylon-wool columns. Unfractionated and nylon-wool nonadherent cells were then sensitized with tumor cells or cell fractions. The cytotoxic activity of sensitized cells was tested against specific tumor cells.

CONCLUSION

It is possible to induce immunity *in vitro* against human lymphoid and nonlymphoid tumor targets using tumor cells or tumor cell fractions. The induction of immunity appears to depend on a variety of factors, e.g. concentration of immunizing cell preparations, subpopulation of immunoreactive responder lymphoid cells, physiologic state of tumor cells, etc. Tumor cells may be antigenic but may not be recognized immunologically due to their suppressive effect, presence of suppressor cells or serum blocking factors. The inhibition of such immunosuppressive factors may thus augment the immune response. Tumor cells which are not able to immunize or are not immunogenic at higher concentrations can become immunogenic following treatment with mitomycin C. Such a treatment presumably blocks the synthesis of the suppressive factor which may be produced by tumor cells. In some cases, even mitomycin treated cells are not able to sensitize and generate killer lymphocytes. The addition of immunomodulator, e.g. mycobacterial cell components, Poly AU or Levamisole, usually restores the ability to respond and generate cytotoxic lymphocytes. These modulators may also potentiate appreciably the elicitation of cytotoxic activity of the sensitized cells against some tumors. Although the mechanisms of their actions is not clear yet, it is possible that these agents amplify response to tumor cells either by augmenting the helper T cell functions or by inhibiting the suppressor cell activity.

Tumor cell-free extracts are immunosuppressive *in vitro*. Fractionation of these extracts tend to separate different cell components. Although most of the tumor cell fractions have different degrees of immunizing and suppressive activity, fractions which sediment at 10-20,000 x g appear to have the most immunizing activity and fractions which sediment at 100,000 x g appear to have the most suppressive activity. The ability of some fractions to immunize seems to be potentiated by the addition of Poly AU or Levamisole.

The various studies discussed here may provide an understanding of induction of immunity against human tumors and guidelines for the immunotherapy and control of cancer.

ACKNOWLEDGMENTS

This investigation was supported by Grant CA 20067-02 awarded by the National Cancer Institute, DHEW and by The Helen S. Fisher Cancer Research Fund of The Children's Hospital.

333

REFERENCES

1. Foley, E.J., "Antigenic Properties of Methylcholanthrene-Induced Tumors in Mice of Strain Origin." *Cancer Res.* 13:835-837, 1953.
2. Prehn, R.T. and Main, J.M., "Immunity to Methylcholanthrene-Induced Sarcomas." *J. Natl. Cancer Inst.* 18:769-778, 1957.
3. Klein, G., Sjorgen, H.O., Klein, E. and Hellstrom, K.E., "Demonstration of Resistance Against Methylcholanthrene-Induced Sarcomas in the Primary Autochthonous Host." *Cancer Res.* 20:1561-1572, 1960.
4. Sjorgren, H.O., Hellstrom, I. and Klein, G., "Transplantation of Polyoma-Induced Tumors in Mice." *Cancer Res.* 21:329-337, 1961.
5. Kikuchi, K., Ishii, Y., Ueno, H. and Koshiba, H., "Cell-Mediated Immunity Involved in Autochthonous Tumor Rejection in Rats." *Ann. N.Y. Acad. Sci.* 276:188-206, 1976.
6. Old, L.J., Boyse, E., Clarke, D.A. and Carswell, E.A., "Antigenic Properties of Chemically Induced Tumors." *Ann. N.Y. Acad. Sci.* 101:80-106, 1962.
7. Klein, E. and Sjorgren, H.O., "Humoral and Cellular Factors in Homograft and Isograft Immunity Against Sarcomas Cells." *Cancer Res.* 20:452-461, 1960.
8. Rouse, B.T., Rollinghoff, M. and Warner, N.L., "Tumor Immunity to Murine Plasma Cell Tumors. II. Essential Role of T Lymphocytes in Immune Response." *Eur. J. Immunol.* 3:218-222, 1973.
9. Rollinghoff, M. and Wagner, H., "*In Vitro* Induction of Tumor Specific Immunity: Requirements for T Lymphocytes and Tumor Growth Inhibition *In Vivo.*" *Eur. J. Immunol.* 3:471-478, 1973.
10. Hellstrom, K.E. and Hellstrom, I., "Lymphocyte-Mediated Cytotoxicity and Blocking Serum Activity to Tumor Antigens." *Advan. Immunol.* 18:209-277, 1974.
11. Cerottini, J.C. and Brunner, T., "Cell-Mediated Cytotoxicity, Allograft Rejection and Tumor Immunity." *Advan. Immunol.* 18:67-132, 1974.
12. Baldwin, R.W., "Immunological Aspects of Chemical Carcinogenesis." *Advan. Cancer Res.* 18:1-75, 1973.
13. Herberman, R.B., "Cell-Mediated Immunity to Tumor Cells." *Advan. Cancer Res.* 19:207-263, 1974.
14. Sharma, B., Tubergen, D.G., Minden, P. and Brunda, M.J., "*In Vitro* Immunisation Against Human Tumor Cells With Bacterial Extracts." *Nature* 267:845-847, 1977.
15. Sharma, B. and Terasaki, P.I., "*In Vitro* Immunization to Cultured Human Tumor Cells." *Cancer Res.* 34:115-118, 1974.
16. Sharma, B., "*In Vitro* Lymphocyte Immunization to Cultured Human Tumor Cells: Parameters for Generation of Cytotoxic Lymphocytes." *J. Natl. Cancer Inst.* 57:743-748, 1976.
17. Sharma, B., "*In Vitro* Immunization Against Human Tumor Cells with Tumor Cell Fractions." *Cancer Res.* 37:4660-4668, 1977.
18. Sharma, B. and Odom, L.F., "Generation of Killer Lymphocytes *in vitro* Against Human Leukemia Cells Using Autologous Leukemia Cells and Bacterial Extracts." Submitted for publication.
19. Sharma, B. and Brunda, M.J., "*In Vitro* Sensitization for Guinea Pig Lymphocytes Against Syngeneic Hepatocarcinoma with Tumor Cells or Bacterial Extracts." *Fed. Proc.* 37:1593, 1978.
20. Quinn, L.A., Woods, L.D., Merrick, S.B., et al., "Cytotoxic Analysis of 12 Human Malignant Melanoma Cell Lines." *J. Natl. Cancer Inst.* 59:301-307, 1977.
21. Semple, T.D., Quinn, L.A., Woods, L.K. and Moore, G.E., "Tumor and Lymphoid Cell Lines from a Patient With Carcinoma of Colon for a Cytotoxicity Model." *Cancer Res.* 38:1345-1355, 1978.
22. Ferber, E., Resch, K., Wallach, D.F.H. and Imm, W., "Isolation and Characterization of Lymphocyte Plasma Membranes." *Biochem. Biophys. Acta.* 266:494-504, 1972.

23. Trizio, D. and Cudkowicz, A., "Separation of T and B Lymphocytes by Nylon Wool Columns: Evaluation of Efficacy by Functional Assay *In Vivo.*" *J. Immunol.* 113:1093-1097, 1974.

24. West, W.H., Cannon, G.B., Kay, H.W., et al., "Natural Cytotoxic Reactivity of Human Lymphocytes Against a Myeloid Cell Line. Characterization of Effector Cells." *J. Immunol.* 118:355-361, 1977.

25. Chedid, L., Parant, F., Gustafson, R.H. and Berger, F.M., "Biological Study of a Nontoxic Water-Soluble Immuno-Adjuvant from Mycobacterial Cell Walls." *Proc. Natl. Acad. Sci.* 69:855-858, 1972.

26. Kotani, S., Hashimoto, S., Matsbara, T., et al., "Lysis of Isolated BCG Cells With Enzymes. 2. Demonstration of Bound Wax D as Component of BCG Cell Walls." *Bikens J.* 6:181-196, 1963.

27. Adam, A., Ciorbaru, R., Petit, J.F. and Lederer, E., "Isolation and Properties of a Macromolecular, Water Soluble, Immunoadjuvant Fraction From Cell Wall of *Mycobacterium smegmatis.*" *Proc. Natl. Acad. Sci.* 69:851-854, 1972.

28. Minden, P., McClatchy, J.K. and Farr, R.S., "Shared Antigens Between Heterologous Bacterial Species." *Infect. Immun.* 6:574-582, 1972.

29. Deckers, P.J., Davis, R.C., Parker, G.A. and Mannick, J.A., "The Effect of Tumor Size on Concomitant Tumor Immunity." *Cancer Res.* 33:33-39, 1973.

30. Whitney, R.A., Levy, J.A. and Smith, A.G., "Influence of Tumor Size and Surgical Reaction on Cell-Mediated Immunity in Mice." *J. Natl. Cancer Inst.* 53:111-116, 1974.

31. Irie, R.F., Iri, R. and Morton, D.L., "A Membrane Antigen Common to Human Cancer and Fetal Brain Tissues." *Cancer Res.* 36:3510-3517, 1976.

32. Roth, J.A., Grimm, E.A. and Morton, D.L., "A Rapid Assay for Stimulation of Human Lymphocytes to Tumor Associated Antigens." *Cancer Res.* 36:3001-3010, 1976.

33. The, T.H., Huiges, H.A., Schraffordt Koops, H., et al., "Surface Antigens on Cultured Malignant Melanoma Cells as Detected by a Membrane Immunofluorescence Method With Human Sera. Lack of Tumor Specific Reactions on Melanoma Cells." *Ann. N.Y. Acad. Sci.* 257:528-540, 1975.

34. Sharma, B. and Terasaki, P.I., "Immunization of Lymphocytes from Cancer Patients." *J. Natl. Cancer Inst.* 52:1925-1926, 1974.

35. Sharma, B., Kohasi, O., Mickey, M.R. and Terasaki, P.I., "Effect of Water-Soluble Adjuvants on *In Vitro* Lymphocyte Immunization." *Cancer Res.* 35:666-669, 1975.

36. Sharma, B. and Odom, L.F., "Generation of Killer Lymphocytes *In Vitro* Against Human Leukemia Cells Using Bacterial Extracts." Submitted for publication, 1978.

37. Kedar, E., Nahas, F., Unger, E. and Weiss, D.W., "*In Vitro* Induction of Cell-Mediated Immunity to Murine Leukemia Cells. III. Effect of the Methanol Extraction Residue (MER) Fraction of Tubercle Bacilli on the Generation of Anti-Leukemia Cytotoxic Lymphocytes." *J. Natl. Cancer Inst.* 60:1097-1106, 1978.

38. Graziano, K.D., Levy, C., Schmukler, M. and Mardiny, M.R., "Parameters for Effective Use of Synthetic Double Stranded Polynucleotides in Amplification of Immunologically Induced Lymphocyte Tritiated Thymidine Incorporation." *Cellular Immunol.* 11:47-56, 1974.

39. Renoux, G., Renoux, M., Teller, M.N., et al., "Potentiation of T-Cell Mediated Immunity by Levamisole." *Clin. Exp. Immunol.* 25(2):288-296, 1976.

40. Faanes, R.B., Dillon, P. and Choi, Y.S., "Levamisole Augments the Cytotoxic T Cell Response Depending on the Dose of Drugs and Antigen Administered." *Clin. Exp. Immunol.* 27:502-506, 1977.

41. Renoux, G. and Renoux, M., "Mechanisms of Action of Levamisole, an Enhancer of Cell-Mediated Immunity." *Ann. Immunol.* (Paris) 128C:275-277, 1977.

42. Kassel, R.L., "Levamisole Plus Antigen: an Immunotherapy Model." *Modulation of Host Immune Resistance in the Prevention or Treatment of Induce Neoplasias,* Fogarty International Center Proceedings No. 28 NIH and John E. Fogarty International Center for Advanced Study in the Health Sciences, Bethesda, MD, 347-348, 1977.

Cell-Mediated Immunity Assays for Breast Cancer-Associated Antigen Recognition

James L. McCoy[1]
J. H. Dean[2]
G. B. Cannon[2]
R. B. Herberman[1]

SUMMARY—Direct and indirect leukocyte migration inhibition LMI assays using allogeneic 3M KC1 extracts of MCF-7 (a breast cancer derived cell line) were performed to detect cell-mediated immunity to tumor-associated antigens of human breast cancer. A large proportion (50-60%) of breast cancer as well as some benign breast disease patients gave positive reactions with the two LMI assays. Low MI reactivity (<10-15% inhibition) was observed with normal donors and patients with cancer of other sites. Analysis of the LMI data as it may relate to disease prognosis indicated that pre-operative breast cancer patients have a higher incidence of reactivity to the MCF-7 antigen than did post-operative patients with no evident disease. Further, LMI reactivity tended to decrease as patients developed clinical recurrence of disease. By using an indirect micro-LMI modified assay it was shown that the LMI reactions were lymphokine-mediated and that this modification has the potential of being semi-quantitated by end-point diluting generated supernatants containing lymphokine. Testing with lymphocyte proliferation assays using 3M KC1 extracts of breast cancer tissue indicated that allogeneic extracts may induce a primary proliferative response to normal alloantigens in addition to TAA. The problems of discrimination between alloantigens and TAA were overcome by the use of autologous whole tumor cells or hypotonic membrane extracts of tumors and normal tissue. Approximately 35% of the breast cancer patients reacted to autologous whole cell membrane extracts of breast cancer tissues, while no appreciable reactivity was seen with normal breast tissue extracts. The results with lymphocyte proliferation also demonstrate its usefulness in *in vitro* detection of cellular immunity of breast cancer patients with autologous materials against breast tumor antigens.

INTRODUCTION

Detection of *in vitro* host reactivity against human tumor-associated antigens (TAA) is largely dependent on the use of reliable and reproducible assays that have the desired specificity and are adequately sensitive to detect weak immunological reactions. Such tests would hopefully have the potential to be used as early diagnostics of cancer with little or no reactivity being

---

[1]Laboratory of Immunodiagnosis, National Cancer Institute, Bethesda, Maryland.
[2]Department of Immunology, Litton Bionetics Research Laboratory, Kensington, Maryland.

demonstrated by normal individuals or individuals with organ related benign lesions. Further, the assays should have the potential to at least be semi-quantitated such that they ultimately might have some predictive value in relation to disease prognosis (including recurrence and magnitude of tumor-burden) and also might provide information on efficacy of chemo-immunotherapy.

Although several laboratories have reported the use of both humoral and cellular immunity assays to detect TAA on human cancer of most organ types (1), many of the studies have been hampered by problems associated with specificity related to normal donor reactivity [e.g., lymphocyte micro-cytotoxicity (2-4)] or with sufficient quantitation or sensitivity to be reliably predictive of disease prognosis and survival.

The purpose of this communication is to report the use of direct capillary tube and indirect agarose microdroplet leukocyte migration inhibition (LMI) and lymphocyte proliferation (LP) assays in measuring host cell-mediated immunity (CMI) reactivity against TAA on human breast cancer. Our approaches in attempting to refine these tests to gain greater specificity and sensitivity as well as attempting to semi-quantitate the immune responses against TAA are discussed.

MATERIALS AND METHODS

Patients. Heparinized whole blood from females with confirmed breast carcinoma or benign breast diesase and from males and females with other diseases was obtained from George Washington University Hospital, the University of South Carolina Medical Center and the Clinical Center of the National Institutes of Health. Patients with all stages of disease were tested at various times before or after surgery.

Leukocytes from normal donors were obtained from the Blood Bank of the National Institutes of Health, from our laboratory and clerical staff and from George Washington University.

Tissue Culture Cells and 3M KCl Extraction. MCF-7 cells (5) from a patient with breast carcinoma were used. The tissue culture line grew as epithelial cells in monolayers and was maintained on antibiotic-free RPMI-1640 medium supplemented with 20% fetal bovine serum (FBS). The bulk-produced cells used for KCl extraction were tested for *Mycoplasma* by the method of Fogh and Fogh (6) and were free of contamination. MCF-7 cells were grown in roller bottles and we harvested the cells by scraping them manually with a rubber policeman and then extracted with 3M KCl (7).

Tumors for MLTI. Single tumor-cell suspensions were prepared under sterile conditions by careful mincing with scissors and scalpel. Intact tumor cells, to be later used as stimulator cells in autologous MLTI, were

338

cryopreserved in 10% dimethyl sulfoxide by controlled-rate ($-1C/min$) freezing in a Planar freezer and were stored in vapor-phase liquid nitrogen. Hypotonic saline membrane extracts (HMP) were prepared, as previously described (8), for use in autologous MLTI studies.

Direct LMI assay. As described in (7), 2×10^7 blood leukocytes obtained by $1 \times g$ sedimentation with Plasmagel were incubated at 37C for 45 minutes with antigen or no antigen. Cell suspensions were drawn into capillaries and placed individually into Sterilin chambers (#308; Sterilin, Surrey, England). McCoy's 5-A medium supplemented with 10% FBS and 100 ug gentamicin/ml was added to the chambers and incubated overnight in a humidified 5% CO_2 atmosphere at 37C.

After incubation of the chambers, the areas of migration were projected onto paper with a Zeiss inverted microscope (x20), drawn, and then measured by planimetry. The MI was calculated by the formula:

$$MI = \frac{\text{mean migration area of 4 replicates in the presence of antigen}}{\text{mean migration area of 4 replicates in the absence of antigen}}$$

Migration indices of patients were compared to those of normals, and the number of positive MIs was determined, as previously described (9), by means of a cut-off value calculated so that 10% of normal MIs fell below this value. MIs falling below this cut-off were considered positive, i.e., below the lower tenth percentile of normals.

Indirect Polymorphonuclear Cell Agarose Droplet Assay—Preparation of Supernatants Containing Leukocyte Inhibitory Factor (LIF). As previously described (10), mononuclear cells from whole blood were prepared by Ficoll-Hypaque separation and the cells resuspended in medium consisting of RPMI 1640 and 10% FBS and adjusted to a concentration of 5×10^5 or 5×10^6 monunuclear cells/ml. Appropriate antigen concentrations or control medium were added to the cells when using 5×10^6 mononuclear cell to generate supernatants, 12 x 75 mm round bottom plastic tubes (Falcon Plastics, #2003) were employed and when 5×10^5 mononuclear cells were used 46 x 5.7 mm conical plastic tubes (Bolab, Derry, New Hampshire, #BB410-450) were employed and the mixtures were incubated at 37C in a humidified 5% CO_2 incubator for 2 hours to initiate lymphocyte triggering. Cells were centrifuged at 200 x g for 10 min and the supernatant containing PPD was aspirated and discarded and the cell pellet was resuspended in complete medium without PPD. They lymphocyte cultures were then incubated at 37C in a humidified 5% CO_2 atmosphere for 24-48 hours to generate the lymphokine, LIF, and then centrifuged at 200 x g for 10 min and the supernatant fluid from each culture was collected and stored at $-96C$ until assaying for LIF.

Testing of LIF Supernatants. Two microliter droplets of 0.2% Seakem agarose containing leukocytes (4 x 10^5 polymorphonuclear cells/droplet) were placed into flat-bottom wells of a micro-test plate and allowed to solidify for 3-5 min at room temperature. Appropriate dilutions of each supernatant were added and the plate was incubated in a humidified 5% CO_2 incubator at 37C for 18-24 hours. After incubation the image of the migration patterns was then projected with a microscope fitted with a Zeiss straight tube photo changer with a prism and a KDL 8X eye piece. The area of the agarose droplet itself was drawn (inner area) and then the dense area of migration of the cells (outer area) was drawn for each well.

The area of each inner agarose droplet and each outer cell migration area for each well was quantitated with a planimeter. The net area of migration of the cells was then obtained by subtracting the inner agarose area from the outer cell migration area for each droplet. A migration index (MI) was calculated as follows:

$$MI = \frac{\text{Mean migration area of replicate droplets in the presence of antigen for each dilution of supernatant}}{\text{Mean migration area of replicate droplets in the absence of antigen for each dilution of supernatant}}$$

Lymphocyte Proliferation Assays. Microculture LP assays with tumor material were performed by a microculture method described previously (11). Mononuclear cells were separated from whole blood by Ficoll-Hypaque and were added to flat-bottom wells of a Cooke microculture plate in medium supplemented with 10% fresh frozen human AB serum and gentamicin (50 ug/ml).

Cryopreserved tumor cells treated with 50 ug mitomycin C/ml (MMC) where then added to the lymphocyte-containing wells. Control cultures with tumor cells alone were included in each assay to determine their residual incorporation. HMP were added to lymphocyte cultures in concentrations ranging from 0.005 to 50 ug/culture. Each microculture was pulse-labeled with [^{3}H]TdR 6 hours before harvest. The cells were harvested after 7 days with the use of a multiple sample harvester and counted in a liquid scintillation counter. Data were analyzed for significance by Welch's modification of Student's t-test.

The SI for MLTI cultures was expressed as the ratio of mean cpm of cultures containing tumor cells minus the cpm of MMC-blocked tumor cells cultured alone, divided by the cpm of control lymphocyte cultures containing no tumor cells. Cultures containing tumor cells alone always had low levels of [^{3}H]TDR incorporation (50-200 cpm). The following formula was used:

$$SI_{MLTI} = \frac{(^{cpm}PBL + \text{tumor cells}) - (^{cpm}\text{tumor cells alone})}{^{cpm}PBL \text{ alone}}$$

340

Table 1—DIRECT CAPILLARY-TUBE LMI REACTIVITIES OF BREAST CANCER, BENIGN BREAST DISEASE, OTHER CANCER PATIENTS AND NORMAL CONTROLS WITH 3M KC1 EXTRACTS OF MCF-7

Leukocyte Donors (Total Positive/Total Tested)

MI Cut-off Value of Positivity	Breast Cancer Patients	Benign Fibrocystic Disease	Benign Fibro-adenoma	Other Cancer	Normal Males	Normal Females
<0.80	25/104 (24%)	5/11 (45%)	0/11-	1/47 (2%)	0/37-	1/49 (2%)
<0.85	57/104 (55%)	5/11 (45%)	3/11 (27%)	3/47 (6%)	1/37 (3%)	1/49 (2%)
<10th Percentile of Normal Donor Females (<0.91)	74/104 (71%)	7/11 (64%)	4/11 (36%)	6/47 (13%)	3/37 (8%)	5/49 (10%)

The SI of cultures containing HMP was expressed as the ratio cpm of experimental cultures containing extract (E) to cmp of control lymphocyte cultures (C) containing no tissue extract:

$$SI(HMP) = \frac{E}{C}$$

RESULTS

Direct Capillary Tube LMI

Direct capillary tube LMI was performed with leukocytes from normal controls and patients with breast cancer, benign breast disease and cancer of other sites using 2 standard batches of 3M KCl extracts of MCF-7 cells (Table 1). Although longitudinal tests have been performed (Figures 1 and 2), only the initial test results of each patient are shown here. The data are presented as a function of three different cut-off values of positivity, i.e., values <0.80, <0.85 and < the 10th percentile of normal donor females' reactivity as described in the Methods section. The purpose of presenting the data in this format was to see if more specificity of the LMI reactivity could be detected with one of these cut-off values, since in essence, all three values are arbitrarily selected and since other investigators using LMI in human cancer studies usually select one arbitary cut-off value (e.g., <0.80) to evaluate the data.

Only 24% of the breast cancer patients reacted to the MCF-7 antigen if an MI cut-off value of <0.80 was used. The proportion of positive reactors increased (55%) if an MI value of <0.85 was considered positive and if the 10th percentile MI value of reactive normal female donors was used then 71% of the breast cancer patients were reactive. Normal males and females and patients with cancer of other sites were consistently negative regardless of the cut-off value used. By contrast, a large proportion of patients with fibrocystic disease and some patients with fibroadenomas were also positive regardless of the cut-off value selected. Thus, the results suggesting that a high proporation of breast cancer patients with breast cancer have a common CMI reactivity against antigens on MCF-7 cells are hampered with specificity problems associated with benign breast disease reactivity with MCF-7 even though normal donors and patients with cancer of other sites are generally unreactive.

Figure 1 presents some of the serial capillary tube LMI test data with one standard batch of MCF-7 extract as a function of time after surgery and in some instances as it relates to disease relapse. Appreciable fluctuations in LMI reactivity with individual patients following surgery were observed. In two patients who relapsed, the early LMI values prior to disease recurrence

342

Figure 1

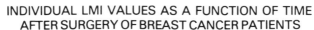

INDIVIDUAL LMI VALUES AS A FUNCTION OF TIME
AFTER SURGERY OF BREAST CANCER PATIENTS

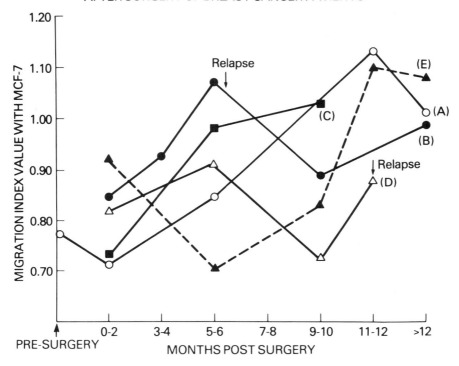

were not useful in predicting relapse. In one patient the MI values increased prior to relapse and in the other patient the values tended to decrease before clinical recurrence of disease. We further evaluated this LMI data by grouping the results as a function of "total percentage positive LMI tests" prior to or following relapse in six patients who had disease recurrence (Figure 2). Although the numbers are small and no statistical meaning can be drawn from this grouped data, there was a trend for patients to become less reactive 1-6 months prior to clinical relapse. These patients maintained about the same degree of reactivity following relapse as the 1-6 month period prior to relapse but were never as reactive as the 12 month time period prior to relapse.

Indirect Agarose Microdroplet Polymorphonuclear Cell Migration Inhibition

The direct LMI assay does not permit analysis of the mechanism of the reaction. We therefore performed indirect assays using human

343

Table 2—INDIRECT AGAROSE MICRODROPLET POLYMORPHONUCLEAR CELL MIGRATION INHIBITION USING SUPERNATANTS GENERATED WITH THE 3M KC1 EXTRACT OF MCF-7 IN ROUND-BOTTOM TUBES[a]

Supernatant Dilutions (Total Positive/Total Tested) [b]

Supernatants Generated with Mononuclear Cells From	undiluted	1:2	1:4	1:8
Breast Cancer Patients	7/14 (50%)	5/14 (36%)	4/14 (29%)	4/14 (29%)
Normal Donors	1/12 (8%)	1/12 (8%)	1/12 (8%)	1/12 (8%)

a)5 x 10[6] mononuclear and 50 μg/ml MCF-7 extract were used to generate supernatants in 12 x 75 mm round-bottom plastic tubes (Falcon Plastics, #2003) with 1 ml media containing 10% FBS.
b)Positive reactions based on 10th percentile or less of the normal donor cut-off values (see Methods section).

polymorphonuclear indicator cells and tested for lymphokine (leukocyte inhibitory factor; LIF) production in supernatants from patient mononuclear cells incubated with the 3M KCl extract of MCF-7 cells (Table 2). We generated the supernatants in 12 x 75 mm "round-bottom" tubes with 5 x 10⁶ cells that are conventionally used by most laboratories in generating LIF containing supernatants. Whereas 7/14 breast cancer patients were reactive with the MCF-7 extract with undiluted supernatants, only 1/12 normal donors gave a positive reaction. Four of the supernatants generated from the breast cancer patients were still positive at 1:8 dilutions. These results suggest that significant levels of LIF are being produced following the interaction of the MCF-7 extract and mononuclear cells from breast cancer patients.

Figure 2

AVERAGE LMI VALUES OF RELAPSED BREAST CANCER PATIENTS AS A FUNCTION OF TIME PRIOR TO OR FOLLOWING RELAPSE

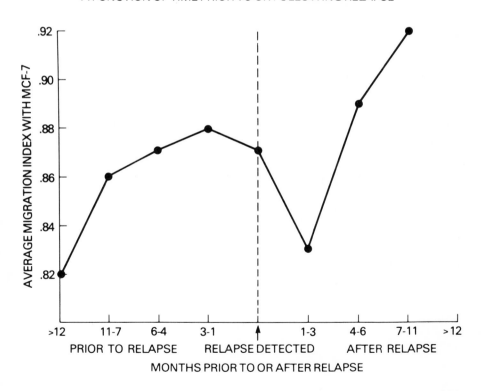

Table 3—INDIRECT AGAROSE MICRODROPLET POLYMORPHONUCLEAR CELL MIGRATION INHIBITION USING SUPERNATANTS GENERATED WITH PPD IN MICRO-CONICAL TUBES

Supernatant Dilutions (Migration Indices)

Supernatants Generated with Mononuclear Cells from [a]	10^{-1}	10^{-2}	10^{-3}	10^{-4}	10^{-5}	10^{-6}
• Tuberculin Skin Reactive Donor A	0.87	0.80*	0.80*	0.86	1.00	—
• Tuberculin Skin Reactive Donor B	0.73*	0.81*	0.81*	0.82*	0.83*	0.90
• Tuberculin Negative Donors	1.18	1.04	1.01	1.06	0.97	1.05

[a] 5 x 10^5 mononuclear cells and 25 µg/ml PPD (Parke-Davis, Detroit, Michigan) were used to generate supernatants in 46 x 5.7 mm conical plastic tubes (Bolab, Derry, New Hampshire, #BB410-450) with 0.2 ml media containing 10% FBS.

*Reactions were arbitrarily considered positive if MI values were ≤0.85.

We have been interested in attempting to semi-quantitate the degree of immune response of patients against TAA using LMI assays. One reasonable approach appeared to be in generating supernatants and then performing end-point dilutions of such supernatants and thus estimating the quantity of LIF produced since patients may vary in their ability to quantitatively produce LIF as a function of their clinical status. The approach used was to generate supernatants in "conical" tubes rather than "round-bottom" tubes. Such a method was previously reported to be successful in the generation of high titered MIF with guinea pig peritoneal exudate cells and PPD (12). In order for assays to ultimately be clincally useful they must also require minimal numbers of leukocytes from small volumes of whole blood. We therefore have developed a microsystem (5 x 10^5 mononuclear cells plus antigen) to generate supernatants using microfuge tubes.

Initially in developing this modified procedure, we used mononuclear cells from tuberculin skin reactive individuals with PPD to generate LIF and then tested these supernatants at log dilutions ($10^{-1}-10^{-6}$) on polymorphonuclear indicator cells in the indirect agarose LMI assay. Representative results of one experiment are shown in Table 3. Reactivity of the two tuberculin positive individuals was detected at $10^{-3}-10^{-5}$ dilutions of the supernatants, whereas no reactivity was detected with the tuberculin skin test negative donor. Physiochemical studies (Braatz, J., McCoy, J.L. and Herberman, R.B., unpublished data) have shown that these supernatant reactive materials have previously reported characteristics of LIF.

Table 4 presents preliminary indirect LMI data of supernatants of breast cancer and benign breast disease patients and normal donors generated with MCF-7 in the microfuge tubes. Four of ten breast cancer patients produced LIF detectable at 10^{-2} dilutions whereas 2/10 were still reactive at 10^{-4} dilutions of the supernatants. None of the normal donors and 1/4 of the benign breast disease patients were reactive. The data are too preliminary to evaluate as a function of disease status and clinical course, but the results do demonstrate that supernatants generated in this fashion with crude breast cancer TAA contain several logs of detectable LIF activity.

Finally, Table 5 shows that patients in a pre-operative state are more reactive than patients tested post-operatively. Both the direct and indirect LMI tests show more reactivity with pre-operative patients.

Allogeneic and Autologous Lymphocyte Proliferation Assays of Breast Cancer Patients

LP data using allogeneic mononuclear cell-tumor antigen combinations are summarized in Table 6. Mononuclear cells from 26 breast cancer

Table 4—INDIRECT AGAROSE MICRODROPLET POLYMORPHONUCLEAR CELL MIGRATION INHIBITION USING SUPERNATANTS GENERATED WITH THE 3M KC1 EXTRACT OF MCF-7 IN MICRO-CONICAL TUBES

Supernatants Generated with Mononuclear Cells from[a]	Supernatant Dilutions (Total Positive/Total Tested) [b]				
	10^{-1}	10^{-2}	10^{-3}	10^{-4}	10^{-5}
• Breast Cancer Patients	4/10 (40%)	4/10 (40%)	2/10 (20%)	2/10 (20%)	0/10 —
• Benign Breast Disease Patients	1/4 (25%)	1/4 (25%)	0/4 —	0/4 —	0/4 —
• Normals	0/8 —	0/8 —	0/8 —	0/8 —	0/8 —

[a] 5×10^5 mononuclear and 50 μg/ml MCF-7 extract were used to generate supernatants in 46 x 5.7 mm conical plastic tubes with 0.2 ml media containing 10% FBS.

[b] Positive reactions based on 10th percentile or less of the normal donor cut-off values (see Methods section).

348

Table 5—PRE-OPERATIVE VERSUS POST-OPERATIVE*
BREAST CANCER REACTIVITY TO THE 3M KCl
EXTRACT OF MCF-7 BY LMI

| Assay | Leukocyte Donors | |
	Pre-operative	Post-operative
Direct LMI	6/12 (50%)	6/28 (21%)
Indirect LMI	5/6 (83%)	5/10 (50%)

*Initial test results only.

patients and 30 normal donors were cultured in the presence of several different 3M KCl extracts of fresh allogeneic breast cancer tissue, normal breast tissue, non-breast tumor tissue and normal blood leukocytes (MLC). Stimulation ratios of ^{3}H-TdR incorporation >3.0 were observed with 4/26 breast cancer patients, while a total of 7/10 benign breast disease patients and 12/30 normal donors demonstrated positive reactivity to the allogeneic breast cancer material. Low reactivity was observed with normal breast tissue, while similar proportions of LP responses were also observed with allogeneic non-breast tumor tissue extracts. A total of 7/12 normal donors were reactive with the allogeneic MLC extract but 0/8 were reactive with similarly prepared extracts of autologous leukocytes. Overall, normal donors and benign breast disease patients responded better to the allogeneic extracts than did breast cancer patients. Thus it appears that the LP assay using allogeneic 3M KCl extracts cannot reliably measure specific TAA reactivity.

We therefore studied whether the LP assay could measure reactivity against TAA in a completely autologous system. Preliminary testing with autologous 3M KCl extracts and breast cancer mononuclear cells did not yield appreciable reactivity. We subsequently tested with intact tumor cells or crude HMP of breast cancer and normal breast tissue as stimulants. The results are presented in Table 7. A total of 41% and 33% of the breast cancer patients reacted with HMP or intact tumor cells, respectively, when 4 x 10^5 responding mononuclear cells were used in the test. None of 15 patients reacted with normal autologous breast cells.

No correlation was found between the LP response to the autologous tumor material and clinical stages of disease (Table 8). More stage 2 and 3 patients were LP positive than stage 1 individuals, but the numbers are too small to be meaningful. Positive reactivity was observed in patients less than 1 month to more than 3 months following surgery. In addition, positive LP responses were observed among patients who received radiation or chemotherapy, as well as untreated patients (data not shown).

Table 6—LYMPHOCYTE STIMULATIONS WITH ALLOGENEIC 3M KC1 EXTRACTS OF CANCER AND NORMAL TISSUES

Extract Used for Stimulation from:	Leukocyte Donor (Total Positive/Total Tested; % Positive)		
	Breast Cancer Patients	Benign Breast Disease Patients	Normal Donors
• Allogeneic Breast Cancer Tissue	4/26 (15%) [5.7] [a]	7/10 (70%) [6.1]	12/30 (40%) [9.1]
• Allogeneic Normal Breast Tissue	1/7 (14%) [3.7]	—	2/10 (20%) [3.5]
• Allogeneic Non-breast Tumor Tissue	2/14 (14%) [4.2]	—	7/8 (39%) [7.7]
• Allgeneic Normal Leukocytes	—	—	7/12 (58%) [18.4]
• Autologous Leukocytes	—	—	0/8-

[a]Mean stimulation index of positive reactors. Stimulation indices were considered positive with SI>3.0.

Table 7—SUMMARY OF LYMPHOCYTE STIMULATION BY AUTOLOGOUS BREAST CANCER CELLS AND EXTRACTS IN MLTI

Form of Stimulator Material	Responding Mononuclear Concentration/well	No. positive (% +) / No. tested	Mean SI of Responders[a]	Mean cpmE-C[b] in Responder
HMP	4×10^5	9/22 (41%)	10.9	7,489
HMP	2×10^5	1/8 (12%)	11.1	653
Intact Breast Cancer Cells	4×10^5	10/30 (33%)	10.9	6,805
Normal Breast Cells	4×10^5	0/15	—	—

[a]SI were considered positive if the value was ≥ 2.0 and $P \leq 0.01$.
[b]E = cultures containing extract; C = control mononuclear cell cultures containing no tissue extract.

351

Table 8—CORRELATION OF LP RESPONSES TO TAA WITH CLINICAL STAGE AND TIME POST SURGERY OF BREAST CANCER PATIENTS

Clinical Stage	No. Positive MLTI/No. Tested (%)	Time Post Surgery		
		1 month	1-3 months	>3 months
1	4/15 (27%)	2/4 (50%)	7/22 (32%)	2/5 (40%)
2	4/11 (36%)			
3	3/5 (60%)			

DISCUSSION

Direct capillary tube LMI (7, 13-18) and LP (13, 19-21) have been used to measure host reactivity against TAA in breast cancer. We further describe here the use of these assays and micro-modifications of them to measure breast TAA recognition by leukocytes of breast cancer patients. LP assays were also useful in detection of TAA recognition by breast cancer mononuclear cells, but appeared to have a requirement for autologous combinations of stimulator tumor materials and patient cells. Both direct and indirect LMI assays were able to detect reasonably specific reactivity using allogeneic materials, with the indirect micro-test appearing to offer potential promise in semi-quantitating CMI responses when using small quantities of whole blood for the generation of LIF.

We have demonstrated the usefulness of standard batches of crude 3M KC1 extracts of MCF-7 cells as antigenic preparations in both direct and indirect LMI assays. The incidence of reactivity obtained was high in patients with breast carcinoma upon initial testing with MCF-7, whereas low reactivity was obtained with normal donors and patients with cancer of other sites. Testing of patients with benign breast disease (largely with fibrocystic disease) using the MCF-7 extract resulted in considerable reactivity of these patients significantly above that of normal controls. Possibly breast tissue antigens are recognized in MCF-7 extracts as well as breast cancer-associated antigens. Hopefully, the LMI assay will be able to discriminate breast cancer from benign breast disease in the future if it is to become promising as an early diagnostic of breast cancer. One approach in attempting to distinguish the two disorders may be to physiochemically fractionate crude breast cancer antigen preparations into "cancer related" and "benign related" reactivities as has been reported by Kadish, et al. (22).

Analysis of direct LMI longitudinal testing with MCF-7 as a function of

352

disease recurrence revealed no clear-cut predictive measure of relapse with individual patients, but if all relapse patient data were grouped then some trends in LMI reactivity versus disease recurrence emerged. LMI reactivity against MCF-7 decreased 1-6 months prior to clinical relapse and generally appeared to plateau at this level following relapse.

It was of interest that pre-operative patients were somewhat more reactive than post-operative patients. Whether this is a function of tumor-burden and antigen-load or due to other factors is only speculative. Further analyses of this data with more patients are required before statistical evaluations are meaningful.

Indirect LMI using supernatants generated by the interaction of breast cancer patient mononuclear cells and 3M KCl extracts of MCF-7 were strongly suggestive of lymphokine association of the reactions, presumably by LIF. Further modification of the indirect technique using a micro-system to both generate and test supernatants appears potentially useful in possibly semi—quantitating patient responses against TAA by performing end-point dilutions of supernatants containing high titered LIF. We are now in the process of using this modified procedure in longitudinal monitoring patient reactivity against a variety of antigenic materials to see if the results of individual patients can be predictive of disease prognosis and whether it will provide useful information related to efficacy of chemo-immunotherapy.

We have demonstrated that patients with carcinoma of the breast responded in a microculture LP assay to either autologous cryopreserved cells or to crude membrane preparations of autologous tumor cells. There appeared to be a definite requirement for autologous tumor cell-lymphocyte combinations since allogeneic antigen materials and patient or normal donor cells yielded nonspecific reactions. The observed autologous proliferative responses appeared to be directed against breast TAA since no reations were observed against autologous normal breast tissue, which did not contain histologically detectable tumor cells in parallel tests where positive results were obtained with tumor materials.

Analysis of autologous LP data as a function of stage of disease did not reveal any predictive information concerning tumor-burden or clinical staging at the time of surgery, although again the number of patients in each staging category is still small.

Although many patients gave positive reactions in MLTI and LMI, many patients tested did not respond to breast-tumor material. This may be due to several factors: a) sensitivity of the assays; b) adequacy of tissue preparation as antigens; c) lack of sufficient antigens in some tumors to elicit immunity or *in vitro* responses; d) presence of inhibitory factors in some tumor preparations; or e) inability of patients to respond at various times during clinical course of disease, either because of depressed immunologic competence or specific depression of reactivity to TAA.

Finally, our results clearly indicate the usefulness of direct and indirect LMI and LP assays in measuring breast TAA recognition by breast cancer patient leukocytes. The full potential of these assays for use in early disease diagnosis and following prognosis of disease is not clear. The indirect micro-LMI assay may emerge as a useful measure of parameters related to disease recurrence, survival and efficacy of therapy by having the capability of semi-quantitating host responses against TAA in sequential testing. One of the major problems remaining with both the LMI and LP studies presented here is to adequately understand the nature of the TAA's being recognized by the CMI response and to distinguish between antigens restricted to neoplastic cells and those associated with benign non-malignant cells.

REFERENCES

1. Herberman, R.B., "Existence of Tumor Immunity in Man." In *Mechanisms of Tumor Immunity*, edited by Ira Green, Stanley Cohen and Robert McCloskey, John Wiley and Sons, New York, 1977.

2. Takasugi, M., Mickey, M.R. and Terasaki, P.I., "Studies on Specificity of Cell-Mediated Immunity to Human Tumors." *J. Natl. Cancer Inst.* 53:1527-1538, 1974.

3. Oldham, R.K., Djeu, J.Y., Cannon, G.B., et al., "Cellular Microcytotoxicity in Human Systems. Analysis of Results." *J. Natl. Cancer Inst.* 55:1305-1318, 1975.

4. Bean, M.A., Bloom, B.R., Herberman, R.B., et al., "Cell-Mediated Cytotoxicity for Bladder Carcinoma. Evaluation of a Workshop." *Cancer Res.* 35:2902-2913, 1975.

5. Soule, H.D., Vazquez, J., Long, A., et al., "A Human Cell Line From a Pleural Effusion Derived from a Breast Carcinoma." *J. Natl. Cancer Inst.* 51:1409-1413, 1973.

6. Fogh, J., and Fogh, H., "Pocedures for Control of Mycoplasma Contamination of Tissue Cultures." *Ann. N.Y. Acad. Sci.* 172:15-30, 1969.

7. McCoy, J.L., Jerome, L.F., Dean, J.H., et al., "Inhibition of Leukocyte Migration by Tumor-Associated Antigens in Soluble Extracts of Human Breast Carcinoma." *J. Natl. Cancer Inst.* 53:11-17, 1974.

8. Fass, L., Herberman, R.B. and Ziegler, J., "Delayed Cutaneous Hypersensitivity Reactions to Autologous Extracts of Burkitt-Lymphoma Cells." *New Eng. J. Med.* 282:3-7, 1970.

9. McCoy, J.L., Jerome, L.F., Anderson, C., et al., "Leukocyte Migration Inhibition by Soluble Extracts of MCF-7 Tissue Culture Cell Line Derived from Breast Carcinoma." *J. Natl. Cancer Inst.* 57:1045-1049, 1976.

10. McCoy, J.L., Dean, J.H. and Herberman, R.B., "Human Cell-Mediated Immunity to Tuberculin as Assayed by the Agarose Micro-droplet Leukocyte Migration Inhibition Technique: Comparison with the Capillary Tube Assay." *J. Imm. Methods* 15:355-371, 1977.

11. Dean, J.H., Silva, J.S., McCoy, J.L., et al., "Lymphocyte Blastogenesis Induced by Potassium Chloride Extracts of Allogeneic Breast Carcinoma and Lymphoid Cells." *J. Natl. Cancer Inst.* 54:1295-1298, 1975.

12. Philp, J.R., Huffman, A.L. and Johnson, J.E., "Amplified Migration Inhibition Effect." *Inf. and Imm.* 14:872-875, 1976.

13. McCoy, J.L., Dean, J.H., Cannon, G.B., et al., "Detection of Cell-Mediated Immunity against Tumor-Associated Antigens of Human Breast Carcinoma by Migration Inhibition and Lymphocyte Stimulation Assays." In *Clinical Tumor Immunology*, edited by Wybran, J. and Staquet, M., Pergamon Press, Oxford, England, p. 77-86, 1976.

14. Anderson, V., Bjerrum, O. and Bendixen, G., "Effect of Autologous Mammary Tumour Extracts on Human Leukocyte Migration *In Vitro*." *Int. J. Cancer* 5:357-363, 1970.

15. Wolberg, W.H., "Inhibition of Migration of Human Autogenous and Allogeneic Leukocytes by Extracts of Patient's Cancers." *Cancer Res.* 31:798-802, 1971.

16. Cochran, A.J., Spilg, W.G., Mackie, R.M., et al., "Postoperative Depression of Tumour Directed Cell-Mediated Immunity in Patients with Malignant Disease." *Br. Med. J.* 2:67-70, 1972.

17. Segal, A., Weiler, O., Genin, J., et al., "*In Vitro* Study of Cellular Immunity Against Autochthonous Human Cancer." *Int. J. Cancer* 9:417-425, 1972.

18. Black, M.M., Leis, H.P., Jr., Shore, B., et al., "Cellular Hypersensitivity to Breast Cancer-Assessment by a Leukocyte Migration Procedure." *Cancer* 33:952-958, 1974.

19. Fisher, P., Golub, E., Holyner, H., et al., "Comparative Effects of Tumor Extracts on Lymphocyte Transformation in Peripheral Blood Cultures of Healthy Persons and Patients with Breast Cancer." *Z. Krebsforsch* 72:155-161, 1969.

20. Mavlight, G.M., Ambus, V., Gutterman, J.V., et al., "Antigen Solubilized from Human Solid Tumors: Lymphocyte Stimulation and Cutaneous Delayed Hypersensitivity." *Nature* (New Biol) 243:188-190, 1973.
21. Robinson, E., Sher, S. and Mekori, T., "Lymphocyte Stimulation by Phytohemagglutinin and Tumor Cells of Malignant Effusions." *Cancer Res.* 34:1548-1551, 1974.
22. Kadish, A.S., Marcus, D.M. and Bloom, B.R., "Inhibition of Leukocyte Migration Inhibition by Human Breast Cancer-Association Antigens." *Int. J. Cancer.* 18:581-586, 1976.

Crispen (ed.): Neoplasm Immunity: Experimental and Clinical

Sensitive Measurement of Immunocompetence and Anti-Tumor Reactivity in Lung Cancer Patients and Possible Mechanisms of Immunosuppression+

J.H. Dean[1]

G.B. Cannon[1]

T.R. Jerrells[1]

J.L. McCoy[2]

R.B. Herberman[2]

SUMMARY—A standardized assay of lymphocyte proliferation (LP) was used to assess the immunocompetence and anti-tumor immunity in lung cancer patients, some of whom were on an immunotherapy protocol receiving BCG or BCG plus irradiated allogeneic lung tumor cells. To measure immunocompetence, lymphocytes were tested in a microculture assay for their responses to the T-cell mitogen phytohemagglutinin (PHA) and to pooled cryopreserved allogeneic stimulating leukocytes in one-way mixed leukocyte cultures (MLC). These data were expressed and analyzed using a relative proliferation index (RPI), with depression defined as RPIs below the 10th percentile of normal donors. An appreciable proportion of lung cancer patients were found to have depressed LP responses on initial testing, and this was somewhat related to clinical stage as follows: Stage I, 18/55 (33%) depressed to PHA and 19/51 (37%) depressed to MLC; Stage II, 7/24 (29%) to PHA and 6/20 (30%) to MLC; Stage III, 17/23 (74%) to PHA and 17/23 (74%) to MLC; Stage IV, 9/16 (56%) to PHA and 8/14 (57%) to MLC. In Stage I lung cancer patients, the disease-free interval of patients who on initial testing had depressed responses to PHA and/or in MLC was compared by life table analysis to that of patients with reactivity in the normal range. The patients with depressed responses had a significantly shorter disease free interval (p < 0.009). To determine the possible mechanism for depressed reactivity, patients previously found to be depressed were studied for suppressor cell activity. A total of 11/21 (52%) of these patients were found to have cells which could suppress the response of normal lymphocytes to PHA. Of these patients with suppressor cell activity, 7/11 (64%) were found to have suppressor cells which were adherent to Sephadex G-10 columns and are presumed to be monocytes.

In LP assays to measure anti-tumor immunity, 28/40 (70%) patients responded to extracts of their autologous lung tumor as evidenced by a stimulation index (SI) of > 2.0 and a significant increase in ^{3}H-thymidine

---

[1]Department of Immunology, Biomedical Research Division, Litton Bionetics, Inc., Kensington, Maryland.

[2]Laboratory of Immunodiagnosis, National Cancer Institute, NIH, Bethesda, Maryland.
+Supported by USPHS contract NO1-CB-63975 from the Division of Cancer Biology and Diagnosis of the National Cancer Institute.

incorporation above the unstimulated controls (p < 0.01). A similar proportion of patients, 8/13 (62%), responded to intact tumor cells. Parallel experiments using both intact tumor cells and HMP demonstrated concordant results. Only 1/16 (6%) patients responded to extracts of autologous normal lung. These results suggest that many lung cancer patients possess cell mediated immunity (CMI) against lung tumor associated antigens which can be detected by LP. The antigenic specificities responsible for reactivity appear to be present on tumor cells, but not in uninvolved lung tissues. The failure of some lung patients to respond to autologous HMP was found to be due to an adherent suppressor cell that suppressed both mitogen and tumor extract-induced LP responses. Removal of the adherent suppressor cell fraction on a Sephadex G-10 column reversed this non-reactivity to autologous tumor antigens. Thus, suppressor cells may account for at least some of the lack of detectable anti-tumor reactivity as well as the immune depression of lung cancer patients.

INTRODUCTION

Assays of LP responses to mitogens or alloantigens offer potentially sensitive indicators of depressed lymphocyte function due to disease or to therapy. These assays may be useful in screening cancer patients, as an aid in staging and prognosis, and to detect those patients with immunologic abnormalities who might be candidates for immunological manipulation. In addition, LP assays might be useful for serial monitoring of patients during the course of their disease and therapy.

Many investigators have reported depression in LP responses in patients with solid tumors (1-13). Most of the studies have been based on differences among patient populations. Until recently, the considerable variability in LP assays has virtually precluded application of the assays to study individual patients in a longitudinal manner. In addition, there have been wide divergences among investigators as to the criteria to be used to express data, to define depressed responses, and to assess biological (as opposed to technical) fluctuations. Most of the criteria used have been adopted arbitrarily, and their relative abilities to discriminate have not been evaluated. This may account for some conflicting reports on the extent of immune depression in some types of cancer or other diseases (14-15). In addition, difficulty has been encountered in attempting to correlate *in vitro* LP data with clinical course, because stable measurements of LP responses to mitogens were not available. We recently published a report (16) in which particular attention was given to problems associated with comparing LP data from different experiments and studying longitudinal responses of individual patients. We proposed the use of a relative proliferation index (RPI), which appeared to be superior to other measures used previously for discriminating between cancer patients and normal donors and for longitudinal monitoring of mitogen or MLC responses. In addition, we observed

358

that LP responses to PHA and to pooled allogeneic cells in MLC gave better discrimination than did the responses to other stimulants.

Cell-mediated immunity (CMI) to tumor-associated (TAA) has been detected in lung cancer patients by the lymphocyte proliferation assay (17-23). It seemed advantageous to have a simple laboratory procedure to determine if lung cancer patients had CMI to TAAs on their autologous tumors, since some have suggested that augmentation of anti-tumor immunity might be translated into an effective and potentially beneficial form of therapy (24).

Most previous studies of LP reactivity against lung tumors have presented convincing evidence of lymphocyte activation, but have not approached the questions of the frequency of these responses in a lung cancer population, their specificity, or the influence of clinical stage or histologic tumor type. The number of patients tested in most studies has been small, and often allogeneic extracts which may not possess a common TAA and which may stimulate because of their foreign alloantigens, were employed.

The present studies were performed to assess LP reactivity in lung cancer patients to PHA and in MLC, and to examine anti-tumor reactivity to autologous TAA. We also studied the relationship between reactivity and clinical status and prognosis, and the possible role of suppressor cells in depressed or undetectable LP responses.

MATERIALS AND METHODS

Blood Specimens

Forty milliliters of heparinized whole blood (20 units/ml of preservative-free heparin) were obtained from lung carcinoma patients who were treated at the Medical University of South Carolina (MUSC), the Clinical Center of the National Institutes of Health, the National Naval Medical Center, Walter Reed Army Hospital and Portsmouth Naval Hospital. Blood from normal volunteers was obtained from the Blood Bank of the Clinical Center of the NIH, and from the laboratory and clerical staff at Litton Bionetics, Medical University of South Carolina, and Portsmouth Naval Hospital.

Blood from patients in all stages of disease was tested prior to and/or more than 1 week following surgery or therapy.

Preparation of Single Cell Suspension and Hypotonic Membrane Extracts

Single cell suspensions (SCS) were prepared from normal and tumor tissue under sterile conditions by careful mincing with scissors and scalpel. Intact tumor and normal lung cells were cryopreserved in medium containing 10% dimethyl sulfoxide and stored in vapor-phase liquid nitrogen for later use as stimulator cells in autologous mixed lymphocyte tumor interaction (MLTI) cultures (10,16).

359

Hypotonic saline membrane preparations (HMP) were prepared from fresh SCS's, as previously described (25). All SCS and HMP were checked for sterility by standard bacteriological methods. All contaminated extracts were discarded. The HMP were again checked for sterility after being dispensed into microtiter plates for patient testing. Selected reactive tumor HMP and/or matched normal lung tissue HMP were tested and found negative for mycoplasma by standard culture methods (Microbiology Section, Bionetics Medical Laboratories) and for evidence of bacterial products using antisera to *Pneumococcus, Streptococcus, Staphylococcus, Pseudomonas* and *E. coli* by Ouchterlony double gel diffusion. In addition, the presence of endotoxin was evaluated and found not to be elevated using a Limulus amebocyte lysate procedure (Microbiological Associates).

Lymphocyte Proliferation (LP) with PHA and in MLC

Peripheral blood mononuclear leukocytes (PBML) from lung cancer patients and normal individuals were isolated by flotation on Ficoll-Hypaque (Litton Bionetics, Inc., Kensington, MD) and washed three times with phosphate-buffered saline (PBS), pH 7.2. PBML were tested in a microculture LP assay, as previously described (26). Briefly, PBML were resuspended at 2×10^6/ml in RPMI 1640 (Grand Island Biologicals, Grand Island, NY) medium supplemented with 25 mM HEPES buffer, 1% glutamine, 20% heat-inactivated, fresh frozen, pooled human serum from donors with blood group AB, (Irvine Scientific, Orange, CA), and 50 μg/ml of gentamicin. Accurate cell counts were obtained using a Cytograph model 6300A (Biophysics Systems, Inc., Mahopac, NY) and cells were added to quadruplicate wells of flat bottom Microtest II plates (Falcon Plastics, Inc., Oxnard, CA) in 0.1-ml volumes at 2×10^5 cells/well using an automatic pipette (Hamilton, Reno, NA) fitted with disposable tips. We examined the response of patient and normal PBML to PHA (0.1-0.5 μg/well; purified grade-Burroughs Wellcome, Co., Research Triangle Park, NC) and to alloantigens, in one-way mixed leukocyte culture (MLC). Pooled allogeneic cells from six normal donors were obtained by leukophoresis and cryopreserved in a programmed rate freezer. For each test, stimulator cells were thawed and treated with 50 μg/ml of MMC for 30 min (37°C) and were added at a concentration of 4×10^5 cells/well to give a stimulator:responder ratio of 2:1. The microtiter plates were incubated at 37°C in a humidified atmosphere with a 5% CO_2 and air mixture. PHA cultures were terminated on day 4 and MLC cultures on day 7, following a 6-h pulse with 1 μCi of ^{3}H-TdR (New England Nuclear, Boston, Mass; specific activity 6.7 Ci/mmol). Cells from all microcultures were harvested onto glass scintillation paper (Grade 934AH, Reeve Angel, Clinton, NJ) with a multiple sample harvester (Brandel, Rockville, MD) followed by precipitation of incorporated label with 5% cold trichloracetic acid. The amount of in-

360

corporated ^{3}H-TdR was determined in a liquid scintillation counter and counted to less than 1% error.

LP response data were expressed as a relative proliferation index (RPI). The RPI, as previously described (16), is defined as the ratio of net CPM (nCPM) [CPM in experimental cultures with stimulant minus baseline CPM] of a test individual (e.g., cancer patient) to the mean nCPM of lymphocytes from normal individuals (three or more) tested simultaneously in the LP assay.

$$RPI = \frac{nCPM \text{ of test individual}}{\text{Mean nCPM of normal individuals}}$$
$$(\geq 3) \text{ tested simultaneously}$$

Thus, the RPI value can be considered as a measure of the degree of responsiveness relative to that of normal individuals tested simultaneously.

RPI data from patient and normal populations were compared by the Wilcoxan two-sample rank-sum test (27).

Depressed responses to PHA or in MLC were defined as those below the lowest tenth percentile of RPI of normal individuals and the cut-offs were: PHA $\leq$ .62, MLC $\leq$ .50. The tenth percentile cut-off point indicates that 90% of the normals tested gave RPI measurements equal to or greater than this value.

In addition, the coefficient of variation (SD/mean) was calculated, which is a good measure of variation relative to the mean.

Lymphocyte Proliferation with Autologous Material

Lymphocyte proliferation (LP) assays with autologous tumor and normal lung tissue were essentially performed as described above and previously in detail (16). PBML were added to quadruplicate wells of microtiter plates at a concentration of 4 x 10^5/wells in a 0.1 ml volume.

Cryopreserved tumor cells were recovered by techniques previously described (12), treated with mitomycin-C (50 μg/ml, MMC, Calbiochem, San Diego, CA), washed 3 times with media to remove excess MMC and added in 0.1 ml quantities to the PBML containing wells. Tumor and normal lung cells were added to give ratios of PBML to tumor cell concentrations ranging from 1:1 to 50:1. Control cultures consisting of tumor cells alone or PBML alone were included in each assay.

Tumor cell HMP or normal cell HMP were diluted in complete media without serum and added in 0.1 ml volumes to quadruplicate lymphocyte cultures (4 x 10^5 cells/well) in concentrations ranging from .005 to 50 μg Lowry protein per well. All cultures were pulse labeled for 6 hours with 1 μCi of ^{3}H-TdR before harvest on day 7. The data were analyzed for significance by Welch's modification of Student's t-test.

The stimulation index (SI) for cultures containing tumor cells was defined as the ratio of mean counts per minute (CPM) of cultures containing tumor

361

cells minus the CPM of mitomycin-C blocked tumor or normal lung cells cultured alone, divided by the CPM of control lymphocyte cultures containing no tumor cells. Cultures containing MMC treated tumor cells alone always had low levels of ^{3}H-TdR incorporation (50-200 CPM).

The SI of cultures containing the HMP was defined as the ratio of the CPM of experimental cultures (E) containing extract to CPM of control lymphocyte cultures (C) containing no tissue extract.

Reactivity to autologous tumor material was considered positive when the SI was greater than or equal to 2.0 and the CPM in the experimental cultures were significantly higher than CPM in the control cultures at $p <$ .01.

Suppressor Cell Studies

Adherent monocytes (MO) were selectively removed, from the PBML of lung cancer patients previously found to be suppressed in the LP assay, by passage through Sephadex G-10 columns, as described in detail by Jerrells (28). In general, this treatment resulted in MO depletion to $< 0.2\%$ (0 positive cells/500 counted) as judged by nonspecific esterase staining (29). In most experiments employing patient PBML, usually 80% of the original cells placed on the column were recovered. Patient MO-depleted PBML, untreated PBML and adherent cells removed from the Sephadex G-10 beads by xylocaine were then studied for suppressor cell activity by co-cultivating with PBML from a normal donor mixed with PHA or allogeneic cells. Cells to be tested for suppressor activity were incubated with MMC (50 μg/10^7 cells) at 37°C for 30 minutes. Following 3 washes with RPMI-1640 to remove excess MMC, the cells were added to the wells of a microtiter plate along with PBL from a normal donor. Patient PBML and MO depleted PBML were tested for suppressor activity by co-cultivating 2 x 10^5 MMC-treated patient cells and 2 x 10^5 normal PBL to achieve a 1:1 ratio. Adherent cells recovered from the G-10 beads were added to normal responder PBML at a final concentration of 20% (i.e., 4 x 10^4 MMC-treated adherent cells were co-cultivated with 2 x 10^5 normal PBML). All co-cultivation experiments were controlled by testing normal PBML with autologous MMC-treated PBML and data were expressed as percent suppression.

RESULTS

Immunocompetence Studies

LP responses to PHA and to alloantigen were studied on a large number of normal individuals and lung cancer patients, over a period of 4 years.

The data of lung cancer patients was expressed as nCPM, SI, and RPI, and the frequency of depressed values below the tenth percentile cut-off are given in Table 1. The RPI and nCPM values for the responses to PHA and

Table 1—LYMPHOCYTE PROLIFERATIVE RESPONSES IN PATIENTS WITH LUNG CARCINOMA TO PHA AND TO ALLOANTIGENS IN ONE-WAY MIXED LEUKOCYTE CULTURES

Stimulant Tested	Number of Patients Tested	Mean Baseline CPM	nCPM Mean Median (CV)		SI Mean Median (CV)		RPI Mean Median (CV)		No. depressed/No. tested (%) nCPM cut-off	SI cut-off	RPI cut-off
PHA	131	935	59,458	53,089**¹ (0.68)	127	76** (1.08)	0.75	0.66** (0.64)	36/131 (27%)	21/131 (16%)	65/131 (50%)
MLC	123	1,530	21,520	15,857** (0.98)	36	20 (1.58)	0.68	0.65** (0.70)	49/123 (40%)	33/123 (27%)	58/123 (47%)

¹Significantly different relative to normal population using Wilcoxon two-sample rank-sum test at $p < 0.05$ (*) or $p < 0.01$ (**).

MLC of lung cancer patients were significantly below those of the normal donors (p < 0.01). The differences in SI values were significant only for PHA. When the frequency of depressed values in cancer patients determined according to SI and RPI measurements, large differences were observed. Only 16% of the patients had depressed SIs to PHA, whereas 50% had depressed RPIs. The nCPM was intermediate in its ability to discriminate normals from cancer patients. These data indicate that SI is probably the least satisfactory of the three measures for defining LP responses and the RPI most satisfactory in discriminating patient responses from normals.

From Table 1, one can observe that of the three measures, nCPM and RPI agree most often. To investigate how closely the three measures were related, a sample of 19 lung cancer patient data were studied and the data are presented in Table 2.

These data are from different patients, assayed on different days, using different lots of mitogens with RPI values based on the responses of PBML of different normal donors. In spite of these variables, close concordance between nCPM and RPI measurements was observed. When the data were analyzed by Kendall's test, the CPM and nCPM values aligned exactly (r = 1.00). Net CPM values agreed with RPI values (r = 0.99), but less well with the SI value (r = 0.60). The SI and RPI values also did not correlate well, (r = 0.58). Note that SI values accompanying the similar RPI values of 0.99 and 1.02 were quite disparate (80.7 and 250.5), while nCPM values were similar (55,463 and 66,858). Furthermore, the RPI values accompanying the similar SI values of 79.3 and 80.7 were quite disparate (0.13 and 0.99, with the first value considered depressed) as were the nCPM values (9,400 and 55,643). There was also a relationship between nCPM values accompanying the RPI values of 0.99 and 2.13 (55,563 and 118,634, respectively), which were approximately double in both RPI and nCPM.

To evaluate sensitivity and reproducibility of our LP assay data and to assess the value of the RPI method for longitudinal monitoring, the coefficient of variation (CV) was calculated for each parameter. Table 3 demonstrates data from four normal individuals (two males and two females) whose LP responses were frequently measured over a period of one year. For each donor, nCPM, SI and the RPI values for PHA and MLC responses were calculated, and RPI and SI values below the tenth percentile cut-off are indicated. An ideal measurement for longitudinally monitoring LP responses would be one which gives a low CV for normal individuals tested over time and the most constant data between test periods. Note that SI values gave a much higher CV than did RPI and nCPM measurements. Very few of the test values by any of the three measures were depressed although, as indicated from the CV values, the nCPM, and especially the SI varied considerably over the testing period. In 8 of 9 cases, RPI had a slightly lower CV. In no case did the SI have a lesser CV.

364

Table 2—LYMPHOCYTE PROLIFERATIVE RESPONSES TO PHA IN LUNG CANCER PATIENTS RANKED BY RELATIVE PROLIFERATION INDEX WITH CORRESPONDING EXPERIMENTAL CPM, BASELINE CPM, NET CPM AND STIMULATION INDEX

Experimental CPM (E)	Baseline CPM (C)	nCPM	SI	RPI
1,415	221	1,195	6.4	0.03
5,492	268	5,224	20.5	0.03
7,517	110	7,407	68.5	0.09
9,520	120	9,400	79.3	0.13
14,703	2,882	11,840	5.1	0.15
10,541	120	10,421	88.2	0.19
17,401	282	17,120	61.2	0.26
20,021	115	19,906	174.6	0.31
35,071	131	34,940	266.7	0.35
36,899	122	36,777	302.4	0.49
45,427	66	45,361	690.9	0.63
46,481	133	46,348	349.5	0.69
56,388	149	56,238	377.0	0.75
56,158	696	55,463	80.7	0.99
67,126	267	66,858	250.5	1.02
77,432	128	77,304	603.8	1.08
73,790	185	73,605	398.9	1.40
84,344	320	84,023	262.8	1.50
120,822	2,189	118,634	55.2	2.13

$r^1 = 0.60$

$r = 0.99$

$r = 0.58$

¹Correlation of similarity determined by Kendall's coefficient of rank correlation (r) test.

We next analyzed CPM and RPI values obtained from over 4 years of LP testing using post-hoc comparisons for Kruskal-Wallis design analysis of variance to determine how these two parameters varied from year to year (Figure 1). As expected CPM values were frequently different ($p \leq 0.05$) between test years while RPI values were more stable. This observation further strengthens our contention that the RPI is a superior method to

Table 3—LONGITUDINAL MONITORING OF LYMPHOCYTE PROLIFERATIVE RESPONSES IN NORMAL DONORS

DONOR	nCMP (CV)	PHA SI (CV)	RPI (CV)	nCPM (CV)	MLC SI (CV)	RPI (CV)
1	141,552	88	0.95	20,856	12	1.05
	55,588	41	0.96	16,881	9	0.89
	70,295	96	0.62[3]	50,617	62	0.92
	111,376	129	1.68	73,471	63	1.25
	161,172	310	1.16	55,485	94	1.05
	(0.42)	(0.78)	(0.36)	(0.55)	(0.76)	(0.14)
2	46,314	64	1.47	31,928	25	1.26
	136,048	773	1.20	22,599	82	0.97
	43,719	86	0.78	78,943	12	1.35
	165,981	199	1.05	81,114	87	1.00
	146,531	384	1.99	21,915	55	1.32
	(0.54)	(0.97)	(0.35)	(0.64)	(0.64)	(0.15)
3	65,279	283	1.00	33,850	60	1.00
	73,256	150	1.03	17,075	13	0.84
	26,613[1]	101	1.71	23,715	98	0.74
	88,202	170	1.02	62,376	125	1.44
	94,059	232	1.01	53,703	89	0.81
	(0.38)	(0.38)	(0.27)	(0.52)	(0.60)	(0.29)
4	122,990	262	1.00	52,343	133	0.92
	106,788	52	1.03	30,613	10	1.00
	47,913	308	1.02	18,541	62	1.01
	94,005	26[2]	1.05	17,239	11	0.86
	50,630	51	0.95	20,358	20	2.65
	(0.40)	(0.96)	(0^4)	(0.53)	(1.11)	(0.59)

[1] nCPM depressed below tenth percentile cutoff value.
[2] SI value for mitogen response depressed below tenth percentile cutoff value.
[3] RPI depressed below tenth percentile cutoff value.
CV = Coefficient of variation. (CV) indicates lowest CV value.

either CPM or SI for expressing data from single determinations and from longitudinal-LP monitoring.

Using the RPI values, we next examined the relationship between depressed LP responses of lung cancer patients and clinical stage. Figure 2 shows the RPI values for LP responses to PHA and MLC on the initial tests of lung cancer patients, prior to therapy besides surgery, grouped by stage of disease. Patients with greater tumor burden, in stages III and IV, had an appreciably higher proportion of depressed responses than did patients with more localized disease.

Since these data suggested that depressed LP responses might be associated with more extensive disease, it was of interest to determine whether

Figure 1- COMPARISON ON VARIATION
IN CPM AND RPI PARAMETERS BY YEARS OF TESTING

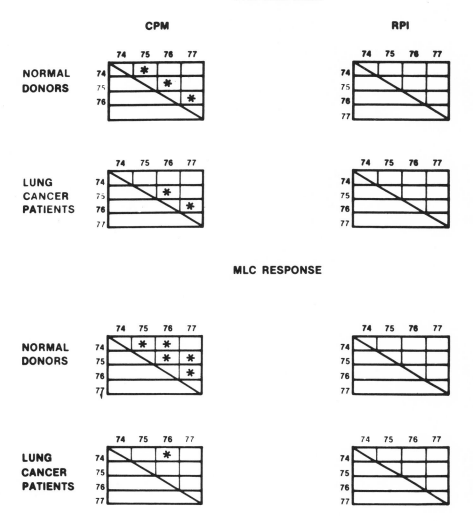

*=Data significantly different at p≤ .05 using the post-hoc comparisons for Kruskal-Wallis design analysis of variance.

Figure 2—RELATIONSHIP OF LYMPHOPROLIFERATIVE RESPONSE OF UNTREATED LUNG CANCER PATIENTS TO STAGE OF DISEASE

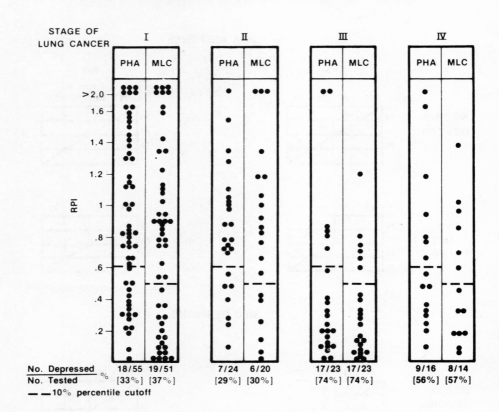

these measures could distinguish within a particular stage of disease, those patients with a greater risk of recurrence. The responses of patients classified as having Stage I disease, by surgical and pathologic criteria, were examined. The disease-free interval of patients with depressed LP responses to PHA and/or MLC in their initial test following surgery was compared by life table analysis to that of patients with responses in the normal range (Figure 3). The patients with depressed PHA or MLC responses had significantly shorter disease-free course (p ≤ 0.009). Thus, the measurement of LP responses to PHA and/or MLC during the perioperative period appears to be able to subclassify patients into separate prognostic categories. Preliminary data from this laboratory also indicate that patients

368

Figure 3—RELATIONSHIP OF LYMPHOPROLIFERATIVE RESPONSES TO PHA AND MLC IN FIRST BLOOD SPECIMEN POST SURGERY TO SURVIVAL FREE OF DISEASE

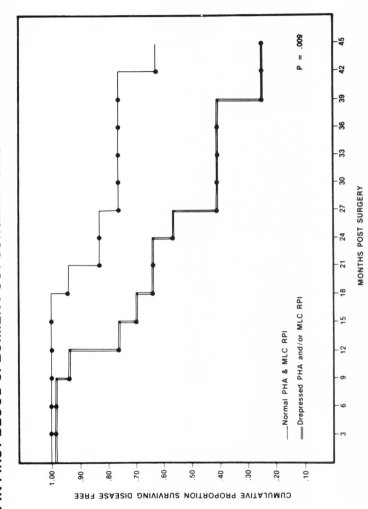

Patient group with normal responses has significantly different (p=.009) disease free interval than group with one or more depressed measurements.

receiving immunotherapy with BCG or BCG plus allogeneic tumor cells may have prolonged disease-free intervals despite depressed LP responses to PHA and MLC (Cannon et al., in preparation).

Anti-Tumor Immunity Studies

The results of the autologous mixed lymphocyte tumor cell interactions (MLTI) of patients with lung cancer are summarized in Figure 4. Significant

Figure 4—LYMPHOPROLIFERATIVE RESPONSES OF LUNG CANCER PATIENTS TO AUTOLOGOUS INTACT TUMOR CELLS

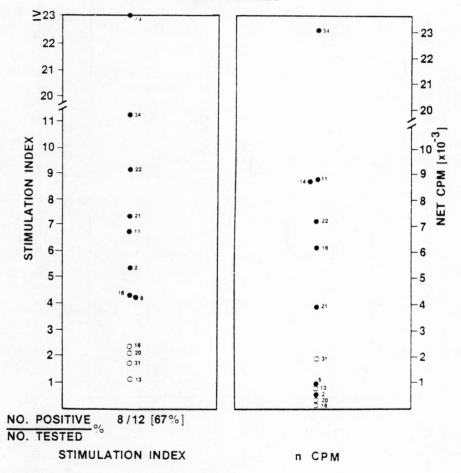

NO. POSITIVE
─────────── %   8 / 12 [67%]
NO. TESTED

STIMULATION INDEX   n CPM

Closed circle (•) indicates positive response (SI ≥ 2.0, p < .01) and open circle (0) indicates negative response. Number to right of data point indicates patient number to allow comparison between SI and nCPM.

370

stimulation (p < 0.01) with SIs greater than 2-fold were observed with 8/12 patients (67%) when their lymphocytes were cultured with their own tumor cells. Data were also expressed as nCPM on the right panel of this figure. Seven of 12 patients were above an arbitrary cut-off of 1000 CPM. The optimal ratio of responding lymphocytes to stimulating tumor cells (R/S) was usually 10:1, although significant proliferation occurred over a broad range of tumor cell concentrations. R/S ratios of 1-2:1 were generally inhibitory or less reactive than ratios of 5-10:1.

To examine the feasibility of using HMP in place of intact tumor cells, eight patients were tested in parallel, using both intact tumor cells and HMP derived from the same tumor. Correlation was obtained in 7/8 paired experiments with both preparations giving either positive (4/8) or negative (3/8) results, with r = .74 comparing SI values (p < 0.001) and r = .61 (p < .001) comparing nCPM. Thus, comparable levels of lymphoproliferation were seen with optimal does of HMP or intact tumor cells.

The generally good agreement between responses to tumor cells and HMP led us to perform subsequent studies with only HMP since HMP extracts are logistically and technically easier to use than frozen tumor cells. A summary of the results of the studies of LP responses to HMP derived from autologous tumor cells is given in Figures 5 and 6. Positive responses were defined as those with greater than 2-fold proliferation, and were observed in 28/40 patients (70%) tested with autologous tumor HMP (Figure 5). Similar results were seen when the data were expressed as nCPM, with 22/40 (55%) patients showing significant levels (p < 0.01) of stimulation with nCPM greater than 1,000 (Figure 6). In some patients it was possible to also assess LP reactivity to HMP prepared from autologous normal lung tissue (Figure 5 and 6). The responses to autologous tumor HMP (nCPM and SI) were significantly different from the responses to normal tissue HMP at p < 0.01 by the Wilcoxon rank-sum test (this statistical procedure was used because of the nonparametric distribution of the data). Of the 16 patients tested with both normal and tumor HMP, only one patient had significant LP greater than 2-fold stimulation by normal lung HMP and then only at the highest concentration of protein tested and with nCPM < 1,000. The reactivity of the majority of patients to autologous tumor, and the low degree of reactivity to similar extracts of normal lung, suggested that TAA were being recognized. However, it was important to rule out the possibility that some of the LP reactivity was directed against contaminating bacterial products or other stimuli. Using antisera against common lung flora, we could find no evidence of bacterial products in the reactive tumor extract. In addition, cultures of these extracts were negative for mycoplasma as well as other bacteria. To rule out the possibility that lung tumor HMPs contained a nonspecific stimulant (i.e., mitogen), a number of normal donors were tested with selected allogeneic tumor

Figure 5—LYMPHOPROLIFERATIVE RESPONSE OF LUNG CANCER PATIENTS TO AUTOLOGOUS TUMOR EXTRACT AND NORMAL LUNG

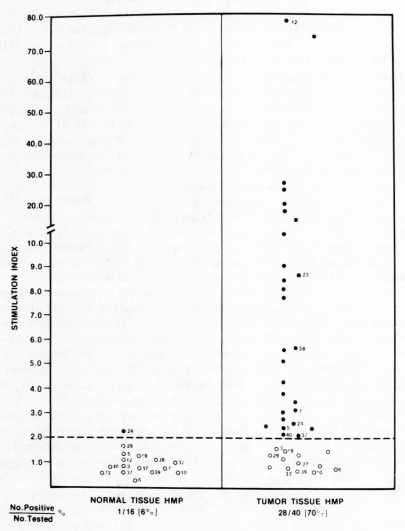

Numbers to the right of the data points are the patient number to allow a direct comparison between the response of each patient to tumor versus normal tissue HMP. Only the results of the initial test on each patient are shown. Data plotted as stimulation index (SI) with SI values ≥ 2.0 (broken line) considered positive when mean CPM of experimental and control cultures different at p < 0.01 level of significance. All data points above the 2 SI cutoff were significant at p < 0.01 in this study.

372

Figure 6—LYMPHOPROLIFERATIVE RESPONSE OF LUNG CANCER PATIENTS TO AUTOLOGOUS TUMOR EXTRACT AND NORMAL LUNG

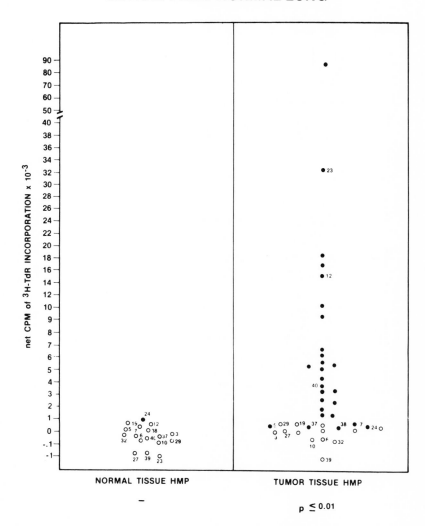

Numbers to the right of the data points are the patient number to allow a direct comparison between the response of each patient to tumor versus normal tissue HMP. Only the results of the initial test on each patient are shown. LP reactivity plotted as net CPM (experimental minus control HMP) with positive responses (SI $\geq$ 2, p < .01) indicated by closed circle (•) and negative responses by open circle (0). Response of lung cancer patients to tumor versus normal lung tissue HMP analyzed by Wilcoxon rank-sum test and significantly different at p < 0.01.

374

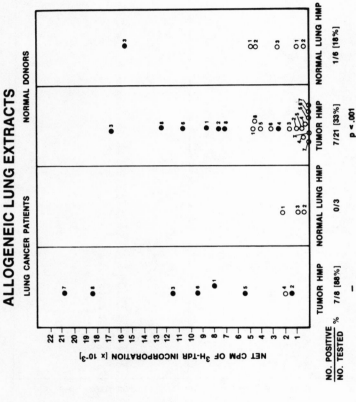

Figure 7—LYMPHOPROLIFERATIVE RESPONSES OF NORMAL DONORS TO ALLOGENEIC LUNG EXTRACTS

Numbers denote separate tumor and/or normal lung extracts . Closed circle (●) indicate positive LP response (SI > 2.0 and p < 0.01) and open circle (0) indicate negative response. Data for responses of lung cancer patients to autologous tumor HMP versus normal donor responses to allogeneic tumor HMP significantly different (p < 0.01) by Wilcoxon rank-sum analysis. No. positive/No. tested (%) shown at bottom of figure.

extracts (Figure 7). The data indicate that 7/8 (88%) of the extracts elicited a positive autologous response by the cancer patients, whereas none of the available paired normal tissue extracts elicited a positive response when allogeneic normal donors were tested with these extracts. Seven of 21 (33%) normal donors responded to tumor HMPs and 1/6 (18%) responded to normal extracts. The substantially lower frequency of reactivity by the normal donors indicated that mitogenic stimulation was not involved, and it seems likely that the reactivity seen was related to recognition of normal alloantigens. The conclusions were strengthened when the data from the testing with some extracts (#3, #4 and #7) were more clearly examined. The autologous patient reacted strongly to extract #7, whereas none of the normal donors were reactive (0/3). In contrast, extract #4 was non-reactive in the patient, whereas 1/3 of the normal donors responded. The one

Figure 8—LP RESPONSES TO TUMOR HMP OF LUNG CANCER PATIENTS WITH VARIOUS STAGES OF DISEASE[1]

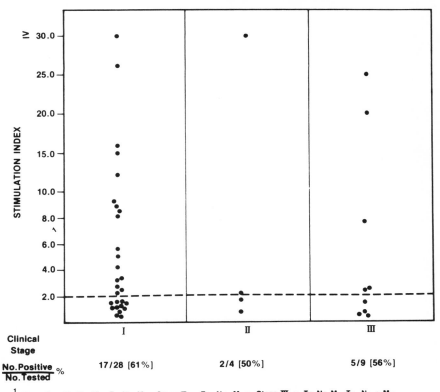

^{1} Stage I = T N_0 M_0, T_2 N_0 M_0; Stage II = T_2, N_1, M_0; Stage III = T_2 N_2 M_0 T_3 N_{1-2} M_0.

375

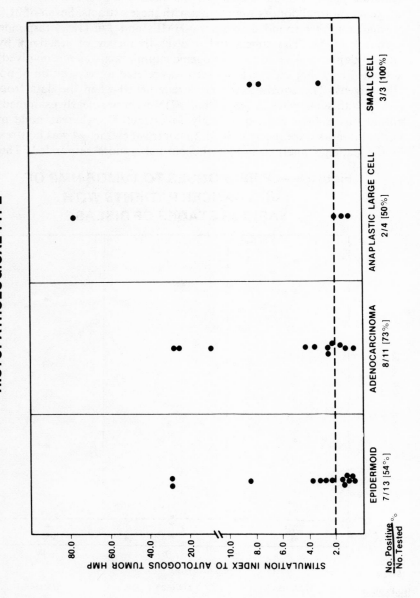

Figure 9—RELATIONSHIP OF LP RESPONSE TO AUTOLOGOUS TUMOR HMP VERSES HISTOPATHOLOGICAL TYPE

normal donor who responded to tumor extract #3 reacted similarly to the matched normal lung HMP. When the overall magnitude of the responses of normal donors to lung tumor HMP was compared to that of the patients by the Wilcoxon rank-sum test, they were found to be significantly different at $p \leq 0.001$.

The data were then examined to determine if the stage of disease influenced the response of lung cancer patients to autologous tumor HMP. Figure 8 shows that the majority of patients with Stage I disease had positive reactions but the incidence of reactivity in the patients with more advanced stages was similar. We also examined the data for a relationship between autologous tumor HMP responses and disease-free interval or survival using the SI (data not shown) but have been unable thus far to discern any correlation.

When responses of patients with different histological types of tumor were examined (Figure 9), the incidence of reactivity was found to be similar in each category.

Since an appreciable number of lung cancer patients were shown to have depressed reactivity in LP assays to PHA or in MLC, it was of interest to determine whether this was a factor in the unreactivity of some patients to their autologous tumor antigen. Figure 10 shows the relationship between LP response to autologous tumor HMP and the LP response to the general stimulant PHA. It should be noted that some patients with depressed LP responses to general stimulants still demonstrated reactivity to autologous tumor HMP (and thus depressed PHA responses appear to be unrelated).

Suppressor Cell Studies

Depressed LP responses in some tumor-bearing rodents and cancer patients (23, 28, 30, 31), have been shown to be due to the presence of suppressor cells, rather than to an intrinsic defect in lymphocyte function. We therefore recalled some patients previously shown to have depressed LP responses to PHA and in the MLC and studied them for suppressor cell activity. Figure 11 demonstrates a representative experiment. Removal of adherent cells by a passage of PBML through Sephadex G-10 columns appreciably enhanced the responses to both PHA and in MLC (left panel). Co-culture of the patients' PBML with normal PBML at a 1:1 ratio significantly suppressed the normal PBML response to PHA and MLC relative to the control of added autologous MMC-treated normal cells (middle panel). In addition, co-cultures of normal PBML and column passed non-adherent PBML from the cancer patient did not produce suppression, while cultures of adherent cells from the patient and normal PBML, at a 20% concentration, had significantly reduced LP responses (right panel). To date, 11/21 (52%) of the lung cancer patients with depressed responses studied had suppressor cell activity and in 7/11 (64%)

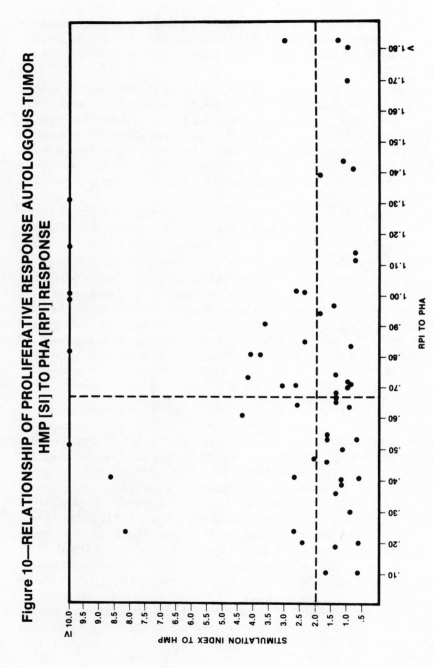

Figure 10—RELATIONSHIP OF PROLIFERATIVE RESPONSE AUTOLOGOUS TUMOR HMP [SI] TO PHA [RPI] RESPONSE

Broken line indicates cutoff for depressed PHA responses (RPI) and positive LP response (SI ≥ 2.0) to tumor HMP.

these cells are adherent to Sephadex G-10 columns and are presumed to be monocytes. With the demonstration of suppressor cells in the circulation of some patients, it seemed possible that some of the unreactivity to autologous tumor antigens was due to suppression. Therefore, a few patients were recalled who had previously been non-reactive to autologous tumor HMP and adherent cells were depleted from their PBML by passage through Sephadex G-10 columns. Figure 12 demonstrates the LP responses to autologous tumor HMP by the PBML of a lung cancer patient, unseparated and after depletion of MO. To provide sufficient MO helper activity, 1% were added to the latter culture. Whereas, the unseparated PBML did not show a detectable response to the tumor extract, the column passaged cells reacted to both concentrations of extract. The addition of 25% esterase staining, Sephadex G-10 adherent autologous cells to the cultures of MO-depleted PBML completely suppressed the LP response.

DISCUSSION

In the present study, lymphocytes from a large group of lung cancer patients were tested for their proliferative responses to PHA and to alloantigens in the MLC. Stimulation indices, which have been most widely used to express the levels of LP responses of cancer patients, were found to be less than satisfactory for mitogen and MLC responses because of: (1) the relative variation of SIs was large for normals; (2) SIs did not correlate well with nCPM and (3) in longitudinal testing there were numerous tests in which RPI and nCPM were depressed but SIs were normal. Baseline CPM (C) values varied widely among individuals and from day to day, and these had an inordinate influence on the SI (E/C). The baseline incorporation of ^{3}H-TdR may be due to the factors quite independent of the ability of the lymphocytes to respond to a stimulus. SI values varied considerably, and although they correlated somewhat with nCPM values, they could not be used accurately to identify depressed patients or to monitor LP responses. In addition, both E and nCPM values were found to vary considerably among experiments, probably due to differences in culture conditions, mitogen or antigen lot, and other technical factors. The RPI, which relates the nCPM value of the test individual to the mean of three or more normal donors tested on the same day, appeared to be more satisfactory than nCPM or SI since the RPI gave a similar CV among normal donors in serial testing of normals than did the other measures (16).

We feel that the RPI calculation is the best parameter for expressing levels of LP responses to mitogens as well as in MLC (16). In addition, since the normal range is narrower, we feel that the use of the RPI will allow a more sensitive discrimination of subtle changes in lymphocyte functions in cancer patients or other individuals. This should also allow more reliable serial

Figure 11—EFFECT OF ADHERENT CELL REMOVAL ON THE LP RESPONSE TO PHA AND IN MLC

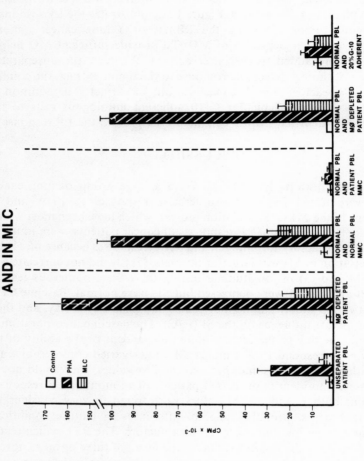

Left panel indicates effect of Sephadex G-10 column passage to deplete MO on LP responses. Middle panel indicates results of co-culture studies in which MMC treated patient PBML were admixed with normal PBML at 1:1 (S/R) ratio. Right panel indicates results of co-culture studies using patient MO depleted PBML or a 20% admix of Sephadex G-10 adherent cells with normal PBML.

Figure 12—EFFECT OF ADHERENT CELL REMOVAL ON THE LP RESPONSE TO AUTOLOGOUS TUMOR HMP

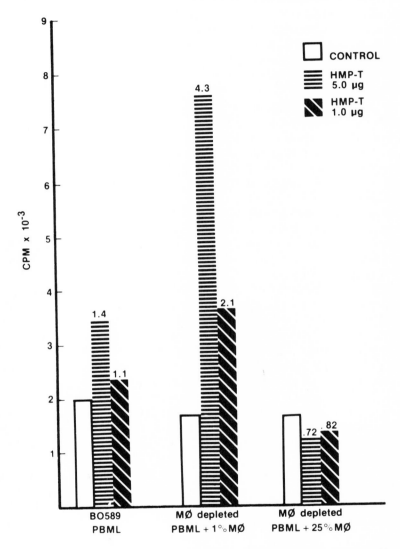

monitoring of cancer patients on immunosuppressive and immunoadjuvant therapy. The main limitation of the RPI is that it must be based on the response of several ($\geq$3) normal individuals tested in each experiment. However, a reasonable alternative to this would be the use of cryopreserved aliquots of PBML from the same normal donor (12).

381

The data presented here confirm that patients with lung carcinoma have significantly impaired LP responses to the T-lymphocyte stimulants, PHA and alloantigens. Impaired lymphocyte function appears to correlate with stage of disease, in that a higher frequency of impaired LP function was observed in patients with more advanced disease.

Initial testing of LP responses to PHA and in the MLC performed on Stage I lung cancer patients following surgery and prior to other therapy was shown to significantly discriminate a group of patients with shorter disease-free intervals on follow-up. This is the first evidence that we are aware of for the predictive value of LP responses in Stage I patients, although others have indicated that mitogen responses were prognostic in more advanced disease patients (13). The depressed values at this time may reflect prolonged post-operative immune depression. This might allow tumor cells, missed or disseminated by surgery, to grow progressively. Alternatively, the depressed responses may be due to latent tumor metastases.

The present study also demonstrated that a high proportion of lung cancer patients have LP reactivity significant even at the stringent $p < 0.01$ level, to autologous tumor material. The levels of lymphocyte blastogenesis induced by the tumor HMP in some patients were as high or higher than seen in cultures with MLC or many bacterial antigens. Therefore, the antigens recognized either on the intact cells or in the extracts appear to be a strong stimuli and/or in some individuals, a considerable proportion of lymphocytes in the circulating population are committed to the antigen.

Although many patients reacted strongly to their autologous lung tumor preparations, others were completely unreactive. We have considered a variety of possible explanations for the lack of reactivity observed in some patients. An easy explanation for lack of reactivity in some patients might be that the tumor was not sufficiently antigenic to elicit an appreciable CMI response. Alternatively, the tumor-associated antigens on some tumors may be very labile and destroyed during the preparation of single cell suspensions or during the extraction procedure. Neither of these hypotheses are easily investigated, but seem quite unlikely for those patients who lost reactivity after initially positive results. One might expect that if patients were depressed in their LP responses to PHA or in MLC, they would be unlikely to react to tumor antigens. However, we failed to find a good correlation between these parameters. It should be noted, however, that some responses to tumor were considerably stronger than others, and without depression, a patient reacting at a given level might react more strongly. In fact, our finding of suppressor cells in some patients, which could inhibit the responses to tumor HMP as well as to PHA and alloantigens, support this possibility. Suppressor cells have also been shown to be one cause of negative or depressed LP responses to mitogens, alloantigens and tumor antigens in rodent tumor systems (22, 23, 30-32). As in the rodent systems, preliminary data indicate that the suppressor cells causing a lack of LP reactivity to autologous tumor material are adherent cells, apparently monocytes. We are currently attempting to confirm these data and to obtain an understanding of the mechanism responsible for this suppression and its frequency in the patient population.

The specificity of the LP reactions appeared in most cases to be directed against tumor-associated antigens (TAA) present in tumor cells or extracts, but not found on normal lung tissue. Some earlier studies on LP responses in lung cancer utilized allogeneic materials as well as autologous materials. Previous studies from this laboratory (26) have demonstrated that allogeneic breast tumor extracts can stimulate the PBML of normal individuals as well as cancer patients and this reactivity appeared to be due to foreign histocompatibility antigens. Since all patient testing in the present study was done with autologous lung cells or extracts, the possible role of foreign histocompatability antigens was virtually eliminated.

In only one case was reactivity to autologous normal lung HMP noted and this occurred at only the highest concentrations tested and involved a low level of nCPM. Vanky, et al. (18) and Roth, et al. (20) likewise reported occasional LP reactivity to autologous normal tissue extracts at high concentrations. It was pointed out by Roth, who noted increased stimulation protein synthesis of one patient to normal lung extract, that normal tissue removed during surgery is of necessity located near the tumor and that this so-called normal tissue could on occasion contain a low concentration of occult tumor cells, TAA or immune complexes.

A major concern regarding the specificity of LP reactivity was the possible role of bacteria or bacterial products. All materials which did not pass both sterility checks were discarded. We also could find no evidence of bacterial products in selected reactive tumor and matched non-reactive normal extracts by Ouchterlony double gel diffusion using antisera against common or pathogenic lung flora. In addition, these extracts were negative upon culture for mycoplasma. The endotoxin levels in these extracts were likewise not elevated and comparable to levels in PBS by the Limulus amebocyte lysate assay. Finally, in tests where cryopreserved single cell suspension were employed, accounting for reactivity due to bacterial products would be less likely since the intact tumor cells were washed multiple times upon thawing and following mitomycin-C treatment. In these tests with single cell suspensions, reactivity was consistently observed against tumor cells and correlated well with reactivity to HMP extracts from these same cells. When normal individuals were tested against selected allogeneic reactive tumor and paired non-reactive normal lung HMP extracts, only a portion of the donors reacted and then at a lower level then some patients. It seems most likely that the occasional LP reactivity observed with these extracts in normal individuals is due to alloantigens rather than to bacterial products or mitogenic stimuli.

The similar reactivity of patients to intact cryopreserved tumor cells and HMP makes it unlikely that different or additional antigens were being recognized in HMP than on intact cells. Thus, additional antigenic determinants do not seem to be introduced during the extraction procedure. The data also suggest that TAA are moderately well preserved during the extraction procedure since the optimal level for maximum LP reactivity in most patients was approximately 1 μg of protein/culture. Extracts have several advantages over intact cells since they are more easily stored and they do not require the cumbersome washing procedures associated with thawing and mitomycin-C treating of cryopreserved cells.

ACKNOWLEDGMENTS

The authors are grateful to B. Baumgardner, F. LeSane, Dr. E. Perlin, Dr. C. Miller, Dr. J. Reid, M. Keels, J. Siwarski, K. Murphy, C. Fox, C. Labash, D. Card, and S. Occhipinti for their assistance.

REFERENCES

1. Garrioch, D.B., Good, R.A., and Gatti, R.A., "Lymphocyte Responses To PHA in Patients With Non-Lymphoid Tumors." *Lancet* 1:618, 1970.
2. McKhann, C.F., Slade, M.S., Gunnarsson, A., and Burk, M.W., "Lymphocyte Responsiveness in Cancer and Transplantation." *Transplant. Proc.* 7:287-290, 1975.
3. Golub, S.H., O'Connell, T.X., and Morton, D.L., "Correlation of *In Vivo* and *In Vitro* Assays of Immunocompetence in Cancer Patients." *Cancer Res.* 34:1833-1837, 1974.
4. Catalona, W.J., Sample, W.F., and Chretien, P.B., "Lymphocyte Reactivity in Cancer Patients: Correlation With Tumor Histology and Clinical Stage." *Cancer* 31:65-71, 1973.
5. Han, T., and Takita, H., "Impaired Lymphocyte Responses to Allogeneic Cultured Lymphoid Cells in Patients With Lung Cancer." *New Engl. J. Med.* 286:605-606, 1972.
6. Rees, J.C., Rossio, J.L., Wilson, H.E., et al., "Cellular Immunity in Neoplasia. Antigen and Mitogen Responses in Patients With Bronchogenic Carcinoma." *Cancer* 36:2010-2015, 1975.
7. Ducos, J., Mingueres, J., Colombies, P., "Lymphocyte Response to PHA in Patients With Lung Cancer." *Lancet* 1:1111-1112, 1971.
8. Mavligit, G.M., Jubert, A.V., Gutterman, J.U., et al., "Immune Reactivity of Lymphoid Tissues Adjacent to Carcinoma of the Ascending Colon." *Surg. Gynec. Obstet.* 139:409-412, 1974.
9. Concannon, J.P., Dalbow, M.H., Eng, C.P., Conway, J., "Immunoprofile Studies for Patients With Bronchogenic Carcinoma I. Correlation of Pre-therapy Studies With Stage of Disease." *Int. J. Radiat. Oncol. Biol. Phys.* 2:447-454, 1977.
10. Dean, J.H., McCoy, J.L., Cannon, G.B., et al., "Cell-Mediated Immune Responses of Breast Cancer Patients to Autologous Tumor-Associated Antigens." *J. Natl. Cancer Inst.* 58:549-555, 1977.
11. Weese, J.L., Oldham, R.K., Tormey, D.C., et al., "Immunologic Monitoring in Carcinoma of the Breast." *Surg. Gynec. Obstet.* In Press, 1977.
12. Oldham, R.K., Dean, J.H., Cannon, G.B., et al., "Cryopreservation of Human Lymphocytes Function as Measured by *In Vitro* Assays." *Int. J. Cancer* 18:145-155, 1976.
13. Wanebo, H.J., Pinsky, C.M., Beattie, E.J., and Oettgen, H.F., "Immunocompetence Testing in Patients With One of the Four Common Operable Cancer—A Review." *Clinical Bulletin* 15-22, 1978.
14. Nelson, H.S., "Delayed Hypersensitivity in Cancer Patients: Cutaneous and *In Vitro* Lymphocyte Response to the Specific Antigen." *J. Nat. Cancer Inst.* 42:765-770, 1969.
15. Paty, D.W., and Bone, G., "Response to PHA in Cancer Patients." *Lancet* 1:668-669, 1973.
16. Dean, J.H., Connor, R., Herberman, R.B., et al., "The Relative Proliferation Index as a More Sensitive Parameter for Evaluating Lymphoproliferative Responses of Cancer Patients to Mitogens and Alloantigens." *Int. J. Cancer* 20:359-370, 1977.
17. Savel, H., "Effect of Autologous Tumor Extracts on Cultures of Human Peripheral Blood Lymphocytes." *Cancer* 24:56-63, 1969.
18. Vanky, F., Klein, E., Stjernsward, J., and Nilsonne, V., "Cellular Immunity Against Tumor-Associated Antigens in Humans: Lymphocyte Stimulation and Skin Reaction." *Int. J. Cancer* 14:277-288, 1974.
19. Roth, J.A., Holmes, E.C., Boddie, A.W., Jr., and Morton, D.L., "Lymphocyte Responses of Lung Cancer Patients to Tumor-Associated Antigens Measured by Leucine Incorporation." *J. Thorac. Cardiovasc. Surg.* 70:613-618, 1975.
20. Roth, J.A., Grimm, E.A., and Morton, D.L., "A Rapid Assay for Stimulation of Human Lymphocytes by Tumor-Associated Antigens." *Cancer Research* 36:3001-3010, 1976.
21. Dean, J.H., McCoy, J.L., Cannon, G.B., et al., "Lymphocyte Proliferation Responses of Patients With Carcinoma of Breast or Lung to Mitogens, Alloantigens and Tumor-Associated Antigens." *Proc. Symp. Detect. and Prevent. of Cancer* In Press, 1978.

385

22. Dean, J.H., Jerrells, T.R., Cannon, G.B., et al., "Demonstration of Specific Cell-Mediated Anti-Tumor Immunity in Lung Cancer to Autologous Tissue Extracts." *Int. J. Cancer* In Press, 1978.

23. Dean, J.H., Padarathsingh, M.L., and Jerrells, T.R., "Application of Immunocompetence Assays for Defining Immunosuppression." *N.Y. Acad. Sci. Workshop* In Press, 1978.

24. Holmes, E.C., "Immunology and Lung Cancer." *Ann. Thorac. Surg.* 21:250-258, 1976.

25. Oren, M.E., and Herberman, R.B., "Delayed Cutaneous Hypersensitivity Reactions to Membrane Extracts of Human Tumors." *Clinical Exptl. Immunol.* 9:45-56, 1971.

26. Dean, J.H., Silva, J.S., McCoy, J.L., et al., "Lymphocyte Blastogenesis Induced by Potassium Chloride Extracts of Allogeneic Breast Carcinoma and Lymphoid Cells." *J. Natl. Cancer Inst.* 54:1295-1298, 1975.

27. Sokal, R.R., and Rohlf, F.J., "The Principles and Practice of Statistics in Biological Research." *Biometry,* W.H. Freeman and Co., San Francisco, 1969.

28. Jerrells, T.R., Dean, J.H., McCoy, J.L., et al., "Role of Suppressor Cells in Depression of *In Vitro* Lymphoproliferative Responses of Lung and Breast Cancer Patients." *J. Natl. Cancer Inst.* In Press, 1978.

29. Koski, I.R., Poplack, D.G., and Blasese, R.M., "A Nonspecific Esterase Stain for the Identification of Monocytes and Macrophages." In *In Vitro Methods in Cell Mediated and Tumor Immunity,* Bloom, B. and David, J.R., eds, Academic Press, New York, 350, 1976.

30. Kirchner, H., Chused, T.M., Herberman, R.B., et al., "Evidence of Suppressor Cell Activity in Spleens of Mice Bearing Primary Tumors Induced by Moloney Sarcoma Virus." *J. Exptl. Med.* 139:1473-1487, 1974.

31. Padarathsingh, M.L., Dean, J.H., McCoy, J.L., et al., "Evidence for and Characterization of Suppressor Cells in BALB/c Mice Bearing ADJPC5 Plasmacytomas." *J. Natl. Cancer Inst.* submitted, 1978.

32. Glaser, M., Herberman, R.B., Kirchner, H., and Djeu, J.Y., "Study of the Cellular Immune Response to Gross Virus-Induced Lymphoma by the Mixed Lymphocyte-Tumor Interaction." *Cancer Res.* 34:2165-2171, 1974.

PANEL DISCUSSION

Chairman: Ray Crispen

Evan Hersh: I have a couple of clarification questions. First, the correlation of the PHA response with prognosis, was that in patients of all stages or stage one?

Jack Dean: It is only in stage one patients.

Hersh: Did you say that the mitomycin treated cells were still capable of suppression?

Dean: Yes, adherent cell types do not seem to be sensitive to mitomycin.

Hersh: That is interesting. We haven't tried mitomycin yet, but in almost every case where we have seen suppression it has been reversed by radiation. I don't know whether those two are analogous or not.
Do you see suppressor cells in patients who are not immunologically incompetent, by, let's say, a PHA assay?

Dean: Actually, that's a little difficult. We select patients for suppressor cell studies that have previously been shown to have depressed PHA and MLC responses.

Hersh: In the data that I showed, there is still a fraction of patients whose PHA responses were in normal range who still showed suppression.

Dean: I suspect that could be possible, we haven't really looked closely.

Hersh: The next question I wanted to ask, relative to the macrophage suppressor, was whether you have used indomethacin in any of the cultures in attempt to reverse this suppression?

Dean: Yes, we have. The data we have, although it is preliminary, does indicate that we can reverse the adherent cell type suppression with indomethacin. We find indomethacin somewhat difficult to work with and it's not as clear as we thought it would be initially, but in some cases it appears to reverse the suppression.
Evan, can I ask you a question? Is it true that about one-third of your lung cancer patients have suppressor cells of the non-adherent type, or the T cell type that are radio sensitive?

Hersh: No. About two-thirds of the patients in each disease category which we looked at showed the suppressor cell. In the majority of patients it is reversed by radiation. Only in one-third has it been reversed, even in part, by thymic hormones.
But, we've only studied about 35 patients, 20 of whom were advanced lung cancer patients.

Dean: Yes, our population would be advanced disease patients too.

Hersh The incidence of suppressor cells is higher than one-third.

Dean: Our incidence of suppressor cells is going to approach 50%. That is a little skewed because we are selectively recalling patients.

Robert Hunter: You showed the difference in suppression of MLC

387

responses with advancing stage, but it didn't look like the means and standard deviations changed very much. However, you did show a big change in survival with the stage I patients. Now, the question is, is there more of a change within a stage that correlates with survival than a change between stages? Is this a test that is better at predicting survival within a particular stage than a staging prediction?

Dean: We did look at other stages as prognosticators and were not satisfied. We really felt the more relevant question was in stage I. Can you sub-categorize survival? We haven't looked closely enough in other stages to know whether that would hold up. It's confounded in those other stages by therapy and that makes it very difficult. Did I miss the question?

Hunter: Maybe I can reword the question. If you take stage one and have long survivors and short survivors, how does the difference between those two groups compare with the difference between stage I and stage III?

Dean: I don't think blastogenesis adds any additional information between stages other than the fact that there is a higher frequency of suppression in the other groups. However, within stage I it appears to sub-categorize. I probably should still discuss this with you, I don't think I've got the point.

Hersh: How many stage I patients are you talking about in this study?

Dean: In the survival study there are 60 patients.

Hersh: How many of them had good intact immune function and how many had bad immune function by your criteria?

Dean: In stage I patients between 30% and 40% of them had depressed immune function.

Hersh: How depressed was depressed?

Dean: Well, it would be around 30% to 40% of that of a normal individual based on a RPI.

Hersh: How well does that correlate with the immune function of those patients who had good survival?

Dean: By the survival table, when we just asked the question if they had a depression to either of the two measures did it change survival, it gave the P value of 0.009.

Hersh: What I mean is, if you look at the immune function of stage I patients who had good survival, how did that compare with the normals, and then how did that, in turn, compare to the group of patients who had poor survival? What kind of differences are you talking about?

Dean: They are really much different. Stage I patients, who had suppressed immune function in the neighborhood of 30% to 40% of normal individuals, based on a RPI were bad survivors.
Those patients, who were within the normal group, would map almost like normals, if you map the RPI.

Hersh: Was there any difference in the age of the two groups?

388

Dean: No, none that was apparent.

Hersh: Are you stating that quite categorically?

Dean: Yes.

Hersh: Even though you had a 30% to 40% in one group and 60% to 70% in the other group?

Dean: We've analyzed the data on the computer by age and we don't see a difference.

Hersh: Is there any difference in terms of histopathologic diagnosis?

Dean: There are three oat cells in the study and they were non-survivals. Otherwise, there was a fairly random distribution of patients.

Hersh: Well, if you excluded your oat cells, how would your data come out?

Dean: It would be the same. By excluding those three patients you are not going to change the P value much.

Hersh: What is your P value?

Dean: The P value is 0.009. The only thing that changes the P value, in the negative direction, although still significant at a 0.05 level or less, is if you include the depressed patients that are receiving BCG. The feeling is, that even through they start out depressed, when you add BCG it enhances their ability to survive. You must remember that the data I am talking about is initial tests only. We are not looking at all of the tests the patient has had.

Hersh: Were there suppressor cells in the stage I patients who had impaired immune function?

Dean: We didn't look that close at stage I patients for supressor cells. We looked primarily in advanced stages for suppressor cells. I don't know the answer yet.

John Miller: In a clinical setting, with the exception of randomized studies, should we be doing routine immune profile studies on patients?

Hersh: Are you talking about cancer patients? I think the prognostic utility of the assays that have been generated thus far is of interest. There are so many patients who are competent and have a poor prognosis and so many patients who are incompetent and have a good prognosis that these assays don't help you tremendously in prognosticating for the patient. If we see an anergic patient at the outset of treatment, it is very unlikely that the patient will respond to any therapeutic modality; but there are responders, and therefore, I don't think that these assays add tremendously to our ability to prognosticate for the patient. They are extremely useful, however, in evaluating almost all of the investigative modalities that are used in cancer. Since there is no established treatment for cancer beyond surgery and radiation, except for a few of the chemotherapeutic regimens, all chemotherapy and certainly all immunotherapy is developmental and research. Furthermore, as these assays become more defined and we develop more sophisticated assays, they will play an increasingly important role in the development of new therapeutic approaches. I think Jack Dean has been involved with assays and he may have a somewhat different point of view and I would love to hear his response.

Dean: I would have to agree with Evan's statement that assays don't assist diagnosis that much. Our emphasis over the past year has been very similar to that of Dr. Hersh and his group, to look at the value of the assays in selecting and developing immuno potentiating therapy, immuno adjuvant therapy. Very little is known about how therapy affects the assays. There is even skepticism over the value of immune therapy in general. So, if we are to improve immune therapy, it would be helpful if we had handles to assist in looking at changes in populations and modulation of immune response by the therapy, so we could select better therapy or better doses.

Hersh: I wish to clarify what I just said. I was referring to assays of immunocompetence or immunodeficiency. When you talk about immunological assays, of course this includes such clinically useful assays like CEA and AFP. In addition, included is what I categorize as immunological assays and that is the determination of whether a leukemia or lymphoma is a T or a B cell disease. These do have clinical implications which need to be taken into account with therapy.

Hunter: One of the problems in this area, which will inhibit the dissemination of this type of assay is that it is very difficult to find two laboratories which will agree on how to do it. These are definitely not cookbook assays and it is very difficult to establish quality control and standards. I believe this is one of the major impediments. You can do it with a great deal of effort within one institution, but you certainly can't set it up as an easy sideline and expect to get any place with any of the assays involving cells.

Hersh: Just one more comment in this area. We had hoped that delayed hypersensitivity skin testing would be useful in this regard because it would obviate some of the problems Dr. Hunter just mentioned. Anyone can put on a skin test with fair accuracy. The problem with delayed hypersensitivity tests, however, is it was not predictive enough. There was too much overlap between the groups of responder and nonresponder subjects.

Brahma Sharma: Evan, I think that there is one test that everybody can do which hasn't been mentioned and that is the total lymphocyte count. It is a very simple test and it has been shown, at least in colorectal cancer, that it can be well applied to survival. What is your thought on this test?

Hunter: May I answer that question. Our university about three years ago bought a new machine from Technicon called the Hemalog, which does differential counts by counting 30,000 cells in a flow-through system. When you count that many cells you get accurate counts of the low frequency cells, monocytes, basophils, and eosinophils. In fact, you can get absolute counts. What we find is that the absolute lymphocyte count doesn't vary very much in patients with lung cancer. It goes down very slightly on the average with an enormous overlap; terminally it tends to go up again, but there are small differences. However, there are two counts that are highly prognostic and they are the absolute monocyte count and the absolute immature myeloid cell count. These increase in a large proportion of the patients about five to six months before death. Patients may still be doing well clinically, but these counts start going up out of the normal range, the statistical probability in their surviving a long time is low.

Hersh: If the absolute monocyte count went up five to six months before death, would not most patients, certainly patients with solid tumors, have been presented with their metastatic disease? In colon cancer, lung cancer, head and neck cancer, breast cancer, five to six months before death is the time when most patients already have had fairly widespread metastatic disease. They may have already been through their front line chemotherapy.

Hunter: This is true. It picks up in patients with metastatic disease, but it also picks up in some of the patients who have been resected before they have clinically obvious metastasis.

James Bennett: It was demonstrated very nicely this afternoon that in advanced disease there were suppressor cells present. Has anyone on the panel had experience with patients with advanced disease after they have received therapy and the tumor load has presumably been reduced. Does the suppressor cell activity then go down?

Hunter: We have had no experience with this yet.

Crispen: Dr. Dean, none of your BCG patients demonstrated recurrent disease. Are you referring to only stage I lung cancer? Was this true in more advanced stages?

Dean: No, that remark ought to be qualified. In the stage I lung cancer patients, who had depressed responses and were then treated with BCG, disease had not recurred. But that group is very small, I am talking about 9 patients.

Crispen: How long were they followed?

Dean: They have been followed beyond two years. We do have a study that Dr. Herberman presented at the World Lung Congress recently, in which we have followed patients on cutaneous BCG, stage I lung cancer patients, randomized to BCG or BCG plus allogeneic tumor cells that is showing significant survival enhancement with BCG therapy. In addition, allogeneic tumor cells do not appear to augment or enhance survival so that BCG alone appears to be adequate.

Crispen: That is similar to the work done at M.D. Anderson. Autologous cells do not seem to add anything to the BCG therapy in these patients. Do you agree with that observation, Dr. Hersh?

Hersh: The only tumor in which we used autologous cells was leukemia. We have not done studies in lung cancer. In leukemia there was no benefit and there was a return to the chemotherapy alone survival when tumor cells were added to BCG in AML.

Crispen: There seems to be a limit to stimulation available for the patient to respond to in whatever method you use. You can not stimulate beyond that. I had another question for Dr. Dean. Do you feel that the response of the patients who are initially depressed and are under immunotherapy with BCG, becomes equal to the response of patients who initially were not depressed and the prognosis becomes the same?

Dean: I wish I had looked at that data more closely, before I left Bethesda. I have been sitting here thinking about the answer to that question because I knew someone was going to ask it, probably you. I don't know the data well enought to answer. One option would be that they may very well stay depressed relative to the peripheral function, that BCG is possibly acting at the macrophage level and that they wouldn't have to have normal T cell function return to show improved survival.

George Mathé: We treated advanced bronchus cancer patients with BCG if they were skin test negative and 50% were restored. The prognosis for the restored patients was the same as the prognosis for the patients who were initially skin test positive. The prognosis for those patients who were not restored was poorer, significantly poorer. May I ask a question? Is there any correlation between the presence of suppressor cells in the blood and negative skin tests?

Hersh: We have that data, but I have not looked at it yet.

Robert Epstein: It has always struck me as paradoxical, that in considering immune responses that there is a rather high incidence of secondary tumors of the same type in patients who have been cured of their original tumor. Breast carcinoma is a very good example, or, carcinoma of the bowel or melanoma. You would think that having a tumor cured of the same type would be the best immunologic protection one could have. I was wondering how this second tumor situation fits into some of the concepts of immuno surveillance and immunologic reactivity to tumors?

Hersh: The incidence of second tumors is, of course, extremely interesting; second tumors of the same histological type as well as second tumors of different histological type. We have seen quite an incidence of melanoma, for instance, in our patients with chronic lymphocytic leukemia and there is an increase in incidence of second primaries, particularly leukemia, in patients who have received chemotherapy and radiotherapy for Hodgkins Disease. This fits in with the concept of immuno surveillance which has been under increasing attack as Prehn, Fidler, and others have demonstrated that lymphocytes can augment as well as depress tumor growth. One also must take into consideration the concept that the carcinogenic event which induced the first tumor, whether it would be a virus or chemical carcinogen, or what have you, presumably has transformed many cells within the body.

392

In fact, you can look pathologically at the tracheal bronchial tree of the smoker and see pre-malignant changes throughout the tracheal bronchial tree. Now, the point you raise about the cure of the primary tumor preventing the induction of the second tumor is an interesting one and to some extent has been approached experimentally. There are a number of studies in which chemotherapy alone has been used to cure an experimental tumor, and it has been demonstrated at least in some of those studies that the animals are not resistant to subsequent challenge with the same tumor cells. In contrast, when immunotherapy has been utilized to cure the experimental tumor, quite frequently there is resistance to subsequent challenge with the same tumor. Now, in the clinical immunotherapy area, except for Prof. Mathé's pioneering work which started in the early sixties, the great thrust in immunotherapy really began around 1971-72, and I don't think those patients who have been cured in association with immunotherapy have been followed long enough. However, perhaps Prof. Mathé would like to comment on whether any of the leukemia patients cured in the 1960's in his clinic have come down with second primaries.

Mathé: No, we have no relapse in our patients who have a long survival with a 16 year follow-up. One thing, however, is they have a significant increase of nerve cells in their bone marrow; and we don't know what this means.

Epstein: Just one other comment, it would seem to me that one of the great problems that arises is what tests correlate, what is the battery and the screen. I wonder whether it might not be useful in, for example, patients who have had a breast removed successfully and have a high incidence of recurrence in the contralateral breast, to see if one can identify by the techniques that we talked about a test that either could select a patient who would develop a second primary or the contrary any level of immuno resistance.

Crispen: There has been some animal model development on tumor dormancy in which the tumors disappear for months or years and then reoccur. It is thought that it might be due to a slight depression of the immune response which allows it to escape and become fully established as a tumor. Whether that depression is due to trauma or other factor is something that we certainly should address. It might be very interesting to look into at another meeting.

IMMUNOLOGIC ASPECTS OF THERAPY

Systemic Administration of BCG Activates Natural Suppressor Cells in the Bone Marrow and Stimulates Their Migration into the Spleen

James A. Bennett[1]
M.S. Mitchell[2]

SUMMARY—Intravenous administration of BCG induces suppressor cells in the bone marrow and spleen that inhibit *in vitro* immunization to alloantigens. Spleen or bone marrow cells from normal or BCG-treated C57BL/6 mice were assayed for suppressor activity by adding them to cultures containing normal syngeneic, killed P815Y tumor cells. Cell-mediated immunity to P815Y was measured by 4-hour ^{51}Cr release and by 48-hour growth inhibition assays. Immunization of normal spleen cells was inhibited by the addition of normal bone marrow cells but not by normal spleen or thymus cells. The suppressive activity of bone marrow cells was enhanced 2 days after BCG and remained elevated at least 14 days. Suppressor cells were found in the spleen 7 days after BCG and continued to increase sharply for another 9 days. BCG did not induce suppressor cells in the thymus. Concomitant with suppression, there was a decrease in bone marrow cell number and an increase in spleen cell number. The splenic suppressor cell was characterized as an adherent, non-T, non-B, non-phagocytic, dense leukocyte which develops independent of the thymus. Suppressor cell development was not inhibited by treatment of mice with an antiproliferative agent such as cytosine arabinside (ara-C) following BCG administration. Moreover, suppressor cells were found in the spleen of thymectomized, irradiated, bone marrow reconstituted mice that had not been treated with BCG. From this evidence it appears that systemic administration of BCG activates natural suppressor cells in the bone marrow and elicits suppressor cells in the spleen through the migration and colonization of the spleen by bone marrow elements.

INTRODUCTION

Bacillus Calmette-Guérin (BCG) is one of the most widely used biological adjuvants in the immunotherapy of malignancy. Although the mechanism of action of BCG is not completely understood, its therapeutic efficacy has been attributed to activation of the lymphoreticular system. Several investigators have found increased immunological reactivity of both T lymphocytes (1, 2) and macrophages (3, 4), as well as nonadherent cells resembling monocytes (5), after BCG administration. However, since the immune system is a tightly regulated network, activation of its components

[1]Department of Pharmacology, Yale University School of Medicine, New Haven, Connecticut.
[2]Department of Medicine, Los Angeles County-University of Southern California Cancer Center, Los Angeles, California.

does not always lead to an increased immune response. Hence, there are several reports where BCG had led to a decrease in immunological responsiveness (6-8). In this report we present evidence that intravenous administration of BCG leads to the induction of suppressor cells in the spleen which inhibit the alloimmunization of normal spleen cells *in vitro*. These splenic suppressor cells, which appear to be immature monocytes, are derived from natural suppressor cells found in normal bone marrow which under the influence of BCG migrate from the bone marrow and colonize the spleen.

MATERIALS AND METHODS

Animals. C57B1/6 (H-2^b female mice were obtained from Charles River Laboratory (Wilmington, Mass., U.S.A.). Experimental mice were 8-12 weeks old and weighed 19-23 grams.

BCG. Mycobacterium bovis, Tice strain, was obtained as a freeze-dried product from the University of Illinois. Each ampule containing $5 \pm 3 \times 10^8$ viable units was reconstituted by adding 1.0 ml of sterile water immediately before use. Except for those experiments reported in Table 1, mice that received BCG were given 2×10^7 viable units intravenously.

Immunization In Vitro. Bone marrow cells (from the femur and tibia) and spleen cells were obtained and suspended under sterile conditions as previously described (9). Spleen cells were immunized *in vitro* according to a modification of the procedure originally described by Mishell and Dutton (10). Briefly, 2×10^7 viable C57B1/6 spleen cells (H-2b) were cultured with 2×10^5 irradiated (4000r) P815 mastocytoma cells (H-2d) in 35 x 10 mm plastic dishes in a total volume of 1 ml. The culture medium was RPMI supplemented with heat inactivated, dialyzed fetal calf serum (5%), glutamine (2mM), sodium pyruvate (1mM), 100x non-essential amino acids (1%), penicillin (100 units/ml), streptomycin (100 μg/ml), and 2 mercaptoethanol (5×10^{-5} M). Cultures were incubated for 4 days at 37° C in an atmosphere of 10% CO_2 in air, and were fed daily with 0.1 ml of RPMI 1640 medium supplemented as previously described (11). At the end of culture, cells were agitated with a rubber policeman, collected, washed, and counted. After viability was assessed by trypan blue dye exclusion, cells were adjusted to appropriate concentrations in fresh culture medium.

Assays for Cell-mediated Immunity (CMI) and Phagocytosis. CMI against P815Y target cells was measured using both the 4 hour ^{51}Cr release assay (12) and the 48-hour growth inhibition assay (13). The percent ^{51}Cr released and the percent growth inhibition were calculated in the following ways:

$$1) \ \%^{51}\text{Cr release} = \frac{\text{CPM in supernatant}}{\text{CPM in pellet} + \text{CPM in supernatant}} \times 100\%$$

2) % growth inhibition = $(1 - T/N) \times 100\%$

where T = number of target cells remaining in the presence of test lymphocytes and N = number of target cells remaining in the presence of normal lymphocytes.

Phagocytosis was measured based on the protection from osmotic lysis of macrophage-engulfed, opsonized sheep red blood cells (SRBC) using the method described by Hersey (14). Briefly 5×10^6 spleen cells were incubated for 16 hours with 1×10^5 ^{51}Cr labeled, opsonized SRBC in a final volume of 0.2 ml. At the end of the incubation period, 1 ml of distilled H_2O was added to the cells for 15 seconds followed by the addition of 1 ml of twice concentrated phosphate-buffered saline. Phagocytosis was measured as the difference after hypotonic shock between $\%^{51}$Cr released from opsonized SRBC incubated with spleen cells and $\%^{51}$Cr released from normal SRBC.

Cell Separation Techniques

(a) Nylon Wool Column. Fractionation of cells over nylon wool columns was performed as previously described (15, 16). Adherent cells were freed from the nylon wool by agitation with forceps in cold phosphate buffered saline. With this procedure we routinely recovered approximately 75% of the total number of cells added to the columns.

(b) Treatment of Spleen Cells with Antisera. Rabbit anti-mouse thymocyte serum was purchased from Microbiological Associates, Bethesda, Md. Rabbit anti-mouse immunoglobulin serum was raised by injecting mouse gamma globulin emulsified in complete Freund's adjuvant into rabbits and repeating the injections at 10 day intervals. After the third injection rabbits were bled and their serum was obtained.

Spleen cells at a final concentration of 10^7 cells/ml were added to the antithymocyte serum (final dilution 1/15) or the anti-immunoglobulin serum (final dilution 1/8 in the presence of 0.2% sodium azide) and mixed slowly for 30 minutes at 4° C. Cells were centrifuged, then resuspended at a concentration of 10^7 cells/ml in guinea pig complement (final dilution 1/15) and incubated at 37° for another 30 minutes. Cells were again centrifuged, resuspended, and the number of trypan blue-excluding cells was adjusted to the desired concentration.

When normal cells were treated under these conditions, antithymocyte serum killed 85% of thymocytes, 4% of bone marrow cells, 75% of nylon wool non-adherent spleen cells, and 14% of nylon wool adherent spleen cells. Moreover, pretreatment of sensitized spleen cells with antithymocyte serum eliminated 88% of their lytic activity in a 4-hour ^{51}Cr release assay. Anti-immunoglobulin serum killed 2% of thymocytes, 31% of whole spleen, 58% of nylon wool adherent spleen, and did not kill nylon wool non-adherent spleen cells.

(c) Treatment of Spleen Cells with Silica (17, 18). Spleen cells were suspended in RPMI 1640 medium in the absence of serum to a concentration of 10^7 cells/ml and incubated for 3 hours at 37° C with 100 μg/ml of silica (Monsanto Co., St. Louis, Missouri). Cells were centrifuged, resuspended and the number of trypan blue-excluding cells were adjusted to the desired concentration in RPMI 1640 medium containing 5% heat inactivated, dialyzed fetal calf serum. Under these conditions the phagocytic activity of normal spleen cells was reduced by more than 50%.

(d) Density Gradient Centrifugation. Discontinuous density gradients were obtained by layering different concentrations of Ficoll-400 (Pharmacia, Piscataway, NJ) into polycarbonate centrifuge tubes (19). Four ml each of 25%, 21%, 16%, and 12% Ficoll were layered into the tubes. Spleen cells at a concentration of 2.5 x 10^7 cells/ml were contained in the 21% fraction. Cells were centrifuged at 20,000 g for 60 minutes at 4°C. Four cell fractions were obtained, washed, and counted.

Unless specified otherwise, the values reported are the mean ± the standard deviation of at least four replicate samples obtained from two or more experiments.

RESULTS

BCG Induced Changes in Spleen, Bone Marrow, and Thymus. When 2 x 10^7 viable units of BCG were given to mice intravenously, the subsequent immunization of their spleen cells against alloantigen *in vitro* was completely suppressed (Table 1). Smaller doses of BCG were less suppressive.

Table 1—THE EFFECT OF I.V. TREATMENT OF MICE WITH BCG ON THE *IN VITRO* GENERATION OF AN IMMUNE RESPONSE BY THEIR SPLEEN CELLS

No. of BCG Organisms	Spleen Cell No. x 10^8	% Specific ^{51}Cr Release	% Specific Growth Inhibition
Control	1.8 ± 0.3	65 ± 3	80 ± 11
1 x 10^6	1.6 ± 0.3	66 ± 4	75 ± 9
5 x 10^6	1.8 ± 0.2	63 ± 4	76 ± 11
1 x 10^7	3.0 ± 0.5	15 ± 7	26 ± 8
2 x 10^7	4.1 ± 0.5	5 ± 2	0
5 x 10^7	Lethal Dose	—	—

C57B1/6 mice were injected intravenously with the indicated doses of BCG. Mice were sacrificed 8 days after treatment. Their spleens were excised and teased into suspension. Twenty million spleen cells from each treatment group were immunized *in vitro* against 2 x 10^5 P815-Y cells. The CMI of the immunized spleen cells was measured by the ^{51}Cr release assay with an effector to target cell ratio of 100:1 and by the growth inhibition assay with an effector to target ratio of 10:1.

400

BCG also had a marked influence on the number of cells not only in the spleen but also in the bone marrow and the thymus (Figure 1). Within two days after the administration of BCG, there was a 40% decrease in the number of bone marrow cells and a 90% decrease in the number of thymus cells. The decrease in bone marrow cells persisted and was still apparent 16 days after BCG, whereas in the thymus a gradual recovery in cellularity began 5 days after BCG, but cellularity did not return to normal levels until 16 days after BCG. In contrast, in the spleen there was no reduction in the number of cells as a result of BCG administration. Rather, a 2-fold, 3-fold, and 6-fold increase in spleen cell number was found respectively on days 7, 11, and 16 after BCG.

Figure 1—THE EFFECT OF BCG ON THE NUMBER OF CELLS IN MOUSE SPLEEN, BONE MARROW, AND THYMUS

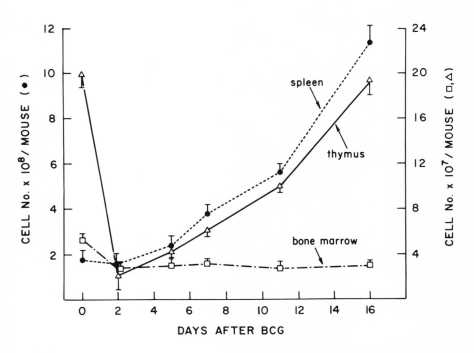

C57Bl/6 mice were injected intravenously with 2×10^7 viable units of BCG. At various times after treatment mice were sacrificed, and their spleen, bone marrow (2 femora and 2 tibiae per mouse), and thymus were excised and teased into single cell suspension. The cell number in each tissue was determined microscopically.

401

Table 2—EFFECT OF SPLEEN, BONE MARROW, AND THYMUS CELLS FROM BCG-TREATED MICE ON THE IMMUNIZATION OF NORMAL SPLEEN CELLS AGAINST ALLOANTIGEN *IN VITRO*.

Days after BCG	% Specific ^{51}CR Release with sensitized spleen cells (65 ± 3); immunized in the presence of:			% Growth Inhibition with sensitized spleen cells (81 ± 7); immunized in the presence of:		
	Spleen	Bone Marrow	Thymus	Spleen	Bone Marrow	Thymus
No BCG	66 ± 2	38 ± 8	62 ± 3	82 ± 8	45 ± 9	74 ± 9
2	64 ± 3	9 ± 4	66 ± 5	88 ± 6	10 ± 5	70 ± 11
7	45 ± 5	5 ± 3	59 ± 4	60 ± 5	8 ± 4	79 ± 8
11	33 ± 6	7 ± 2	67 ± 3	37 ± 11	19 ± 10	85 ± 8
16	31 ± 5	3 ± 2	64 ± 3	31 ± 8	12 ± 4	80 ± 12

C57B1/6 mice were given 2 x 10⁷ viable units of BCG intravenously. At the indicated times after treatment spleen, bone marrow, and thymus were excised, and single cell suspensions from each tissue were prepared. Six million of these cells were added to 2 x 10⁷ normal C57B1/6 spleen cells, and this mixture was cultured for 4 days with 2 x 10⁵ killed P815-Y cells. At the end of the culture period the CMI of the sensitized spleen cells was determined using an effector to target cell ratio of 100:1 in the ^{51}Cr release assay and 10:1 in the growth inhibition assay.

The suppressive influence of cells in the spleen, bone marrow, or thymus was determined by adding them to cultures of normal spleen and immunizing this mixture against P815Y. As shown in Table 2, significant suppression of CMI occurred as a result of adding 6×10^6 normal syngeneic bone marrow cells to splenic lymphocytes before immunization *in vitro*. No suppression resulted from the addition of normal spleen or normal thymus cells. Treatment of mice with BCG markedly enhanced the suppressive activity in bone marrow and induced suppressive activity in spleen. Three-fold enhancement in suppression by bone marrow cells occurred two days after administration of BCG, and this enhancement was still apparent 14 days later. However, in spleen suppression was not apparent until 7 days after BCG, and was further increased 11 and 16 days after BCG. Although not shown, the suppressor cell activity as well as the cell number found in the spleen on day 60 was approximately the same as that found on day 16. Unlike bone marrow and spleen, thymus cells from BCG treated mice did not suppress the immunization of normal spleen cells.

Characterization of the BCG-Induced Splenic Suppressor Cell

(A) Adherence. There are approximately 70% nylon wool adherent and 30% nylon wool nonadherent cells in a normal mouse spleen. When nylon wool adherent and nonadherent spleen cells from normal and BCG treated-mice were mixed in this 70%:30% proportion and then immunized, dramatic suppression in the development of CMI occurred when adherent cells from BCG mice were mixed with nonadherent cells from normal mice (Table 3).

Table 3—*IN VITRO* IMMUNIZATION OF MIXTURES OF NYLON WOOL FRACTIONATED SPLEEN CELLS FROM NORMAL AND BCG TREATED MICE

Cell Population(s)	%Specific ^{51}Cr Release	% Specific Growth Inhibition
Normal Whole	69 ± 2	83 ± 8
BCG Whole	4 ± 4	0
Norm N.A. + Norm A.	62 ± 5	80 ± 11
Norm N.A. + BCG A.	9 ± 3	12 ± 7
BCG N.A. + BCG A.	5 ± 4	0
BCG N.A. + Norm A.	54 ± 4	70 ± 8

Spleen cells were obtained from normal mice or from mice treated eight days earlier with 2×10^7 viable units of BCG. Cells from each group were fractionated through nylon wool, and the nonadherent (NA) and adherent cell fractions were obtained. Cell fractions obtained from normal mice were mixed with each other as well as with cell fractions obtained from BCG-treated mice in a proportion of 30% NA cells with 70% A cells to a total cell number of 2×10^7. These mixtures were immunized against P815-Y *in vitro*, and the immunized cells were tested in the CMI assays as already described.

In contrast no deficit in the ability to be immunized was noted when non-adherent cells from BCG mice were mixed with adherent cells from normal mice. Thus, suppressor cell activity was concentrated in the adherent fraction of spleen from BCG treated mice.

(B) *Investigation of the Involvement of T Cells in Suppression.* Suppression of the immunization of normal spleen cells by adherent spleen cells from BCG mice was directly proportional to the number of the suppressor adherent cells added to the mixture (Figure 2). Although not shown in the Figure, 1×10^7 adherent cells from BCG treated mice completely prevented immunization of 2×10^7 normal spleen cells. Pretreatment of the adherent cells with anti θ serum and complement did not reduce their suppressive activity (Figure 2). Although these data indicated that the suppressor cells were not T cells, it was possible that T cells were required for the development of suppressor activity. To test this point, mice that had been

Figure 2—THE EFFECT OF ANTI θ SERUM TREATMENT OF NYLON WOOL-ADHERENT SPLEEN CELLS FROM BCG-TREATED MICE ON THEIR ABILITY TO SUPPRESS THE *IN VITRO* GENERATION OF AN IMMUNE RESPONSE BY NORMAL MOUSE SPLEEN CELLS

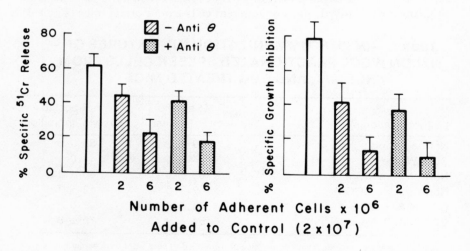

Spleen cells were obtained from mice given 2×10^7 BCG organisms *i.v.* eight days earlier. The nylon wool-adherent fraction was obtained and was either added to normal spleen cell cultures directly or treated with anti θ serum and complement and then added to normal spleen cell cultures. These cultures were immunized against P815-Y, and the sensitized cells were tested for CMI as already described.

404

Table 4—EFFECT OF NYLON WOOL-ADHERENT SPLEEN CELLS FROM UNTREATED OR BCG-TREATED "B" MICE ON THE *IN VITRO* IMMUNIZATION OF SPLEEN CELLS FROM NORMAL MICE AGAINST ALLOANTIGEN

Additional Adherent Cells	% Specific ^{51}Cr Release 100:1	% Specific Growth Inhibition 10:1
None	64 ± 2	84 ± 6
Normal Spleen (1 x 10^7)	63 ± 2	80 ± 5
"B" Spleen (6 x 10^6)	67 ± 3	78 ± 4
"B" Spleen (1 x 10^7)	51 ± 5	60 ± 8
BCG "B" Spleen (6 x10^6)	15 ± 3	30 ± 5
BCG "B" Spleen (1 x 10^7)	7 ± 2	0

Twenty million spleen cells from normal C57B1/6 mice were cultured with 2 x 10^5 killed P815 cells for 4 days. Additional cells were obtained from the spleen of normal mice, "B" mice, or BCG-treated "B" mice and added in the number indicated in the parentheses. Mice that had been thymectomized, lethally irradiated, and bone marrow-reconstituted were considered "B" mice. Nylon wool-adherent spleen cells were obtained from BCG-treated "B" mice 10 days after the IV administration of 2 x 10^7 viable units of BCG. Values reported are the mean ± the standard deviation of 4 replicate samples obtained from two experiments.

thymectomized, irradiated and protected with syngeneic bone marrow ("B" mice) were treated with BCG. It is apparent from Table 4 that admixture of adherent spleen cells from these mice significantly inhibited the immunization of normal cells. It should be pointed out, however, that the suppressor cells in "B" mice did not develop until 10 days after treatment with BCG, whereas in normal mice splenic suppressor cells were detected 7 days after treatment. It is also of interest that addition of 10^7 adherent cells from "B" mice that had not been treated with BCG caused a significant reduction in the immunization of normal spleen cells. Addition of a similar number of adherent cells from normal spleen had no effect.

(C) *Activity of BCG-Induced Suppressor Cells Following Treatment with Anti-Mouse Immunoglobulin Serum Plus Complement.* Pretreatment of adherent spleen cells from BCG mice with anti-mouse Ig serum and complement did not diminish their capacity to inhibit the immunization of normal spleen cells (Table 5).

(D) *Further Separation of Suppressor Activity in Adherent Spleen Cells from BCG Mice by Centrifugation through a Discontinuous Ficoll Density Gradient.* Four cell fractions were obtained following density gradient centrifugation of adherent spleen cells. The two lighter fractions found near

405

Table 5—THE EFFECT OF ANTI Ig SERUM TREATMENT OF NYLON-WOOL ADHERENT SPLEEN CELLS FROM BCG MICE ON THEIR ABILITY TO SUPPRESS THE *IN VITRO* IMMUNIZATION OF NORMAL SPLEEN CELLS

Additional Adherent Cells	% Specific ^{51}Cr Release	% Specific Growth Inhibition
None	61 ± 2	81 ± 7
Normal Spleen	60 ± 2	82 ± 8
BCG Spleen	29 ± 4	36 ± 5
BCG Spleen + Anti Ig	31 ± 5	29 ± 9
BCG Spleen + Anti Ig + C^1	28 ± 4	33 ± 5

Mice were treated intravenously with 2 x 10^7 viable units of BCG. Eight days after treatment mice were sacrificed and their spleen cells were obtained. Nylon wool-adherent spleen cells were incubated at 4°C with rabbit anti mouse Ig serum for 30 minutes, washed, and then incubated at 37°C for another 30 minutes in RPMI medium alone or in RPMI medium containing guinea pig complement (C). Six million additional cells were added to 2 x 10^7 normal spleen cells and this mixture was immunized *in vitro*.

Table 6—EFFECT OF NYLON WOOL-ADHERENT SPLEEN CELLS OF DIFFERENT DENSITY FROM BCG MICE ON THE *IN VITRO* IMMUNIZATION OF NORMAL SPLEEN CELLS

Additional Adherent Cells	%Specific ^{51}Cr Release	% Specific Growth Inhibition
None	65 ± 2	79 ± 8
Normal Spleen	63 ± 4	82 ± 10
BCG Spleen	32 ± 5	20 ± 11
BCG Spleen "Light"	53 ± 3	47 ± 10
BCG Spleen "Medium"	34 ± 5	22 ± 8
BCG Spleen "Dense"	40 ± 4	30 ± 12

Adherent spleen cells were obtained from BCG-treated mice and were centrifuged through a discontinous Ficoll density gradient. Three cell fractions were obtained. The "Light" fraction were those cells found near the top of the gradient. The "Medium" fraction were those cells found near the middle of the gradient. The "Dense" fraction were those cells found in the pellet. 6 x 10^6 of these cells were added to 2 x 10^7 normal, unfractionated spleen cells, and this mixture was immunized *in vitro* against P815-Y.

the top of the gradient had very few cells in each fraction and thus were pooled. When this pooled population was stained with Wright's stain and examined microscopically, 50% of the population were large cells that had

Table 7—EFFECT OF SILICA TREATMENT OF NYLON WOOL-ADHERENT SPLEEN CELLS FROM BCG MICE ON THEIR ABILITY TO SUPPRESS THE *IN VITRO* IMMUNIZATION OF NORMAL SPLEEN CELLS

Additional Adherent Cells	% Phagocytic Activity	% Specific ^{51}Cr release	% Specific Growth Inhibition
None		63 ± 2	80 ± 9
Normal Spleen	50	61 ± 4	84 ± 7
BCG Spleen	59	35 ± 5	27 ± 8
BCG Spleen (no silica)	65	21 ± 2	12 ± 5
BCG Spleen (silica)	31	31 ± 4	24 ± 7

Adherent spleen cells were obtained from BCG-treated mice. These cells were incubated at 37° C for 3 hours in the absence of silica or with 100 μg/ml of silica. Cells were harvested, washed, and 6 x 10⁶ of these cells were added to 2 x 10⁷ normal, unfractionated spleen cells and this mixture was immunized *in vitro* against P815-Y.

Phagocytic activity was measured as the difference after hypotonic shock between the % ^{51}Cr released from opsonized SRBC incubated with the indicated spleen cell preparation and the % ^{51}Cr released from normal SRBC.

the appearance of activated macrophages, whereas the other 50% consisted of smaller lymphocytic cells. The two heavier cell fractions, one recovered near the bottom of the gradient and the other in the pellet, were similar to each other. Twenty-five percent of each population were cells of the macrophage monocyte series, but these were smaller than those found in the pooled "light" fractions. The other 75% of the "medium" and "dense" populations consisted of small lymphocytes. The effects of these fractions on the immunization of normal spleen cells were shown in Table 6. Suppressor activity was found in all the cell fractions, but was greatest in the "medium," slightly less in the "dense," and least in the "light" fraction.

(E) *The Effect of Silica on Suppressor Activity.* Phagocytosis of opsonized SRBC by adherent spleen cells from BCG-treated mice appeared to be slightly increased over that found with adherent cells from normal mice (Table 7). However, since this data represents the mean of only two samples, its significance remains to be determined. Incubation of adherent spleen cells from BCG-treated mice with 100μg/ml of silica for 3 hours at 37° C resulted in a 50% inhibition in their phagocytic activity. In spite of this reduction, silica pretreatment had no effect on the suppressive activity of this population on normal spleen cell immunization (Table 7). It is of interest that 3 hour incubation of adherent cells from BCG-treated mice in the absence of silica increased the suppressor activity in this population. The basis for this increase is currently under investigation.

(F) *Quantitative Cellular Changes within the Spleen of BCG-Treated Mice.*
As shown previously in Table 2, systemic BCG treatment resulted in a
dramatic increase in both the size and the number of cells in the spleen. The
types of cells responsible for this increase were analyzed by determining
their susceptibility to treatment with either anti Ig serum or anti θ serum
plus complement. According to this analysis the percentage of both B cells
and T cells was decreased by more than 50% in the spleen of BCG-treated
mice (Table 8). Concomitantly there was about a 3-fold increase in the
percentage of cells lacking markers detectable by the antisera. However,
when the actual cell number was calculated, a three-fold increase in the
number of both B cells and T cells and a 15-fold increase in the number of
cells not categorized as B or T was found.

Table 8—CHANGES IN THE CELL POPULATION WITHIN THE SPLEEN OF MICE TREATED WITH BCG

	Normal Spleen	BCG Spleen (Day 14)
Cell No./Spleen	1.8×10^8	11.2×10^8
% B cells	31	14
% T cells	42	19
% other cells	27	67
B cell No./spleen	5.6×10^7	1.6×10^8
T cell No./spleen	7.6×10^7	2.1×10^8
Other cell No./spleen	4.9×10^7	7.5×10^8

Spleen cells were obtained from mice given 2×10^7 BCG organisms *i.v.* 14 days earlier. B Cells were
those that were killed by incubation with rabbit anti mouse Ig serum and complement. T cells were
those that were killed by incubation with anti θ serum and complement. Other cells were those that
lacked markers detectable by the above antisera.

*The Effect of Ara-C on the Development of BCG-Induced Splenic Suppressor
Cells.* The above increase in cell number as well as in suppressor cell activity
in the spleen were most apparent between days 7 and 16 after BCG
treatment (Figure 1 and Table 2). Treatment of mice with ara-C following
BCG administration resulted in only a slight reduction of the BCG-induced
increase in spleen cell number and did not affect the induction of splenic
suppressor cells by BCG (Table 9).

Table 9—THE EFFECT OF SPLEEN CELLS FROM MICE TREATED WITH BCG OR WITH BCG FOLLOWED BY ARA-C ON THE *IN VITRO* IMMUNIZATION OF NORMAL SPLEEN CELLS AGAINST ALLOANTIGEN

Additional Spleen Cells from Mice Treated with:		Cell No. x 10^8 per mouse spleen	% Specific ^{51}Cr release	% Specific Growth Inhibition
Control		1.8 ± 0.3	68 ± 3	80 ± 7
BCG	Day 0	10.2 ± 1.1	36 ± 5	40 ± 8
BCG	Day 0	7.8 ± 0.9	43 ± 6	36 ± 11
Ara-C	Days 1-7			
BCG	Day 0	7.3 ± 1.4	34 ± 6	30 ± 12
Ara-C	Days 7-13			

C57B1/6 mice were injected intravenously with 2×10^7 viable units of BCG. On the indicated days mice were given Ara-C, 20 mg/kg *i.v.* Mice were sacrificed on day 14, and 6×10^6 spleen cells from these mice were added to 2×10^7 normal spleen cells. This mixture was cultured for 4 days with 2×10^5 killed P815-Y cells.

DISCUSSION

It is clear from the data presented that spleen cells from mice treated with large doses of BCG could not be immunized against alloantigen *in vitro*. This was apparently due to the presence of suppressor cells which were generated during the BCG-induced increase in spleen cell number. These suppressor cells were adherent to nylon wool but did not carry markers detectable by antisera which were specific for B or T lymphocytes. Since BCG has been shown to activate macrophages (3, 4, 20) and since macrophages play a pivotal role in modulating immunological responses (21), it is attractive to postulate that the BCG-induced splenic suppressor cell is a macrophage. However, the density of the suppressor cell population and its lack of phagocytic activity are not typical of a classical macrophage. Thus, it would appear that the suppressor cell is either a monocyte or an atypical lymphocyte.

The marked increase in spleen cell number induced by BCG seemed to correlate with the level of suppressor cell activity in the spleen. The basis for this increase could be due either to an increase in spleen cell proliferation or to a migration of cells into the spleen or to a combination of both of these possibilities. The fact that an antiproliferative agent such as ara-C inhibited only slightly the increase in spleen cell number and did not influence the induction of suppressor cells brought about by BCG suggests that proliferation did not play a significant role in the induction of suppressor cells. Thus, migration of cells into the spleen seems to be the basis for the suppressive activity concentrated there after BCG. Based on the data the bone marrow seems to be the source of these migratory suppressor cells. As shown in Table 2, there were cells resident in normal bone marrow that suppressed the immunization of normal spleen cells. These "natural" suppressor cells were almost as inhibitory as the splenic suppressors induced by BCG. BCG further activated the suppressor activity in bone marrow and led to a persistent decrease in bone marrow cell number. The gradual increase in spleen cell number and splenic suppressor cell activity after BCG is consistent with the idea of emigration of suppressor cells from the bone marrow into the circulation and gradual colonization of the spleen with these bone marrow elements. The absence of suppressor activity in normal spleen and the presence of such activity in spleen of bone marrow reconstituted "B" mice lends further credence to this idea of colonization of the spleen by bone marrow suppressor cells. The increase in this activity under the influence of BCG could be due to its stimulation of chemotaxis (22), hematopoiesis (23, 24) or a combination of both of these phenomena as well as stimulation of other biochemically mediated events. The exact mechanism is not clear at this time.

It should be mentioned that BCG also induced a substantial decrease in the number of thymus cells. However, since no suppressor cells were found in the thymus and since BCG induced the development of splenic suppressor cells in "B" mice, it is clear that neither the thymus nor T-cells were necessary for the induction of splenic suppression. However, this does not rule out the possibility that these thymic changes play a significant role in the mediation of some other event stimulated by BCG *in vivo*.

In summary it appears that systemic administration of BCG activates natural suppressor cells resident in normal bone marrow and stimulates the migration of these cells into the spleen. Under the influence of a large number of these suppressor cells, spleen cell immunization *in vitro* is completely prevented. It is most likely that these BCG-induced splenic suppressor cells are immature monocytes, but the possibility of them being atypical lymphocytes cannot be ruled out. While the overall effect of BCG *in vivo* is usually one of adjuvancy, these results underscore its ability to stimulate intrinsic suppressor elements of immunity as well. It is conceivable that adjuvancy itself may always to the resultant of concomitant stimulation of both helper and suppressor forces.

REFERENCES

1. Mokyr, M.B., and Mitchell, M.S., "Activiation of Lymphoid Cells by BCG *In Vitro.*" *Cell. Immunol.* 15:264-273, 1975.

2. Mackaness, G.B., Auclair, P.J., and Lagrange, P.H., "Immunopotentiation with BCG. Immune Response to Different Strains and Preparations." *J. Natl. Cancer Inst.* 51:1655-1667, 1973.

3. Mitchell, M.S., Kirkpatrick, D., Mokyr, M.B., and Gery, I., "On the Mode of Action of BCG." *Nature New Biol.* 243:216-218, 1973.

4. Cleveland, R.P., Meltzer, M.S., and Zbar, B., "Tumor Cytotoxicity *in Vitro* by Macrophages from Mice Infected with Mycobacterium Bovis Strain BCG." *J. Natl. Cancer Inst.* 52: 1887-1895, 1974.

5. Murahata, R.I., and Mitchell, M.S., "Antagonism of Immunosuppression by BCG." In *The Macrophage in Neoplasia,* ed. by M.A. Fink, Academic Press, New York, pp. 263-265, 1976.

6. Klimpel, G.R., and Henney, C.S., "BCG-Induced Suppressor Cells. 1. Demonstration of a Macrophage-Like Suppressor Cell that Inhibits Cytotoxic T-Cell Generation *in Vitro.*" *J. Immunol.* 120:563-569, 1978.

7. Geffard, M., and Orbach-Arbouys, S., "Enhancement of T Suppressor Activity in Mice by High Doses of BCG." *Cancer Immunol. Immunother.* 1:41-43, 1976.

8. Florentin, I., Huchet, R., Bruley-Rosset, M., et al., "Studies on the Mechansim of Action of BCG." *Cancer Immunol. Immunother.* 1:31-39, 1976.

9. Bennet, J., Ehrke, J., Fadale, P., et al., "Immunosuppressive Effects of Methylglyoxal-Bis (Guanylhydrazone) on Mouse Bone Marrow and Spleen Cells and their Antagonism by Spermidine." *Biochem. Pharmacol.* In Press, 1977.

10. Mishell, R.I., and Dutton, R.W., Immunization of Dissociated Spleen Cell Cultures from Normal Mice." *J. Exp. Med.* 126:423-442, 1967.

11. Orsini, F., Pavelic, Z., and Mihich, E., "Increased Primary Cell Mediated Immunity in Culture Subsequent to Adriamycin or Daunorubicin Treatment of Spleen Donor Mice." *Cancer Res.* 37:1719-1726, 1977.

12. Brunner, K.T., Mauel, J., Cerottini, J.C., and Chaupis, B., "Quantitative Assay of the Lytic Action of Immune Lymphoid Cells *in Vitro:* Inhibition by Isoantibody and by Drugs." *Immunol.* 14:181-196, 1968.

13. Brunner, K.T., Mauel, J., and Schindler, R., "*In Vitro* Studies of Cell Bound Immunity: Cloning Assay of the Cytotoxic Action of Sensitized Lymphoid Cells on Allogeneic Target Cells." *Immunol.* 11:499-506, 1966.

14. Hersey, P., "Macrophage Effector Function." *Transplantation* 15:282-290, 1973.

15. Julius, M.H., Simpson, E., and Herzenberg, L.A., "A Rapid Method for the Isolation of Functional Thymus-Derived Murine Lymphocytes." *European J. Immunol.* 3:645-649, 1973.

16. Trizio, D., and Cudkowicz, G., "Separation of T and B Lymphocytes by Nylon Wool Columns. Evaluation of Efficacy by Functional Assays *in Vivo.*" *J. Immunol.* 113:1093-1097.

17. Allison, A.C., Harrington, J.S., and Birbeck, M., "An Examination of the Cytotoxic Effects of Silica on Macrophages." *J. Exp. Med.* 124:141-154, 1966.

18. Allison, A.C., "Fluorescence Microscopy of Lymphocytes and Mononuclear Phagocytes and the Use of Silica to Eliminate the Latter." In: *In Vitro Methods in Cell-Mediated and Tumor Immunity,* ed., by B.R. Bloom and J.R. David, pp. 395-404, Academic Press, New York, 1976.

19. Zembala, M., and Asherson, G.L. "The Rapid Purification of Peritoneal Exudate Macrophages by Ficoll (Polysucrose) Density Gradient Centrifugation." *Immunology* 19:677-682, 1970.

411

20. Schultz, R.M., Papamatheakis, J.P., Luetzeler, J., and Chirigos, M.S., "Association of Macrophage Activation with Antitumor Activity by Synthetic and Biological Agents." *Cancer Res.* 37:3338-3343, 1977.

21. Nelson, O.S., editor *Immunobiology of the Macrophage,* Academic Press, New York, 1976.

22. Poplack, D.G., Sher, N.A., Chaparas, S.D., and Blaese, M.R., "The Effect of Mycobacterium bovis (Bacillus Calmette-Guérin) on Macrophage Random Migration, Chemotaxis, and Pinocytosis." *Cancer Res.* 36:1233-1237, 1976.

23. Buhles, W.C., and Shifrine, M., "Increased Bone Marrow Production of Granulocytes and Mononuclear Phagocytes Induced by Mycobacterial Adjuvants: Improved Recovery of Leukopoiesis in Mice after Cyclophosphamide Treatment." *Infection and Immunity* 20:58-65, 1978.

24. Fisher, B., Taylor, S., Levine, M., et al., "Effect of Mycobacterium bovis (Strain Bacillus Calmette-Guérin) on Macrophage Production by the Bone Marrow of Tumor-bearing Mice." *Cancer Res.* 34:1668-1670, 1974.

Augmentation of Anti-Tumor Cytotoxicity in Spleen Cells of MOPC-315 Tumor-Bearers[†]

Margalit B. Mokyr[1]
D. Braun[1]
S. Dray[1]

SUMMARY—Spleen cells from BALB/c mice bearing various sizes of MOPC-315 plasmacytoma tumors were not cytotoxic *in vitro* or *in vivo*. These noncytotoxic spleen cells became cytotoxic upon *in vitro* education with stimulator tumor cells. The level of *in vivo* anti-tumor cytotoxicity exhibited by these educated spleen cells from tumor-bearing mice, regardless of tumor size, was at least equal to, but usually superior to that of educated spleen cells from normal mice. On the other hand, the level of *in vitro* anti-tumor cytotoxicity exhibited by these educated spleen cells from tumor-bearing mice was dependent on tumor size; compared to the cytotoxicity exhibited by educated normal spleen cells, the level for educated tumor-bearer spleen cells was similar when the spleen donors bore small tumors (12 mm) but lower when the donors bore large tumors (20 mm). The decrease in the level of *in vitro* cytotoxicity obtained with educated tumor-bearer spleen cells as tumor growth progressed correlated with an increase in the percentage of splenic macrophages. Removal of glass wool adherent tumor-bearer spleen cells resulted in a decrease in the percentage of macrophages as well as in the expression of *in vitro* anti-tumor cytotoxicity. Combining removal of glass adherent cells with *in vitro* education led to higher levels of anti-tumor cytotoxicity than the sum of the levels exhibited by spleen cells subjected to either process alone.

INTRODUCTION

The effectiveness of adoptive cellular immunotherapy of cancer depends on the ability of the infused cells to survive in the recipient host and to implement a potent anti-tumor response. The ready availability and histocompatibility of the tumor-bearer's own lymphoid cells would make them an ideal source of cells for adoptive therapy provided methods can be developed to potentiate their anti-tumor cytotoxicity. Previous work from this laboratory has demonstrated that murine lymphoid cells which became unresponsive to tumor antigen during lethal plasmacytoma growth can be converted by immune-RNA to a state of immunological responsiveness as assessed *in vitro* by the macrophage migration inhibition assay (1).

In the present study, *in vitro* education with stimulator tumor cells and/or

[1]Departments of Microbiology and Immunology, University of Illinois at the Medical Center, Chicago, Illinois.
[†]Supported in part by NIH grant PHS CA-18241

413

depletion of glass adherent cells were employed as other methods to evoke anti-tumor activity in noncytotoxic spleen cells from mice bearing plasmacytoma tumors. Anti-tumor activity was evaluated *in vitro* by the Cr^{51} release assay and *in vivo* by the local adoptive transfer assay.

METHODS

In Vitro Generation of Cytotoxic Spleen Cells. The *in vitro* method for generating anti-tumor cytotoxicity was described previously (2, 3). Briefly, responder spleen cells (75 x 10⁶) were cultured with or without Mitomycin C-treated stimulator tumor cells (2 x 10⁶) at 37°C in a humidified atmosphere of 5% CO_2 in air for 4-7 days.

Anti-Tumor Cytotoxicity Assays. The cell-mediated lysis elicited by uneducated or educated tumor-bearer spleen cells was determined *in vitro* in the Cr^{51} release assay (4) and *in vivo* in the Winn assay (5). The percentage specific Cr^{51} release was assessed by the following formula:

$$\% \text{ Sp. } Cr^{51} \text{ release} = \frac{\% \text{ lysis with test spleen cells} - \% \text{ lysis with uneducated normal spleen cells}}{\% \text{ maximal lysis (freeze thaw)} - \% \text{ lysis with uneducated normal spleen cells}} \times 100$$

and the percentage reduction in tumor incidence was calculated by the following formula:

$$\% \text{ reduction} = 1 - \frac{\text{tumor incidence with test spleen cells}}{\text{tumor incidence with uneducated normal spleen cells}} \times 100$$

The data presented is representative of the data obtained in 3-6 individual experiments.

Depletion of Cells Adherent to Glass Wool. Tumor-bearer spleen cells (6 x 10⁸) suspended in 30 ml warmed MEM supplemented with 20% fetal calf serum were applied to individual 50 ml sterile glass wool columns. Columns were incubated at 37°C for 45 minutes with occasional rotation. Non-adherent spleen cells were eluted in 100 ml of warmed MEM. The yield of cells recovered from the columns was about 15-25% with a marked decrease in macrophages as judged by morphological criteria.

EXPERIMENTAL PLAN AND RESULTS

Spleen Cells from MOPC-315 Tumor-Bearing Mice Are Not Cytotoxic at Any Stage of Tumor Growth. BALB/c mice were injected subcutaneously

414

with 1 to 4 x 10⁶ MOPC-315 plasmacytoma cells, a dose which leads to progressively growing tumors that kill the mice in 20 ± 3 days. On various days post-tumor inoculation, including days 3, 7 (when palpable tumor nodules first appear), 10 (when tumor diameter is 9-12 mm) or 14 (when tumor diameter is 16-20 mm), mice were sacrificed, their spleens removed, and single cell suspensions prepared by mechanical disruption (2). These spleen cells were assayed for their anti-tumor activity *in vitro* by the Cr^{51} release assay and *in vivo* by the local adoptive transfer assay (Table 1). Spleen cells from mice bearing the MOPC-315 tumors for 3-14 days were unable to lyse target cells *in vitro* (less than 5% Cr^{51} release) at a spleen/tumor ratio of 100/1 and did not reduce tumor incidence *in vivo* in the Winn assay at a spleen/tumor cell ratio of 50/1.

Table 1—ASSESSMENT OF ANTI-TUMOR IMMUNITY IN SPLEEN CELLS OF BALB/c MICE BEARING MOPC-315 TUMORS

Source of spleen cells	% specific[a] Cr^{51} release	Tumor[b,c] incidence	% reduction of tumor incidence
Normal mice	0	5/5	0
day 3 tumor-bearers	-0.9±1.2	5/5	0
day 7 tumor-bearers	-0.4±0.9	5/5	0
day 10 tumor-bearers	3.7±0.3	5/5	0
day 14 tumor-bearers	-2.1±1.2	5/5	0

[a]Cr^{51} release was performed at an effector/target cell ratio of 100:1.
[b]Winn assay was performed at an effector/target cell ratio of 50:1.
[c]Numbers of mice showing tumor/total mice inoculated.

In Vitro Anti-Tumor Cytotoxicity can be Generated in Noncytotoxic Tumor-Bearer Spleen Cells Upon In Vitro Education. Noncytotoxic spleen cells from mice injected 3, 7, 10, or 14 days earlier with 1 to 4 x 10⁶ MOPC-315 cells were cultivated with or without MOPC-315 stimulator tumor cells for 4-7 days and subsequently tested in the Cr^{51} release assay. No significant anti-tumor cytotoxicity was observed with normal or tumor-bearer spleen cells cultured without stimulator tumor cells (less than 5%). *In vitro* education led to the generation of anti-tumor cytotoxicity in both normal and tumor-bearer spleen cells (Figure 1). High levels of anti-tumor cytotoxicity were seen with educated spleen cells from normal mice on days 4-6 of the education culture with maximal levels on the fifth day of the culture. Similar

415

**Figure 1—ANTI-TUMOR CYTOTOXICITY IN BOTH
NORMAL AND TUMOR-BEARER SPLEEN CELLS**

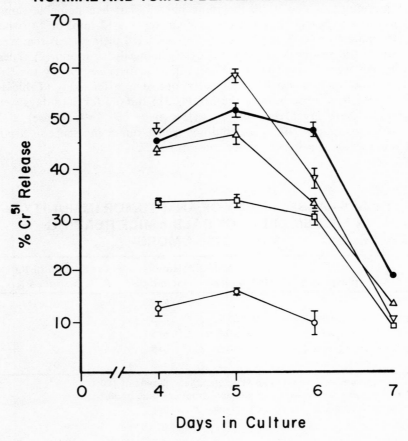

Development of *in vitro* anti-MOPC-315 tumor cytotoxicity in spleen cells from normal BALB/c mice (•) and mice bearing MOPC-315 tumors for 3 (□), 7 (△), 10 (▽), and 14 (○) days upon *in vitro* education with MOPC-315 stimulator cells for 4-7 days.

kinetics of development of anti-tumor cytotoxicity was observed with educated spleen cells from tumor-bearing mice regardless of tumor size. Therefore, for the sake of simplicity, only data obtained on the fifth day of the *in vitro* education culture will be presented for the remainder of this report. The levels of anti-tumor cytotoxicity obtained with educated spleen cells from mice bearing tumors for up to 10 days were similar to the levels obtained with educated normal spleen cells. On the other hand, the levels of anti-tumor cytotoxicity exhibited by educated spleen cells from mice bearing large tumors were substantially lower.

416

Table 2—*IN VIVO* ANTI-TUMOR ACTIVITY (WINN ASSAY) EXHIBITED BY EDUCATED SPLEEN CELLS FROM NORMAL MICE AND FROM MICE BEARING LARGE SIZE TUMORS

Responder spleen cells	Stimulator tumor cells	Tumor incidence[a,b]	% reduction of tumor incidence
Normal	None	5/5	0
day 13 tumor bearer	None	5/5	0
Normal	MOPC-315	3/5	40
day 13 tumor bearer	MOPC-315	0/5	100

[a]Winn assay was performed at an effector/target cell ratio of 15/1.
[b](Numbers of mice showing tumor)/(total mice inoculated).

In Vivo Anti-Tumor Cytotoxicity can be Generated in Noncytotoxic Tumor-Bearer Spleen Cells Upon In Vitro Education. The ability of educated tumor-bearer spleen cells to reduce tumor incidence *in vivo* was evaluated in the Winn assay at a spleen/tumor cell ratio of 15/1 (Table 2). Normal spleen cells or tumor-bearer spleen cells that were cultured in the absence of stimulator tumor cells did not reduce tumor incidence, while normal spleen cells that were educated *in vitro* led to 40% reduction in tumor incidence. On the other hand, educated spleen cells from day 13 tumor-bearing mice which exhibited low levels of *in vitro* anti-tumor cytotoxicity were very effective in mediating *in vivo* anti-tumor activity and led to complete prevention of tumor growth. Similar levels of *in vivo* anti-tumor cytotoxicity were obtained with educated spleen cells from mice bearing the tumors for 3-14 days regardless of tumor size.

The compiled results obtained in all the experiments performed to date regarding the level of *in vivo* anti-tumor activity exhibited by educated normal and educated tumor-bearer spleen cells are shown in Table 3. Uneducated normal and uneducated tumor-bearer spleen cells did not reduce tumor incidence while educated spleen cells from normal mice reduced tumor incidence by 69%. Educated spleen cells from tumor-bearing mice were superior to educated normal spleen cells in mediating *in vivo* anti-tumor activity and led to 89% reduction in tumor incidence.

The Percentage of Macrophages in Spleen Cells from MOPC-315 Tumor-Bearers Increases During Tumor Growth. Studies were performed to determine how splenic weight, macrophage percentage, and nucleated cell

417

Table 3—COMPILED RESULTS OF THE *IN VIVO* ANTI-TUMOR ACTIVITY (WINN ASSAY) EXHIBITED BY EDUCATED SPLEEN CELLS FROM NORMAL AND FROM TUMOR-BEARING MICE

Responder[a] spleen cells	Stimulator tumor cells	Tumor[b,c] incidence	% reduction of tumor incidence
Normal	None	40/40	0
Tumor[b] Bearer	None	50/50	0
Normal	MOPC-315	14/45	69
Tumor[b] Bearer	MOPC-315	5/45	89

[a]Winn assay was performed on effector/target cell ratio.
[b]Spleen cells from mice bearing the tumors for 6-14 days.
[c](Numbers of mice showing tumor)/(total mice inoculated).

Figure 2—CORRELATION OF SPLENIC WEIGHT, MACROPHAGE PERCENTAGE, AND NUCLEATED CELL NUMBER WITH TUMOR SIZE

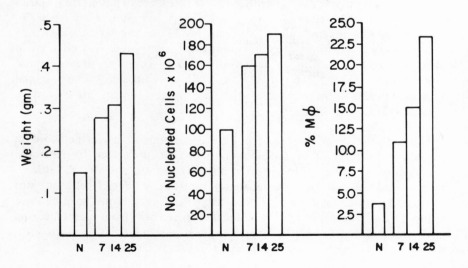

Weight, number of nucleated cells, and percentage of macrophages of spleens from normal mice (N) and from mice bearing MOPC-315 tumors with diameters of 7, 14 and 25 mm.

418

number correlated with tumor size (Figure 2). Baseline studies demonstrated that the average spleen weight of normal mice was 0.15 gm, yielding approximately 100 million nucleated cells, 3.6% of which were morphologically identified as macrophages. When spleens of tumor-bearing mice were evaluated, an increase in tumor size resulted in an increase in spleen weight (ranging from 0.28 gm/spleen for 7.1 mm tumors to 0.43 gm/spleen for 25.5 mm tumors) and a slight increase in nucleated cell number (ranging from 160 million for 7.1 mm tumors to 185 million for 25.5 mm tumors). Increased tumor size also resulted in an increase in splenic macrophage percentage, reaching 23% of total splenic nucleated cells for 25.5 mm tumors. These results suggest that the decreased ability of educated spleen cells from day 14 tumor-bearing mice to mediate *in vitro* anti-tumor cytotoxicity (Figure 1) might be due to an increase in the percentage of macrophages in the spleens of tumor-bearing mice.

Depletion of Macrophages from Tumor-Bearer Spleen Cells Leads to Augmented Anti-Tumor Cytotoxicity. Adherence of spleen cells from mice bearing large tumors to glass wool columns reduced the percentage of macrophages from 20-25% to less than 4% in the eluted, nonadherent cells. Fractionated, nonadherent spleen cells as well as unfractioned spleen cells from mice bearing 19 mm tumors were cultured in the presence or absence of stimulator tumor cells and subsequently tested for their anti-tumor cytotoxicity in the Cr^{51} release assay (Figure 3). Unfractionated tumor-bearer spleen cells cultured in the absence of stimulator cells did not exhibit anti-tumor cytotoxicity whereas fractionated, nonadherent spleen cells exhibited significant levels of anti-tumor cytotoxicity. Unfractionated, tumor-bearer spleen cells became cytotoxic upon *in vitro* education exhibiting similar levels of anti-tumor cytotoxicity as did uneducated, nonadherent cells (30% vs 29%, respectively). *In vitro* education of nonadherent, tumor-bearer spleen cells led to a substantial augmentation of anti-tumor cytotoxicity resulting in 96% Cr^{51} release even at an effector/target cell ratio of 20/1. The level of anti-tumor cytotoxicity exhibited by educated, nonadherent tumor-bearer spleen cells, at both effector/target cell ratios tested, was greater than the sum of the levels of cytotoxicity seen with spleen cells subjected to glass wool adherence or *in vitro* education alone (100% vs 29% + 30% at an effector/target cell ratio of 100/1 and 96% vs 16% + 13% at an effector/target cell ratio of 20/1).

DISCUSSION

The *in vitro* generation of cytotoxic cells is being widely studied for possible use in immunotherapy (6-9). The advantages of utilizing *in vitro* educated cells over *in vivo* sensitized cells for therapeutic purposes are: a) the

419

risk of immunizing hosts with malignant cells is eliminated; b) the levels of cell-mediated lysis produced are significantly higher (7, 10, 11); c) antigens which are weakly immunogenic *in vivo* can evoke high levels of cell-mediated lysis upon *in vitro* education (10); and d) a more rapid generation of cytotoxicity (5 days) occurs (2, 3).

Several attempts have been made to alter tumor growth in the local adoptive transfer assay with cells obtained *in vitro* education of spleen cells from normal (8, 12-15) or tumor-immune animals (16). The capacity of such cells to mediate systematic anti-tumor activity was also evaluated. Burton and Warner (8) obtained marginal anti-tumor activity when *in vitro* activated spleen cells from normal mice were injected intravenously, even though the cells were "fully active" in the Cr^{51} release assay and in the Winn assay. Such results are consistent with results obtained by Bernstein (7) who showed that transfer of systemic tumor immunity against Gross Virus-induced rat lymphomas is successful only with *in vitro* reactivated immune spleen cells but not with *in vitro* educated normal spleen cells. However, the possibility of using *in vitro* education for human immunotherapy would be greatly facilitated by the ability to sensitize the lymphocytes from tumor-bearing individuals. Treves, et al., (6) compared the ability of educated spleen cells from normal mice or from mice bearing progressively growing tumors to protect against lethal lung metastases following excision of the primary tumors. Educated spleen cells from normal mice led to 71% survival as compared to 44% survival of the control animals. Educated tumor-bearer spleen cells were less effective than educated normal cells and led to 57% survival. Our data indicate that *in vitro* educated tumor-bearer spleen cells are more cytotoxic than *in vitro* educated normal spleen cells in the local adoptive transfer assay. Thus, they might also prove to be more efficient in transferring systemic anti-tumor immunity.

Spleen cells from MOPC-315 tumor-bearing mice did not exhibit *in vitro* or *in vivo* anti-tumor cytotoxicity at any stage of tumor growth. This failure might reflect an insufficiency in the number of cytotoxic cells in tumor-bearer spleens (17) or the presence of suppressor mechanisms which prevent the expression of cytotoxicity (18). In light of these considerations, our demonstration that noncytotoxic tumor-bearer spleen cells exhibit anti-tumor cytotoxicity upon *in vitro* education may be explicable by 1) the sensitization of potentially reactive cells within the unreactive population, 2) the derepression of suppressed cytotoxic cells, 3) a shift in the balance between suppressor and cytotoxic cells in favor of cytotoxicity, and 4) a combination of these effects.

Studies into the regulation of the immune response have revealed that the balance between immunostimulation and immunosuppression can be subject to the actions of macrophages. The nature of this regulation appears to be dependent upon the ratio between macrophages and immunocompetent

420

lymphocytes. Low ratios augment the response of purified lymphocytes while high ratios suppress their response (19-21). Our results are consistent with these observations in that an increase in the percentage of splenic macrophages during progressive tumor growth is associated with a decrease in anti-tumor cytotoxicity upon *in vitro* education of tumor-bearer spleen cells. Adherence of tumor-bearer spleen cells to glass wool columns results in 1) a reduction in the percentage of splenic macrophages to a percentage approximating that of normal spleen cells; 2) expression of *in vitro* anti-tumor cytotoxicity in cultured nonadherent spleen cells; and 3) augmented anti-tumor cytotoxicity upon *in vitro* education. These results suggest that the anti-tumor cytotoxicity exhibited by tumor-bearer spleen cells is subject to suppression by macrophages. Pellis, et al., (22) have also implicated high

Figure 3—*IN VITRO* CYTOTOXIC ACTIVITY IN UNFRACTIONATED AND NONADHERENT TUMOR-BEARER SPLEEN CELLS

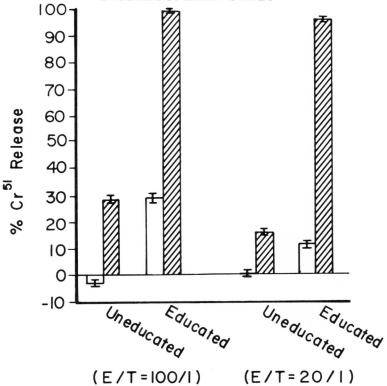

In vitro cytotoxic activity exhibited by unfractionated (□) and glass wool depleted (nonadherent) (▨) tumor-bearer spleen cells (19 mm tumor diameter) that were cultured *in vitro* in the presence or absence of stimulator tumor cells.

421

percentages of macrophages in the suppression of *in vivo* anti-tumor cytotoxicity by spleen cells from mice immunized with supraoptimal doses of soluble fibrosarcoma tumor antigen. Still, the possibility that the suppression seen in MOPC-315 tumor-bearer spleen cells is mediated by an adherent cell different than macrophages cannot be ruled out. Folch and Waksman have shown that T cells which inhibit the response of normal rat spleen cells to supraoptimal doses of mitogen are also removed by glass adherence (23). In an attempt to identify the nature of the adherent suppressor cell that operates in the MOPC-315 tumor system, experiments are now being performed to evaluate the effect of removing phagocytic cells on anti-MOPC-315 cytotoxicity. However, to prove that this suppression is mediated by macrophages, the effect of adding an increasing number of purified macrophages to nonadherent tumor-bearer spleen cells and to normal spleen cells will be evaluated.

Other investigators have reported marked increases in macrophages in the spleens of tumor-bearing animals and have indicated their involvement in the suppression of the following: 1) mitogenic responsiveness (24, 25); 2) lymphocyte proliferation in mixed leukocyte-tumor cell interactions (24, 26); and 3) generation of cells cytotoxic to alloantigens (24, 27). Our results extend these findings by suggesting that the generation of *anti-tumor* cytotoxicity in spleen cells of tumor-bearing mice is also subject to negative regulation by macrophages.

The level of *in vitro* anti-tumor cytotoxicity exhibited by educated, nonadherent tumor-bearer spleen cells was greater than the sum of the levels of cytotoxicity seen with spleen cells subjected to glass wool adherence or education alone. In view of this, we would anticipate that the *in vivo* anti-tumor activity of educated, *nonadherent* tumor-bearer spleen cells might prove to be even greater than the activity of educated, unfractionated tumor-bearer spleen cells. Thus educated, nonadherent tumor-bearer lymphoid cells might become useful in immunotherapeutic regimens requiring histocompatible cells with agumented anti-tumor cytotoxicity.

ACKNOWLEDGMENTS

We wish to acknowledge the expert technical assistance of Miss Katherine Siessmann whose efforts were invaluable in the performance of this work, as well as assistance of Mrs. Mitzi B. Sabato in the preparation of this manuscript.

REFERENCES

1. Braun, D., Dray, S., "Immune RNA-Mediated Transfer of Tumor Antigen Responsiveness to Unresponsive Peritoneal Exudate Cells from Tumor-Bearing Animals." *Cancer Res.* 37:4138, 1977.

2. Burton, R., Thompson, J., Warner, N.L., *"In Vitro* Induction of Tumor-Specific Immunity." *J. Immunol. Methods* 8:133, 1975.

3. Mokyr, M.B., Braun, D.P., Usher, D., et al., "The Development of *In Vitro* and *In Vivo* Anti-Tumor Cytotoxicity in Noncytotoxic, MOPC-315-Tumor-Bearer, Spleen Cells 'Educated' *In Vitro* with MOPC-315 Tumor Cells." *Cancer Immunol. Immunother.* (In press.)

4. Brunner, K.T., Mauel, J., Rudolf, H., Chapuis, B., "Studies on Autograft Immunity in Mice. I. Induction, Development and *In Vitro* Assay of Cellular Immunity." *Immunology* 18:499, 1970.

5. Winn, H.J., "The Immune Response and the Homograft Reaction." *Nat. Cancer Inst. Monogr.* 2:113, 1959.

6. Treves, A.J., Cohen, I.R., Feldman, M., "Immunotherapy of Lethal Mestastases by Lymphocytes Sensitized Against Tumor Cells *In Vitro."* *J. Nat. Cancer Inst.* 54:777, 1975.

7. Bernstein, I.D., "Passive Transfer of Systemic Tumor Immunity with Cells Generated *In Vitro* by a Secondary Immune Response to a Syngeneic Rat Gross Virus-Induced Lymphoma." *J. Immunol.* 118:122, 1977.

8. Burton, R.C., Warner, N.L., *"In Vitro* Induction of Tumor-Specific Immunity. IV. Specific Adoptive Immunotherapy with Cytotoxic T Cells Induced *In Vitro* to Plasmacytoma Antigens." *Cancer Immunol. Immunother.* 2:91, 1977.

9. Cheever, M.A., Kempf, R.A., and Fefer A., "Tumor Neutralization, Immunotherapy and Chemoimmunotherapy of a Friend Leukemia with Cells Secondarily Sensitized *In Vitro. J. Immunol.* 119:714, 1977.

10. Berke, G., Clark, W.P., Feldman, M., *"In Vitro* Induction of a Heterograft Reaction. Immunological Parameters of the Sensitization of Rat Lymphocytes Against Mouse Cells *In Vitro."* *Transplantation* 12:237, 1971.

11. Feldman, M., Cohen, I.R., Wekerle, H., "T-Cell-Mediated Immunity *In Vitro:* An Analysis of Antigen Recognition and Target Cell Lysis." *Transplant. Rev.* 12:57, 1972.

12. Rouse, B.T., Wagner, H., Harris, A.W., *"In Vivo* Activity of *In Vitro* Immunized Lymphocytes. I. Tumor Allograft Rejection Mediated by *In Vitro* Activated Mouse Thymocytes." *J. Immunol.* 108:1353, 1972.

13. Rollinghoff, M., Wagner, H., *"In Vitro* Induction of Tumor Specific Immunity: Requirements for T Lymphocytes and Tumor Growth Inhibition *In Vivo."* *Europ. J. Immunol.* 3:471, 1973a.

14. Rollinghoff, M., Wagner, H., *"In Vivo* Protection Against Murine Plasma Cell Tumor Growth by *In Vitro* Activated Syngeneic Lymphocytes." *J. Nat. Cancer Inst.* 51:1317, 1973b.

15. Kedar, E., Schwartzbach, M., Raanan, Z., Hefetz, S., *"In Vitro* Induction of Cell-Mediated Immunity to Murine Leukemia Cells. II. Cytotoxic Activity *In Vitro* and Tumor Neutralizing Capacity *In Vivo* of Anti-leukemia Cytotoxic Lymphocytes Generated in Macrocultures." *J. Immunol. Methods* 16:39, 1977.

16. Bernstein, I.D., Wright, P.W., and Cohen, E., "Generation of Cytotoxic Lymphocytes *In Vitro:* Response of Immune Rat Spleen Cells to a Syngeneic Gross Virus-induced Lymphoma in Mixed Lymphocyte-tumor Culture." *J. Immunol.* 116:1367, 1976.

17. Padarathsingh, M.L., McCoy, J.L., Dean, J.H., et al., "Examination of General and Tumor-specific Cell-mediated Immune Responses in Mice Bearing Progressively Growing Plasmacytomas." *J. Nat. Cancer Inst.* 58:1701, 1977.

423

18. Fujimoto, S., Greene, M.I., Sehon, A.H., "Regulation of the Immune Response to Tumor Antigens. I. Immunosuppressor Cells in Tumor-bearing Hosts." *J. Immunol.* 116:791, 1976.

19. Mokyr, M.B. and Mitchell, M.S., "Activation of Lymphoid Cells by BCG *In Vitro.*" *Cellular Immunol.* 15:264, 1975.

20. Wing, E.J. and Remington, J.S., "Studies on the Regulation of Lymphocyte Reactivity by Normal and Activated Macrophages." *Cell. Immunol.* 30:108, 1977.

21. Allison, A.C., "Mechanisms by Which Activated Macrophages Inhibit Lymphocyte Responses." *Immunological Rev.* 40:3, 1978.

22. Pellis, N.R., Mokyr, M.B. and Kahan, B.D., "Cell Mediated Immunity to Solubilized Antigens of a Methylcholanthrene (MCA) Induced Fibrosarcoma." *Proc. Amer. Assoc. Cancer Res.* 18:138, 1977.

23. Folch, H. and Waksman, B.H., "Regulation of Lymphocyte Responses *In Vitro* V. Suppressor Activity of Adherent and Nonadherent Rat Lymphoid Cells." *Cell. Immunol.* 9:12, 1973.

24. Kirchner, H., Chused, T.M., Herberman, R.B., et al., "Evidence of Suppressor Cell Activity in Spleens of Mice Bearing Primary Tumors Induced by Moloney Sarcoma Virus." *J. Exp. Med.* 139:1473, 1974.

25. Elgert, K.D. and Connolly, K.M., "Macrophage Regulation of the T-Cell Allogeneic Response During Tumor Growth." *Cell. Immunol.* 35:1, 1978.

26. Glaser, M., Kirchner, H. and Herberman, R., "Inhibition of *In Vitro* Lymphoproliferative Response to Tumor Associated Antigens by Suppressor Cells from Rats Bearing Progressively Growing Gross Leukemia Virus Induced Tumors." *Int. J. Cancer* 16:384, 1975.

27. Fernbach, B., Kirchner, H., Bonnard, G. and Herberman, R., "Suppression of Mixed Lymphocyte Responses in Mice Bearing Primary Tumors Induced by Murine Sarcoma Virus." *Transplant.* 21:381, 1976.

The Use of Bacteria for the Identification of Functionally Different Lymphocyte Subpopulations in Blood Smears†

Marius Teodorescu[1]
R. Kleinman[1]
E. Mayer[1]
A. Bratescu[1]
K. DeBoer[1]

SUMMARY—We developed a new methodology that uses bacteria for the identification of lymphocyte subpopulations in blood smears or in cell suspensions. Some bacteria bind to the lymphocytes via purified antibody chemically coated on the bacteria, whereas other bacteria (fixed) have the natural ability to bind to lymphocyte subpopulations. To label the cells in whole blood, the blood cells (including erythrocytes) were washed, one or two strains of bacteria were added in excess and the mixture was centrifuged. The excess bacteria were then washed out by low-speed centrifugation, and smears were prepared. B cells were identified by using *Brucella melitensis* and/or anti-light chain antibody coated *E. coli*. Four T cell subpopulations (T_1, T_2, T_3, T_4) and two B cell subpopulations (B_1, B_2) were identified by using the natural binding of various strains of bacteria. The relative proportion of these lymphocyte subpopulations was found to be similar in normal donors but to vary in some cancer patients. Some of these subpopulations appeared to be functionally different: T_1T_2 cells responded to mitogens and allogeneic cells, were specifically cytotoxic and appeared to contain suppressor cells. The T_3T_4 cells responded to allogeneic cells, did not develop into specific cytotoxic cells and responded poorly to mitogens. The T_4 cells were naturally cytotoxic for allogeneic lymphocytes and for established lymphoblastoid cell lines. We concluded that bacteria are useful, stable, shelf reagents that can be used to identify and enumerate functionally different lymphocyte subpopulations in clinical laboratories.

INTRODUCTION

Lymphocytes are morphologically alike but functionally heterogeneous; i.e., subpopulations have been described with specialized functions (1,2). Human B and T lymphocytes, and their subpopulations, have been shown

---

[1]Department of Microbiology and Immunology, University of Illinois at the Medical Center, Chicago, Illinois.
†Supported by the grants 2R01AM19414 from the National Institute of Arthritis, Metabolism and Digestive Diseases and R01CA21399 from National Cancer Institute.

to have different surface markers by a variety of procedures (3-6). However, none of these procedures has been used for the routine identification of lymphocyte subpopulations in stained blood smears. As a consequence, very little knowledge has been accumulated regarding the changes in lymphocyte subpopulations under various physiologic or pathologic conditions. Since experimental evidence has been accumulated on the different roles of lymphocyte subpopulations in the evolution of tumors it would be useful to have a routine procedure to determine changes in lymphocyte subpopulation in cancer patients.

We showed, in rabbits, that B and T lymphocytes could be identified simultaneously in blood smears by using antibody-coated bacteria (7). We also demonstrated that B cells and subpopulations of T cells could be identified by their natural binding of different strains of bacteria (8). Here we describe a simple and reproducible methodology for the identification of human lymphocyte subpopulations in blood smears. This methodology uses the antibody-mediated and natural binding of bacteria to lymphocytes subpopulations. Evidence that these subpopulations are functionally different is also presented.

MATERIALS AND METHODS

Antibody-coated bacteria were prepared as previously described (8). Briefly, a strain of *Escherichia coli (E. coli 0)* which does not bind spontaneously to lymphocytes was fixed with glutaraldehyde, and chemically coated with purified antibody against either κ or λ chains was covalently coupled to the bacterial cell wall.

Bacterial suspensions were prepared as previously described (8). The bacteria were grown in Difco antibiotic III medium (DIFCO, Detroit, MI.) and were fixed with formaldehyde. Out of 53 strains of different genuses and species, 13 were selected that bound to lymphocytes (8). However, only 8 were used in this study: *Arizona hinshawii* (ATCC-31241),[1] *Escherichia coli-2* (NRRL-B-11010),[2] and 3 (NRRL-B-11011), *Bacillus globigii* (NRRL-B-11007), *Brucella melitensis* (ATCC-31242), *Sarcina lutea* (NRRL-B-11012), *Staphylococcus aureus* 1 (ATCC-31240) and 2 (UI-57)[3].

Labeling the lymphocytes with bacteria and the preparation of smears were carried out as follows. The blood was collected in heparinized tubes and the blood cells were washed three times at 4°C in Eagle's MEM supplemented with 6% bovine serum albumin (BSA) and 0.02% sodium azide. The cell suspension was adjusted with the same medium up to the

---

[1]American Type Culture Collection, Rockville, Maryland.
[2]Northern Regional Research Center, U.S. Department of Agriculture, Peoria, Illinois.
[3]University of Illinois Medical Center, Department of Microbiology, Chicago, Illinois.

initial volume of blood. To each sample of 0.2 ml of blood cell suspension we added 0.05 ml or 0.05 ml from each of two bacterial strains (double labeling) of one bacterial strain (single labeling) to reach a ratio of about 10 bacteria/red cell. The mixture was centrifuged at 900 X g at 4°C for 6 minutes to promote the binding of bacteria to lymphocytes. The pelleted cells were resuspended in 2.5 ml of MEM-BSA and recentrifuged three times at 150 X g at 4°C for 10 minutes. After each centrifugation, the supernatant layer which contained the unbound bacteria was discarded. After the final centrifugation, the pellet was resuspended in MEM-BSA to give a final volume of 0.2 ml. Smears were prepared and stained with Wright stain. Lymphocytes with bacteria attached were easily scored (Figure 1).

The background of unbound bacteria in the blood smears was usually very low and the number of bacteria associated with each cell was relatively high (Figure 1). To provide a standard which corrects for the random association of bacteria with blood cells, a cell was considered labeled based on the following criterion. Two hundred erythrocytes of each slide (1-2 microscopic fields) were screened for their association with bacteria. The largest number of bacteria (X) associated with a single erythrocyte on a measure of random association; thus, a lymphocyte associated with X + 1 or more bacteria was scored as labeled. Three separate counts of one hundred lymphocytes were performed (unless otherwise specified).

The separation of lymphocyte subpopulations by bacterial adherence was carried out as described elsewhere (10). Briefly, the bacteria were covalently coupled to gelatin layers by using gluteraldehyde. The lymphocyte suspensions were centrifuged against these bacterial monolayers for 10 minutes, and the cells that adhered were separated from those that did not adhere.

The lymphocyte cultures were set up as previously described. Briefly, peripheral blood lymphocytes were separated by centrifugation on Ficoll Hypaque. The mitogen response of the lymphocytes was determined by ^{3}H-TdR incorporation in cultures set up in microtiter plates (10). The mixed lymphocyte cultures were carried out according to O'Leary, et al., (11) and the cytotoxic assays according to Lightbody (12). When specified, the monocytes and/or the Ig-bearing cells were removed from the lymphocyte population as described previously (10).

RESULTS

1. *Identification of Ig-Bearing Lymphocytes in Blood Smears.* One of the advantages of labeling the lymphocyte subpopulations in whole blood smears is that the selective loss of a particular subset may be avoided. Our major manipulation of the cells involved numerous washings. To determine the effect of these washings on the lymphocyte population, we counted

427

Figure 1—LYMPHOCYTES LABELED BY BACTERIA IN BLOOD SMEARS

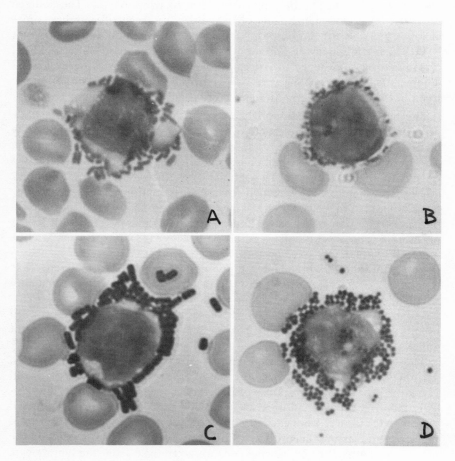

A: *E. coli*, B: *A. Hinshawii*, C: *B. globigii*, D: *S. aureus*.

(automatic cell counter, Coulter Counter) the leukocytes before and after the cells were washed six times. On the average, the total number of leukocytes was reduced by about 15%. However, the percentage of lymphocytes was increased by about 16% suggesting that whatever loss might have occurred was at the expense of polymorphonuclear cells. Thus, we concluded that any significant loss of lymphocytes during the labeling procedure was unlikely.

428

The percentage of Ig-bearing lymphocytes (B cells) in the blood of donors with normal leukocyte and differential counts, determined by labeling them with a mixture of anti-κ and anti-λ antibody coated *E. coli,* ranged from 14 to 19% with an average of 16.3% (Table 1). When each of these donors was assayed for the percentage of κ-bearing and λ-bearing cells, the values ranged from 8 to 11% for κ-bearing cells, with an average of 9.3%, and 5 to 11% for λ-bearing cells (16.3%) (Table 1). Even on an individual basis, the sum of the κ-bearing and λ-bearing cells agreed well with the total number of Ig-bearing cells.

To investigate whether or not the bacteria were binding to the lymphocytes via the Fc receptor of B cells *E. coli* coated with normal rabbit IgG was used. Very few (0-3%) of the lymphocytes were labeled, which indicated that essentially all of the bacterial binding was dependent on the antibody-combining site of the anti-κ and anti-λ antibodies. If the anti-κ and anti-λ antibodies were not specific for κ or λ light chains and/or if some of the Ig-bearing cells had passively absorbed surface Ig, some or all of the B cells would have bound both to the anti-κ and anti-λ Ab-*E. coli.* This would have resulted in the sum of the κ-bearing and λ-bearing cells, being greater than the actual number of Ig-bearing cells. The fact that the sum of the κ-bearing and λ-bearing cells was essentially equal to the total number of Ig-bearing cells indicated that the anti-κ and anti-λ antibodies were specific and that there was no passively absorbed Ig on normal B cells. However, both κ and λ chains may be formed on the same cell in pathologic conditions. In a preliminary study on five patients with rheumatic diseases we found that both κ and λ chains were present on the same cell, suggesting either passive attachment of Ig through Fc receptors or the existence of autoantibodies aganst determinants on the lymphocyte membrane.

Table 1—PERCENTAGES OF NORMAL B LYMPHOCYTES LABELED BY ANTI IG-LIGHT CHAIN ANTIBODY-COATED *E. COLI* IN BLOOD SMEARS

Bacteria	Mean value[a]	Range[b]
Anti κ-Ab-Ec[c]	9.3	8-11
Anti λ-Ab-Ec	6.7	5-11
Anti κ+anti λ-Ab-Ec	16.3	14-19
Expected exclusion	≥16 (9.3+6.7)	—
Expected inclusion	<16	—

[a]The values in the controls/cells labeled with *E. Coli* coated with natural IgG were subtracted (0%-3%).
[b]Range of values from seven individual tests.
[c]Anti κ (λ) Ab-Ec=*E. Coli* coated with anti κ (or anti λ) purified antibody prepared in rabbits.

Table 2—PERCENTAGES OF LYMPHOCYTES BINDING BACTERIA IN BLOOD SMEARS

Bacteria	Average normal donors (9 donors)	Range normal donors	Average in cord blood	Range in cord blood (5 samples)
Ab-E. coli 0	16	13-20	17	10-23
B. melitensis	16	14-18	24	17-32
A. hinshawii	54	49-62	54	42-59
E. coli 2	51	42-61	63	57-69
E. coli 3	51	45-55	ND	ND
B. globigii	25	18-32	40	33-48
S. lutea	15	11-20	ND	ND
S. aureus 1	16	12-20	18	11-31
S. aureus 2	18	10-23	17	10-31

2. *Percentages of Normal Lymphocytes Naturally Binding in Blood Smears.*
In a previous study, we demonstrated that several bacteria bound naturally
to various percentages of purified lymphocytes in suspensions examined by
phase contrast microscopy. Here we determined the percentage of lymphocyte labeled by eight different strains in blood smears. This study was
done to establish the individual variability of bacterial binding. On the
average, 16% of the lymphocytes bound Ab-*E. coli* or *B. melitensis*. This
result was expected, based on our previous study which showed that *B.
melitensis* binds to B cells (8,9). To determine whether the percentage of
lymphocytes which bind bacteria in blood smears is a biological constant,
the binding of the eight strains of bacteria and of Ab-*E. coli* to the
lymphocytes from nine normal donors was studied. Since the percentage of
Ig-bearing cells may be expected to be a biological constant, the individual
variation in the percentage of lymphocytes which bound various bacteria
was compared with the individual variations in the percentage of Ig-bearing
cells. Based on this criterion, the bacteria were subdivided into three groups:
a) those in which the individual variation was equal to or less than that of
Ig-bearing cells; i.e., *B. melitensis, A. hinshawii, E. coli* 2 and 3 and *S. aureus*
1 (Table 2); b) those in which the individual variation was slightly higher
than that of Ig-bearing cells; i.e., *S. lutea, S. aureus*-2 and *B. globigii;* and c)
those which showed too large a variability to be of any use as constant
markers (data not shown). Thus, only those in the first two groups were
used in the "mapping" of lymphocyte subpopulations.

Although the percentages of lymphocytes binding bacteria was too high to be due to immune receptors, we performed the same assay on five samples of cord blood (Table 2). We found that the number of lymphocytes binding *B. melitensis* was slightly higher than that binding Ab-*E. coli* 0. In general, the other percentages were similar or slightly higher than in adult blood smears. Thus, taken together these data indicate that the percentages of lymphocytes binding bacteria are biological constants and that the binding does not involve any "immune" mechanism.

3. *"Mapping" Lymphocyte Subpopulations in Blood Smears.* The "mapping" was carried out to determine whether the percentages of lymphocytes binding various bacteria in blood smears relfect the existence of cell subpopulations as they did in cell suspensions (8). The percentages of lymphocytes which bound one bacterial strain (single labeling) or various combinations of two bacterial strains (double labeling) were determined. The results obtained from three normal donors were arranged in "chessboard" tables and maps were constructed: one example is presented here (Table 3, Figure 2). When the two strains were morphologically different (Figure 1) the percentages of lymphocytes which bound each strain of bacteria, or both strains, were determined.

(a) *Identification of Ig$^+$ Cells (B Cells) and Ig$^-$ Cells (T Cells).* The percentages of lymphocytes which bound *B. melitensis* alone was 18%, and Ab-*E. coli* alone 18%. When both bacteria were used simultaneously, 19% of the lymphocytes had bacteria attached. This suggested that these two bacteria bound to the same cells. Of these, 19% obtained in double labeling tests, 14 had both bacteria attached to the same cell, 2 had only Ab-*E. coli* and 3 had only *B. melitensis.* The few lymphocytes (2% and 3%) which bound only one bacterial strain in the double labeling test could have been due to competition for space on the lymphocyte membrane and, for all practical purposes, were disregarded. We concluded that *B. melitensis* and Ab-*E. coli* identified the same lymphocyte subpopulation, namely B cells, a fact in agreement with our previous studies (8,9). Thus, in Figure 2, we considered both Ig-bearing cells and *B. melitensis* binding cells as the same population, namely B cells, and the Ig$^-$ cells and Bm$^-$ cells as T cells.

(b) *Identification of T cell Subpopulations.* The next bacteria considered was *A. hinshawii* which, when used alone, identified 50% of the lymphocytes. When used together with *B. melitensis,* 16% of the cells had both bacteria attached, a percentage close to that obtained when *B. melitensis* was used alone. Thus, we considered that practically all B cells and a large part of the T cell populations were identified by *A. hinshawii.* For the reasons given above, the relatively small percentage of cells which bound only *B. melitensis* was disregarded. Also, the fact that the total percentage of labeled cells when the two bacteria were used together was greater than the percentage of labeled cells when *A. hinshawii* was used alone could have been due to counting variation.

Figure 2—THE MAP OF THE LYMPHOCYTE SUBPOPULATIONS IDENTIFIED IN BLOOD SMEARS BY NATURAL BINDING OF BACTERIA.

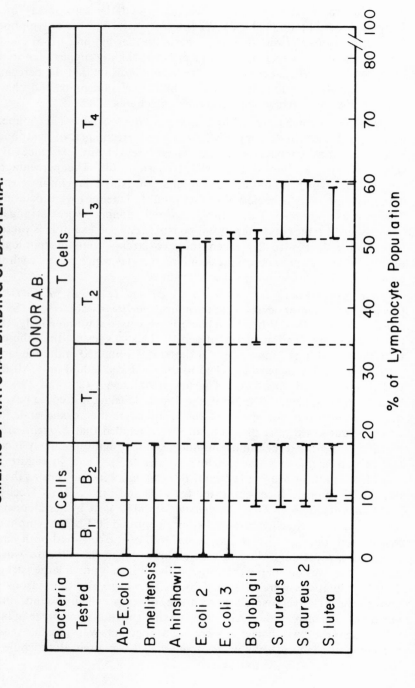

DONOR A.B.

Table 3—PERCENTAGES OF LYMPHOCYTES LABELED WITH ONE OR COMBINATIONS OF TWO BACTERIA

Bacteria used for Labeling (x)	None	Ab-E. coli 0	simultaneous labeling with (y): B. melitensis	A. hinshawii	B. globigii	S. aureus 1
Ab-E. coli	18		2^x 3^x 14^y	4 34 16	12 29 3	—
B. melitensis	18	19		7 31 6	6 17 11	9 11 9
A. hinshawii	50	54	54		23 0 25	35 15 10
B. globigii	29	44	34	49		24 12 1
S. aureus 1	20	—	30	60	33	

The upper right of the table: First value (x) = % cells labeled by bacteria on the left side of the table.
Second value (y) = % cells labeled by the bacteria shown at the top of the table.
Third value (xy) = % cells with bacteria on the same lymphocyte.

The lower left = the total % of cells labeled by bacteria (x+y).

433

B. globigii alone bound to 29% of the lymphocytes, *A. hinshawii* to 50%, and when used together, to 49%. Out of these 49%, 25 were labeled by both bacteria, 23 by *A. hinshawii* alone, and none by *B. globigii* alone (Table 3). Thus, it appears that only part of *A. hinshawii* positive cells (Ah$^+$) cells were also *B. globigii* positive (Bg$^+$), suggesting that *B. globigii* bound to a subpopulation of lymphocytes identified by *A. hinshawii*. Thus, the Bg marker divided the Ah$^+$ cells into two subsets: Ah$^+$Bg$^-$ (T$_1$ cells) and Ah $^+$Bg$^+$ (T$_2$ cells) (Figure 2). The placement of a Bg marker on T$_2$ instead of T$_1$ cells was rather arbitrary since we did not find any bacteria which could identify only Ah$^+$Bg$^-$ cells in blood smears. However, we found such a marker in an individual map for cell suspensions in a previous study (8) and the mapping here was done for consistency. *A. hinshawii* alone bound to 50% of the lymphocytes, *S. aureus*-1 to 20% and when used together to 60%. Thus, 10% (60-50) of the lymphocytes were identified by *S. aureus*-1 but not by *A. hinshawii* so another subset of T cells that was Ah$^-$Sal$^+$ was identified (T$_3$ cells). The remaining lymphocytes which did not bind any of these bacteria were called T$_4$ cells. Thus, by bacteria adherence, we identified B cells and four T cell subpopulations.

(c) *Subpopulations of B Lymphocytes.* The relatively small percentage of B cells of the total lymphocyte population makes the task of identifying B cell subpopulations difficult. However, based on the labeling performed with the four bacteria (*B. melitensis, A. hinshawii, B. globigii,* and *S. aureus* -1), we subdivided the B cell into B$_1$ and B$_2$ using the same rationale.

(d) *The Use of Other Bacteria for Mapping.* In a previous study, we mapped the lymphocyte subpopulations by using 13 different strains of bacteria. Here, as shown above, only four were sufficient to identify four T and two B cell subpopulations. We also used the other bacterial strains (see Materials and Methods) to map the lymphocyte subpopulations and the same results were obtained (Figure 2).

Table 4—THE RESPONSE OF T$_1$T$_2$ and T$_3$T$_4$ LYMPHOCYTES TO MITOGENS AND ALLOGENEIC CELLS MEASURED BY ^{3}H-TdR INCORPORATION AND EXPRESSED AS PERCENTAGE OF THE RESPONSE OF PBL[a]

| Cells | PHA | Mitogens | | | Allogeneic Cells |
		PWM	Con A	SLo	Cells
T$_1$T$_2$	NA	ND	133	—	106
T$_3$T$_4$	22	33	10	17	105

[a]The response of PBL was considered 100%.

434

4. *The Response to Mitogens and Allogeneic Cells of PBL Separated by Bacterial Adherence.* The response to mitogens of the following three cell populations was compared: 1) cells purified only by Ficoll-Hypaque (PBL); 2) cells that did not bind to *E. coli*-2 monolayers (T_3T_4); 3) cells that bound to *E. coli*-2 and were removed by vigorous shaking; and 4) cells "sham-depleted" using *E. coli*-0 monolayers.

The T_3T_4 cells gave greatly reduced responses to the four mitogens tested as compared to the unseparated cell populations (Table 4). At the same time, cells recovered from monolayers of *E. coli*-0 gave, on the average, almost the same response as the original PBL; i.e., only a slight reduction was observed (data not shown).

In order to determine whether the blast transformation was also affected, a morphological examination of Con-A-stimulated lymphocytes was performed. We found that about 50% of the stimulated PBL were in blast form after 3 days of cultivation (compared to λ% in the unstimulated control), but only about 10% blast cells appeared in stimulated cultures of T_3T_4 cells (4% in the unstimulated control). The viability of the depleted cell populations was not affected since, after three days in culture, both the original cell population and the cells submitted to the depletion procedure with either *E. coli*-0 or *E. coli*-2 had approximately the same viability, as determined by trypan blue exclusion (over 90%).

The removal of monocytes and/or B cells did not change the pattern of the results obtained. For example, the T_3T_4 lymphocytes responded much less than purified T cells at any concentration of Con A.

Although the viability, determined by trypan blue exclusion, of cells depleted by either *E. coli*-2 (T_3T_4 cells) or *E. coli*-0 monolayers (PBL) was similar to the viability of the unseparated cell populations (PBL), further proof was needed that the unattached cells recovered from *E. coli*-2 monolayers were not functionally impaired.

For this, we compared the response in one-way mixed lymphocyte cultures of PBL with the response of T_1T_2 and T_3T_4 cells. We found that the T_3T_4 cells gave a response similar to that of PBL or T_1T_2 cells (Table 4).

5. *Induction of Specifically Cytotoxic Lymphocytes in MLC.* Since both T_1T_2 and T_3T_4 lymphocytes responded to MLC, we proceeded to determine whether both these cell populations became cytotoxic for allogeneic lymphocytes. We compared the cytotoxic activity of PBL with that of T_1T_2 and T_3T_4 cells (Table 5). The PBL and T_1T_2 cells, which were not cultured with allogeneic cells, did not become cytotoxic. However, the T_3T_4 cells were cytotoxic, i.e., manifested a "spontaneous" killing activity. All three cell populations (PBL, T_1T_2 and T_3T_4) were cytotoxic when activated by allogeneic cells; but when the spontaneous cytotoxic effects were subtracted, it appeared that only PBL and T_1T_2 cells had this property. Thus, although

both T_1T_2 and T_3T_4 cells responded in MLC only T_1T_2 became specifically cytotoxic.

Table 5—SPECIFIC CYTOTOXIC ACTIVITY GENERATED IN ONE WAY MLC BY PBL, T_1T_2 and T_3T_4 cells against allogeneic cells (^{51}Cr release)

Effector[a] Cells	Per Cent specific ^{51}Cr release		
	Unstimulated (A)	Stimulated by Allogeneic PBL (B)	Specific cyto-toxic effect (A-B)
PBL	0.7 (-4-7)[b]	37.2 (18-50)[b]	36.5
T_1T_2	1.0 (0-2)[c]	39.0 (33-45)[c]	38.0
T_3T_4	19.2 (4-29)[b]	31.7 (13-51)[b]	12.5

[a]The effector cells were incubated with mitomycin C treated allogeneic PBL for 6 days. The allogeneic target cells were prepared by PHA stimulation and labeled with ^{51}Cr.
[b]Range of results from four experiments.
[c]Range from two experiments.

6. *Natural Killer Activity of Lymphocyte Subpopulations.* The above-mentioned observation that T_3T_4 lymphocytes killed allogeneic target cells without being stimulated by them led to the hypothesis that these cells might have natural or spontaneous killer function, a function considered particularly important in tumor immunology. To assess this hypothesis, we used a procedure commonly applied for the study of natural cytotoxicity; namely, the induction of ^{51}Cr release from established malignant lymphoblastoid cells lines (13).

The PBL showed low spontaneous killing (SK) activity against the B cell lines and relatively high SK activity against the T cell lines, confirming earlier reports of others (13). When the PBL was separated into T_1T_2 cells and T_3T_4 cells, differences in the SK activity were observed. Compared with PBL, the T_3T_4 cells had a significantly higher SK activity against the T cell lines and also a 2- to 3-fold higher SK activity against the B cell lines (Table 6). The T_1T_2 cells had an SK activity which was similar to that of the unseparated PBL. By further separating the T_3T_4 cells into two subpopulations (T_3 and T_4 cells) by using monolayers of *S. aureus*-1, the SK activity of the T_4 subpopulation was significantly higher than that of the T_1T_2, T_3 or PBL populations. The relatively low SK activity in the T_1T_2 or T_3 cell populations might have been due to their own SK activity or to contamination with T_4 cells.

The possible role played by monocytes and/or B cells in the SK activity of T_3T_4 cells was also considered. Purified T cells were prepared by

436

Table 6—SPONTANEOUS CYTOTOXICITY OF LYMPHOCYTE SUBPOPULATIONS AGAINST LYMPHOBLASTOID CELL LINES DETERMINED BY ^{51}Cr RELEASE IN A 4 h ASSAY

Target Cells[a]		Effector Cells			
	PBL	T_1T_2	T_3T_4	T_3	T_4
B cell lines	7[b](22)[c]	8 (12)	16 (13)	4 (3)	29 (3)
T cell lines	27 (25)	30 (12)	46 (15)	20 (3)	44 (3)
Mean values[d]	17	19	31	12	36

[a]B cell lines: RPMI-7666; Raji, SB; T cell lines: HSB2, CEM, Jurkat, Molt 3.
[b]Mean value calculated from percentages of specific ^{51}Cr release.
[c]The number of assays on different lines.
[d]*Statistical analysis*. The differences between the mean values for all lines were analyzed using the *t* test. Significant differences in SK activity were found between PBL and T_3T_4 cells (p=0.004), between T_1T_2 and T_3T_4 cells (p=0.0096), and between T_3 and T_4 cells (p=0.002). No significant differences were found between PBL and T_1T_2 cells (p =0.380) or between T_3T_4 and T_4 cells (p=0.355).

removing the monocytes and the B cells from PBL; the T_1T_2 cells were separated from T_3T_4 cells and their SK activity was tested against both T and B lymphoblastoid cell lines. Under these conditions, the SK activity of T_3T_4 cells was significantly higher than that of T_1T_2 cells (p=0.0002) or that of T cells (p=0.0002). Thus, the T_4 lymphocytes appear to be primarily responsible for the SK phenomenon.

DISCUSSION

We showed here the Ig-bearing cells can be enumerated in blood smears by using antibody-coated bacteria and that normal B cells do not appear to have passively adsorbed surface Ig. Several strains of bacteria were shown to bind the lymphocytes in human blood smears in a reproducible manner. By labeling the lymphocytes with a single strain of bacteria or with two strains simultaneously, four T cell subpopulations and at least two B cell sub-populations could be identified. The functions of these subpopulations appeared to be different with respect to mitogen responsiveness and to specific and natural killing activity for allogeneic cells or malignant lymphoblastoid cell lines.

In this study, we considered B cells as those cells which had surface Ig, identified here by anti-light chain antibody-coated *E. coli*-0. Based on this criterion, *B. melitensis* appeared to identify only B cells, for the following reasons: First, when suspensions of lymphocytes were treated with either Ab-*E. coli*, *B. melitensis*, or both, essentially the same percentage of lymphocytes were labeled. Second, when the blood smears were treated simultaneously with Ab-*E. coli* and *B. melitensis*, practically all lymphocytes were double labeled, as previously described (10). Third, when Ig-bearing cells were removed, the remaining cells (Ig⁻ cells) did not bind either *B. melitensis* or Ab-*E. coli* (unpublished observations). Fourth, the binding of *B. melitensis* to lymphocytes did not reduce the percent of E-rosette forming cells, but the binding of *E. coli*-2 did (unpublished observations). Fifth, when B cells were enriched by E-rosette formation and Ficoll-Hypaque centrifugation to about 60% Ig-bearing cells, the same enrichment occurred in Bm^+ cells. Finally, in chronic lymphocytic leukemia, about 90% of the lymphocytes bind *B. melitensis* (14). Thus, in this study we considered as B cells those lymphocytes that bound *B. melitensis* (Bm^+), and/or Ab-*E. coli* -0 (Ig^+), and those which did not bind (Ig^-Bm^-) as T cells. Our assumption that the Ig⁻ cells in normal peripheral blood were essentially all T cells was supported by our data which showed that thymus cell antigen and surface Ig were mutually exclusive (7). This assumption was also supported by recent reports which showed that, in normal human peripheral blood, about 20% of the lymphocytes were Ig^+ (15), a figure similar to our data, and about 80% were E-rosette-forming (T cells), thereby accounting for essentially all the lymphocytes. Thus, for all practical purposes, the so-called "null" cells were ignored.

The B cells have been subdivided by others into two subpopulations, one of which was claimed to have passively attached surface Ig (16). Our results here clearly show that B cells have only one kind of light chain, κ or λ, strongly suggesting that it is not absorbed from the serum. However, in five patients with colagen diseases having circulating immune complexes, we found, by using the same test, that both κ and λ chains were in the same lymphocytes. This suggests that our test may have valuable application in clinical laboratory. It appears that the methods used by Lobo, et al., (16) to remove the passively adsorbed surface Ig, in fact, makes some of the B cells to lose their own surface Ig in the absence of mitogen stimulation, as we have previously demonstrated (17).

The subpopulations of lymphocytes identified by bacterial adherence appeared to be biological constants. Moreover, even the cord blood lymphocytes were similar with the adult subpopulations. Therefore, it may be expected that changes under physiologic or pathologic conditions occur. For example, in an on-going study on cancer patients (Teodorescu and Das Gupta), we found both decreases and increases in the binding of bacteria by lymphocytes. Particularly noticeable was a reduction in the proportion of T_1T_2 cells.

It is difficult at this moment to make good correlations between the lymphocyte subpopulations identified here by bacterial adherence and those identified by other investigators using different procedures (18). This is especially true for blood smears since there is practically no other comparable method to identify subpopulations of B and T cell subpopulations. The methods based on immunofluorescence are limited only to B and T cells even when applied to blood smears (19). So far, all the evidence for B and/or T cell subpopulations has been obtained by using purified lymphocyte suspensions and either rosette formation with erythrocytes or staining with fluorescent antibody. These procedures are tedious, highly variable and difficult to reproduce. Since the same subpopulation of approximately similar size can be identified in suspensions and in blood smears, we are currently attempting to correlate the subpopulations identified by bacterial adherence with those identified by various rosette techniques by using cell suspensions. The high strength of binding of bacteria to lymphocytes makes the results obtained much more reliable and reproducible and less dependent on handling than other procedures (e.g., E rosettes). Moreover, by labeling the cells in blood smears, the variability which results from purification may also be eliminated and a permanent record is obtained.

The fact that the same reagents may be used to identify and enumerate the lymphocyte subpopulations and to separate them offers another advantage. Correlations may be established between numbers and particular functions by using this methodology. For example, the response to mitogens of T_1T_2 cells was different from that of T_3T_4 cells. The T_4 lymphocytes appeared to be particularly involved in natural cytotoxicity; the T_3T_4 cells responded to allogeneic cells without becoming specifically cytotoxic. Therefore, the T_3T_4 cells may be the T helper cells for the allogeneic reactions, cells which respond to LD antigens while the T_1T_2 cells, or only one of these subpopulations, may be specifically cytotoxic or cells responded to SD antigens. The T_1T_2 cells also appear to have suppressor functions since the T_3T_4 cells become naturally cytotoxic for allogeneic cells, or for lymphoblastoid cell lines, in the absence of T_1T_2 cells (Table 5). Studies underway are focused on this topic. The simple and rapid separation procedure will allow a good functional characterization of lymphocyte subpopulations.

The mechanism of natural binding of bacteria to lymphocytes is not yet known. However, we know that *B. melitensis* binds to a determinant on the B cells which is not an immunoglobulin g. Preliminary evidence based on the study of mutants of *E. coli* which bind to lymphocytes suggest that the interaction between bacteria and lymphocytes involves a "lectin" on the lymphocyte membrane and a carbohydrate on the bacterial cell wall (20). The role of lectins on cell membranes in the recognition process has been recently pointed out in a comprehensive review (21).

We may conclude that by identifying functionally different lymphocyte subpopulations in a reproducible manner bacteria will become useful reagents for clinical laboratories. The monitoring of chemo and radio-therapy of cancer patients will probably benefit from the development of this new methodology.

REFERENCES

1. Huber, B., Devinsky, O., Gershon, R. K. and Cantor, G., "Cell-mediated Immunity: Delayed-type Hypersensitivity and Cytotoxic Responses are Mediated by Different T-Cell Subclasses." *J. Exp. Med.* 143:1534, 1976.
2. Boyse, E.A. and Cantor, H., "Surface Characteristics of T-Lymphocyte Subpopulations." *Hospital Practice* 12:81, 1975.
3. Pellegrino, M.A., Ferrone, S. and Theofilopoulos, N.J., "Rosette Formation of Human Lymphoid Cells with Monkey Red Blood Cells." *J. Immunol.* 115:1065, 1977.
4. Forbes, I.J., and Zalewski, P.D., "A Subpopulation of Human B Lymphocytes that Rosette with Mouse Erythrocytes." *Clin. Exp. Immunol.* 26:99, 1976.
5. Sandilands, G.P., Gray, K., Coonery, A., et al., "Formation of Auto-rosettes by Peripheral Blood Lymphocytes." *Clin Exp. Immunol.* 22:493, 1975.
6. Wybran, J., Chantler, S., and Fundenberg, H.H., "Human Blood T Cells: Response to Phytohemagglutinin." *J. Immunol.* 110:1157, 1973.
7. Teodorescu, M., Mayer, E.P. and Dray, S., "Simultaneous Identification of T and B Cells in Blood Smears Using Antibody-coated Bacteria." *Cell Immunol.* 24:90, 1976.
8. Teodorescu, M., Mayer, E.P. and Dray, S., "Identification of Five Human Lymphocyte Subpopulations by Their Differential Binding of Various Strains of Bacteria." *Cell Immunol.* 29:353, 1977.
9. Mayer, E.P., Bratescu, A., Dray, S. and Teodorescu, M., "Enumeration of Human B Lymphocytes in Stained Blood Smears by Their Binding of Bacteria." *Clin. Immunol. Immunopathol.* G:37, 1978.
10. Kleinman, R. and Teodorescu, M., "The Response to Mitogens and Allogeneic Cells of Human Lyphocyte Subpopulations Separated by Their Differential Binding to Monolayers of Bacteria." *J. Immunol.* 120:2020, 1978.
11. O'Leary, J., Reinsmoen, N. and Yunis, E.J., "Mixed Lymphocyte Reaction." In: *Manual of Clinical Immunology,* Ed. by N.R. Rose and H. Friedman, American Society for Microbiology, 820, 1976.
12. Lightbody, J., "Use of Cell-mediated Lympholysis Test in Transplantation Immunity." In: *Manual of Clinical Immunology,* Ed. by N.R. Rose and H. Friedman, American Society for Microbiology, 851, 1976.
13. Callawaert, D.M., Kaplan, J., Peterson, W.D. (jr.) and Lightbody, J.J., "Spontaneous Cytotoxicity of Human Lymphoblast Cell Lines Mediated by Normal Peripheral Blood Lymphocytes." *Cell. Immunol.* 33:11, 1976.
14. Teodorescu, M., Mayer, E.P. and Dray, S., "Enumeration and Identification of Human Leukemic Lymphocytes by Their Natural Binding of Bacteria." *Cancer Res.* 37, 175, 1977.
15. Haegert, D.G., Hurd, C. and Coombs, R.R.A., "Comparison of the Direct Antiglobulin Rosetting Reaction With Direct Immunofluorescence in the Detection of Surface Membrane Immunoglobulin on Human Peripheral Blood Lymphocytes." *Immunology,* 34:533, 1978.
16. Lobo, P.I., Westerwelt, F.B. and Horwitz, D.A., "Identification of Two Populations of Immunoglobulin-bearing Lymphocytes in Man." *J. Immunol.* 114:116, 1975.
17. Teodorescu, M., Buchholz, D.M. and Dray, S., "Maintenance of Lymphocyte Surface Ig by Mitrogen Stimulation *in vitro.*" *J. Immunol.* 115, 1584, 1975.
18. Dwayer, J.M., "Identifying and Enumerating T and B Lymphocytes." *Progr. Allergy.* 21:178, 1976.
19. Pepys, M.B., Stegna-Guidetti, C., Mirjah, D.D., et al., "Enumeration of Immunoglobulin-bearing Lymphocytes in Whole Peripheral Blood." *Clin. Exp. Immunol.* 26:91, 1976.
20. Mayer, E.P. and Teodorescu, M., "Selection of Lymphocyte Binding Mutants of *Escherichia coli* for the Identification of Lymphocyte Subpopulations." *Fed. Proc.* 37:1654, 1978.

21. Simpson, D.L., Tharne, D.R., Lah, M.M., "Lectins: Endogenous Carbohydrate Binding Proteins from Vertebrate Tissues: Functional Role in Recognition Process." *Life Sciences* 22:727, 1978.

Human Spontaneous Cell-Mediated Cytotoxicity

Bonita Bundy[1]
D. Nelson[1]

SUMMARY—Destruction of target cells *in vitro* by lymphocytes from non-immunized donors is termed spontaneous cell-mediated cytotoxicty (SCMC) or natural cytotoxicity (NC). We have compared SCMC with two other *in vitro* cytotoxicity reactions using Chang liver cell targets: mitogen-induced cellular cytotoxicity (MICC) and antibody-dependent cellular cytotoxicity (ADCC). When peripheral blood mononuclear cells (PBM) were employed as effectors, the rate of target cell damage due to SCMC was significantly less than that due to MICC and ADCC; and tenfold greater effector to target cell ratios were required to produce equivalent target cell damage in SCMC as in MICC or ADCC. In order to define the surface characteristics of the SCMC effector cell, we have used a variety of cell separation techniques and have found the SCMC effector cell in human peripheral blood to be a non-phagocytic, surface-immunoglobulin (sIg) negative, Fc receptor positive lymphocyte. Organ distribution studies revealed comparable SCMC, MICC and ADCC effector activity in PBM and spleen cells, tonsillar cells mediated only MICC, and thymocytes did not mediate cytotoxicity. Pretreatment of effector cells with trypsin significantly inhibited SCMC but not ADCC and this inhibition was not reversible by short-term incubation in autologous plasma. Thus, although SCMC and ADCC are both functions of sIg negative, Fc receptor positive lymphocyte(s) which possess indentical organ distribution, separate mechanisms are involved in SCMC and ADCC. Studies undertaken to measure the SCMC effector cell potential of PBM from a variety of patients with immunodeficiency diseases showed SCMC activity to be normal in the majority of these patients. These results suggest that SCMC activity may be a very primitive effector function which is maintained in immunodeficiency diseases and also that the increased incidence of neoplasia in these patients may not be due to defective SCMC-mediated immunological surveillance.

INTRODUCTION

The phenomenon of spontaneous cell-mediated cytotoxicity (SCMC) or natural cytotoxicity (NC) has recently been described in a variety of experimental animals (1-5) and in humans (6-12). This form of cytotoxicity

---

[1]Metabolism Branch, National Cancer Institute, National Institutes of Health, Bethesda, Maryland.

443

involves the lysis of cell line targets by lymphoid cells from non-immunized donors. We have investigated SCMC in humans and the nature of the human SCMC effector cell. SCMC was compared with two other cytotoxicity reactions mediated by lymphoid cells from donors which have not been intentionally sensitized: mitogen-induced cellular cytotoxicity (MICC) and antibody-dependent cellular cytotoxicity (ADCC). In all three assays, human effector cells were reacted with the same ^{51}Cr labeled human Chang liver cell targets. For comparative purposes, MICC was employed as a model of T-cell mediated cytotoxicity, while ADCC was utilized as a model for the type of cellular cytotoxicity mediated by K cells (13).

In the present studies, the kinetics, mechanisms, organ distribution and the identity of the effector cell for SCMC will be compared with these same parameters for MICC and ADCC. In addition, the results of clinical studies on SCMC in immune deficient patients will be present and speculations will be made about the implications of the finding for the role of SCMC in immune surveillance.

MATERIALS AND METHODS

Media and Reagents

RPMI medium 1640 (1640), balanced salt solution (BSS) and 2.5% trypsin in normal saline were obtained from the Media Section, National Institutes of Health. RPMI medium 1640 containing 25mM Hepes buffer (1640 Hepes), heat-inactivated fetal calf serum (FCS), penicillin-streptomycin and L-glutamine were obtained from Grand Island Biological Company, Grand Island, New York. Supplements to 1640 were: 4mM glutamine, 100 units/ml penicillin and 100 μg/ml streptomycin. Phytohemagglutinin-W (PHA), obtained from Burroughs and Wellcome, Beckenham, England, was diluted in 1640 and stored frozen at $-20°C$ until used.

Isolation of Effector Cell Populations

Peripheral blood mononuclear cells from normal individuals and immunodeficiency patients were isolated from heparinized venous blood by Ficoll-Hypaque density centrifugation at 2250 x G for 5 minutes. Interface PBM were washed three times with 1640 5% FCS before cytotoxicity testing.

The methods of obtaining macrophage-depleted lymphocytes, the separation of lymphocytes on Sephadex anti-Fab immunoabsorbent columns, and depletion of Fc receptor positive lymphocytes on antigen-antibody coated flasks, have been previously described in detail (10, 13, 14). Briefly, PBM were depleted of macrophages by incubation with iron-carbonyl for 45 minutes at 37°C, treatment with a magnet, and recentrifugation over Ficoll-Hypaque. These macrophage-depleted lymphocytes were washed and suspended in RPMI 1640 containing 25mM Hepes, buffer, 2.5mMEDTA, 0.3% NaHCO$_3$ and 5% FCS for filtration thru a Sephadex anti-Fab column (purified rabbit anti-human (Fab')$_2$ covalently linked to Sephadex G-200).

After collection of sIg negative lymphocytes, sIg positive lymphocytes were competitively eluted from the column with human gamma globulin (Cohn Fr II, Miles-Pentex Labs, Elkhart, Indiana). A portion of the sIg negative lymphocyte fraction was depleted of Fc receptor bearing cells on insolubilized antigen-antibody coated (TNP-FCS, rabbit anti-TNP) plastic flasks. All subpopulations were washed three times with 1640 5% FCS before cytotoxicity testing.

Spleen cells from a patient undergoing splenectomy for trauma, tonsils from patients undergoing elective tonsillectomy and thymuses from patients with non-malignant thymic enlargements were teased in BSS 10% FCS, centrifuged over Ficoll-Hypaque to obtain mononuclear cells and were washed three times in the same manner used for all other effector cells.

Cytotoxicity Assay

A microcytotoxicity assay utilizing ^{51}Cr labeled Chang cells was performed as previously described (10, 13). In brief, Chang liver cells adapted to spinner culture (Microbiological Associates, Bethesda, Maryland) were labeled with ^{51}Cr (5 x 10^6 viable cells with 100 μCi ^{51}Cr) at 37°C for 30 minutes and washed 3 times with 1640 5% FCS. Effector cells (at various concentrations) and Chang targets (at 1 x 10^5/ml) were all suspended in 1640 supplemented with penicillin-streptomycin, glutamine and 5% FCS for the cytotoxicity assay. Cultures were established in triplicate in U or V bottomed microplates containing 100 μl of effector cells, 100 μl of target cells and 20 μl of one of the following: 1) 1640 alone for SCMC; 2) PHA at a final concentration of 1 μg/ml for MICC; or 3) 10^{-3} final concentration of rabbit anti-Chang serum for ADCC. Values for SCMC, MICC and ADCC represent the mean ± 1 S.E. of the % lysis, calculated as:

$$\frac{\text{Experimental Release—Background Release}}{\text{Maximum Release—Background Release}} \times 100$$

where the background release represents target cells incubated with medium alone and maximum release is determined by freezing and thawing target cells three times.

Trypsin Treatment and Plasma Incubation

To remove trypsin-sensitive cell surface structures, macrophage-depleted lymphocytes were incubated at concentration of 10^7 cells/ml in BSS alone or 1.0% trypsin in BSS for 45 minutes at 37°C. An aliquot of each cell population was subsequently incubated for one hour at 4°C with heat-inactivated autologous plasma to allow possible re-arming of effectors to take place. All fractions were then washed before cytotoxicity testing.

445

RESULTS

Kinetics of Cytotoxicity Reactions

Experiments were undertaken to compare the rates of target cell damage due to SCMC, MICC and ADCC. With Ficoll-Hypaque separated normal human peripheral blood mononuclear effectors and different intervals of incubation ranging from 5 minutes to 24 hours, target cell damage due to SCMC, MICC and ADCC was evident even at 5 minutes (Figure 1). Target cell damage due to MICC and ADCC, however, proceeded at a more rapid rate than that due to SCMC over the entire time course. Thus, of the three cytotoxicity assays, target cell damage due to SCMC proceeds at a slower

Figure 1

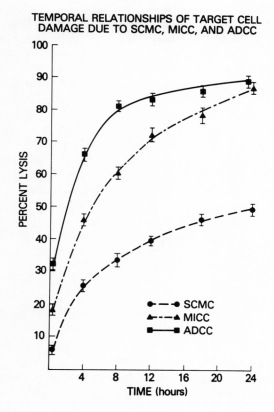

TEMPORAL RELATIONSHIPS OF TARGET CELL DAMAGE DUE TO SCMC, MICC, AND ADCC

Time course of SCMC, MICC and ADCC. Cytotoxicity cultures were established and incubated at 37°C for various time periods ranging from 5 minutes to 24 hours. Effector to target cell ratio in all cases was 100:1. PHA concentration for MICC was 1μg/ml final in cultures. Antibody for ADCC was 1:1000 final of rabbit anti-Chang serum.

446

Figure 2

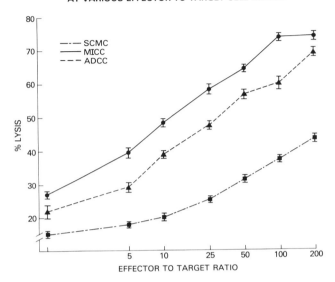

SCMC, MICC, AND ADCC
AT VARIOUS EFFECTOR TO TARGET CELL RATIOS

SCMC, MICC and ADCC at varying effector to target cell ratios. A constant number of Chang target cell (10^4 per culture) was incubated with varying numbers of normal peripheral blood mononuclear cells for 18 hours at 37°C. Values represent mean % lysis ± 1 S.E. of triplicate cultures.

rate than that due to MICC or ADCC (10). All subsequent experiments were done with an optimum 18 hour incubation period.

Studies were next undertaken to assess SCMC, MICC and ADCC at varying effector to target ratios. Figure 2 shows the result of a dose-response experiment in which a constant number of target cells was incubated with increasing numbers of human peripheral blood mononuclear effector cells. As can be seen, target cell damage due to SCMC only becomes significant at an effector to target ratio (E/T) of 10:1 or greater, while significant cytotoxicity due to MICC and ADCC is apparent at an E/T of 1:1. Moreover, effectors are less efficient at target cytolysis in SCMC in that 10 to 30 times more effectors are required to produce the same % lysis in SCMC as in ADCC or MICC. Thus SCMC requires greater numbers of effector cells than does MICC or ADCC to produce an equivalent amount of cytotoxicity.

447

Effector Cell Identities

Studies were next undertaken to identify the effector cells mediating these forms of cytotoxicity, as shown in Figure 3. Normal peripheral blood mononuclear cells were depleted of macrophages by iron-carbonyl and then separated into surface immunoglobulin (sIg) positive and sIg negative fractions using Sephadex anti-Fab immunoabsorbent columns. The sIg negative fraction was further depleted of Fc receptor bearing cells by repeated adherence to antigen-antibody complex plates. SCMC and ADCC were shown to be mediated solely by sIg negative, Fc receptor positive lymphocytes, MICC could be mediated by sIg negative Fc receptor negative cells (10, 11).

Figure 3—SCMC, MICC AND ADCC EFFECTOR CELL CHARACTERIZATION

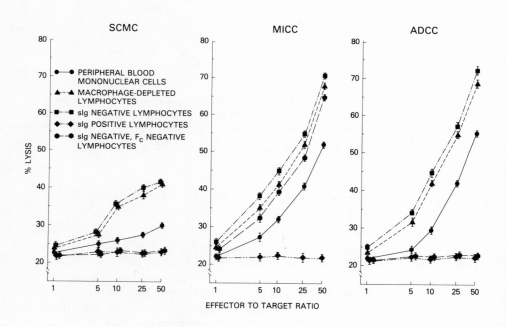

Subpopulations of normal peripheral blood were isolated and incubated at various E/T ratios with a constant number of Chang cell targets (10^4 per culture). Determinations of SCMC, MICC and ADCC were made simultaneously. Values represent mean % lysis ± 1 S.E. of triplicate cultures.

448

Figure 4

ORGAN DISTRIBUTION OF EFFECTOR CELLS
MEDIATING SCMC, ADCC AND MICC

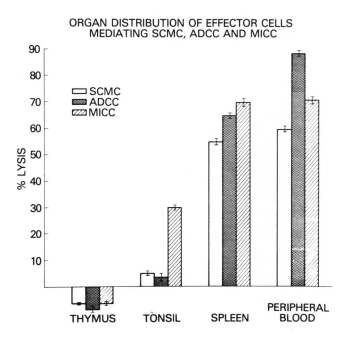

Organ distribution of effector cells mediating SCMC, ADCC and MICC. Spleen and peripheral blood mononuclear cells were from the same individual. Thymus and tonsillar cells were from two other individuals. Values represent mean % lysis ± 1 S.E.

Organ Distribution of Cytotoxic Effectors

Since both SCMC and ADCC were functions of sIg negative, Fc receptor positive cells (K-cells) while MICC was mediated by sIg negative, Fc receptor negative cells (T-cells), further studies were undertaken to ascertain whether the organ distribution of SCMC, ADCC and MICC effector cell activities would be the same or different. In a comparison of the effector cell activity in human lymphoid organs, Ficoll-Hypaque separated mononuclear cells from peripheral blood, tonsil, thymus and spleen were studied at varying effector to target ratios (Figure 4). As can be seen, SCMC, MICC and ADCC effector functions detected in spleen were comparable to those seen in peripheral blood. However, tonsillar mononuclear cells mediated MICC but functioned poorly in SCMC and ADCC. Thymus did not mediate either SCMC, MICC or ADCC. Thus SCMC and ADCC effector

449

cell activities occurred in parallel in these organs, both being present in spleen and peripheral blood and both being absent in tonsil and thymus. MICC, however, was present in all of the tissues except thymus.

Trypsin Treatment and Reincubation in Autologous Plasma

Thus, since both SCMC and ADDCC were mediated by sIg negative Fc receptor positive cells and effector cells occurred in similar organ distributions, further studies were undertaken to determine whether the mechanisms of SCMC and ADCC were different. Since ADCC is mediated by Fc receptor bearing cells (13), and Fc receptors are known to be trypsin-resistant (15), peripheral blood effector cells were treated with trypsin prior to cytotoxicity testing. Macrophage-depleted normal peripheral blood lymphocytes were incubated with 1.0% trypsin for 45 minutes at 37°C and tested at varying effector to target cell ratios in SCMC and ADCC (Figure 5). As can be seen, trypsin treatment has no effect on ADCC, while the

Figure 5

EFFECTS OF TRYPSIN TREATMENT AND SUBSEQUENT INCUBATION
IN AUTOLOGOUS PLASMA ON SCMC AND ADCC

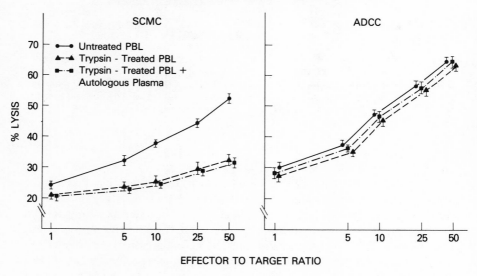

Effect of trypsin treatment with subsequent incubation in autologous plasma on SCMC and ADCC. Normal peripheral blood lymphocytes were treated with 1.0% trypsin for 45 minutes at 37°C prior to cytotoxicity testing. Subsequent to trypsin treatment, a portion were incubated with heat-inactivated autologous plasma for one hour at 4°C and tested in SCMC and ADCC assays. Values represent mean % lysis ± 1 S.E. of triplicate cultures.

450

cytotoxic capacity in SCMC of these treated effector cells is significantly diminished. Thus, the mechanisms of SCMC and ADCC were shown to be different. It could be argued that SCMC merely represents a type of ADCC in which cytophilic anti-target cell antibody occurring naturally in plasma is passively absorbed onto the effector cell, and that trypsin is merely destroying this antibody. If this were true, however, the inhibition caused by trypsin treatment should be reversed by re-arming the cell through exposure to autologous plasma. As can be seen in Figure 5, the effect of trypsin is not reversible by subsequent incubation in autologous plasma. Thus, the mechanisms of SCMC and ADCC are different and, furthermore, the mechanism of SCMC is probably not due to antibody passively absorbed onto the effector cell from plasma.

Clinical Studies

Because SCMC has been proposed as a mechanism for immune surveillance *in vivo* (7) in experimental animals and in man, studies were undertaken to measure the SCMC effector cell potential of peripheral blood mononuclear cells from a variety of patients with immunodeficiency diseases, who are known to have an increased incidence of neoplasia. In spite of profound functional deficiencies in T and B-cells *in vivo* and *in vitro,* SCMC activity was found to be normal in patients with hypogammaglobulinemia (N=26), selective IgA deficiency (7), Wiskott-Aldrich Syndrome (5), ataxia-telangiectasia (3) and dysgammaglobulinemia (5). SCMC was normal in one patient with severe combined immunodeficiency and absent in a second such patient. This suggests that a chronic defect in SCMC-dependent immune surveillance may not be the cause of increased neoplasia in these patients.

DISCUSSION

Cytotoxicity occurring *in vitro* when lymphoid cells from non-immunized donors are added to a variety of cell-line derived targets in the presence of nutrient medium is termed natural cytotoxicity (NC) or spontaneous cell-mediated cytotoxicity (SCMC). Recently much interest has arisen in the phenomenon of SCMC because of the potential relevance of this "naturally" occurring *in vitro* cytolytic mechanism to *in vivo* immunologic surveillance against tumor cells. Recent studies in our laboratory have centered on the analysis of SCMC in humans and experimental animals and the comparison of SCMC with two other forms of *in vitro* cytotoxicity mediated by non-immunized effector cells: mitogen-induced cellular cytotoxicity (MICC) and antibody-dependent cellular cytotoxicity (ADCC). Allogeneic ^{51}Cr labeled human Chang liver cells are employed for all cytotoxicity reactions, making such comparisons valid. While SCMC occurs in the absence of any known inductive stimulus other than effector-target cell contact, plant lectins such as PHA and anti-target cell antibodies represent inducing agents added to cytotoxicity cultures for MICC and ADCC, respectively. Our studies have involved several aspects of these cytotoxicity reactions including kinetics, effector cell identity, mechanisms of lysis, and the cytotoxic effector potential of peripheral blood mononuclear cells from both normal individuals and patients with a variety of primary and secondary immunodeficiency diseases.

With regard to kinetics, SCMC occurs relatively quickly with as little as five minutes of effector and target cell contact being required for cytolysis to be observed. However, target cell damage due to SCMC proceeds more slowly than that due to MICC and ADCC. As to the efficiency of the cytolytic reactions, SCMC requires considerably higher (at least 10-30 fold higher) effector to target cell ratios to produce target cytolysis equivalent to that in MICC and ADCC. This requirement for high numbers of effectors for SCMC could reflect a less efficient cytolytic mechanism, perhaps indicating a paucity of effector cell surface receptors or other constituents required for this form of cytotoxicity. On the other hand, the lower levels of target cell damage seen for SCMC may be due to smaller numbers of SCMC effector cells in peripheral blood compared to MICC or ADCC effectors. It should be emphasized that although SCMC requires higher effector to target ratios and proceeds more slowly than MICC and ADCC, these differences are relative; and, in fact, SCMC possesses similar kinetics to the cytotoxicity observed in human immune cell-mediated lympholysis *in vitro* (16). SCMC probably occurs during MICC and ADCC reactions as well and contributes to the % target cell lysis observed in MICC and ADCC. With regard to kinetics, our data for SCMC are in general accord with those of Peter, et al., (9) and Pross and Jondal (17).

In the present studies the effector cell(s) mediating SCMC and ADCC was shown to be present in a lymphocyte sub-population lacking surface immunoglobulin (sIg), but possessing Fc receptors. In addition, sIg negative Fc receptor negative T-cells mediated MICC but not ADCC. B-cells possessing surface immunoglobulin did not mediate cytotoxicity. In prior studies SCMC, MICC and ADCC effector activity against cell-line targets was shown to be absent from neutrophils and adherent monocytes, complement receptor positive PBM, and DRw antigen bearing lymphoctyes (10, 12, 18). Recent studies have shown that cells capable of binding neuraminidase coated sheep erythrocytes (T-cells) possess SCMC, MICC and ADCC activity while non T-cells mediate only SCMC and ADCC. When T-cells were separated into subsets based on the expression of Fc receptors for IgG (Tγ) and IgM (Tμ), SCMC and ADCC occurred solely in Tγ cell enriched subsets while MICC was mediated by both Tμ and Tγ cells (19). Thus all lymphocyte fractionation procedures resulted in a co-purification

452

of effectors for SCMC and ADCC but not MICC. These results for cell surface characteristics for the SCMC effector have in general been corroborated by the studies of others.

Since the effector(s) mediating SCMC and ADCC was not separable on the basis of surface characteristics, studies were undertaken to determine if the organ distribution of these activities was different. However, it was found that SCMC and ADCC but not MICC effector activities occurred in parallel distributions in spleen, tonsil, thymus and peripheral blood. To investigate the mechanism of SCMC, effector cells were treated with trypsin which abrogated SCMC but not ADCC. Thus, although SCMC and ADCC effectors were inseparable based on surface characteristics and organ distributions, the mechanism of cytotoxicity was shown to be different. One possible explanation for these results for trypsin treatment on SCMC might be that SCMC represents ADCC due to passively absorbed naturally occurring anti-target cell antibodies which are removed by trypsin treatment. However, our inability to re-arm SCMC by incubation of trypsin-treated cells in autologous plasma and the reappearance of SCMC in trypsin-treated cells following culture in the absence of human plasma (10) makes "natural" ADCC an unlikely mechanism for SCMC.

Having thus defined the indentity of the effector cell mediating SCMC and gained some insight into the mechanism of cytotoxicity, studies were undertaken to investigate SCMC in patients with various immunodeficiencies affecting T-cells, B-cells and macrophages. These patients are known to have an increased risk of neoplasia and if SCMC as assessed *in vitro* related to *in vivo* immunologic surveillance, then these patients might be expected to have diminished SCMC effector function. In extensive studies in our laboratory, SCMC by PBM was normal in patients with common variable hypogammaglobulinemia, selective IgA deficiency, Wiskott-Aldrich Syndrome, ataxia telangiectasia and dysgammaglobulinemia. SCMC was absent only in one of two patients studied with severe combined immunodeficiency. In virtually all of these patients SCMC was present in spite of profound functional deficiencies of T-cells and B-cells as assessed both *in vitro* and *in vivo*. Thus SCMC appears to be a basic effector mechanism preserved in all but the most profoundly immunodeficient patients. While these results do not exclude the possibility of defects in SCMC in these patients at some critical time or in some location other than peripheral blood, they suggest that SCMC as assessed *in vitro* does not correlate with the risk of cancer in humans and that defects in other immune surveillance mechanisms may be the critical deficiencies leading to neoplasia in these patients.

REFERENCES

1. Herberman, R.B., Nunn, M.E. and Lavrin, D.H., "Natural Cytotoxic Reactivity of Mouse Lymphoid Cells Against Syngeneic and Allogeneic Tumors. I. Distribution of Reactivity and Specificity." *Int. J. Cancer* 16:216-229, 1975.

2. Kiessling, R., Klein, E. and Wigzell, H., "Natural Killer Cells in the Mouse. I. Cytotoxic Cells with Specificity for Mouse Moloney Leukemia Cells. Specificity and Distribution According to Genotype." *Eur. J. Immunol.* 5:112-117, 1975.

3. Nunn, M.E., Djeu, J.Y., Glaser, M., et al., "Natural Cytotoxic Reactivity of Rat Lymphocytes Against Syngeneic Gross Virus-Induced Lymphoma." *J. Natl. Cancer Inst.* 56:393-399, 1976.

4. Arnaud-Battandier, F., Bundy, B.M. and Nelson, D.L., "Natural Killer Cells in Guinea Pig Spleen Bear Fc Receptors." *Eur. J. Immunol.* In press, 1978.

5. Arnaud-Battandier, F., Bundy, B.M., O'Neil, M., et al., "Cytotoxic Activities of Gut Mucosal Lymphoid Cells in Guinea Pigs." *J. Immunol.* In press, 1978.

6. Takasugi, M., Mickey, M.R. and Terasaki, P.I., "Reactivity of Lymphocytes from Normal Persons on Cultured Tumor Cells." *Cancer Res.* 33:2898-2902, 1973.

7. Kay, H.D. and Sinkovics, J.G., "Cytotoxic Lymphocytes from Normal Donors." *Lancet* 2:296-297, 1974.

8. Rosenberg, E.B., McCoy, J.L., Green, S.S., et al., "Destruction of Human Lymphoid Tissue Culture Cell Lines by Human Peripheral Lymphocytes in ^{51} Cr Release Cellular Cytotoxicity Assays." *J. Natl. Cancer Inst.* 52:345-352, 1974.

9. Peter, H.H., Pavie-Fischer, J., Fridman, W.H., et al., "Cell-Mediated Cytotoxicity *in vitro* of Human Lymphocytes Against a Tissue Culture Melanoma Cell Line (IGR3)." *J. Immunol.* 115: 539-548, 1975.

10. Nelson, D.L., Bundy, B.M. and Strober, W., "Spontaneous Cell-Mediated Cytotoxicity by Human Peripheral Blood Lymphocytes *in vitro.*" *J. Immunol.* 119:1401-1405, 1977.

11. Nelson, D.L., Bundy, B.M., and Strober, W., "Spontaneous Cytotoxicity by Human Peripheral Blood Lymphocytes." In *Regulatory Mechanisms in Lymphocyte Activation,* edited by Lucas, D.O., Academic Press, New York, 518-520, 1977.

12. Vierling, J.M., Steer, C.J., Bundy, B.M., et al., "Studies of Complement Receptors on Cytotoxic Effector Cells in Human Peripheral Blood." *Cell. Immunol.* 35:403-413, 1978.

13. Nelson, D.L., Bundy, B.M., Pitchon, H.E., et al., "The Effector Cells in Human Peripheral Blood Mediating Mitogen-Induced Cellular Cytotoxicity and Antibody-Dependent Cellular Cytotoxicity." *J. Immunol.* 117:1472-1481, 1976.

14. Nelson, D.L. and MacDermott, R.P., "Modifications of Anti-Fab Immunoabsorbent Separation of Human Peripheral Blood Mononuclear Cells." In *Regulatory Mechanisms in Lymphocyte Activation,* edited by Lucas, D.O., Academic Press, New York, 587-590, 1977.

15. Eden, A., Bianco, C. and Nussenzweig, V., "Mechanism of Binding Soluble Immune Complexes to Lymphocytes." *Cell. Immunol.* 7:459-466, 1973.

16. Bonnard, G.D., Lemos, L. and Chappuis, M., "Cell-Mediated Lympholysis After Sensitization in Unidirectional Mixed Lymphocyte Culture in Man." *Scand. J. Immunol.* 3:97-106, 1974.

17. Pross, H.F. and Jondal, M., "Cytotoxic Lymphocytes From Normal Donors. A Functional Marker of Human Non-T Lymphocytes." *Clin. Exp. Immunol.* 21:226-235, 1975.

18. Nelson, D.L., Strober, W., Abelson, L.D., et al., "Distribution of Alloantigens on Human Fc Receptor-Bearing Lymphocytes: The Presence of B-Cell Alloantigens on sIg-Positive but Not sIg-Negative Lymphocytes." *J. Immunol.* 118:943-946, 1977.

19. Pichler, W.J., Gendelman, F.W. and Nelson, D.L., "Fc-Receptors on Human T-Lymphocytes II. Cytotoxic Capabilities of Human Tγ, Tμ, B and L Cells." Submitted for publication, 1978.

454

In Vitro Approaches for Generating Cytotoxic Lymphocytes Against Autologous Human Leukemia Cells[†]

Joyce M. Zarling[1]

L. Eskra[1]

R. Kloop[1]

P. Raih[1]

F. Bach[1]

SUMMARY—Three different approaches were taken aimed at generating cytotoxic T lymphocytes (CTLs) capable of lysing autologous human leukemia cells. Firstly, since lymphoblastoid cell lines and human leukemia cells often express cross-reactive serologically detectable antigens, lymphocytes were sensitized to x-irradiated autologous lymphoblastoid cell lines (LCL) and tested for their ability to lyse human leukemia cells. Although lymphocytes sensitized to autologous LCL cells lyse autologous and allogeneic LCL cells, cytotoxicity for human leukemia cells was rarely detected indicating that LCL cells and leukemia cells generally do not share cross-reactive target antigens for CTLs. Secondly, since lymphocytes cultured with x-irradiated autologous leukemia cells do not differentiate into anti-leukemic CTLs (possibly because the leukemia cells induce only weak lymphocyte proliferative responses), x-irradiated allogeneic normal cells (as a proliferation inducing stimulus) were added to a mixture of remission lymphocytes and x-irradiated autologous leukemia cells. This approach resulted in CTLs that lysed autologous leukemia cells and not remission bone marrow cells. Thirdly, T cells were sensitized to x-irradiated allogeneic cells pooled from 20 normal individuals since such "pool" sensitized lymphocytes lyse virtually all allogeneic cells and because transformed cells reportedly express antigens cross-reactive with alloantigens. "Pool" sensitized T cells lysed autologous LCL cells as well as autologous hairy cell leukemia cells but not autologous normal T cells, B cells nor mitogen induced blasts.

INTRODUCTION

Although it has been clearly demonstrated in most experimental animal tumor systems that tumor associated transplantation antigens (TATA) are expressed on tumors and are capable of inducing cell mediated immune responses (for review, see 1), it has been difficult to establish whether human

[1]Immunobiology Research Center and the Departments of Human Oncology, Medicine, Medical Genetics and Surgery, University of Wisconsin, Madison, Wisconsin.
[†]Supported by NIH grants CA-20409, CA-14520, CA-16836, AI-11576 and AI-08439.

455

malignant cells likewise express TATA against which beneficial host immune responses may be mounted. We (2,3) and others (4) have been unsuccessful at generating lymphocytes cytotoxic for autologous leukemia cells by stimulating remission lymphocytes with x-irradiated autologous leukemia cells in mixed leukocyte culture. It is possible, however, that leukemia cells that are not immunogenic on their own may express target antigens against which cytotoxic T lymphocytes (CTLs) can be directed after appropriate immune stimulation. Our studies have thus been focused on alternative approaches towards generating cytotoxic lymphocytes capable of lysing leukemia cells in order to provide evidence that human leukemia cells express target antigens that can be recognized by autologous CTLs and also to provide new approaches towards immunotherapy of human leukemia.

Three different approaches were taken in attempts to generate CTLs capable of lysing leukemia cells. First, since Epstein-Barr (EB) virus transformed lymphoblastoid cell lines (LCL) express serologically cross-reacting antigens with many human leukemia cells (5,6), we hypothesized that these cells may also share target antigens against which CTLs are directed. Thus, experiments were performed to determine whether sensitization of lymphocytes with autologous LCL cells would give rise to CTLs capable of lysing human leukemia cells. Second, for maximal generation of CTLs against alloantigens, responding lymphocytes must be stimulated with allogeneic cells that express different target antigens (or CD antigens) detected by CTLs as well as lymphocyte defined (LD) antigens that induce proliferative responses in helper cells (for review, see 7). Human leukemia cells usually induce only minimal proliferative responses (8-12 Zarling *et al.*, unpublished) and no cytotoxic responses in autologous lymphocytes (2-4). We thus asked whether the addition of x-irradiated allogeneic cells (as a strong proliferation inducing stimulus) to a mixed culture of remission lymphocytes and x-irradiated autologous leukemia cells in a "three cell" experiment would result in the generation of lymphocytes cytotoxic for autologous leukemia cells (2). Third, many transformed cells and tumor cells reportedly express antigens cross-reactive with histocompatibility antigens expressed on normal cells of unrelated members of the species (13-18). We thus asked whether sensitization of lymphocytes with x-irradiated normal cells pooled from 20 individuals (a procedure that results in the generation of CTLs capable of lysing virtually all allogeneic target cells) (19) would give rise to CTLs cytotoxic for autologous LCL cells (20) and autologous leukemia cells (3). We report here that lymphocytes cytotoxic for autologous leukemia cells and not autologous normal cells can be generated by the "three cell" approach and by the allogeneic "pool" sensitization approach.

456

METHODS AND MATERIALS

Establishment of LCL Lines

LCL cells were generated in our laboratory by infecting peripheral blood lymphocytes from normal individuals with Epstein-Barr virus as previously described (21) and passaging the cells in medium consisting of RPMI-1640 plus 25 mM Hepes buffer and 10% heat inactivated normal human serum. The LCL cells were free of mycoplasma contamination.

Purification of Lymphocytes and Leukemic Cells

Lymphocytes were isolated from heparinized peripheral blood by Ficoll-Hypaque sedimentation and resuspended in medium consisting of RMPI-1640 plus 25 mM Hepes buffer and 20% heat inactivated normal human serum. This medium is referred to as "culture" medium. T cells were separated from the Ficoll-Hypaque purified lymphocytes by rosetting with sheep red blood cells as previously described (22). Leukemic cells from most patients were isolated from heparinized peripheral blood or from bone marrow. Leukemic cells were isolated from portions of spleen removed from the hairy cell leukemia patients. The leukemia cells from the blood and spleen of the hairy cell leukemia patients were isolated by depletion of T cells by rosetting with sheep red blood cells (22). Leukemia cells and normal lymphocytes were stored in liquid nitrogen after control-freezing of cells suspended in "freezing medium" that consists of RPMI-1640 plus 25 mM Hepes buffer, 25% heat inactivated normal human serum and 10% DMSO.

Preparation of Pooled Allogeneic Cells

Lymphocytes insolated from Ficoll-Hypaque sedimentation from the peripheral blood of 8 to 20 normal unrelated individuals were pooled in equal numbers (19) and resuspended in "freezing medium" as described above. The pooled cells were stored frozen in liquid nitrogen.

In Vitro Sensitizations

Responding lymphocytes (1×10^5) were cultured in Linbro round bottom microwells with 1×10^5 x-irradiated (2500 R) allogeneic stimulating cells as previously described (23). Allogeneic stimulating cells were from a single individual or from a "pool" of 8 to 20 normal individuals (19). Responding lymphocytes were also stimulated with 2×10^4 x-irradiated (4000 R) autologous LCL cells as previously described (20). Alternatively, sensitizations were performed in 25 ml tissue culture flasks using 8×10^6 responding lymphocytes and 8×10^6 allogeneic stimulating cells (2500 R) or 1.5×10^6 autologous LCL cells (4000R). The sensitization wells or flasks were fed with fresh culture medium on days 2 and 5 and on day 7 cell mediated lysis assays were performed.

Cell Mediated Lysis (CML) Assays

CML assays were performed on day 7 as previously described (23) using as target cells, normal lymphocytes cultured in the absence of mitogens for 7 days, phytohemagglutinin (PHA) induced blasts, LCL cells or leukemic cells (that were thawed and cultured for 2 days prior to their use as targets). The target cells were labeled with 250 μCi ^{51}Cr for 1 hour, followed by 3 washes with cold medium. The target cells were resuspended in culture media at a concentration of 2 x 10^5 cells/ml and 0.05 ml target cells were added to each of several replicate culture wells containing the effector cells that were generated in the wells or placed in wells after harvesting from flasks. The CML assays were terminated after 6 to 8 hour incubations at 37°C and the percent specific ^{51}Cr release was calculated as previously described (23).

Cell "blocking" experiments were performed by adding varying numbers of unlabeled "blocking" cells to microwells containing the effector cells prior to the addition of ^{51}Cr labeled target cells. The % specific ^{51}Cr released from target cells in the presence and absence of unlabeled "blocking" cells was compared.

RESULTS AND DISCUSSION

Generation of Anti-Leukemic Cytotoxic Lymphocytes by Sensitization to Lymphoblastoid Cell Lines

Lymphocytes sensitized to autologous EB virus transformed lymphoblastoid cell lines (LCL) differentiate into cytotoxic lymphocytes that lyse autologous as well as allogeneic LCL cells (20, 24-26). In order to determine whether LCL cells may share common target antigens with human leukemic cells against which cytotoxic lymphocytes can be directed, lymphocytes were sensitized with autologous LCL cells and tested for their ability to lyse a variety of human leukemia cells. Lymphocytes from individual A, after sensitization with autologous x-irradiated LCL cells (A A-L$_x$, were cytotoxic for autologous and allogeneic LCL cells, however these same effector cells were not significantly cytotoxic for the leukemia cells from the patients tested (Table 1). Most of these leukemia cells were, however, sensitive to cell mediated lysis, as shown on the right hand side of Table 1; lymphocytes from individual A sensitized to pooled allogeneic normal cells (pool$_x$ lysed the ^{51}Cr labeled leukemia cells from 9 of 11 patients.

Results of cell blocking experiments shown in Figure 1 further suggest that human leukemia cells and LCL cells rarely share common target antigens. Lymphocytes sensitized with autologous LCL cells were tested for their ability to lyse ^{51}Cr labeled autologous LCL cells in the presence of varying numbers of unlabeled LCL cells and leukemia cells. Whereas

458

Table 1—FAILURE OF LYMPHOCYTES SENSITIZED WITH AUTOLOGOUS LCL CELLS TO LYSE HUMAN LEUKEMIA CELLS

Target cells	Effectors:**	% Specific ^{51}Cr Release* ($\pm$S.D.)	
		A A-L$_x$	A Pool$_x$
AML-1†		8.4 ($\pm$ 9.3)	21.1 ($\pm$ 3.8)
AML-2		-2.5 ($\pm$ 6.6)	28.6 ($\pm$ 6.0)
AML-3		-4.9 ($\pm$ 1.3)	30.1 ($\pm$ 10.8)
AML-4		11.3 ($\pm$ 9.1)	64.3 ($\pm$ 10.5)
AMMoL-1		-0.1 ($\pm$ 2.4)	43.5 ($\pm$ 13.5)
AMMoL-2		-1.7 ($\pm$ 3.8)	3.3 ($\pm$ 1.5)
ALL-1		4.9 ($\pm$ 5.8)	33.5 ($\pm$ 14.3)
ALL-2		0.6 ($\pm$ 1.1)	84.6 ($\pm$ 10.9)
CLL-1		-0.3 ($\pm$ 2.8)	33.0 ($\pm$ 3.8)
CLL-2		1.2 ($\pm$ 1.5)	8.0 ($\pm$ 1.6)
AUL-1		-4.1 ($\pm$ 1.9)	10.9 ($\pm$ 0.6)
Autologous LCL		41.9 ($\pm$ 2.4)	17.5 ($\pm$ 2.1)
Allogeneic LCL		20.2 ($\pm$ 6.7)	31.8 ($\pm$ 2.8)

*Effector: target cell ratio=30:1.
**Lymphocytes from individual A were sensitized to autologous LCL cells (A-L$_x$) or to pooled allogeneic normal cells from 20 individuals (pool$_x$) as described in the methods. The ^{51}Cr release assays were performed 7 days after the onset of mixed leukocyte culture.
†AML=acute myelogenous leukemia; AMMoL=acute myelomonocytic leukemia; ALL= acute lymphocytic leukemia; CLL=chronic lymphocytic leukemia; AUL=acute undifferentiated leukemia. The numbers following the abbreviations for the leukemias refer to the patients' numbers.

unlabeled autologous and allogeneic LCL cells blocked cell mediated lysis of the ^{51}Cr labeled autologous LCL cells, unlabeled leukemia cells from the majority of the 17 patients with various types of leukemia failed to block cell mediated lysis of the ^{51}Cr labeled LCL cells. It is of interest to note that leukemic blasts from patient 9, who has been in unmaintained stable condition with >60% undifferentiated leukemic blasts in the peripheral blood for 5 years, blocked lysis of the LCL cells to the same extent as did autologous or allogeneic LCL cells indicating that these leukemia cells share antigens cross-reactive with LCL cells. Chronic lymphocytic leukemia cells from patient 17 blocked, to a lesser extent, lysis of the LCL cells. Our findings that LCL cells and human leukemia cells rarely share cross-reactive target antigens against which cytotoxic lymphocytes can be generated, despite the known cross-reactivity between serologically detected antigens

459

Figure 1—ABILITY OF UNLABELED LEUKEMIA CELLS TO BLOCK LYSIS OF ^{51}CR LABELED LCL CELLS BY LYMPHOCYTES SENSITIZED TO AUTOLOGOUS LCL CELLS

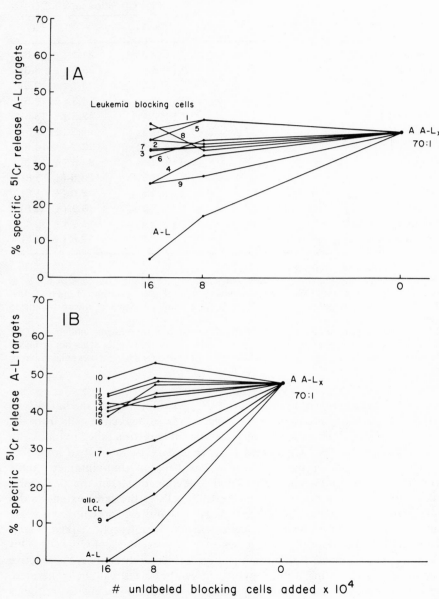

◄

Lymphocytes from individual A, sensitized to autologous LCL cells (A-L$_x$), were tested for their ability to lyse ^{51}Cr labeled autologous LCL targets (A-L) in the presence and absence of varying numbers of unlabeled "blocking" cells from leukemic patients 1-17 or varying numbers of unlabeled autologous LCL cells (A-L) or allogeneic LCL cells (allo-LCL). Chronic lymphocytic leukemia cells from patient 17 and acute undifferentiated leukemia cells from patient 9 significantly blocked cell mediated lysis of the LCL cells. The patients' leukemic cells that failed to significantly block cell mediated lysis of the LCL cells were as follows:

   3 patients with chronic lymphocytic leukemia
   5 patients with acute lymphocytic leukemia
   2 patients with acute myelomonocytic leukemia
   1 patient with lymphosarcoma cell leukemia
   4 patients with acute myelogeneous leukemia

on these cells (5,6) would suggest that immunization of leukemic patients with LCL cells would be unlikely to enhance cell-mediated immune responses against autologous leukemia cells.

Generation of Lymphocytes Cytotoxic for Autologous Leukemia Cells by a "Three-Cell" Approach

We (2,3) and others (4,27) have found that lymphocytes stimulated in mixed leukocyte culture with autologous leukemia cells or leukemia cells from HLA identical siblings, do not differentiate into CTLs capable of killing the leukemia cells. Leukemia cells may express target antigens that differ from those expressed on the patient's normal lymphocytes but cytotoxic responses are not generated against these leukemia associated target antigens. One explanation for the failure of cytotoxic responses to be generated could be that the leukemic cells usually induce only minimal proliferative responses in autologous helper lymphocytes. We thus asked whether the addition of normal allogeneic lymphocytes (as a helper inducing stimulus) to a mixed culture of remission lymphocytes and x-irradiated autologous leukemia cells would result in the generation of lymphocytes cytotoxic for autologous leukemia cells. The results in Table 2 show that stimulation of lymphocytes, from a patient in remission from acute myelomonocytic leukemia, in a "three-cell" protocol resulted in the production of cytotoxic lymphocytes that lysed autologous leukemia cells but not autologous remission bone marrow cells. Stimulation of the patient's lymphocytes with neither the autologous leukemia cells alone nor the allogeneic cells alone resulted in significant cytotoxicity against the leukemic cells.

461

Table 2—IN VITRO GENERATION OF LYMPHOCYTES CYTOTOXIC FOR AUTOLOGOUS ACUTE MYELOMONOCYTIC LEUKEMIA CELLS BY A "THREE-CELL" PROTOCOL

Responding lymphocytes		Stimulating cells	Effector/target cell ratio	% Specific ^{51}Cr Release ±S.D.			
				Leukemic cells	Remission marrow cells	Normal lymphocytes from A	Normal lymphocytes from B
C (patient's lymphocytes)	L_x	(patient's leukemia cells)	40:1	17.8 ± 6.5	3.5 ± 1.4	44.0 ± 4.1	1.8 ± 2.3
C + A_x		normal allogeneic lymphocytes					
C	L_x		40:1	0.0	0.0		
C	A_x		40:1	2.9 ± 1.1	0.45 ± 1.6	60.7 ± 10.1	2.2 ± 2.2
B (normal individual)	L_x		20:1	17.5 ± 12.0	14.7 ± 2.0	-0.7 ± 3.4	-0.4 ± 2.8
B	A_x		20:1			27.7 ± 2.3	-0.2 ± 3.4

Effector cells were collected 7 days after stimulation, and incubated with 1 x 10^4 ^{51}Cr-labelled target cells at the designated effector: target cell ratios. The % specific ^{51}Cr release was measured after a 6 hour incubation of effector cells and target cells at 37°. [Reprinted from Zarling, et al., *Nature* 262:691-693, 1976 (2)].

The efficacy of the "three-cell" approach for generating anti-leukemic cytotoxic lymphocytes has been confirmed in a series of patients with acute myelogenous leukemia (4) and also in certain cases where lymphocytes from siblings HLA identical with the leukemic patient were used as responding cells (26). These results suggest that leukemia cells from at least some patients express target antigens capable of inducing cytotoxic responses in autologous lymphocytes provided that a helper stimulus (in this case, allogeneic stimulating cells) is provided.

Generation of Anti-Leukemic Cytotoxic Lymphocytes by Sensitization to Pooled Allogeneic Cells

It has been previously demonstrated in this laboratory (19) that sensitization of lymphocytes against normal cells pooled from 20 randomly chosen individuals gives rise to cytotoxic T lymphocytes (CTLs) that lyse all allogeneic target cells differing from the responding cells with regards to CD antigens. Since transformed cells and tumor cells often express cell surface antigens cross-reactive with histocompatibility antigens expressed on normal allogeneic cells (13-18), we hypothesized that a method for generating CTLs capable of lysing autologous tumor cells may be to sensitize lymphocytes with a "pool" of allogeneic cells (17).

The results shown in Table 3 indicate that lymphocytes from two of the three individuals tested, after sensitization to the "pool," were cytotoxic for autologous LCL cells but not autologous normal cells. The normal lymphocytes were, however, sensitive to lysis by allogeneic lymphocytes sensitized to the pool. In Table 4 are shown the findings that pool sensitization of T cells gives rise to CTLs cytotoxic for autologous LCL cells but not for autologous normal T cells, B cells nor phytohemagglutinin (PHA) induced blasts.

Shown in Table 5 are results indicating that sensitization of lymphocytes from individual S with pooled cells from 8 or 18 individuals was as efficacious, in terms of generating CTLs against autologous LCL cells, as was sensitization with x-irradiated autologous LCL cells. However, sensitization with none of the 8 single members of the pool (A through H) resulted in CTLs that lysed autologous LCL cells although, as expected, sensitization with cells from these single individuals resulted in CTLs cytotoxic for the sensitizing allogeneic cells. The finding that sensitization of lymphocytes to cells from single allogeneic individuals does not give rise to CTLs capable of lysing autologous LCL cells is a reproducible finding; in only one of 18 cases did sensitization with single allogeneic cells give rise to a significant cytotoxic response against autologous LCL cells.

The results of these experiments thus indicate that sensitization to pooled allogeneic normal cells is an effective means for generating CTLs capable of lysing EB virus transformed autologous LCL cells but not autologous

Table 3—LYSIS OF AUTOLOGOUS AND ALLOGENEIC LCL CELLS FOLLOWING POOL SENSITIZATION*

Responder cells	Stimulating cells	Number of effector cells per target cell	% Specific ^{51}Cr release (±S.D.) Target cells					
			A-LCL	A	S-LCL	S	C-LCL	C
A	Pool[20]x	35	46.7 ± 5.7	-2.8 ± 3.7	92.3 ± 7.6		87.4 ± 6.5	
A	A-LCLx	60	41.1 ± 19.1					
S	Pool[20]x	35	82.4 ± 9.2		17.9 ± 3.3	2.8 ± 7.3	85.9 ± 7.2	64.5 ± 3.4
S	S-LCLx	60			33.4 ± 2.4			
C	Pool[20]x	35	94.0 ± 11.8	70.1 ± 9.1	91.4 ± 7.6	44.3 ± 5.4	5.3 ± 3.2	
C	C-LCLx	60					70.2 ± 3.5	-2.8 ± 1.6

*Lymphocytes from individuals A, S, and C were stimulated with x-irradiated autologous LCL cells (designated A-LCL, S-LCL or C-LCL) or a pool of 20 allogeneic stimulating cells (designated pool[20]x) and lysis of the LCL cells and normal lymphocytes (A, S, and C) was measured on day 7. Lymphocytes from A, S, and C cultured in media alone caused -3.0 to 2.3% [51]Cr release from autologous LCL cells. [Reprinted from Zarling and Bach, *J. Exp. Med.* 147:1334-1340, 1978 (20)].

Table 4—ABILITY OF POOL SENSITIZED T LYMPHOCYTES TO LYSE AUTOLOGOUS LCL CELLS AND THEIR FAILURE TO LYSE AUTOLOGOUS B CELLS, T CELLS AND PHA BLASTS*

% specific ^{51}Cr release ($\pm$ S.D.)
Target cells

Responding T lymphocytes	Stimulating cells	H-LCL	H-T cells	H-B cells	allogeneic LCL
Exp. 1					
H	Pool^{20}x	20.8 ± 8.9	-1.8 ± 9.4	2.9 ± 9.7	35.9 ± 5.2
D	H x		61.9 ± 6.9	65.2 ± 11.6	

Responding T lymphocytes	Stimulating cells	S-LCL	S-cultured lymphocytes	S-PHA blasts	M-cultured lymphocytes	M-PHA blasts
Exp. 2						
S	Pool^{20}x	15.3 ± 3.1	-2.7 ± 2.0	-1.3 ± 3.9	23.9 ± 5.0	13.3 ± 4.7
M	Pool^{20}x		43.0 ± 5.6	47.2 ± 4.8	-0.5 ± 3.7	-4.3 ± 1.7

*Responding T lymphocytes were stimulated with x-irradiated pooled cells from 20 individuals (pool^{20}x) or x-irradiated cells of individual H (H$_x$). CML assays were performed on day 7 using 40 effector cells: target cells. T-enriched and B-enriched cells from individual H (designated H-T and H-B) were isolated as described in the methods and cultured for 7 days before use as target cells. PHA blasts were used 60 hours after incubating lymphocytes with PHA. [Reprinted from Zarling and Bach, J. Exp. Med. 147:1334-1340, 1978 (20)].

465

Table 5—LYSIS OF AUTOLOGOUS LCL CELLS AND ALLOGENEIC CELLS FOLLOWING ALLO- OR POOL-SENSITIZATION

| | | % specific ^{51}Cr release ± S.D.* | | | | | |
| | | Target cells | | | | | |
Effector cells**	S's LCL cells	A	B	D	E	G	H
S (A)	0.0 ± 2.7	33.5					
S (B)	1.9 ± 3.0		43.7				
S (C)	2.8 ± 3.9						
S (D)	1.9 ± 4.3			50.9			
S (E)	3.7 ± 4.4				92.9		
S (F)	0.1 ± 2.7						
S (G)	-0.8 ± 3.8					39.3	
S (H)	2.3 ± 5.0						37.1
S (Pool[8])	18.7 ± 3.2						
S (Pool[18])	23.0 ± 2.6	18.5	30.3	53.9	101.6	45.9	112.9
S (S-LCL)	24.6 ± 3.1						

*S.D. ranged from 1.1 to 6.2% ^{51}Cr release.
**Lymphocytes were sensitized with x-irradiated normal lymphocytes from single individuals (A through H), with pooled cells from 8 to 18 individuals (pool[8] and pool[18]), or with autologous LCL cells (S-LCL). Cytotoxicity on the allogeneic target cells derived from members of the pool and on autologous LCL cells was assayed on day 7 using a ratio of 25 effector cells: target cell. [Reprinted from Zarling and Bach, J. Exp. Med. 147:1334-1340, 1978 (20)].

normal B or T cells nor autologous PHA induced blasts. In order to determine whether pool sensitization may be an approach for generating CTLs capable of lysing fresh autologous malignant cells that have not been adapted to tissue culture, T cells from two patients with hairy cell leukemia were sensitized to the "pool" and tested for their ability to lyse autologous leukemia cells. The results of these experiments are shown in Table 6. T cells, isolated from the spleen or peripheral blood of the patients, after stimulation with the pool, lysed autologous splenic and circulating hairy cell leukemia cells but not autologous normal T cells. Stimulation of the patients' T cells with x-irradiated autologous leukemia cells failed to give rise to CTLs cytotoxic for autologous leukemia cells and stimulation with allogeneic cells from single individuals resulted in only minimal cytotoxic responses against autologous leukemia cells.

466

Further evidence was obtained suggesting that hairy cell leukemia cells, but not normal cells, express target antigens cross-reactive with those expressed on pooled allogeneic cells. T cells from patient 1, after pool sensitization, lysed ^{51}Cr labeled autologous leukemia cells and this cytotoxicity was inhibited by the addition of unlabeled autologous leukemia cells but not by autologous normal T cells (Table 7). That the leukemia cells do not nonspecifically inhibit cell mediated lysis was demonstrated by the finding that leukemic cells inhibit only minimally (and to the same extent as do the patient's normal cells) cytotoxicity against unrelated target cells (3).

The mechanism whereby sensitization of lymphocytes to pooled allogeneic normal cells gives rise to CTLs capable of lysing autologous LCL cells or leukemic cells is not clear at present. However, in view of previous reports indicating that abnormal cells often express antigens cross-reactive with alloantigens (13-18), it is most probable that LCL cells and the leukemic cells, that were lysed by autologous CTLs following pool sensitization, express target antigens cross-reactive with alloantigens expressed on the pooled allogeneic stimulating cells. It would seem that there are at least three possibilities to explain why antigens expressed on LCL cells and leukemic cells might cross-react with alloantigens. First, as a result of morphological transformation there may be derepression of genes coding for antigens that are expressed on normal cells of other members of the species (28,29). Second, EBV (or in the case of leukemic cells, an as yet undefined virus) may code for cell membrane determinants that partially cross-react with many alloantigens. Third, any genetic or phenotypic modification of normal histocompatibility CD antigens might result in expression of target antigens that would be cross-reactive with alloantigens (17). Despite our present lack of knowledge as to whether the target antigens detected on LCL cells and leukemia cells by "pool" activated CTLs are transformed cell "specific" transplantation antigens, derepressed normal histocompatibility antigens or conceivably differentiation antigens, use of the "pool" may have general applicability in terms of generating effector cells cytotoxic for autologous malignantly transformed cells of various histological types.

Studies are currently underway in our laboratory to determine whether immunization of mice with weakly immunogenic syngeneic tumor cells together with allogeneic normal cells in an "*in vivo* three-cell" protocol will be successful in terms of inducing resistance to challenge with the viable syngeneic tumor cells. Additionally, experiments are being performed to determine whether *in vivo* immunization of mice with pooled allogeneic normal mouse cells will be a successful approach for conferring resistance to the development of transplantation tumors and to the development of spontaneous leukemias in mice.

Table 6—LYSIS OF AUTOLOGOUS HAIRY CELL LEUKEMIA CELLS BY T CELLS SENSITIZED TO POOLED ALLOGENEIC NORMAL CELLS*

Responding T Cells	Stimulating Cells	% ^{51}Cr Release ± S.D. Target Cells			
		Patient I's Splenic Leukemic Cells	Patient I's Peripheral Leukemic Cells	Patient I's Peripheral T Cells	Individual A's Peripheral T Cells
Exp. a					
PI (patient 1)	P1-L$_x$ (patient 1's leukemia cells)	1.7 ± 2.3		0.5 ± 3.0	
P1	pool$_x$	24.5 ± 1.8		0.8 ± 2.5	
Exp. b					
P1 (Patient 1)	P1-L$_x$ (patient 1's leukemic cells)	-1.0 ± 0.5			
P1	A$_x$	5.3 ± 2.6			37.7 ± 3.9
P1	pool$_x$	19.0 ± 3.7	21.1 ± 0.8	-1.5 ± 2.7	36.4 ± 5.6
A (normal individual)	P1-L$_x$	32.8 ± 2.6			
A	pool$_x$	29.5 ± 2.8	45.5 ± 3.1	15.8 ± 2.7	-9.2 ± 3.4
		Patient 2's Splenic Leukemic Cells	Patient 2's Peripheral Leukemic Cells	Patient 2's Peripheral T Cells	Individual A's Peripheral T Cells

Exp. c

		(patient 2's leukemic cells)			
P2 (patient 2)	P2-L$_x$	-2.6 ± 1.7			
P2	pool$_x$	18.1 ± 5.6	27.2 ± 3.6		
A (normal individual)	P2-L$_x$	25.2 ± 4.1	21.0 ± 2.6	16.8 ± 4.9	-3.6 ± 2.0

Exp. d

P2 (patient 2)	pool$_x$	18.9 ± 1.5	-0.3 ± 2.5
B (normal individual)	pool$_x$	32.7 ± 2.9	41.0 ± 5.4

*T cells from normal individuals A and B and from the patients with hairy cell leukemia (P1 and P2) were isolated as described in the methods and the T cells were stimulated with the leukemia cells (P1-L$_x$ and P2-L$_x$), with cells from a single normal individual (A$_x$) or with normal cells pooled from 20 individuals (pool$_x$). The ratio of stimulating leukemic cells to responding T cells was 1:1 in this experiment, however, in no case when the patients' T cells were stimulated with autologous leukemia cells at ratios of .1:1 to 2:1 was cytotoxicity against the leukemia cells detected (data not shown). T cells from the normal individuals and the patients that were cultured in the absence of stimulating cells, were not cytotoxic for the leukemic cells (-2.3 ± 1.4 to 0.6 ± 2.0% ^{51}Cr release). [Reprinted from Zarling, et al., Nature, in press (3)].

Table 7—ABILITY OF UNLABELED LEUKEMIC AND NORMAL CELLS TO BLOCK LYSIS OF ^{51}CR LABELED AUTOLOGOUS LEUKEMIC CELLS BY T CELLS SENSITIZED TO THE POOL*

Effector Cells	Unlabeled Blocking Cells	% ^{51}Cr Release ± S.D.	% Inhibition of Lysis
		P1 leukemic cells	
P1 (patient 1) pool $_x$	none	16.8 ± 3.8	—
	P1 splenic leukemic cells	2.4 ± 1.3	86
	P1 peripheral leukemic cells	0.8 ± 0.9	95
	P1 peripheral T cells	17.3 ± 3.8	0

*T cells from patient 1 (P1) were sensitized to the pooled allogeneic cells (pool$_x$) and on day 7, the effector cells were tested for their ability to lyse ^{51}Cr labeled autologous splenic leukemic cells at a ratio of effector:target cells of 20:1 in the presence or absence of 20 unlabeled "blocking cells" per ^{51}Cr labeled target cell. The ^{51}Cr release assay was terminated after 7 hours. The % inhibition of lysis was determined by comparing the % cell-mediated ^{51}Cr released from target cells in the presence and absence of unlabeled blocking cells. [Reprinted from Zarling et al., *Nature,* in press (3)].

470

REFERENCES

1. Ristow, S. and McKhann, C.F., "Tumor-Associated Antigens." In *Mechanisms of Tumor Immunity,* edited by I. Green, S. Cohen and R. T. McCluskey, pp. 109-146, John Wiley and Sons, New York, 1977.

2. Zarling, J.M., Raich, P.C., McKeough, M. and Bach, F.H., "Generation of Cytotoxic Lymphocytes *In Vitro* Against Autologous Human Leukaemia Cells." *Nature* 262:691-693, 1976.

3. Zarling, J.M., Robins, H.I., Raich, P.C., et al., "Generation of Cytotoxic T Lymphocytes to Autologous Human Leukemia Cells by Sensitization to Pooled Allogeneic Normal Cells." *Nature* 1978, in press.

4. Lee, S.K. and Oliver, R.T.D., "Autologous Leukemia-Specific T-Cell-Mediated Lymphocytotoxicity in Patients With Acute Myelogenous Leukemia." *J. Exp. Med.* 147:912-922, 1978.

5. Halterman, R., Leventhal, B.G. and Mann, D.L., "An Acute Leukemia Antigen: Correlation With Clinical Status." *N Engl. J. Med.* 287:1272-1274, 1972.

6. Mann, D.L., Leventhal, B. and Halterman, R., "Human Antisera Detecting Leukemia-Associated Antigens on Autochthonous Tumor Cells." *J. Natl. Cancer Inst.* 54:345-347, 1975.

7. Bach, F. H., Bach, M.L. and Sondel, P.M., "Differential Function of Major Histocompatibility Complex Antigens in T Lymphocyte Activation." *Nature* 259:273-281, 1976.

8. Bach, M.L., Bach, F.H. and Joo, P., "Leukemia-Associated Antigens in the Mixed Leukocyte Culture Test." *Science* 166:1520-1522, 1969.

9. Fridman, W.H. and Kourilsky, F.M., "Stimulation of Lymphocytes by Autologous Leukaemic Cells in Acute Leukaemia." *Nature* 224:277-278, 1969.

10. Leventhal, B.G., Halterman, R.H., Rosenberg, E.B. and Herberman, R.B., "Immune Reactivity of Leukemia Patients to Autologous Blast Cells." *Cancer Res.* 32:1820-1825, 1972.

11. Gutterman, J.V., Hersh, E.M., McCredie, K.B., et al., "Lymphocyte Blastogenesis to Human Leukemia Cells and Their Relationship to Serum Factors, Immunocompetence, and Prognosis." *Cancer Res.* 32:2524-2529, 1972.

12. Fefer, A., Michelson, E. and Thomas, E.D., "Stimulation of Lymphocytes in Mixed Culture by Cells from HL-A Identical Siblings." *Clin. Exp. Immunol.* 23:214-218, 1976.

13. Invernizzi, G. and Parmiani, G., "Tumour Associated Transplantation Antigens of Chemically Induced Sarcomata Cross Reacting With Allogeneic Histocompatibility Antigens." *Nature* 254:713-714, 1975.

14. Garrido, F., Schirrmacher, V. and Festenstein, H., "Studies on H-2 Specificities on Mouse Tumour Cells by a New Microradioassay." *J. Immunogenetics* 4:15-27, 1977.

15. Parmiani, G. and Invernizzi, G., "Alien Histocompatibility Determinants on the Cell Surface of Sarcomas Induced by Methylcholanthrene. I. *In Vitro* Studies." *Int. J. Cancer* 16:756-767, 1975.

16. Martin, W.J., Gipson, T.G., Martin, S.E. and Rice, J.M., "Derepressed Alloantigen on Transplacentally Induced Lung Tumor Coded for by. H-2 Linked Gene." *Science* 194:532-533, 1976.

17. Bach, M.L., Bach, F.H. and Zarling, J.M., "Pool-Priming: A Means of Generating T Lymphocytes Cytotoxic to Tumour or Virus-Infected Cells. *Lancet* 1:20-22, 1978.

18. Sasportes, M., Dehay, C. and Fellous, M., "Variations of the Expression of HL-A Antigens on Human Diploid Fibroblasts *In Vitro.*" *Nature* 233:332-334, 1971.

19. Martinis, J. and Bach, F.H., "HLA CD Antigen Crossmatching—The Pool Cell-mediated Lympholysis Test." *Transplantation* 25:39-41, 1978.

471

20. Zarling, J.M. and Bach, F.H., "Sensitization of Lymphocytes Against Pooled Allogeneic Cells. I. Generation of Cytotoxicity Against Autologous Human Lymphoblastoid Cell Lines." *J. Exp. Med.* 147:1334-1340, 1978.

21. Sugden, W. and Mark, W., "Clonal Transformation of Adult Human Leukocytes With Epstein-Barr Virus." *J. Virology* 23:503-508, 1977.

22. Hoffman, T. and Kunkel, H.G., "The E Rosette Test." In: *In Vitro* Methods in Cell-Mediated and Tumor Immunity, edited by B.R. Bloom and J.R. David, pp. 77-81, Academic Press, New York, 1976.

23. Zarling, J.M., McKeough, M. and Bach, F.H., "A Sensitive Micromethod for Generating and Assaying Allogeneically Induced Cytotoxic Human Lymphocytes." *Transplantation* 21:468-476, 1976.

24. Golub, S., Svedmyr, E., Hewetson, J., et al., "Cellular Reactions Against Burkitt Lymphoma Cells. III. Effector Cell Activity of Leucocytes Stimulated *In Vitro* With Autochthonous Lymphoma Cells." *Int. J. Cancer* 10:157-164, 1972.

25. Svedmyr, E., Wigzell, H. and Jondal, M., "Sensitization of Human Lymphocytes Against Autologous or Allogeneic Lymphoblastoid Cell Lines: Characteristics of the Reactive Cells." *Scand. J. Immunol.* 3:499-508, 1974.

26. Zarling, J.M. and Bach, F.H., "Alloantigen Induced Enhancement and Suppression, of Human Cytotoxic Lymphocyte Responses to Autologous Lymphoblastoid Cell Lines." *Scand J. Immunol.* 1978, in press.

27. Sondel, P.M., O'Brien, C., Porter, L., et al., "Cell-Mediated Destruction of Human Leukemic Cells by MHC Identical Lymphocytes: Requirement for a Proliferative Trigger *In Vitro*." *J. Immunol.* 117:2197-2203, 1976.

28. Bodmer, W.F., "A New Genetic Model for Allelism at Histocompatibility and Other Complex Loci: Polymorphism for Control of Gene Expression." *Transpl. Proc.* 5:1471-1475, 1973.

29. Silver, J. and Hood, L., "Preliminary Amino Acid Sequences of Transplantation Antigens: Genetic and Evolutionary Implications." *Contemp. Top. Mol. Immunol.* 5:35-68, 1976.

472

Phase I-II Study of Immunotherapy of Malignant Effusions With BCG Cell Wall Skeleton-P3†

Stephen P. Richman[1]
E.M. Hersh[1]
J.U. Gutterman[1]
A. Rios[1]
E.E. Ribi[2]

SUMMARY—Twenty seven patients with 28 malignant effusions were treated with intracavitary BCG cell wall skeleton and trehalose dimycolate attached to mineral oil microdroplets. Toxicity and efficacy were studied over a dose range from 150 to 4500 μg. Response was CR = 11%, PR= 18%, stabilization = 39%, and failure = 32%. Toxicity consisted of fever = 64%, pain = 54% and increase in effusion = 32%. One patient developed liver dysfunction and pulmonary infiltrates, probably as a result of vaccine toxicity.

INTRODUCTION

The demonstration that viable BCG injected into tumor nodules was capable of causing necrosis of the tumor (1) has resulted in efforts to exploit this modality in treating visceral tumor and in efforts to develop nonviable preparations which would have the potential of increased efficacy and decreased toxicity compared with that of the viable parent vaccine. One such preparation is BCG cell wall skeleton (CWS). This is obtained by disruption, proteolytic enzyme digestion, and organic solvent extraction of the intact organism (2). Cell wall skeleton attached to oil microdroplets is active in the suppression of tumor growth in the guinea pig line 10 hepatoma but does not cause tumor regression unless combined with the trehalose dimycolate known as P3 (3). However, in the clinical setting, Yamamura and his associates have demonstrated that CWS attached to mineral oil is capable of causing necrosis when injected into tumor nodules (4). It has prolonged the survival of lung carcinoma patients, when combined with conventional therapy, compared with patients treated with conventional therapy alone (5). In addition, patients with lung carcinoma and malignant pleural effusion treated with intrapleural CWS have a prolonged survival over those treated with conventional therapy alone (5).

Because of its greater activity over CWS alone in the guinea pig hepatoma

[1]Section of Immunology, Department of Developmental Therapeutics, The University of Texas System Cancer Center, M.D. Anderson Hospital and Tumor Institute, Houston, Texas
[2]National Institute of Allergy and Infectious Diseases, Rocky Mountain Laboratory, Hamilton, Montana.
†Supported by PHS grants CA-05831 and CA-14984 and NCI and NIH contract NO1-33888.

system (3), we have chosen to evaluate BCG cell wall skeleton plus P3 (BCG CWS-P3). We have completed a phase I-II evaluation of the activity and toxicity of this material when injected into cutaneous tumor nodules. It is capable of causing tumor necrosis which is manifested histologically by a granulomatous reaction similar to that caused by viable BCG vaccine (6). This paper reports the phase I-II evaluation of this material in the treatment of active malignant pleural and peritoneal effusions in patients with advanced malignancy. The clinical activity and toxicity have been studied over a dose-range from 150 μg to 4,500 μg of CWS-P3.

PATIENTS AND METHODS

All patients had histological proof of malignancy and cytological proof of the presence of a malignant effusion. Criteria for eligibility consisted of the presence of a malignant effusion, refractory to chemotherapy, and recurring after at least one thoracentesis or paracentesis.

Almost all patients were receiving chemotherapy for visceral disease concurrent with this study (see results). Immunotherapy was intercalated between courses of chemotherapy, allowing at least one week from the last dose of chemotherapy until the administration of the vaccine and at least two weeks from vaccine administration to the next dose of chemotherapy to permit initial evaluation of vaccine effects. Patients receiving chemotherapy were called responders to the immunotherapy only when the effusion itself responded and other measurable disease did not.

For patients with pleural effusion, an attempt was made to drain as much of the effusion as possible by needle or catheter. The vaccine was then injected back through the drainage device in 20 to 50 cc of normal saline. The patients then changed position every five minutes for 30 minutes to distribute the vaccine. For patients with peritoneal effusions, no attempt was made to completely drain the effusion. Usually one to three liters were removed, the vaccine was injected in 15 to 20 cc of saline and the patient was directed to change positions as done for pleural effusions. Patients were serially questioned and examined for fever and pain. Fever was considered present when temperature was in excess of 100°F. Pleural effusions were examined by upright and decubitus x-rays. Abdominal effusions were followed by physical examination and abdominal circumference measurements.

A complete response was defined as no recurrence of the effusion following drainage and instillation of the vaccine for at least two months. A partial response was defined as less than a 50% recurrence and stable disease was defined as more than a 50% recurrence followed by stabilization and no further accumulation for at least two months. Some patients experienced a rapid reaccumulation of the fluid within 72 hours following administration

474

of the vaccine (see results). This was interpreted as an inflammatory response to the vaccine, was drained, and did not influence interpretation of the response.

The BCG CWS-P3 was prepared as previously described (3). The components were combined at a concentration of 750 μg of CWS and 750 μg P3 (total 1500 μg)/ml vaccine. The vaccine was stored at 4° C, tested for sterility, and unused portions were discarded after two weeks.

Table 1—INTRACAVITARY CWS-P3.
PATIENT POPULATION

PRIMARY DIAGNOSIS	SITE OF EFFUSION	
	PLEURAL	PERITONEAL
Breast carcinoma	14	3
Adenocarcinoma—Abd. primary	0	4
Sarcoma	1	1
Mesothelioma	1	1
CLL	1	0
Other	2	0
TOTAL	19	9

RESULTS

Twenty-seven patients were treated (Table 1). Eighteen patients had malignant pleural effusion, eight patients had malignant ascites, and one patient had both and was counted twice, giving a total of 28 effusions treated. The majority of patients had breast carcinoma. Twenty-six patients were receiving concurrent chemotherapy or hormonal therapy. Twenty patients had visceral disease in addition to the effusion involving brain, lung, bone, liver and other abdominal organs. Two patients had novisceral disease consisting of nodal or dermal involvement. Nineteen of the 27 patients were women, reflecting the preponderance of breast carcinoma patients.

A dose range between 150 μg and 4,500 μg of CWS plus P3 was studied. For convenience, the patients have been grouped into four dose groups as indicated in Table 2. Patients who received more than one dose are categorized by the highest dose they received. For the 28 effusions, the response rate was complete remission: 11%; partial remission: 18%; stabilization for at least two months: 39%; and failure: 32%. The response rate did not appear to be clearly dose-related. In addition to the clinical responses,

475

Table 2—THERAPEUTIC RESULTS OF INTRACAVITARY CWS-P3

DOSE CWS-P3	RESPONSE				
(µg)	N	CR	PR	STABLE	FAIL
150-300	8	1	1	6	0
600-1000	9	0	2	2	5
1200-1500	8	1	2	3	2
2250-4500	3	1	0	0	2
TOTAL (%)	28	3 (11)	5 (18)	11 (39)	9 (32)

(N = number; CR = complete response; PR = partial response)

a conversion in cytology from consistently positive to negative was seen in seven patients. Three of these patients had a complete response and four had stabilization of disease.

If complete response, partial response, and stabilization are grouped together as "responding patients," the median survival of this group was nine months with a range of 2 to 24+ months. The median survival of the nine patients who failed treatment was one month, with a range of less than one-to-three months.

Toxicity (Table 3) consisted of fever (64% of patients) and serosal pain (54% of patients). Neither form of toxicity was clearly dose-related. In addition to fever and pain, five of the patients with ascites experienced nausea and vomiting and two experienced diarrhea. This was usually of 24 to 72 hours duration. There was a positive correlation between the development of fever and pain and response but this was not significant by Chi square testing. Nine patients experienced increases in their effusion within 72 hours after the treatment which were attributed to the treatment itself rather than to the disease process. Six of these nine later had

Table 3—TOXICITY OF INTRACAVITARY CWS-P3

DOSE CWS-P3				
(µg)	N	FEVER	PAIN	EFFUSION
150- 300	8	6	5	4
600-1000	9	3	3	3
1200-1500	8	6	4	2
2250-4500	3	3	3	0
TOTAL (%)	28	18 (64)	15 (54)	9 (32)

stabilization of their disease with loculation of fluid. One had a partial response and two of these patients failed treatment.

One patient had an unusually prolonged and severe toxic reaction which was attributed to the vaccine. This patient had a prior history of active tuberculosis. His intermediate PPD prior to therapy, however, was negative. He received 4,500 μg intraperitoneally for ascites. Within three days, he developed an elevation in bilirubin, alkaline phosphatase, and SGOT which resolved within one week. The cytology of the effusion converted from negative to positive and CEA levels in the effusion decreased from 539 to 123. In the next month, the effusion resolved but the patient developed fever and bilateral interstitial pulmonary infiltrates. These infiltrates persisted for four months and progressed to the point of causing dyspnea. It was felt that the patient had a hypersensitivity reaction and prednisone 40 mg/day was administered with rapid resolution of the fever and infiltrates. A lung biopsy was not obtained.

DISCUSSION

This study has shown that BCG CWS-P3 can safely be given to cancer patients. Toxicity consisting primarily of fever and pain was similar to that caused by conventional agents. Although the patients treated intraperitoneally did experience nausea and vomiting, this toxicity was transient and no evidence of obstruction developed. A recent report demonstrating the activity of *C. parvum* in the treatment of pleural and peritoneal effusions (8) demonstrated an inflammatory response in the treated cavity but no clinical evidence of obstruction developed in these patients.

Since the patients in this study were receiving chemotherapy concurrent with the CWS-P3, it is not possible to be absolutely certain that the responses observed were due to the vaccine. There is little doubt, however, that there was, at a minimum, a sclerosing inflammatory reaction and that this activity alone would justify a controlled phase II study.

It will probably be necessary in the future to consider separate therapeutic strategies for pleural and peritoneal effusions. It is likely that the optimal treatment for pleural effusion requires complete drainage via a chest tube. However, in the case of peritoneal effusions, fairly large volumes may be necessary to properly distribute the vaccine (7), regardless of the amount of effusion which is first removed. This therapeutic setting is somewhat unusual in that it is one of the few situations in which experimental immunotherapy abuts on some form of standard treatment. In particular, tetracycline (9, 10, 11) has shown a high activity in the treatment of pleural effusion and an acceptable level of toxicity. It will be valuable to determine

477

whether or not the immunotherapeutic agents have an efficacy in this setting comparable to that of the conventional agents, whether or not the mechanism of action is different, and whether or not the therapeutic agent might have a "systemic effect" beyond the local inflammatory effect.

REFERENCES

1. Morton, D.L., Eilber, F.R., Malmgren, R.A. and Wood, W.C., "Immunological Factors Which Influence Response to Immunotherapy in Malignant Melanoma." *Surgery* 68:158-164, 1970.
2. Azuma, I., Ribi, E.E., Meyer, T.J., et al., "Biologically Active Components from Mycobacterial Cell Walls. I. Isolation and Composition of Cell Wall Skeleton and Component P3." *J. Natl. Cancer Inst.* 52: 95-101, 1974.
3. Meyer, T.J., Ribi, E.E., Azuma, I. and Zbar, B., "Biologically Active Components from Mycobacterial Cell Walls. II. Suppression and Regression of Strain-2 Guinea Pig Hepatoma." *J. Natl. Cancer Inst.* 52: 103-111, 1974
4. Yamamura, Y., Yoshizaki, K., Azuma, I., et al., "Immunotherapy of Human Malignant Melanoma With Oil-Attached BCG Cell Wall Skeleton." *Gann* 66: 355-363, 1975.
5. Yamamura, Y., "Immunotherapy of Lung Cancer With Oil-Attached Cell Wall Skeleton of BCG." In *Immunotherapy of Cancer, Present Status of Trials in Man,* edited by Terry, W.D., and Windhorst, D., Raven Press, New York, p. 173, 1978.
6. Richman, S.P., Gutterman, J.U., Hersh, E.M. and Ribi, E.E., "Phase I-II Study of Intratumor Immunotherapy With BCG Cell Wall Skeleton Plus P3." *Cancer Immunol. Immunother.* In press.
7. Rosenshein, N., Blake, D., McIntyre, P.A., et al., "The Effect of Volume on the Distribution of Substances Installed into the Peritoneal Cavity." *Gynecol. Oncol.* 6: 106-110, 1978.
8. Webb, H.E., Oaten, S.W. and Pike, C.P., "Treatment of Malignant Ascitic and Pleural Effusion with *Corynebacterium parvum.*" *Br. Med. J.* 1: 338-340, 1978.
9. Rubinson, R.M. and Bolooki, H., "Intrapleural Tetracycline for Control of Malignant Pleural Effusion: A Preliminary Report." *South. Med. J.* 65: 847-849, 1972.
10. Wallach, H.W., "Intrapleural Tetracycline for Malignant Pleural Effusions." *Chest* 68: 510-512, 1975.
11. Bayly, P.C., Kisner, D.L., Sybert, A., et al., "Tetracycline and Quinacrine in the Control of Malignant Pleural Effusion." *Cancer* 41: 1188-1192, 1978.

Adjuvant Chemoimmunotherapy for Malignant Melanoma

Joseph G. Sinkovics[1]
C. Plager[1]
M. McMurtrey[1]
N.E. Papadopoulos[1]
R. Waldinger[1]
S. Combs[1]
J. Romero[1],
M. M. Romsdahl[1]

SUMMARY—Patients with malignant melanoma received chemoimmunotherapy. Two modalities of immunotherapy were compared: BCG (Chicago) *versus* BCG (Chicago) and allogeneic melanoma viral oncolysates. Two major modalities of chemotherapy were administered: dacarbazine and semustine; or vincristine, actinomycin D and dacarbazine. There appears to be no significant difference in response to the 2 chemotherapeutic modalities; these data will be analyzed elsewhere.

Patients at risk with stage I (primary tumor), II (satellitosis and in-transit metastases) and III B-C (grossly evident regional lymph nodes metastases [B] breaking through the capsule of lymph nodes [C]) were treated after rendered clinically tumor-free surgically. Patients with stage IV (distant visceral metastases) disease were treated with clinically evident disease (except for 2 patients). The median follow-up for this analysis falls between 16 and 22 months. Eighty-one patients were treated with chemotherapy and BCG; 39 patients (48%) are alive without disease. Fifty patients were treated with chemotherapy, BCG and melanoma viral oncolysates; 20 patients (40%) are alive without disease. A trend for slower progression of disease or for longer duration of "no evidence of disease" clinical status for patients receiving chemoimmunotherapy can be recognized in comparison to patients receiving chemotherapy only (or as expected from the natural history of the disease), but administration of melanoma viral oncolysates did not improve results obtained with chemotherapy and BCG. Several patients with expected relapse remain tumor-free after adequate length of chemoimmunotherapy for poor prognosis stage III B-C disease. With stage IV disease, 86% of patients receiving adequate length of chemotherapy progressed eventually; 73% of patients receiving adequate length of chemoimmunotherapy progressed within the same period of observation.

---

[1]Section of Clinical Tumor Virology and Immunology and Solid Tumor Clinics (Service), Departments of Medicine and Surgery, University of Texas System Cancer Center, M.D. Anderson Hospital and Tumor Institute, Houston, Texas.

481

INTRODUCTION

Natural History and Major Prognostic Factors

In the natural history of malignant melanoma there are several well established prognostic factors (1-5). Among the histological subtypes of this tumor, nodular melanoma carries the worse prognosis. The depth of invasion of the primary lesion over Clark's level 3 or Breslow's thickness 1 mm is directly correlated with the incidence of metastases in the regional lymph nodes, and thus survival (Tables 1-3). Prognostication based on levels of invasion as given in Table 1 is applicable to extremity lesions; primary lesions on trunk carry worse prognosis. Large ulcerated primary tumors, tumors invading blood vessels or tumors excised with tumor cells at the surgical margins often disseminate. Melanoma located on trunk, in the head and neck region or in the mucous membranes carries much worse prognosis than melanoma of the extremities. Exceptions exist: melanoma of the sole or subungual melanomas are of bad prognosis. The course of the disease is more malignant in men than in women.

After removal of the primary melanoma (stage I), 18% of patients experience local recurrence such as satellitosis or in-transit metastases close to the primary site (stage II); in 19%, the tumor disseminates (stage IV) through hematogenous routes by-passing regional lymph nodes; 23% will develop regional lymph node metastases (stage III) and 40% remain disease-free (6). Of the 23% with regional lymph node metastases (stage III), 6% will remain-tumor free after surgical dissection, but 17% will have postoperative recurrence or dissemination (6).

When the regional lymph nodes are clinically positive, the 5 year survival rate remains well under 20%. All patients with grossly positive regional lymph nodes eventually die with metastatic melanoma (7). When the regional lymph nodes are only microscopically involved, the 5 year survival rate (not necessarily tumor-free) after surgical dissection is in the range of 50%.

Since the rate of regional lymph node metastases varies from 13 to 59% for Clark's level 4, and from 41 to 75% for Clark's level 5 primary lesion with high mortality for deep lesions (Table 2), patients at high risk can readily be identified at the diagnosis of the primary tumor. Indeed, overall 5 year survival rates for Clark's level 4 and 5 primary melanoma are often set at about 50%, but 2 recent analyses arrived at 15 and 37% survival rates, respectively, for Clark's level 5 primary tumors (4,8).

Advanced disease is difficult to treat. Dacarbazine, actinomycin D, the nitrosoureas, hydroxyurea, mitomycin C, vincristine, cyclophosphamide, 5-fluorouracil and procarbazine alone or in combination can elicit objective tumor response in controlled trials in less than 30% of patients (9). Combination of dacarbazine with various other drugs has not significantly

482

Table 1—LEVELS, THICKNESS, REGIONAL LYMPH NODE METASTASES AND SURVIVAL

Levels	Primary Melanoma			Recurrence and/or Metastases	% Regional Lymph Node Metastases	% Five Year Survival
	Thickness mm	Diameter mm	Surface mm²			
	<0.76	5	6	0		
	>5	>30	40	100		
2					4	100
3					7	88
4					25	60
5					70	15
	0.6-2				9	
	2.1-3				22	
	>3				>39	
	<1					100
	1.1-2					82
	2.1-3					58
	>3					<55

References (1, 2, 3, 4)

Table 2—LEVELS OF INVASION OF PRIMARY MELANOMA AND REGIONAL LYMPH NODE METASTASES

Clark's Levels	% Regional Lymph Node Metastases	
1-2	5-25	
3	5.5-26.1	32
4	12.8-58.6	67
5	40.9-75	66
	(1)	(5)

References (1, 5)

Table 3—PROGNOSTICATION OF PRIMARY MELANOMA AS BASED ON LEVELS OF CLARK

Level	% Mortality	% 5 Year Survival
2	5-8.3	81-100
3	13-35.2	75-100
4	25-46.1	45- 70
5	42.1-88	15- 57

Reference (1)

improved response rate. Newer drugs (peptichemio: hexapeptides of di-2-chloroethyl-amino-1-phenylalanine; maytansine; vindesine: 3-4 dehydrovinblastine; AMSA: 4'-9-acridinyl-amino methane sulfon-m-anisidine; and PALA: N-phosphonacetyl L-aspartate) so far did not offer major improvement in the treatment of advanced disease. Thus, efforts to prevent the advancement of micrometastatic disease to gross stage III or stage IV disease appears to be well justified.

IMMUNOLOGY

Melanoma-specific immunity depends on the existence of tumor-specific antigens. Autologous (individually specific) and allogeneic (shared) melanoma cell surface and cytoplasmic antigens have been recognized (10-12), but clear distinction of these antigens from fetal antigens has not been accomplished (13). However, the melanoma associated antigen could be clearly distinguished from HL antigens (14). Antibodies reacting with antigens derived from cultured melanoma cells occurred in the sera of 84%

of melanoma patients, 66% of sarcoma and carcinoma patients and 8% of controls (15). A solubilized melanoma antigen has been isolated, but fetal cells could absorb antibodies from immune sera reacting with this antigen (16). The excretion in the urine of melanoma-associated antigens in patients with melanoma has been repeatedly demonstrated (17).

Patients with malignant melanoma react with antibody-production and with the generation of cytotoxic lymphocytes to autochthonous and allogeneic melanoma cells. However, these patients also react similarly to tumor cells other than melanoma; and control individuals without malignant melanoma also may react immunologically to melanoma cells. The antibody-mediated immune reactions directed toward melanoma cells include: 1. reactions in immunofluorescence and hemadsorption tests to cell membrane and cytoplasmic antigens; 2. complement-dependent cytolytic antibodies; 3. antibody-antigen complexes blocking lymphocyte-mediated cytotoxicity; 4. antibodies counteracting blocking serum factors (unblocking serum factors); and 5. antibodies potentiating lymphocyte-mediated cytotoxicity or rendering noncommitted lymphocytes cytotoxic to melanoma cells (antibody-dependent, lymphocyte-mediated cytotoxicity) (18-21).

Patients immunized with autologous or allogeneic melanoma cells and BCG develop cross-reacting, melanoma-specific complement-fixing IgG antibodies (22).

Lymphocyte-mediated cytotoxicity may be selective (directed to melanoma cells only) and nonselective (directed to various different histologic types of tumors) (18, 23). Both T and non-T lymphocytes produce cytotoxicity. Lymphocytes of patients with melanoma acquired increased cytotoxity after incubation *in vitro* with cultured autologous or allogeneic melanoma cells (24). These lymphocytes express selective cytotoxicity directed to melanoma cells only; autologous fibroblasts or allogeneic breast carcinoma or sarcoma cells are spared. Lymphocytic infiltration of melanomas has been correlated with better prognosis (25), but this parameter is also known to have failed to correlate with better prognosis (26).

The immunological assessment of patients with early stages of malignant melanoma seldom reveals defects of prognostic significance; in advanced disease delayed hypersensitivity reactions are often decreased, espeically as measured by the *de novo* acquired sensitization to DNCB (27).

"SPONTANEOUS" REGRESSION

This rare phenomenon is considered to be immunologically mediated (28, 29), but endocrine and metabolic mechanisms are also possible. Cutaneous melanomas regress more often than visceral metastases. Primary melanomas may regress, while visceral metastases continue to grow. Two patients attended by us appear to have experienced "spontaneous" tumor regression.

The first patient is a now 59 year old woman (ML, MDAH# 36090) with a melanoma of primary configuration removed from the left scapular region in 1956. Left frontal lobe metastases were surgically removed in April and August, 1960 and in January, 1961. At the last surgery, 50 gm tumor tissue was resected. The patient received perfusion through the internal carotid artery with L-phenylalanine mustard 15 mg 6-times. In 1961 a left axillary lymph node containing metastatic malignant melanoma was removed. All surgical specimens were verified histologically to contain metastatic melanoma. The patient survived without further evidence of tumor growth. In 1969 bilateral carotid arteriograms showed complete occlusion of the left middle cerebral artery with collateral circulation from the left anterior and posterior cerebral arteries (30). There is right-sided hemiparesis and motor dysarthria. The patient raised her children and attends her household chores without help. She is without clinically evident tumors in 1978. She never received systemic chemotherapy or immunotherapy. Her present medication is phenytoin, propoxyphen and chlordiazepoxide.

The second patient is a man (RH MDAH# 103442) now 56 years old who in 1973 developed an anal lesion diagnosed as fistula. The non-healing lesion was biopsied in 1974 revealing an "undifferentiated malignant tumor". The patient had an indurated anal canal and bilateral inguinal lymphadenopathy consisting of 1.5x2 cm firm nodes. In June 1974 he underwent an abdominoperineal resection with colostomy. In July 1974 the right groin was dissected: 10 of 15 nodes were positive for tumor. Both surgical specimens contained "undifferentiated malignant tumor suggestive of amelanotic malignant melanoma" (Figure 1), but electron microscopy failed to reveal melanosomes. The inguinal surgical area became infected with *Serratia liquefaciens* but healed. The chest film, liver and brain scans were negative. The patient returned in September for dissection of clinically highly positive left groin. However, between July and September all enlarged lymph nodes receded and in September he was found to be without clinically detectable disease. He was strongly reactive in skin tests to recall antigens. He remains clinically tumor-free in July 1978.

The lymphocytes of this patient were tested in September 1974 for cytotoxicity in the LabTek chamber/slide assay, as described elsewhere (31, 32), and were found to exert very strong, non-selective cytotoxicity to a battery of established human tumor cell lines (Figure 2). Thereafter, the patient received scarifications with 10^8 Chicago BCG and intracutaneous inoculations of allogeneic melanoma cell viral oncolysates (33) (Figure 2). Both lymphocyte-mediated and antibody-potentiated and lymphocyte-mediated cytotoxicity declined when tested against non-melanoma tumor cells (rhabdomyosarcoma and squamous cell carcinoma of the uterine cervix), but remained highly active when tested against melanoma target cells; in particular, reactions to the allogeneic melanoma cell line with which the

486

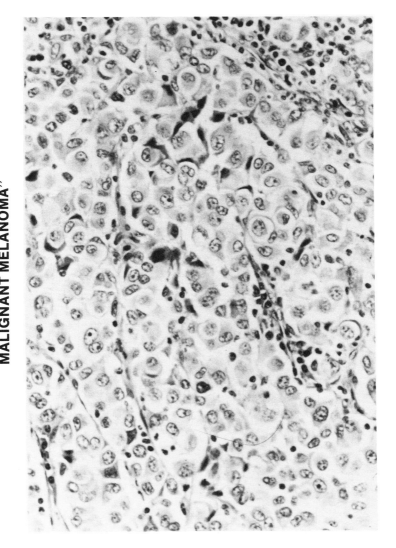

Figure 1—SECTION OF ORIGINAL TUMOR FROM ANAL CANAL INTERPRETED AS
"UNDIFFERENTIATED MALIGNANT TUMOR SUGGESTIVE OF AMELANOTIC
MALIGNANT MELANOMA"

Figure 2—PATIENT CIRCULATED NON-SELECTIVELY CYTOTOXIC LYMPHOCYTES AT THE TIME OF TUMOR REJECTION

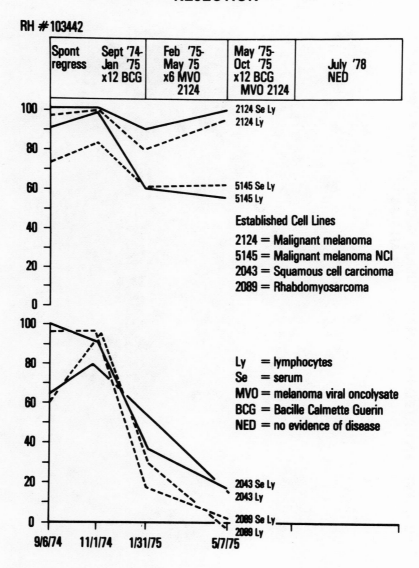

RH #103442

Spont regress	Sept '74-Jan '75 x12 BCG	Feb '75-May 75 x6 MVO 2124	May '75-Oct '75 x12 BCG MVO 2124	July '78 NED

2124 Se Ly
2124 Ly

5145 Se Ly
5145 Ly

Established Cell Lines

2124 = Malignant melanoma
5145 = Malignant melanoma NCI
2043 = Squamous cell carcinoma
2089 = Rhabdomyosarcoma

Ly = lymphocytes
Se = serum
MVO = melanoma viral oncolysate
BCG = Bacille Calmette Guerin
NED = no evidence of disease

2043 Se Ly
2043 Ly

2089 Se Ly
2089 Ly

9/6/74   11/1/74   1/31/75   5/7/75

Non-selective cytotoxicity rapidly subsided. Melanoma cell-directed cytotoxicity persisted. Cytotoxicity was especially strong against the allogeneic human melanoma cell line (#2124) with which the patient was immunized.

488

patient was immunized remained high (Figure 2). These assays indicate that the patient possessed very vigorous "natural killer cell" activity at the time of tumor rejection which rapidly declined despite administration of BCG. Further, this patient could be immunized against an allogeneic melanoma cell line. The assays do not indicate that the patient possessed melanoma-specific immunity at the time of tumor rejection and before immunotherapy. Thus, while it is possible, there is no evidence that tumor-specific immune reactions were responsible for the rejection of this tumor.

DESIGNS OF CHEMOIMMUNOTHERAPY

The design of an effective adjuvant chemoimmunotherapy regimen is very difficult, because of several unknown factors involved. Some of the major unanswered questions are as follows:

1. Is chemotherapy immunosuppressive, so that it may negate the efficacy of immunostimulation? In this context, the 2 major drugs, dacarbazine and the nitrosoureas, were found to be not overtly immunosuppressive: in patients with melanoma, DTIC did not suppress either delayed hypersensitivity reactions to DNCB or to recall skin test antigens or antibody production to Vi antigen or to tetanus toxoid (34). Semustine (methyl CCNU) also spared both cell-mediated and humoral immune reactions in patients with melanoma (35).

2. When interferon is combined with chemotherapy, would the cytostatic effects of interferon alter the chemotherapy-senstivity of the tumor cells? Interferons act as powerful regulators of cell growth. The growth of human osteogenic sarcoma cells and some lymphoblasts is inhibited by human interferons (36, 37). Cell growth inhibition by interferon is selective; for example, elongated (fibroblastic) cells were inhibited more than epithelial cells in cultures of human prostate glands (38). By reducing the growth fraction of tumor cell populations, interferons may also reduce radio- and chemotherapy-sensitivity of tumor cells. By inhibiting desmoplastic (fibroblastic) cells more than epithelial cells, interferons may decrease the size of a tumor nodule but without true antitumor effect. Conceivably, in breast carcinoma where extensive desmoplastic reaction is common, the decrease of the desmoplastic reaction may lead to misinterpretation of the effect as if tumor size reduction were due to true antitumor effect.

When injected directly into melanoma nodules of patients, human interferon was able to elicit tumor size reduction with biopsy-proven lymphocytic reaction (39). This latter effect can be explained by activation of cytotoxic lymphocytes by certain preparations of human interferon. Thus, with caution and moderation in expectations, interferon may possibly be useful as an adjunct to chemotherapy. Because of possible adverse effects, as envisioned above, prospectively randomized trials will be required.

489

3. Is immunotheraphy effective because of its specific antitumor effects or because of activation of macrophages and natural killer lymphocytes without engendering specific antitumor immunity? 4. Would the addition of tumor-specific active immunization intensify the efficacy, if any, of non-specific immunostimulation? The clinical trial reported herein was initiated in seeking answer to this last question.

Previous claims for significant success in prolonging remission in regional or visceral metastatic disease by the use of *nonspecific immunostimulation* have not generally been accepted, mainly because 1. the difference in favor of immunotherapy existed only when treated patients were compared with historical controls; 2. in some trials the response rate of historical controls to dacarbazine was unusually low and thus the response rate to dacarbazine and BCG in the investigated group of patients appeared better, even though this latter response rate was achieved in other trials by dacarbazine alone; and 3. the prospectively randomized trial of the SWOG could not confirm that BCG added any benefits beyond what was achieved by chemotherapy only (40). BCG was ineffective 1. against large, growing tumors; 2. against visceral metastases outside the anatomical region of BCG application; 3. in improving the rate of remission induction when combined with chemotherapy; and 4. in preventing the development of brain metastases (41). In some trials, augmented tumor growth after BCG vaccination is believed to have occurred (42).

In contrast, regression of approximately 65% of intracutaneous metastatic melanomas occurs after intralesional injection of BCG. Regression of injected tumors takes place in 90% of PPD-reactive patients. Occasionally (up to 21%), noninjected lesions may also regress; however, visceral metastases do not regress as a rule (43). A woman with skin metastases experienced complete remission following repeated BCG vaccinations applied at distant noninvolved areas of skin (44). On rare occasions, plumonary metastasis regressed after injection of BCG into skin metastases (45). BCG vaccination of patients after dissection of regional lymph node metastases is claimed to have reduced recurrence rates or prolonged either survival and/or the time interval from surgery to recurrence (46).

Tumor-specific immunization of patients with X-irradiated autologous or allogeneic melanoma cells was claimed to have increased melanoma-directed immune reactions as measured *in vitro* and decreased the level of circulating serum blocking factors (18, 47). An occasional patient thus immunized was observed to show temporary tumor response (48). Further, remissions have been reported in patients with recurrent melanoma treated with purified tumor-specific antigen without or with dacrabazine (49).

The combination of nonspecific immunostimulation with BCG and X-irradiated melanoma cells were first reported to increase the rate of chemotherapy-induced remissions in stage IV disease (47), but without

490

survival benefits (50). In later trials, an alarming trend of tumor growth enhancement in patients immunized with BCG and X-irradiated melanoma cells was observed (42, 51-53).

Adjuvant chemotherapy with dacarbazine alone did not prevent recurrences (54), but either combination chemotherapy (55) or dacarbazine and BCG were claimed to have significantly reduced the rate of recurrent disease (56).

In the original design of the clinical trial reported herein, the following principles were observed:

1. Subcategories of patients in stages I-III with prognostically bad disease would receive chemoimmunotherapy after being rendered surgically tumor-free by clinical criteria.

2. Patients with stage IV disease will have surgically accessible tumors removed and will receive chemoimmunotherapy even when tumor-free state could not be achieved.

3. Dacarbazine and a nitrosurea (semustine) in one regimen; vincristine, actinomycin D and dacarbazine in another regimen will be the major chemotherapeutic modalities. This second regimen originally included also cyclophosphamide, but the protocol was amended in favor of removal of cyclophosphamide.

4. For immunotherapy, Chicago BCG scarified on days 17 and 24 in between courses of chemotherapy spaced at 28 days was chosen. The contents of one amp were scarified in a rotating fashion on the 4 extremities proximally and occasionally on the trunk next to the excised lesion. In addition, into the same lymph node draining area where BCG was scarified, intracutaneous inoculations of melanoma viral oncolysates were given (but injections through scarified areas were avoided in order to prevent slow healing BCG ulcerations). These lysates were prepared from a characterized melanoma cell line #2124 (57). Cell cultures were infected with the PR8 influenza A virus (Figures 3 and 4), were harvested, disintegrated, inactivated with ultraviolet light, stored deep frozen and used after extensive tests for bacteriological sterility (33, 58). Viral oncolysates were chosen because of evidence provided by work with animal tumors that tumor antigens remain highly immunogenic in these lysates (59, 60) and by laboratory assays of immunized patients showing intensification of anti-tumor immune reactions as measured *in vitro* after immunizations with viral oncolysates (33, 60).

5. Patients with stage I disease were to receive treatment for 1 year, patients with all other stages for 2 years. Originally, all patients were to be treated for 2 years (or to relapse and/or progression), but the amended protocol reduced treatment time for patients with stage I disease to 1 year.

6. Patients receiving chemoimmunotherapy and surgically treated control patients were to undergo extensive immunological monitoring, in

491

Figure 3—ESTABLISHED HUMAN TUMOR CELL LINE INFECTED WITH PR8 INFLUENZA A VIRUS

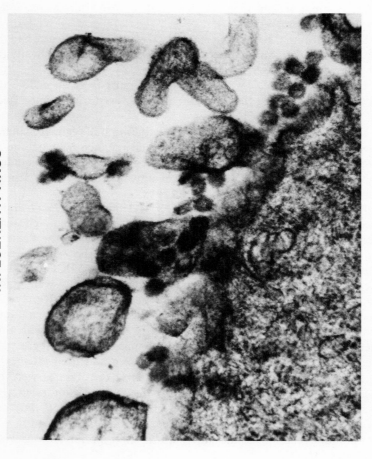

Virus particles are released. Cytopathic effect is minimal. (Electron microscopy was made possible by the generosity of the Lippman Fund).

492

Figure 4—HEMADSORPTION TEST

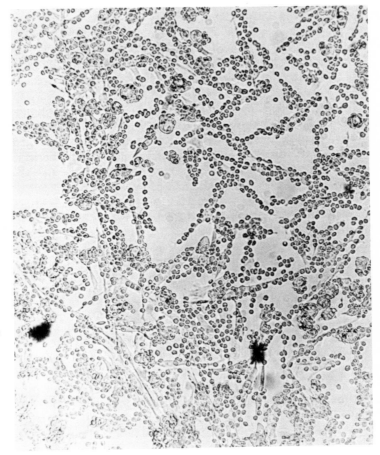

Erythrocytes adhere to elongated cells of melanoma cell line #2124 infected with PR8 influenza A virus. No hemadsorption takes place in un-infected cultures or in cultures pre-treated with anti-influenza virus immune sera (not shown).

particular *in vitro* assays measuring melanoma-directed immune reactions. For the first 3 months only viral oncolysates, for the second 3 month period only BCG and both viral oncolysates and BCG thereafter were to be given, so that immune reactions to each and then to both of these modalities of immunotherapy could be determined (Figure 5). All patients were to be skin tested with recall antigens (purified protein derivative, dermatophytin, mumps, monilia).

7. Patients receiving chemotherapy and BCG were to be compared with patients receiving chemotherapy, BCG and melanoma viral oncolysates. Both groups were to be compared to concurrent and past control patients treated only surgically (stages I-III) or with chemotherapy only (stages II-IV); a few patients who refused chemotherapy would be treated with immunotherapy only.

The trial could not be conducted as designed. No major granting agency provided support. Thus, immune monitoring was done only exceptionally. All patients signed informed consent. Residents of the state of Texas received most often (but not always) the full treatment (chemotherapy, BCG and melanoma viral oncolysates). Out-of-state patients received chemotherapy and BCG, so that shipment of viral oncolysates across state lines was avoided. Some informed patients accepted only parts of the treatment regimen. Others refused to continue either the full chemotherapy part and opted for BCG only, or accepted one chemotherapeutic agent and immunotherapy. Because of lack of funds necessary for the preparation of viral oncolysates, a larger number of patients received chemotherapy and BCG than chemotherapy, BCG and melanoma viral oncolysates. Patients received either BCG only or both BCG and viral oncolysates at the same time.

Patients under observation on the program for more than 6 months are included in the tabulations. The results of this clinical trial were previously analyzed twice before. It appeared that progression of disease was retarded in the groups of patients receiving chemotherapy, BCG and melanoma viral oncolysates (Tables 4-5) (61-63). The present report contains the results of analysis done in July and August 1978. This is an incomplete interim report with median observation time for all patients between 16 and 22 months. It is to be followed by a series of reports up to 5 years or more.

CHEMOIMMOTHERAPY: INTERIM REPORT

Stages I-II Disease

Tables 6 and 7 detail patients who received adjuvant chemiom-munotherapy for stage I disease and Table 8 summarizes the results as of July-August, 1978. In this patient population a few patients had tumors with relatively benign prognosis, but the prognosis was worsened by the fact that

Figure 5—CHEMOIMMUNOTHERAPY REGIMEN FOR MALIGNANT MELANOMA

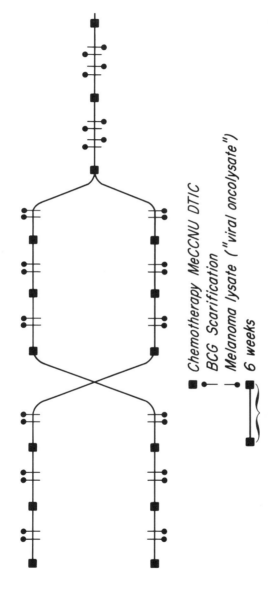

■ Chemotherapy MeCCNU DTIC
• BCG Scarification
| Melanoma lysate ("viral oncolysate")
■ 6 weeks

Immunological monitoring was contemplated before, during and after each modality of immunotherapy (BCG or melanoma lysates) separately and after the combined modalities. In the actual clinical trial time interval between courses of chemotherapy was 28 days; semustine and dacarbazine or vincristine, actinomycin D and decarbazine were given; both modalities of immunotherapy were used together on days 17 and 24; and immunological monitoring of patients was done only exceptionally.

Table 4—PROGRESSIVE DISEASE IN PATIENTS OF ALL STAGES TREATED FOR MALIGNANT MELANOMA

Treatment	Progressors Patients treated		and % of Progressors	
	Oct. '76		Apr '77	
Chemotherapy & BCG	6/12	50%	14/27	52%
Chemotherapy, BCG & MVO	7/28	25%	14/36	39%

References (61-64)

Table 5—PRELIMINARY EVALUATION OF CHEMOIMMUNOTHERAPY REGIMENS FOR MALIGNANT MELANOMA

Treatment	Progressors (Apr '77) Patients Treated	Progressors %
Semustine, dacarbazine, BCG	7/11	64
Semustine, dacarbazine, BCG, MVO	5/14	36
Vincristine, cyclophosphamide*, actinomycin D, dacarbazine, BCG	7/16	44
Vincristine, cyclophosphamide*, actinomycin D, dacarbazine, BCG, MVO	9/22	41

*Omitted from amended protocol; patients who started on full regimen continued without cyclophosphamide. References (61-64).

some of these tumors occurred on the trunk of male patients. These patients with shallow lesions would now be excluded from the amended protocol. Two patients in the chemotherapy, BCG and melanoma lysate group died of widely metastatic disease. These 2 patients do not have matching patients in the chemotherapy plus BCG group. Both patients (E.B. and B.C.) had very deep primary lesions. A patient (E.K.) with a deep lesion also progressed in the chemotherapy plus BCG group, but he could be salvaged by surgical dissection of regional lymph node metastases. Table 9 shows that Clark levels were comparable between the 2 groups, but the thickness of penetration suggests worse prognosis for the group receiving chemotherapy, BCG and melanoma viral oncolysates. Most concurrent control patients treated with BCG only, or held under observation without treatment (Table 10) had shallow and prognostically favorable lesions, thus their clinical

Table 6—PATIENTS WITH STAGE I MALIGNANT MELANOMA RECEIVING CHEMOTHERAPY AND BCG

Patient	Tissue Type	Primary Tumor Site	Clark's Level	Thickness mm	Date	Treatment	State
RA m	SSN	Tr	4	3.1	5/76	VCR (CTX) Act D DTIC BCG 1 1/2 y (16 courses) 5/76-11/77	NED 6/78
TB m	SS	Tr	3	0.9	11/75	MeCCNU DTIC BCG 12/75-12/77	NED 8/78
AB m	N	Tr	3	4	8/76	VCR (CTX) Act D DTIC BCG (16 courses) 9/76-2/78	NED 7/78
AC f	N	Tr	3	2	6/76	VCR (CTX) Act D DTIC BCG 9/76-	NED 7/78
GC m	N	Tr-	4	2	1/78	VCR Act D DTIC BCG 2/78-4/78	NED 8/78
RD m	N	Tr-	4	2.5	1/77	MeCCNU DTIC HU BCG 2/77-1/78	NED 8/78
FD m		Tr	4	2.5	12/75	VCR (CTX) Act D DTIC BCG 1/76-12/77	NED 8/78
AD m	SS	HN	4	1.2	1/77	DTIC BCG 4/77-3/78	NED 8/78
JH m		Tr	4	2.8	9/77	DTIC BCG 11/77-	NED 8/78
OJ f	SS	Tr	3	1	11/75	MeCCNU DTIC BCG 12/75-11/77	NED 6/78
JK m	SS	GU	3	2.5	11/75	VCR Act D DTIC BCG 1/78-	NED 7/78 Ing. Dissect
EK m	N	Leg	4	5	5/76	VCR (CTX) Act D DTIC BCG] 8/7610/76 Progr. St. III 7/77	NED 8/78
JM m	SSN	Tr	4	1.7	9/77	DTIC BCG 11/77-	NED 7/78
EM m	SS	Tr	3	0.7	10/76	VCR Act D DTIC] 1/77-3/77 BCG 1/77-10/77	NED 8/78
CM f	SSN	Tr	3	2	12/76	DTIC BCG 2/77-1/78	NED 8/78
JM m	SSN	HN	3	1.5	8/76	VCR (CTX) Act D DTIC 9/76-1/77] BCG 9/76-	NED 8/78
PS f	N	Tr	3	2	10/76	VCR (CTX) Act D DTIC 1/77-1/78	NED 7/78
GT f	SS	Tr	3-4		1/76	VCR (CTX) Act D DTIC 2/76] BCG 2/76-	NED 4/78
JV m	N	Tr	3	1.4	2/77	VCR (CTX) Act D DTIC] BCG 4/77-11/77	NED 4/78
JW m	SS	Tr	3	0.5	9/76	DTIC BCG 10/76-11/77	NED 8/78

GU = genitourinary tract
] = patient interrupted treatment
f = female
m = male

SS = superficial spreading
N = nodular
Tr = trunk
HN = head & neck

VCR = vincristine
CTX = cyclophosphamide
Act D = actinomycin D
DTIC = dacarbazine
MeCCNU = semustine

HU = hydroxyurea
NED = no evidence of disease

Table 7—PATIENTS WITH STAGE I MALIGNANT MELANOMA RECEIVING CHEMOTHERAPY, BCG AND MELANOMA VIRAL ONCOLYSATES

Patient	Tissue Type	Site	Clark's Level	Thickness mm	Date	Treatment	State
JC m	N	Tr	3	2	5/77	VCR Act D DTIC] BCG MVO 7/77-8/77] BCG 8/77-7/78	NED 7/78
EC m	SSN invasive, margins positive	Tr	4	6	12/75	VCR CTX Act D DTIC BCG MVO 2/76-2/77 Progr: BCNU HU 5FU	Dead 9/77
BC f	N	HN	3	4.5	6/76	VCR CTX Act D DTIC BCG MVO 7/76-10/77 Progr: BCNU HU cis-plat	Dead 3/78
DMcC m	N	Tr	3	2.2	11/76	VCR (CTX) Act D DTIC] BCG MVO 4/77-6/77 BCG 1/77-1/78	NED 7/78
BO f	N	Tr	3	1.8	5/76	VCR (CTX) Act D DTIC BCG MVO 7/76-6/77	NED 7/78
AS f	SS	Tr		0.5	3/76	VCR (CTX) Act D DTIC BCG MVO 5/76-11/76	NED 8/78
CW m	SS	Tr	4	0.8	2/76	VCR (CTX) Act D DTIC BCG MVO 4/76-11/77	NED 7/78
JW m	N deep ulcerated	Tr	5		6/76	VCR (CTX) Act D DTIC BCG MVO 8/76-6/78	NED 7/78

Abbreviations: See Table 6
MVO = melanoma viral oncolysates

498

Table 8—PATIENTS WITH STAGE I MALIGNANT MELANOMA

Treatment Category	Number of Patients	Alive NED	Progressing	Dead with Tumor	Relapsed Interrupted Treatment	Relapsed Adequately Treated
Chemotherapy BCG	20	19	1*	0	1*/4	0/16
Chemotherapy BCG MVO	8	6	0	2	0/2	2/6
——BCG——	6	6	0	0	—	—
Chemotherapy	2	1	1	1	—	—
None (after surgery)	8	7	1†	0	—	—
All	44	39	5	3	1/6	2/22

*Advanced to stage III but rendered surgically NED
†Has stage IV Hodgkin's disease treated with MOPP and XRt

course can not be readily compared with that of the patients receiving chemotherapy. Among the treated tumor-free patients there are several who by current prognostic criteria were expected to relapse: A.B., A.C., G.C., R.D., F.D., J.H., J.K., C.M., P.S. and G.T. in the chemotherapy plus BCG and J.C., D. McC. and J.W. in the chemotherapy, BCG and melanoma lysate group. When compared with "matched historical controls", these patients appear to have so far benefited from the treatment program, but the contribution of immunotherapy, if any, to the effects of chemotherapy can not be determined (see Appendix). These 2 groups contain several newly entered patients. Further analyses will be reported periodically.

Table 9—LEVELS AND THICKNESS OF PRIMARY MELANOMAS OF THE COMPARED GROUPS OF PATIENTS

Treatment	Level*	Thickness*
Chemotherapy BCG	3.4	2.06 mm
Chemotherapy BCG MVO	3.5	3.34 mm
Other (Table 10)	3.0	1.48 mm

*Average

Patients under treatment for stage II disease are few in this trial and have received much diversified modalities of treatment (Table 11). Patients T.K., Y.S., H.S. and T.T. should be listed among those with stage III A disease because their in-transit metastases were farther than 3 cm from the primary lesion. However, they did not have at the beginning of treatment clinically evident regional lymph node metastases. Since all other patients with stage III disease had grossly evident disease in the regional lymph nodes, these 2 groups of patients are analyzed separately.

Stage III Disease

Patients in this category all carry an extremely grave prognosis, because clinically palpable gross disease in the regional nodes of the primary tumor was always present before surgical dissection. In agreement with data in the literature (7), the rate of death with recurrent tumors is close to 100% in this group of patients.

In many cases the capsules of the lymph nodes were broken through and melanoma cells infiltrated the soft tissues in between lymph nodes. These patients should be recognized as of stage III C and at the highest risk for recurrence and distant metastases. Many of these patients certainly had subclinical stage IV disease. Table 12 and 13 give the details of 2 groups of

500

Table 10—PATIENTS WITH STAGE I MALIGNANT MELANOMA RECEIVING NO TREATMENT (AFTER WIDE EXCISION), BCG OR CHEMOTHERAPY

Patient	Primary Tumor					Treatment	State
	Tissue Type	Site	Clark's Level	Thickness mm	Date		
SA f	N	R arm			8/73	—	NED 3/78
JC f	SS	Breast	2	0.8	9/76	—	NED 7/78
CC m		Tr	4	4	11/75	MOPP for stage IV HD	Progr 7/78
JG m	SS	Tr	3	1	5/76	—	NED 8/78
WH m		Tr	2		7/76	—	NED 5/78
RR f	N	R thigh	4	1.4	8/77	—	NED 6/78
VS f	SS	R shoulder	3	0.75	6/76	INH & rifampin for TB	NED 5/78
JW m		Tr	2	0.5	12/75	—	NED 10/77
MB f	SS	Tr	3	0.7	1/77	BCG	NED 7/78
RG f	SS	Tr	3	0.8	11/76	BCG	NED 6/78
Rl m	SS	Tr	3	1.1	1/77	BCG	NED 6/78
DK m	SS	L shoulder	2	0.8	4/78	BCG	NED 8/78
C McN m		HN	invasive (52)		4/75	BCG	NED 8/78
NS f	N	Tr	3	0.8	2/77	BCG	NED 7/78
MH f	N	Tr	3	5	3/76	BCNU HU DTIC	Dead 3/78
LJ f	SS	R arm	4		9/77	DTIC 3 courses	NED 8/78

axilla dissected: negative

INH = isoniozid
MOPP = mechlorethamine, vincristine (oncovin), procarbazine, prednisone
HD = Hodgkin's disease
For abbreviations, see Table

Table 11—LIST OF PATIENTS WITH STAGE II DISEASE

Patient	Primary Tumor		Treatment for Stage II Disease	State
LB m	SSN HN level 3	3 mm 6/77	BCG 8/77	NED 7/78
AH f	SS (ulcer) L leg level 4	1.2 mm 10/76	Perfusion L-PAM Act D 4/77	NED 3/78
Ph f	Seen first with stage II disease (satellitosis)		Perfusion L-PAM TF Levamisole*	LR 7/78
TK m	SSN Tr level 3	2.5 mm 1/77	Excision VCR Act D DTIC BCG MVO 2/77-6/77 Progression: axillary nodes, liver	Dead 12/77
JS m	N Tr	1.5 mm 6/75	VCR Act D DTIC BCG 3/77-6/78 LR excision BCNU HU	NED 7/78
HS f	N L leg level 3	10/74	MeCCNU DTIC] BCG 11/75 LR perfusion L-PAM 1/76 Regional node & distant metastases	Dead 7/77
TT m	N L thigh	9/75	Perfusion L-PAM Act D LR DTIC BCG LR Repeated excisions	Progr 6/78 NED 8/78

*Treated by Dr. L. Spitler, San Francisco, California
LR=local recurrence

patients: those who received chemotherapy plus BCG and those who received chemotherapy BCG and melanoma lysates. After regional lymph node metastases had occurred, it is of little meaning to detail the features of the primary lesion. For sake of simplification, the features of primary lesion have been omitted from these tables. Although the chemotherapeutic regimens varied (semustine and dacarbazine *versus* vincristine, actinomycin D and dacarbazine), there appears to be no difference between these regimens; both contained dacarbazine. Therefore, specific reference to chemotherapeutic regimens have also been omitted from these tables, but differences, if any, between these chemotherapeutic regimens will be analyzed in future reports (Plager, C. et al., in preparation, 1979). The time interval between the primary melanoma and its metastases to the regional lymph nodes may reflect the tumor's growth kinetics and the host-tumor relationship. Therefore, this information has been included in the tables. Patients who failed in these regimens received further treatment with hydroxyurea, 5-fluorouracil, procarbazine, mitomycin C, high-dose (bolus) actinomycin D and dacarbazine, cis-platinum and high dose methotrexate with leucovorin rescue. Responses to these treatment regimens were rare and only partial; no major impact on survival benefits appeared; this information will be analyzed in future reports. This information is irrelevant to the present aim, therefore it will not be given here. However, the time interval between beginning of treatment and failure and the time of death are presented. Table 14 gives an overview of the clinical state of patients with stage III (gross regional lymph node metastases) disease as of July-August, 1978. Table 15 shows time intervals between stages I and III and between beginning of treatment and its failure. It is apparent that invervals between beginning of treatment and its failure are not different for the 2 compared groups. The time for women without recurrent disease is the longest in the chemotherapy, BCG and melanoma viral oncolysate group (over 22 months), but the time interval between stage I and III disease is also the longest in this group (45 months). Thus, this difference may reflect host-tumor relationship rather than significant difference in treatment.

The major aim of the trial, *i.e.* whether or not melanoma cell extracts (antigens) intensify the efficacy of chemotherapy and non-specific immunostimulation with BCG, can be answered in the negative. This trial does not demonstrate any benefit or harm from the addition of melanoma viral oncolysates to the chemotherapy plus BCG regimen. Earlier reports suggested a delay of disease progression in those patients who received chemotherapy, BCG and melanoma viral oncolysates (61-64). After the inclusion of larger numbers of patients and extending the observation period for over 1-1/2 years, this trend is not evident anymore; but surviving patients remain available for further analysis.

Table 12—PATIENTS WITH STAGE III MALIGNANT MELANOMA RENDERED TUMOR-FREE SURGICALLY AND RECEIVING CHEMOTHERAPY AND BCG FOR SUBCLINICAL DISEASE

Patient	Time from Stage I to III	Treatment	State
JB f	6/75-1/77	3/77-	NED 7/78
JB f	6/76-7/76	8/76-11/76) Progr	Dead 3/77
KC m	10/76-10/76	12/76-6/78	NED 8/78
RC f	9/72-11/76	12/76-12/78	NED 8/78
JC m	10/75-2/77	3/77-]	NED 8/78
WC m	2/73-10/75	11/75-]	Dead 6/77
VC f	2/77-8/77	10/77-] BCG—3/78	NED 6/78
CC m	4/75-5/75	6/75-1/76]	NED 8/78
CE m	4/75-12/75	1/76-8/76) Progr	Dead 10/76
MF m	9/75-9/75	1/76-3/76) Progr	Dead 6/76
GG m	3/63-10/76	3/77-6/78	NED 6/78
SH m	5/75-9/77	12/77-6/78) Progr	Progr 6/78
VH m	1/74-12/75	1/76-5/77) Progr	Dead 1/78
HJ m	2/77-2/78	3/78-7/78) Progr	Progr 7/78
RK m	3/77-11/77	12/77-2/78) Progr	Dead 5/78
DK m	1/77-2/77	3/77]	NED* 8/78
DL m	/68-6/76	7/76] Hepatitis	Dead 10/76
		Autopsy: no melanoma	
EL f	4/76-9/77	10/77-	NED 7/78
CMcM m	7/75-8/77	10/77	NED 7/78
MM f	10/72-11/74	4/76-10/76) Progr	Dead 12/76
LM f	9/76-11/77	1/78-	NED 7/78
SM f	-3/76	4/76-10/76) Progr	Dead 2/77
MN f	6/73-9/73	1/75-1/76) Progr	Dead 12/76
CN m	6/76-4/77	6/77-1/78] BCG—4/78	NED 7/78
AR m	5/67-10/74	12/74-12/75 Progr 4/77	Dead 8/77
MR f	5/72-12/77	2/78-	NED 8/78
KR f	9/77-9/77	12/77-	NED 6/78
PS f	11/63-5/74	12/74-11/76	NED 7/78
AS m	5/74-8/76	9/76-2/77) Progr	Dead 4/77
OS m	12/73-11/76	1/75] BCG—11/75	Dead
JS m	5/64-5/77	6/77-11/77) Progr	Dead 3/78
VS f	9/73-11/75	12/75-7/76) Progr	Dead 6/77
WW m	10/76-8/77	9/77-	NED 8/78
DW m	10/76-11/76	1/77-8/77) Progr	NED 7/78

f=female
m=male
]=patient interrupted treatment
)Prog=progression of disease while on treatment

504

Table 13—PATIENTS WITH STAGE III MALIGNANT MELANOMA RENDERED TUMOR-FREE SURGICALLY AND RECEIVING CHEMOTHERAPY, BCG AND MELANOMA VIRAL ONCOLYSATES FOR SUBCLINICAL DISEASE

Patient	Time from Stage I to III	Treatment	State
LB f	6/63-12/75	2/76-9/76]	NED 8/78
NB f	/75-3/77	6/77-	NED 8/78
MB m	-3/76	4/76-6/76]	Dead 2/77
MC f	/65-4/77	6/77-	NED 6/78
MC m	/71-8/75	10/75-5/76) Progr	Dead 11/76
MC f	4/76-6/76	7/76-6/78	NED 7/78
RC m	8/73-6/76	7/76-2/77) Progr	Dead 4/77
WD m	1/74-9/74	11/74-	NED 8/78
RF m	6/74-12/75	2/76-12/77	NED 6/78
MG f	/73-4/77	6/77-7/77] BCG-9/77	Dead 3/78
NG f	12/74-7/76	7/76-10/76) Progr	Dead 11/76
BH m	2/77-3/77	4/77-	NED 6/78
OH m	7/74-8/74	8/74-5/75) Progr	Dead 7/76
JH m	11/75-3/77	7/77-11/77]	Dead 3/78
AK m	-4/74	4/76-8/76) Progr	Dead 12/76
GL f	3/75-4/76	4/76-4/77) Progr	Dead 6/77
GM m	3/76-9/76	10/76-10/77) Progr	Progr 6/78
FP m	7/74-8/76	9/76-12/76]	NED 8/78
BP f	8/74-12/74	4/75-3/76) Progr	Dead 8/76
FP m	5/67-2/74	2/75-12/76) Progr	Progr 7/78
MS f	8/73-1/74	10/75-9/77	NED 5/78
ES m	-8/75	11/75-10/77	NED 7/78
ES m	5/76-7/76	8/76-10/76) Progr	Dead 11/76
LS f	12/71-3/75	3/75-1/76]	Dead 3/77
RT f	7/73-8/76	9/76-8/78	NED 8/78
GT f	12/73-12/76	2/77-4/77]	Dead 8/77
AW m	10/74-8/75	8/75-6/77	NED 6/78
AMcW f	/68-10/75	10/76-10/77	Dead 4/78
FW m	/67-3/75	4/76-3/78	NED 8/78
JY m	12/74-4/76	5/76-8/76) Progr	Dead 11/76
W			

Abbreviations: See Table 12

Table 14—PATIENTS WITH GROSSLY POSITIVE STAGE III DISEASE RECEIVING CHEMOIMMUNOTHERAPY AFTER SURGICAL DISSECTION

Treatment	Patients	Alive		Dead		Progressing in <3 Treatments	Relapsed Inadequately Treated (%)	Relapsed Adequately Treated (%)
		NED (%)	Progressing	with Tumors	without Tumors			
Chemotherapy BCG	34	17 (48.5)	2 16	14	1	2	2/8 4/10	12/24 (50)
Chemotherapy BCG MVO	30	13 (43.3)	2 17	15	0	4	5/7 9/11	8/19 (42)
All	64	30 (46)	4 33	29	1		13/21 (62)	20/43 (46.5)

Table 15—TIME INTERVALS FROM STAGE I TO STAGE III DISEASE, FROM BEGINNING OF TREATMENT TO FAILURE OR FROM BEGINNING OF TREATMENT TO LAST CLINICAL EVALUATION (JULY-AUGUST 1978) FOR NED PATIENTS

Gender of Patients & Treatment		Patients	Stages I→III months	Treatment→Failure months	NED months	Progressors & Dead Patients
Females	Ch BCG	13	29.5	7	16.4+	5/13
	Ch BCG MVO	14	44.9	9.75	22.3+	8/14
Males	Ch BCG	21	35.8	8.4	17.3+	11/21
	Ch BCG MVO	16	24.3	7.3	29.1+	9/16
All	Ch BCG	34	33.4	8	15.9+	16/34
	Ch BCG MVO	30	35	8.4	26+	17/30

Many patients (practically all) in these groups were expected to relapse, if prognostic criteria based on "matched historical controls" and the known natural history of the disease are applied (1, 7). It appears that all tumor-free patients (see Appendix) benefited from the chemoimmunotherapy regimen in as much as they remained alive clinically tumor-free despite very bad prognostic features. However, the contributions of immunotherapy, if any, to the efficacy of chemotherapy, can not be determined. These 2 groups contain several newly entered patients and patients who received only chemotherapy; only BCG; or no treatment other than surgical dissection of positive regional lymph nodes. These patients may serve as a concurrent control group to those shown in Table 14 and will be presented in future tabulations. Further analyses will be periodically reported.

Stage IV Disease

It is estimated that patients with metastatic malignant melanoma live less than 2 years, usually less than 16 months, irrespective of any treatment modality that is currently available. These patients seldom can be rendered clinically tumor-free by surgical procedures. Thus, their chemotherapy or chemoimmunotherapy is not administered in an adjuvant (prophylactic) fashion. Most patients treated in our trial had rapidly advancing visceral disease and failure of treatment was evident in less than 3 months from beginning of treatment, i.e. there was no time to deliver "adequate" treatment, in many. Only 2 patients (Mrs. E.D.M. and Mrs. E.S., see Appendix) were without clinically evident disease at the beginning of treatment; both patients remained in remission. All other patients had evidence for clinical disease. Table 16 summarizes the clinical state of these patients as compared to a third, concurrent group of patients receiving chemotherapy only. All chemotherapy regimens included dacarbazine, either with a nitrosourea, or with vincristine and actinomycin D. For failing patients, hydorxyurea was added. For further failures, several other regimens (as listed in connection with advancing stage III patients) were administered. Response rates were poor and will be analyzed elsewhere (Sinkovics, J.G.: *Proceedings of the Thirteenth International Cancer Congress,* Pergamon Press, London, 1979, in preparation; Plager, C. et al., in preparation, 1979). Differences in survival between the 3 groups of patients as shown in Table 16 are not significant, but smaller numbers of patients succumbed to advancing disease in the chemotherapy plus BCG group, when adequately treated, than in other groups. Table 17 shows that the time interval from beginning of treatment to death was the longest in the chemotherapy, BCG and melanoma viral oncolysate group. Patients with progressing disease appear to live longer in the chemotherapy plus BCG group than in the chemotherapy only group, but this difference is not evident for patients with partial remission or stable disease status. There are no tumor-free patients in the chemotherapy only group.

Table 16—PATIENTS WITH STAGE IV DISEASE RECEIVING CHEMOTHERAPY OR CHEMOIMMUNOTHERAPY

Treatment	Patients	Alive NED	Alive PR/Stable	Alive Progressing	Dead	Progressing & Dead Inadequately Treated	Progressing & Dead Adequately Treated (%)
Chemotherapy BCG	24	2*	3	3	16	6/6	13/18 19/26 (73)
Chemotherapy BCG MVO	11	1*	1	0	9	3/3	6/8
Chemotherapy	19	0	3	5	11	4/5	12/14 (86)

*Two patients treated after rendered surgically NED. One patient treated with bilateral lung matastases and entered complete remission.

Table 17—TIME INTERVALS FOR PATIENTS RECEIVING CHEMOTHERAPY OR CHEMIOIMMUNOTHERAPY FOR STAGE IV DISEASE*

Categories of Response or Lack of Response	Treatment Modalities		
	Ch BCG	Ch BCG MVO	Ch — —
Dead	6.25	12.8	5.1
Progressing	>15.3	—	>4.2
PR/Stable	>9	>14	>14.6
NED	>17	>17	—

*Time, mean in months, from beginning of Treatment to Death, Length of Progressive Disease, Partial Remission or Stable Disease Status and Duration of NED Status.

DISCUSSION

Lymphocyte- and monocyte-macrophage-mediated cytotoxicity as measured against cultured human melanoma target cells appears to correlate directly with the clinical course of malignant melanoma: patients with decreased activity relapsed, patients with increased activity remained in remission (65). While BCG-induced cell-mediated immunity did not always correlate with remission, those patients who failed to express cell-mediated immunity always relapsed (66). Measures aimed at the intensification of cell-mediated immunity have been widely accepted as reasonable and potentially useful in the treatment of malignant tumors. Vaccination with BCG is expected to intensify cell-mediated immune reactions (but in mice, not only macrophages and natural killer cells but also suppressor cells are activated by BCG). In addition, BCG may activate cells of the reticuloendothelial system and thus removal of those antigen-antibody complexes that block cell-mediated immune reactions can be facilitated. Such blocking serum factors are well recognized in advanced malignant melanoma and can be measured also within phagocytic cells, i.e. polymorphonuclear leukocytes (67). Despite these expectations, some laboratory assays failed to demonstrate clearly that vaccination with BCG achieved these favorable effects (68). Nevertheless, the majority of new reports still credit BCG with favorably altering the course of malignant melanoma (69-72), even though this trend is seldom, if ever, shown to be statistically significant in prospectivity randomized trials (73).

Tumor-specific immunization in man remains of unproven value. In itself, it could produce exceptional remissions in patients with melanoma (47, 48), but when combined with nonspecific immunostimulation (46, 69) or with chemotherapy and nonspecific immunostimulation (50, 74), tumor-specific immunization has not, thus far, added significantly to survival.

Better defined human tumor antigen preparations and laboratory assays more reliable than lymphocyte-mediated cytotoxicity (for example: migration inhibition; immune adherence) for the measurement of immune reactions to these antigens are needed. At the clinical level, prospectively randomized trials should compare the value of adjuvant chemotherapy alone, immunotherapy alone, and combined chemoimmunotherapy in prognostically bad stages of malignant melanoma. Deep primary disease on the trunk and head and neck region; and metastatic disease in the regional lymph nodes after surgical dissection form the categories most amenable for this type of treatment. Short term effects on disease progression are of limited value; long-term effects on survival advantage should be evaluated. Should certain modalities of adjuvant chemotherapy become carcinogenic in man, it will be of great value to observe whether or not concomitant immunotherapy will have reduced the rate of this complication.

The clinical trial reported herein is incomplete. It indicates benefit in terms of relapse-free survival for some patients at high risk with prognostically bad disease. However, these patients are compared to historical controls and their poor prognosis is based on the known natural history of the disease. These benefits are especially impressive in many patients with grossly evident stage III disase. Practically all patients in this category have subclinical stage IV disease and long tumor-free survival in this category is practically unknown. All patients with stage III disease in this trial fall in this category. Within this short observation period, there appears to emerge a sizeable number of patients who remain alive relapse-free despite expectations to the contrary. It is not possible to determine the contribution of BCG to this effect; chemotherapy might have achieved this effect alone. A great disavantage of this trial is that no funds were provided for the laboratory monitoring of these patients. However, it is possible to state that the addition of allogeneic melanoma cell lysates (in the form of viral oncolysates) has not significantly improved the response rate to chemotherapy and BCG within the time limits of this analysis.

The treatment of most patients with stage IV disease was not of adjuvant modality in as much as most of these patients had rapidly advancing clinically evident tumors. Time intervals from beginning of treatment to death and length of survival with progressing disease were longer for patients receiving chemoimmunotherapy than for patients receiving chemotherapy only (Table 17).

Table 18 summarizes for all stages the 2 compared groups of patients who received chemoimmunotherapy. There is no evidence that the administration of melanoma viral oncolysates improved response rate. The delay in disease progression reported at the time of earlier analyses (Tables 4 and 5) is evident now as a trend only; there is no significant gain at this point of analysis from the administration of melanoma viral oncolysates.

510

Table 18—SUMMARY OF PATIENTS OF ALL STAGES RECEIVING TWO MAJOR MODALITIES OF CHEMOIMMUNOTHERAPY

Stage	Treatment	Patients	NED (%)	Alive PR/Stable	Progressing (%)	Dead (%)
I	Ch BCG	20	19	0	1	0
	Ch BCG MVO	8	6	0	0	2
II	Ch BCG	3	1	0	1	1
	Ch BCG MVO	1	0	0	0	1
III	Ch BCG	34	17	0	2	15
	Ch BCG MVO	30	13	0	2	15
IV	Ch BCG	24	2	3	3	16
	Ch BCG MVO	11	1	1	0	9
All	Ch BCG	81	39 (48)	3	7 39 (48)	32
	Ch BCG MVO	50	20 (40)	1	2 29 (56)	27

This trial may be comparable with the British chemoimmunotherapy trial for acute myelogenous leukemia where early analyses indicated retardation of disease progression for patients receiving chemotherapy, BCG and active tumor-specific immunization with leukemic cells, but after 2 years of follow-up this difference was not evident anymore (75).

APPENDIX

Selected Case Histories

Case 1. PAS, female (born 1938) had nodular malignant melanoma, Clark level 4, thickness 2 mm excised from her back in 1976. From January 1977 to January 1978 she received 12 courses of chemotherapy (vincristine 1 mg, actinomycin D 1.5 mg and dacarbazine 2450 mg per course) and 24 BCG (Chicago) scarifications. She remains tumor-free in July 1978. *Comment:* Longer observation is warranted; this primary melanoma was expected to metastasize to axillary lymph nodes, but within the period of 2 years no such metastases occurred.

Case 2. DEMcC, male (born 1945) developed nodular malignant melanoma, Clark level 3, thickness 2.2 mm on his trunk in 1976. After wide excision, chemotherapy was given with vincristine 2 mg on day 1, cyclophosphamide 925 mg on day 2, actinomycin D 0.37 mg daily on days 1-5 and dacarbazine 460 mg daily on days 1-5. After 3 courses (April, May, June, 1977), the patient interrupted treatment, but accepted the continuation of immunotherapy with BCG (Chicago) and allogeneic melanoma viral oncolysates. Immunotherapy was given from April 1977 to January 1978, twice monthly. Patient remains tumor-free in July, 1978. *Comment:* This primary melanoma was expected to metastasize rapidly, but no metastases occurred. Longer observation is recommended.

Case 3. OB, male (born 1932) developed nodular malignant melanoma on the trunk in 1976; the tumor penetrated to Clark level 3 and its thickness was 1.8 mm. After wide excision, patient received chemotherapy (vincristine 2 mg on day 1, actinomycin D 0.5 mg daily on days 3, 4 and 5 and dacarbazine 500 mg daily on days 1-5) and immunotherapy with BCG (Chicago) and allogeneic melanoma viral oncolysates. He received 10 courses of chemotherapy and 20 immunizations from July 1976 to June 1977. He remains tumor-free in July 1978. *Comment:* this tumor was expected to have spread to regional lymph nodes, but no metastases are detectable. Longer observation is warranted.

Case 4. JLW, male (born 1957) developed malignant melanoma in a birthmark on his trunk in 1976; the tumor invaded the dermis and residual tumor was found in the cicatrix at wide excision. Patient began chemotherapy (vincristine 2 mg on day 1, actinomycin D 0.5 mg daily days 1-5, dacarbazine 425 mg daily days 1-5) and immunotherapy (Chicago BCG and allogeneic melanoma viral oncolysates on days 17 and 24) in August

1976. He received 13 courses of chemotherapy and 41 immunizations. Patient remains tumor-free in July 1978. *Comment:* This was a deeply invasive primary tumor with high probability of subclinical spread at the beginning of chemoimmunotherapy. Longer observation is warranted.

Case 5. MS, female (born 1925) had primary malignant melanoma excised from her left arm in 1973. Developed left axillary metastases in 1974. After excision, left axillary metastases recurred in 1975. Tumor cells were found in between lymph nodes in fibroadipose tissue. From October 1975 to September 1977 the patient received 18 courses of chemoimmunotherapy at about 6 weeks intervals with semustine 175 mg on day 1 and dacarbazine 425 mg daily days 1-5 and BCG (Chicago) and allogeneic melanoma viral oncolysates on days 17 and 24. She remains tumor-free in July 1978. *Comment:* Extremely poor prognosis was predicted for this patient. Even though she is approaching the end of her 3rd year tumor-free, longer observation is warranted.

Case 6. MC, female (born 1927) developed a 6 mm thick primary malignant melanoma on the right side of her neck in 1976. Metastases to right neck and parotid lymph nodes developed in the same year and were dissected. From July 1976 to June 1978 patient received 24 courses of chemotherapy (vincristine 2 mg day 1, cyclophosphamide 950 mg day 2, actinomycin D 0.4 mg daily days 1-5 and dacarbazine 500 mg daily days 1-5) and 48 immunizations with BCG (Chicago) and allogeneic melanoma viral oncolysates. She remains tumor-free in July 1978. *Comment:* Extremely poor prognosis was predicted for this patient whose stage I disease rapidly advanced to stage III in 1976. Her 2 year tumor-free state is an excellent result but clearly longer follow-up is needed.

Case 7. JS, male (born 1900) developed primary malignant melanoma on left chest wall penetrating to Clark level 4 in 1970. In 1975 multiple left axillary and supraclavicular lymph node metastases developed, despite BCG (Chicago) scarifications. Patient received semustine 150 mg day 1 and dacarbazine 360 mg daily days 1-3 in 7 courses at monthly intervals with complete regression of lymph node metastases. In 1976 patient refused further chemotherapy. Shortly thereafter he died with recurrent disease. *Comment:* The lymph node metastases were not biopsied for histological proof but were clincally positive for tumor. Rapid recurrence and death after discontinuation of chemotheraphy is proof that chemotherapy alone was effective in this case to contain disease.

Case 8. FW, male (born 1904) developed superficial spreading type malignant melanoma penetrating to Clark level 3 and thickness 0.8 mm in his right upper arm in 1967. In 1975 metastases occurred in subcutaneous tissues and lymph nodes of right axilla. At dissection, 18 of 36 lymph nodes were positive. Patient received chemoimmunotherapy from April 1976 to March 1978 with dacarbazine 480 mg daily days 1-5 at monthly intervals and BCG (Chicago) scarifications with allogeneic melanoma viral on-colysates on days 17 and 24 of each course. At the same time, patient received 5 mg diethylstilbestrol daily for stage C prostatic carcinoma. In August 1978 he was stable with prostatic carinoma and tumor-free with melanoma. *Comment:* Hormone-sensitivity of melanoma is a possible contributing factor to the good result; for example, abstract C-113 of the 1978 ASCO Meeting (American Society for Clinical Oncology) contains information concerning estrogensensitivity of human melanoma.

Case 9. TC, male (born 1910) had a large left temporal tumor resected repeatedly in 1973-7. The area received radiotherapy with 5000 r plus 1500 r with 11 MEV electrons. In 1975 cervical lymph node metastases developed. After neck dissection, patient received further radiotherapy (5600 r with 18 MEV electrons and photons and 5500 r with 7 MEV electrons). In 1976 lung metastases developed. By light microscopy, this tumor was thought to be a "neurogenic" sarcoma. Electron microscopy equivocally showed abundant melanosomes. The tissue diagnosis was revised to malignant melanoma, "sarcomatoid" subtype. Patient receives chemoimmunotherapy since May 1977 with vincristine, cyclophosphamide, actinomycin D, dacarbazine, BCG (Chicago) and allogeneic melanoma viral oncolysates. He is alive with partial remission (or stable disease) in July 1978. *Comment:* This most unusual case of sarcomatoid melanoma will be reported elsewhere with illustrations of histology and chest films.

Case 10. EDM, female (born 1917) had "nevi" removed from her nose in 1959. In 1969 metastatic malignant melanoma was excised from the nasal cavity. In 1976 metastatic malignant melanoma was excised from a lymph node in the left arm. From October 1976 to June 1978 patient received chemoimmunotherapy (vincristine, actinomycin D, dacarbazine and BCG) and remains NED in July 1978. *Comment:* Head and neck malanoma carries bad prognosis but the naturally slow progression of the patient's disease warrants much longer observation.

Case 11. Mr. EG (born 1948) had a "lesion" at right calf in 1975-6 which spontaneously regressed. Patient developed large fist-sized palpable right inguinal lymph node metastasis of an unclassifiable malignant neoplasm, probably amelanotic malignant melanoma. The right groin received radiotherapy with 7000 r in a twice daily treatment schedule with regression of the metastatic tumor. The patient had multiple bilateral pulmonary metastases. He received chemotherapy with vincristine 2 mg on day 1, actinomycin D 0.5 mg daily on days 1-5, decarbazine 500 mg daily on days 1-5 and hydroxyurea 1 gm daily on days 1-3; BCG (Chicago) was scarified on days 17 and 24. This regimen was repeated monthly (every 28 days) beginning in December 1977 and continuing in August 1978 (9 courses). After the third course, all pulmonary metastases regressed. Patient remains in complete remission and continues the same regimen. *Comment:* Tissue diagnosis of

514

melanoma has not been firmly established, but amelanotic malignant melanoma remains the most likely category for this tumor. This patient remains in complete remission early in 1979. The value of this regimen is documented further in the next case.

Case 12. JE, female (born 1923) had nodular melanoma removed from right leg in 1977. Local recurrences necessitated re-excisions, perfusion with melphalan and finally amputation in 1978. Later in 1978 patient was admitted with metastases in stomach, small intestine, liver, lungs and bone marrow. She had urinary tract infection with *E. coli* and septicemia with *Staphylococcus aureus*. Disseminated intravascular coagulation developed with platlets 63,000/mm³, prothrombin time > 100 sec, fibrinogen 54 mg% and fibrin split products 422 μg/ml. Vitamin K, fresh frozen plasma and oxacillin were given with platelet count rising to 186,000/mm³ and other values normalizing (prothrombin time 12 sex, fibrinogen 130 mg%, fibrin split products 87 μg/ml. Chemotherapy consisted of vincristine 2 mg on day 1; actinomycin D 0.5 mg daily on days 1-5; dacarbazine 300 mg daily on days 1-5; and hydroxyurea 1 gm daily for 5 days. Abdominal masses rapidly decreased in size and lungs cleared. Liver scans documented decrease in size of metastases. After 4 courses early in 1979, patient has no blood in stool, remains in excellent nutritional state, restores her blood count promptly after chemotherapy, her chest film is negative for metastases, the size of the liver is normal with small residual metastatic nodules shown by scan. She achieved partial remission and continues the same chemotherapy with increased doses of dacarbazine (500 mg per day x 5) within each course at 28 days intervals. *Comment:* This newly acquired patient has not been included in the tabulations. Her case shows that the regimen used may be drastically effective for certain patients with stage IV disease.

ACKNOWLEDGMENTS

Supported by Kelsey-Leary Foundation, Don & Sybil Harrington Foundation and the Baker and Taylor Drilling Co. of Texas. The authors are grateful to K. Hill and Z. Mouton for secretarial assistance and to D. Gaines for laboratory assistance. Dr. D. Groschel performed bacteriological sterility assays of viral oncolysates. Dr. R. Crispen evaluated the original design of this trial and contributed advice and support.

REFERENCES

1. Veronesi, U., Bajetta, E., Cascinelli, N., et al., "New Trends in the Treatment of Malignant Melanoma." *International Advances in Surgical Oncology* 1:113-156, 1978.
2. Breslow, A., "Problems in the Measurement of Tumor Thickness and Level of Invasion in Cutaneous Melanoma." *Human Pathology* 8:1-2, 1977.
3. Breslow, A., "Tumor Thickness, Level of Invasion and Node Dissection in Stage I Cutaneous Melanoma." *Ann. Surg.* 182:572-575, 1975.
4. Wanebo, H.J., Woodruff, J. and Fortner, J.G., "Malignant Melanoma of the Extremities: A Clinicopathological Study Using Levels of Invasion (Microstage)." *Cancer* 35:666-676, 1975.
5. Holmes, E.C., Clark, W., Morton, D.L., et al., "Regional Lymph Node Metastases and the Level of Invasion of Primary Melanoma." *Cancer* 37:199-201, 1976.
6. DeVita, V.T. and Fisher, R.I., "Natural History of Malignant Melanoma as Related to Therapy." *Cancer Treatm. Rep.* 60:153-157, 1976.
7. Geelhoed, G.W., Breslow, A. and McCune, W.S., "Malignant Melanoma: Correlation of Long-Term Follow-Up with Clinical Staging, Level of Invasion and Thickness of Primary Tumor." *Am. Surg.* 43:77-85, 1977.
8. Davis, N., McLeod, R., Beardmore, G., et al., "The Henry Joseph Windsor Lecture: Melanoma is a Word, not a Sentence." *Austral. New Zealand J. Surg.* 46:188-196, 1976.
9. Sinkovics, J.G., *Medical Oncology, an Advanced Course,* Marcel Dekker, New York, 1979 (in press).
10. Shiku, H., Takahashi, T., Oettgen, H.F. and Old, L.J., "Cell Surface Antigens of Human Malignant Melanoma." *J. Exp. Med.* 1-4:873-881, 1976.
11. Roth, J.A., Holmes, E.C., Resifeld, R.A., et al., "Isolation of a Soluble Tumor-Associated Antigen from Human Melanoma." *Cancer* 37:104-110, 1976.
12. Kerney, S.E., Montague, P.M., Chretien, P.B., et al., "Intracellular Localization of Tumor-Associated Antigens in Murine and Human Malignant Melanoma." *Cancer Res.* 37:1519-1524, 1977.
13. Siebert, E., Sorg, C., Hopple, R. and Macher, E., "Membrane Associated Antigens of Human Malignant Melamona. III. Specificity of Human Sera Reacting with Cultured Melanoma Cells." *Internat. J. Cancer* 19:172-178, 1977.
14. McCabe, R.P., Ferrone, S., Pellegrino, M.A., et al., "Purification and Immunologic Evaluation of Human Melamona-Associated Antigens." *J. Nat. Cancer Inst.* 60:773-777, 1978.
15. Grimm, E.A., Silver, H.K.B., Roth, J.A., et al., "Detection of Tumor-Associated Antigen in Human Melanoma Cell Line Supernatants." *Internat. J. Cancer* 17:559-564, 1976.
16. Bystryn, J.C. and Smalley, J.R., "Identification and Solubilization of Iodinated Cell Surface Human Melanoma-Associated Antigens." *Internat. J. Cancer* 20:165-172, 1977.
17. Volkers, C., Cooke, K., Bennett, C. and Whitfield, P., "Urinary Melanoma Antigen Exretion." Abstracts in *Internat. Cancer Research,* Data Bank Series CB05 No. 6, P. 9, abstract 37, June, 1978.
18. Sinkovics, J.G. and Harris, J.E., In *The Immunology of Malignant Disease.* pp. 471-479 and p. 526, C.V. Mosby, St. Louis, 1976.
19. Embleton, M.J., Ransom, J.H. McIllmurray, M.B. and Reeves, W.G., "Immunological Monitoring in a Controlled Trial of Immunotherapy in Stage II B Malignant Melanoma." *Brit. J. Cancer* 37:497-504, 1978.
20. Hershey, P., Edwards, A., Milton, G.W. and McCarthy, W.H., "Relationship of Cell-Mediated Cytotoxicity Against Melanoma Cells to Prognosis in Melanoma Patients." *Brit. J. Cancer* 37:505-513, 1978.
21. Murray, E., Ruygrok, S., Milton, G.W. and Hershey, P., "Analysis of Serum Blocking

516

Factors Against Leukocyte-Dependent Antibody in Melanoma Patients." *Internat. J. Cancer* 21:578-587, 1978.

22. Leong, S.P.L., Sutherland, C.M. and Krementz, E.T., "Immunofluorescent Detection of Common Melanoma Membrane Antigen by Sera of Melanoma Patients Immunized Against Autologous or Allogeneic Cultured Melanoma Cells." *Cancer Res.* 37:4035-4042, 1977.

23. Thota, H., Sinkovics, J.G., Carrier, S.K., et al., "Cytotoxic Lymphocytes. III. Cross-reactions Between Melanoma and Sarcoma Cells as Expressed by Lymphocytes and Serum Factors of Patients with Melanoma and Sarcoma and of Normal Healthy Donors." *Pigment Cell,* edited by, V. Riley, Karger, Basel, 2:124-133, 1976.

24. Golub, S.H. and Morton, D.L., "Sensitization of Lymphocytes *in vitro* Against Human Melanoma-Associated Antigens." *Nature* 251:161-163, 1974.

25. Smith, J.L., Jr., "Histopathology and Biologic Behavior of Malignant Melanoma." In *Neoplasms of the Skin and Malignant Melanoma.* Year Book Medical Publishers, Chicago, pp. 293-330, 1976.

26. Beardmore, G.L., Quinn, R.L. and Little, J.H. "Malignant Melanoma in Queensland: Pathology of 105 Fatal Cutaneous Melanomas." *Pathology* 2:277-286, 1970.

27. Lui, V.K., Karpuchas, J., Dent, P.B., et al., "Cellular Immunocompetence in Melanoma: Effect of Extent of Disease and Immonotherapy." *Brit. J. Cancer* 32:323-330, 1975.

28. Bulkley, G.B., Cohen, M.H., Banks, P.M., et al., "Long Term Spontaneous Regression of Malignant Melanoma with Visceral Metastases." *Cancer* 36:485-494, 1975.

29. Bodurtha, A.J., Berkelhammer, J., Kim, Y.H., et al., "A Clinical Histologic and Immunoglic Study of a Case of Metastatic Melanoma Undergoing Spontaneous Remission." *Cancer* 37:735-742, 1976.

30. McNeel, D.P. and Leavens, M.E., "Long-term Survival with Recurrent Metastatic Intracranial Melanomia." *J. Neurosurg.* 29:91-93, 1968.

31. Sinkovics, J.G., "Monitoring *in vitro* of Cell-mediated Immune Reactions to Tumors." *Methods in Cancer Research,* H. Busch, editor, p. 107-175, 1973.

32. Kay, H.D., Thota, H. and Sinkovics, J.G., "A Comparative Study on *in vitro* Cytotoxic Reactions of Lymphocytes from Normal Donors and Patients with Sarcomas to Cultured Tumor Cells." *Clin. Immun. Immunopathol.* 5:218-234, 1976.

33. Sinkovacs, J.G., Loh, K.K. and Shullenberger, C.C., "Use of Viral Oncolysates for Tumor-Specific Immunotherapy in Man." In *Modulation of Host Immune Resistance in the Prevention or Treatment of Induced Neoplasias,* Fogarty International Center, Bethesda, Maryland, pp. 235-236, 1977.

34. Bruckner, H.W., Mokyr, M.B. and Mitchell, M.S., "Effect of Imidazole-4-Carboxamide 5-(3, 3-dimethyl-l-triazeno) on Immunity in Patients with Melanoma." *Cancer Res.* 34:181-183, 1974.

35. Berd, D., Wilson, E., Bellet, R.E. and Mastrangelo, M.J., "Methyl CCNU Adjuvant Chemotherapy of Malignant Melanoma is not Immunosuppressive." *Proc. 14th Ann. Meet. Am. Assoc. Clin. Oncol.* 19:349, 1978.

36. Strander, H., Cantell, K., Ingimarsson, S., et al., "Interferon Treatment of Osteogenic Sarcoma: A Clinical Trial." In *Modulation of Host Immune Resistance in the Prevention or Treatment of Induced Neoplasis,* Fogarty International Center, Bethesda, Maryland, pp. 377-381, 1977.

37. Hilfenhaus, J. and Karges, H.E., "Growth Inhibition of Human Lymphoblastoid Cells by Human Interferon Preparations." In *Molecular Base of Malignancy,* E. Deutsch, K. Moser, H. Rainer and A. Stacher, editors, Georg Thieme, Stuttgart, pp. 73-79, 1976.

38. Job, L. and Horoszewicz, J.S., "Differential Effects of Interferon on Human Prostatic Fibroblasts and Epithelial Cells." *Am. Assoc. Cancer Res.* 18:205, 1977.

39. Check, W., "Immunoadjuvants in Cancer Therapy: Some Benefits, Many Questions." *JAMA* 239:1945-1947, 1978.

40. Costanzi, J.J., "Chemotherapy and BCG in the Treatment of Disseminated Melanoma." *Am. Assoc. Cancer Res.* 18:114, 1977.

41. Grooms, G.A. Eilber, F.R. Morton, D.L., "Failure of Adjuvant Immunotherapy to Prevent Central Nervous System Metastases in Malignant Melanoma Patients." *J. Surg. Oncol.* 9:147-153, 1977.

42. Gerner, R.E. and Moore, G.E., "Feasibility Study of Active Immunotherapy in Patients with Solid Tumors." *Cancer* 38:131-143, 1976.

43. Mastrangelo, M.J., Berd, D., Bellet, R.E., "Critical Review of Previously Reported Clinical Trials of Cancer Immunotherapy with Nonspecific Immunostimulants." *Ann. New York Acad. Sci.* 277:94, 1976.

44. Coates, A.S. and Peters, M., "Complete Remission of Metastatic Malignant Melanoma Following Immunotherapy with Bacillus Calmette-Guerin (BCG): Report of a Case." *Austral. New Zealand J. Surg.* 47:362-365, 1977.

45. Mastrangelo, M.J., Bellet, R.E., Berkelhammer, J. and Clark, W.H., "Regression of Pumonary Metastatic Disease Associated with Intralesional BCG Therapy of Intracutaneous Melanoma Metastases." *Cancer* 36:1305-1308, 1975.

46. Eilber, F.R. Morton, D.L., Holmes, E.C., et al., "Adjuvant Immunotherapy with BCG in Treatment of Regional Lymph Node Metastases From Malignant Melanoma." *New England J. Med.* 294:237-240, 1976.

47. Currie, G.A., McElwain, T.J., "Active Immunotherapy as an Adjuvant to Chemotherapy in the Treatment of Disseminated Malignant Melanoma: A Pilot Study." *Brit. J. Cancer* 31:143-156, 1975.

48. Laucius, J.F., Bodurtha, A.J., Mastrangelo, M.J. and Bellet, R.E., "A Phase II Study of Autologous Irradiated Tumor Cells Plus BCG in Patients with Metastatic Malignant Melanoma." *Cancer* 40:2091-2093, 1977.

49. Arlen, M., Hollinshead, A. and Scherer, J., "Tumor-Specific Immunity in Patients with Malignant Melanoma." *Surgical Forum* 28:168-169, 1977.

50. Newlands, E.S., Don, C.J., Roberts, J.T., "Clinical Trial of Combination Chemotherapy and Specific Active Immunotherapy in Disseminated Melanoma." *Brit. J. Cancer* 34:174-179, 1976.

51. McIllmurray, M.B., Embleton, M.J., Reeves, W.G. et al., "Controlled Trial of Active Immunotheraphy in Management of Stage II B Malignant Melanoma." *Brit. Med. J.* 1:540-542, 1977.

52. Embleton, M.J., Ransom, J.H., McIllmurray, M.B. and Reeves, W.G., "Immunological Monitoring in a Controlled Trial of Immunotherapy in Stage II B Malignant Melanoma." *Brit. J. Cancer* 37:497-504, 1978.

53. Hedley, D.W., McElwain, T.J. and Currie, G.A., "Specific Active Immunotherapy Does Not Prolong Survival in Surgically Treated Patients with Stage II B Malignant Melanoma and May Promote Early Recurrence." *Brit. J. Cancer* 37:491-496, 1978.

54. Hill, G.J., Moss, S., Fletcher, W. et al., "DTIC Melanoma Adjuvant Study: Final Report." *Am. Soc. Clin. Oncol.* 19:309, 1978.

55. Banzet, P., Jacquillat, C. Civatte, J., et al., "Adjuvant Chemotherapy in the Management of Primary Malignant Melanoma." *Cancer* 41:1240-1248, 1978.

56. Wood, W.C., Cosimi, A.B., Carey, R.W. and Kaufman, S.D., "Randomized Trial of Adjuvant Therapy for "High Risk" Primary Malignant Melanoma." *Surgery* 83:677-681, 1978.

57. Sinkovics, J.G., Gyorkey, F., Kusyk, C. and Siciliano, M., "Growth of Human Tumor Cells in Established Cultures." *Methods in Cancer Research* 14:243-323, 1978.

58. Romero, J.J., Sinkovics, J.G., Plager, C., et al., "Preparation and Immunogeneic Value of Viral Oncolysates for the Immunotherapy of Human Tumors." *Am. Soc. Microbiol.* p. 85, 1977.

59. Sinkovics, J.G., "Immunotherapy of Human Tumors." *Pathobiology Annual* 8:241-284, 1978.

518

60. Cassel, W.A., Murray, D.R., Torbin, A.H., et al., "Viral Oncolysate in the Management of Malignant Melanoma. I. Preparation of the Oncolysate and Measurement of Immunologic Responses." *Cancer* 40:672-679, 1977.

61. McMurtrey, M.J., Campos, L.T., Sinkovics, J.G., et al., "Chemoimmunotherapy for Melanoma: Preliminary Clinical Data and Difficulties with *in vitro* Monitoring of Tumor-Specific Immune Reactions." In *Neoplasmas of the Skin and Malignant Melanoma,* Year Book Medical Publ., Chicago, pp. 471-484, 1976.

62. Sinkovics, J.G., Plager, C., McMurtrey, M.J., et al., "Viral Oncolysates for the Immunotherapy of Human Tumors." *Am. Assoc. Cancer Res.* 18:86, 1977.

63. Sinkovics, J.G., Plager, C., McMurtrey, M.J., et al., "Active Immunization with Viral Oncolysates Integrated in the Chemoimmunotherapy of Human Tumors (Melanoma and Sarcoma)." *Abstracts of 17th Interscience Conference on Antimicrobiol. Agents and Chemotherapy,* abstract 460, 1977.

64. McMurtrey, M.J., Sinkovics, J.G., Plager, C., et al., "Adjuvant Chemoimmunotherapy for Stage III (Regional Lymph Node Metastases) Malignant Melanoma." *Am. Soc. Clin. Oncology* 18:308, 1977.

65. Saal, J.G., Riethmuller, G., Rieber, E.P. et al., "Regional BCG-Therapy of Malignant Melanoma: *in vitro* Monitoring of Spontaneous Cytolytic Activity of Circulating Lymphocytes." *Cancer Immunol. Immunother.* 3:27:33, 1977.

66. Trapeznikov, N.N., Iavorskii, V.V., Kadagidze, Z.G. et al., "Immune Response in Patients with Skin Melanoma Treated with Nonspecific and Adoptive Immunotherapy." *Vopr. Onkol.* 23:27-33, 1977.

67. The, T.H., Huiges, H.A., Schraffordt Koops, H. and van Wingerden, I., "Immune Complexes in PMN Cells of Malignant Melanoma Patients." *Scand. J. Immunol.* 6:754, 1977.

68. Gersten, M.J., Hadden, E.M., Kaplan, M.H., et al., "Immunologic Defects in Melanoma Patients: Lack of Effect of BCG Therapy." *Clin. Bullet.* 7:63-69, 1977.

69. McCulloch, P.B., Dent, P.B.,Blajchman, M., et al., "Recurrent Malignant Melanoma: Effect of Adjuvant Immunotherapy on Survival." *Canad. Med. Assoc. J.* 117:33-36, 1977.

70. Paterson, A.H.G., Watson, M., Williams, D. and McPherson, T.A., "Bacille Calmette-Guerin (BCG) Immunotherapy in Stage I, Clark's Level (CL) 3-5 Malignant Melanoma." *Am. Soc. Clin. Oncology* 19:389, 1978.

71. Deutschmann, K.M., Peter, H.H., Schultheis, W. and Deicher, H., "Experience with BCG Adjuvant Immunotherapy in Stage II Malignant Melanoma." *Tumori* 63:303-307, 1977.

72. ElDomeiri, A.A., Dasgupta, T.F., Trippon, M., et al., "Adjuvant Chemotherapy and Immotherapy in High Risk Patients with Melanoma." *Surg. Gyn. Obstet.* 146:230-232, 1978.

73. Windhorst, D. and Terry, W.D., editors, *Immunotherapy of Cancer: Present Status of Trials in Man,* Raven Press, New York, 1978.

74. Hedley, D.W., McElwain, T.J. and Currie, G.A., "Tumor Regression and Survival of Patients with Disseminated Malignant Melanoma Treated ·with Chemotherapy and Specific Active Immotheraphy." *Europ. J. Cancer* 13:1169-1173, 1977.

75. Powles, R.I., Russell, J., Lister, T.A., et al., "Immunotherapy for Acute Myelogenous Leukemia: A Controlled Clinical Study 2 1/2 Years after Entry of the Last Patient." *Brit. J. Cancer* 35:265-272, 1977.

From BCG to More Quantifiable Immunity Systemic Adjuvants in Active Immunotherapy of Cancer Minimal Residual Disease

Georges Mathé[1]
L. Olsson[1]
I. Florentin[1]
N. Kiger[1]
M. Bruley-Rosset[1]
S. Orbach-Arbouys[1]
J. Schulz[1]

SUMMARY—BCG was the first immunity systemic adjuvant used in experimental and cancer immunotherapy.

There is today a dozen of clinical randomized trials in which BCG has given a significant benefit, but there are also trials where the BCG branch was not different from the control one. It appears from our experimental analysis that these negative results may be due to several factors: a) the preparation of BCG used; b) the modality applied; c) the dose: a dose smaller than the optimal one does not induce any effect (which may be the case of many negative trials); and a higher than optimal dose may induce immunodepression via the amplification of suppressor cells. Hence the necessity for the immune monitoring of the patients submitted to immunotherapy and of attracting the attention to dosimetry.

As dosimetry is very difficult for BCG, we have conducted a series of experiments on the *second generation of immunity adjuvants* for which the dosimetry is easy, searching for those and/or their dosages which do not induce suppressor cells and at the same time possess some of the favorable effects of BCG for the antitumor activity without the amplification of suppressor cells.

At present time, we have shown that in the case of T-cell immunodepression, thymosin and levamisole may restore T-cell immunity.

In the absence of immunodepression, aziridine amplifies mainly the null cells and the T-cells, Pseudomonas aeruginosa the B cells, glucan and glucan analogs the macrophages.

Several combinations are presented.

INTRODUCTION

Even with the most extensive surgery and radiotherapy, malignant cells remain behind, having already left the site of the primary tumor, as is the

---

[1]Institut de Cancérologie et d'Immunogénétique, Hôpital Paul-Brousse and Departement d'Hematologie de l'Institut Gustave-Roussy, Villejuif, France.

521

Figure 1—CORRELATION BETWEEN THE CHEMOTHERAPY DOSE AND NUMBER OF CELLS KILLED

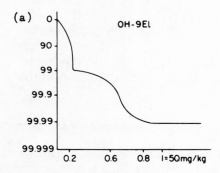

(a)

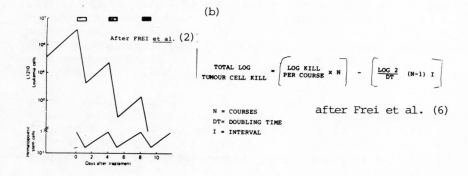

(b)

$$\text{TOTAL LOG TUMOUR CELL KILL} = \left[\text{LOG KILL PER COURSE} \times N\right] - \left[\frac{\text{LOG } 2}{DT}\ (N-1)\ I\right]$$

N = COURSES
DT = DOUBLING TIME
I = INTERVAL

after Frei et al. (6)

(c)

RESISTANT CELLS $1/10^6$

RESISTANT DAUGHTER CELLS PRODUCED $1/10^4$

after Frei et al. (6)

[a]Chemotherapy does not kill the last cell (1);
[b]This is due to the fact that chemotherapy obeys first order kinetics (2, 3, 4, 5); hence the effect of an intermittent chemotherapy depends on the number of cells killed in a cycle, the number of cycles, the intervals and the doubling time (6);
[c]and on the primary and secondary resistances (6).

522

case in more than 70% of solid tumors.

Although chemotherapy provides for a correlation between the dose and the number of cells killed, it is not capable of eliminating "the last cells" (Figure 1a) (1). This phenomenon is related to the fact that it obeys first order kinetics (Figure 1b) (2, 3, 4, 5) and to both primary and secondary resistances (Figure 1c) (6).

Today, the results of adjuvant chemotherapy in post-menopausal breast cancer ceases to be significant after 3 years' follow-up (7) and the results in osteosarcoma (8) (the difference in the patients' curves in both the treated and the non-treated was large after 2 years, but markedly diminished after four years) seem to follow a similar path.

Hence, when chemotherapy cures the patients, it is probably by reducing the number of neoplastic cells to the number eradicable or controllable by natural (immune) resistance.

Salmon (9) established a remarkable curve for operated breast cancer patients showing that all patients in whom 10^9 cells remain will relapse, while only those carrying 10 neoplastic cells or less have 100% chance of being cured (Figure 2a).

These 10 neoplastic cells seem to be of great importance, since that is precisely the mean inductive number of most murine grafted tumors, especially that of L1210 leukemia (Figure 2b). We have observed that 10 cells of this murine leukemia were needed to kill 50% of normal mice, while 1 cell only was necessary to obtain the same mortality in immunodepressed animals, in which this natural immune resistance is decreased.

I: This observation led us to search for ways to augment the number of cells in immunoprophylactic experiments where, using BCG as a non-specific immuno-adjuvant and irradiated tumor cells as specific stimulus, we succeeded in increasing it to 10^5. We have treated L1210 leukemia (10, 11) and other neoplasias (12) with the same immunomanipulation applied after the establishment of the neoplasia (immunotherapy), and were able to cure animals carrying $\leq 10^5$ leukemic cells (Figure 2c) (10).

We conducted our first trial of active immunotherapy in man in patients with acute lymphoid leukemia (ALL) because, in 1962, it was one of the rare diseases in which we were able to maintain long remission with chemotherapy. We thought that we might be able to reduce the number of post-chemotherapy residual leukemia cells to a number accessible to active immunotherapy (13). This randomized trial in which 7 patients out of 20 in the immunotherapy branch are still in remission 16 years later, versus 0 in the control group, induced, despite criticism to which we responded (14), many clinical trials on active immunotherapy with BCG ± cells in this disease. Some are in favour of our conclusions (15, 16) while others could not confirm it (17).

The same phenomenon has occurred with trials concerning other diseases.

Figure 2—THE NEOPLASTIC CELL NUMBERS KILLED BY NATURAL (IMMUNE) RESISTANCE

(a)

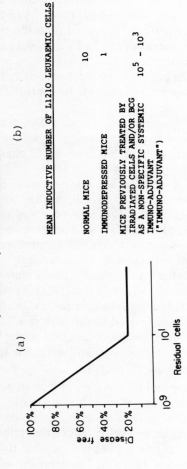

(b)

MEAN INDUCTIVE NUMBER OF L1210 LEUKAEMIC CELLS	
NORMAL MICE	10
IMMUNODEPRESSED MICE	1
MICE PREVIOUSLY TREATED BY IRRADIATED CELLS AND/OR BCG AS A NON-SPECIFIC SYSTEMIC IMMUNO-ADJUVANT ("IMMUNO-ADJUVANT")	$10^5 - 10^3$

(c)

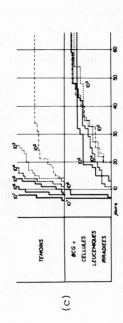

[a] According to Salmon's (9) calculation, post-surgical minimal residual disease needs to be reduced to 10 cells by chemotherapy in order to achieve 100% cure;

[b] this number corresponds to the mean inductive number of L1210 leukemia in mice; it can be increased to 10^5 in an immunoprophylactic experiment employing BCG and a specific vaccine made of irradiated tumor cells;

[c] it is also this number, 10^5 cells, which immunotherapy, i.e., immunomanipulation applied *after* the tumor is established, can eradicate (10).

524

Table 1 contains some of the currently significant results obtained in randomized trials with BCG and cells in ALL (13, 14, 15, 16) or with BCG alone in lymphosarcoma (18, 19), carcinoma of the bronchus (20, 21) and melanoma (22, 23, 24). One of the objects of this paper will be to explain the coexistence of positive and negative (17) trials, and to evaluate the factors of immunotherapy application which determine the types of results obtained.

In the first experiment quoted on L1210 leukemia (10), we used cells as specific immunotherapy and/or BCG as non-specific immunotherapy. We had shown in another experiment (11) that this combination was superior to the use of cells or BCG as single agents only.

However, this does not allow us to conclude that cells or adjuvants alone could not be, in some circumstances, sufficient to exert a significant action.

We showed that when the inoculated neoplastic cell population was very small (10^2), in the case of EAkR leukemia, irradiated cells alone were able to cure the animals which later resisted the challenge with the same tumor (Figure 3) (25).

There are several critical factors determining the effect of specific immunotherapy, i.e., the dose factor (Table 2) (26), and some substances, such as solubilized cell antigens, may differ in their preparation and which may lead to the opposite results (27).

On the other hand, immunity adjuvant alone may also be efficient as demonstrated with BCG given after cell reduction by chemotherapy in L1210 leukemia (Figure 4) (28). Here also, there are factors which determine the effect of BCG, such as the preparation used (only the living Pasteur BCG is efficient in our screening [29]), and the route used (only the i.v., the scarification and heaf gun administrations are efficient in our mice experiments [30]). BCG can also be applied before surgery, between the tumor and the lymph nodes, as in the cases of EAkR lymphosarcoma (31) and B16 melanoma (32) (regional active immunotherapy).

The dose of BCG might be the most important factor, as shown in our experiment in EAkR leukemia. There is an optimal dose, below which the effect is insignificant and over which it is diminished as well (Table 3) (26). In 1975, we also described the dose-effect correlation on the hemolytic plaque forming test. The dose of 1 mg of BCG per mouse increased the response, 0.2 mg, and 3mg/mouse did not affect it, while 10 mg decreased it (Table 4) (33).

We presume that doses smaller than the optimal one are insufficient to induce the septicemia shown to be necessary by Khalil et al., (34) for an optimal action on murine leukemia. We used a modality of application in man (shown in Table 5), which adapts the dose to the immune status of the patient.

Table 1—MINIMAL RESIDUAL DISEASE IMMUNOTHERAPY RANDOMIZED TRIALS WITH PRESENTLY SIGNIFICANT FAVORABLE RESULTS

	Immunotherapy Alone			
	Cells + BCG	BCG	Levamisole	Krestin
Acute Lymphoid Leukaemia Lymphosarcoma	Mathé et al. (13, 14, 15) Eortc H.W.P. (16)		Pavlovsky et al. (68)	
Acute Myeloid Leukaemia		Hoerni et al. (18) Cabanillas et al. (19)		
Bronchus		Pouillart el al. (20) McKneally et al. (21)	Amery (70)	
Melanoma		Ikonopisov (22) Kaufman et al. (23) Paterson et al. (24)	Gonzales & Spitler (72)	
Breast			Rojas et al. (69)	
Head & Neck			Wanebo et al. (71)	
Stomach				Taguchi (65)
Ovary				

	Immunotherapy + Chemotherapy > Chemotherapy			
	BCG +Cells	Cells or "Purified" Antigen	BCG	BCG and C. *Parvum*
Acute Lymphoid Leukaemia Lymphosarcoma				
Acute Myeloid Leukaemia	Powles et al. (44) Uden et al. (45, 46)	Bekesi & Holland (53)	Vogler et al. (47, 48) Whittaker & Slater (49)	
Bronchus		Stewart et al. (54)		
Melanoma			Kaufman et al. (23)	Jacquillat et al. (50)
Breast				
Head & Neck				
Stomach				
Ovary	Hudson et al. (51)		Alberts (52)	

527

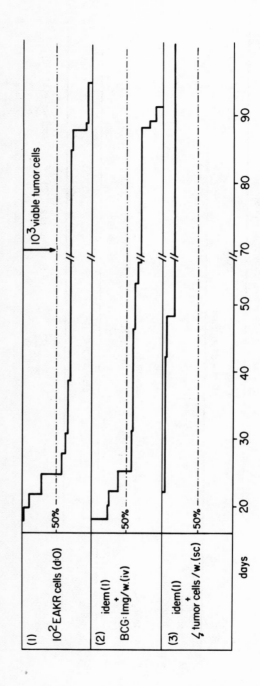

Figure 3—ATTEMPT AT ACTIVE SYSTEMIC IMMUNOTHERAPY OF EAkR MURINE LEUKEMIA INOCULATED WITH ONLY 10^2 TUMOR CELLS, WITH EITHER BCG ALONE (NOT EFFECTIVE) OR WITH IRRADIATED TUMOR CELLS ALONE (EFFECTIVE)

Table 2—THE ANTI-TUMORAL EFFECT OF IRRADIATED TUMOR-CELLS INJECTED S.C. EVERY WEEK WITH START AT DAY +1 AFTER TUMOR-CELL INOCULATION AND GIVEN MAXIMALLY 8 TIMES

Treatment	No. of tumor-cells inoculated	Mean survival time of dying mice in days (range)	Non-tumor bearing mice>90 days after tumor-inoculation (%)	Statistics†
None (controls)	10^2	28.0±1.8 (21-34)	10	—
	10^3	25.5±2.0 (20-29)	5	—
	10^5	16.8±1.6 (13-19)	0	—
	10^6	14.7±1.4 (12-16)	0	—
10^5 irradiated tumor-cells injected s.c. per week start day +1	10^2	35.2±3.8 (27-42)	10	N.S.
	10^3	32.0±3.6 (28-37)	5	N.S.
	10^5	15.8±2.0 (12-20)	0	N.S.
	10^6	15.0±1.6 (12-19)	0	N.S.
10^7 irradiated tumor-cells injected s.c. per week start day +1	10^2	47.4±6.5 (36-61)	70	$P<0.01$
	10^3	42.7±5.6 (33-54)	45	$P<0.01$
	10^5	17.8±1.4 (14-22)	0	N.S.
	10^6	15.6±2.0 (11-20)	0	N.S.
10^9 irradiated tumor-cells injected s.c. per week start day +1	10^2	43.1±7.0 (34-62)	65	$P<0.01$
	10^3	46.4±4.1 (37-55)	50	$P<0.01$
	10^5	16.3±1.9 (13-22)	0	N.S.
	10^6	14.6±1.1 (12-17)	0	N.S.
10^9 irradiated normal lymphoid cells injected s.c. start day +1	10^2	25.0±2.5 (16-31)	10	N.S.
	10^3	22.6±2.0 (17-28)	0	N.S.
	10^5	15.3±1.7 (13-21)	0	N.S.
	10^6	14.3±2.2 (12-21)	0	N.S.

†Statistics have been performed with Wilcoxon's non-parametric test comparing survival of all control mice with the survival of the various immune-stimulated groups.

The problem of immunosuppression due to the dose higher than the optimal one was totally obscure until we demonstrated with Geffard et al., (35) that this was due to the stimulation of suppressor cells by such doses (Table 6). This problem arises during the chronic as well as after single or short-term administration (Table 7) (36).

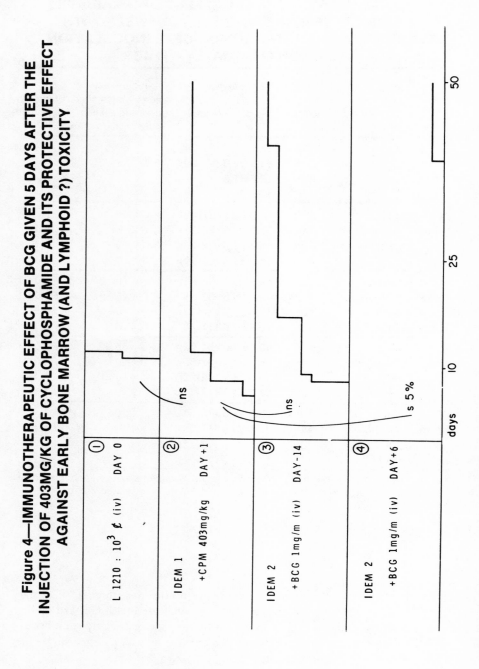

Figure 4—IMMUNOTHERAPEUTIC EFFECT OF BCG GIVEN 5 DAYS AFTER THE INJECTION OF 403MG/KG OF CYCLOPHOSPHAMIDE AND ITS PROTECTIVE EFFECT AGAINST EARLY BONE MARROW (AND LYMPHOID ?) TOXICITY

530

Table 3—THE ANTI-TUMORAL EFFECT OF VARIOUS DOSES OF BCG INJECTED I.V. EVERY WEEK WITH START AT DAY +1 AFTER TUMOR-CELL INOCULATION AND GIVEN MAXIMALLY 8 TIMES

Treatment	No. of tumor-cells inoculated	Mean survival time of dying mice in days (range)	Non-tumor bearing mice >90 days after tumor-inoculation (%)	Statistics*
None (controls)	10^2	26.8±2.3 (19-32)	15	—
	10^3	23.1±1.9 (18-32)	5	—
	10^5	16.5±2.0 (12-20)	0	—
	10^6	15.3±1.6 (12-18)	0	—
1.4 × 10^6 viable units BCG i.v. per week start day +1	10^2	25.1±2.9 (18-31)	20	N.S.
	10^3	24.0±1.8 (19-30)	5	N.S.
	10^5	15.6±2.1 (11-19)	0	N.S.
	10^6	14.9±1.7 (11-18)	0	N.S.
7 × 10^6 viable units BCG i.v. per week start day +1	10^2	32.3±4.7 (26-41)	45	$P<0.01$
	10^3	29.3±3.6 (24-36)	35	$P<0.01$
	10^5	17.8±1.9 (13-21)	25	$P<0.01$
	10^6	14.9±2.0 (11-19)	0	N.S.
21 × 10^6 viable units BCG i.v. per week start day +1	10^2	22.5±1.3 (17-25)	0	$P<0.01$
	10^3	20.3±1.8 (15-24)	0	$P<0.01$
	10^5	14.1±2.0 (11-18)	0	N.S.
	10^6	14.2±2.3 (10-18)	0	N.S.

*Statistics have been performed with Wilcoxons' non-parametric test comparing the survival of all mice in the control group with the survival of the various immune-stimulated groups.

Table 4—INFLUENCE OF THE DOSE OF FRESH LIVING BCG (INJECTED I.V. 14 DAYS BEFORE ANTIGEN) ON THE HUMORAL RESPONSE OF MICE SHEEP RED BLOOD CELLS (JERNE TEST)

Dose (mg)	Index of stimulation		
10	I^a = 0.06 ↘	S^b>	1%
5	I = 1.3	NS	
1	I = 4.01 ↗	S>	2%
0.5	I = 4.01 ↗	S>	1%
0.1	I = 1.64	NS	
Control	I = 1		

a Mean No. of PFC/spleen of experimental mice / Mean No. of PFC/spleen of controls

b Student Fisher test. S, significant; NS, not significant.

Table 5—MODALITY OF BCG APPLICATION

1. DELAYED HYPERSENSIBILITY +
    ONE DOSE OF 75mg ON ONE SCARIFIED AREA/WEEK
2. DELAYED HYPERSENSIBILITY—
    FOUR DOSES OF 75mg ON FOUR SCARIFIED AREAS/WEEK
3. IF TEMPERATURE < 38°C, THE APPLICATION IS REPEATED THE FOL-
    LOWING DAY

Figure 5—A SIMPLISTIC SCHEME DEPICTING THE PROCESS OF NATURAL RESISTANCE AGAINST TUMORS AND ITS MODULATION BY IMMUNOTHERAPY

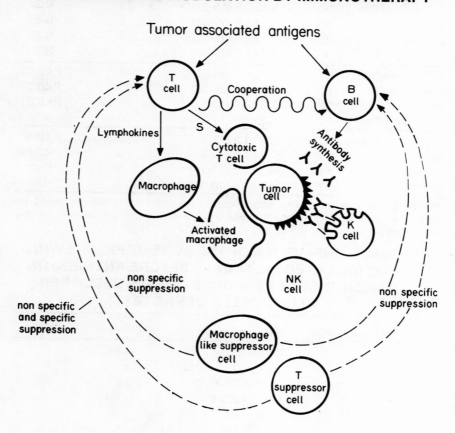

Table 6—STIMULATION OF SUPPRESSOR CELLS WITH HIGH DOSE OF BCG

Mixed lymphocyte reaction between $C_{57}B1/6$ Normal or BCG-treated spleen cells and irradiated DBA/2 spleen cells

Dose of BCG injected to $C_{57}B1/6$	CPM in cultures with irradiated $C_{57}B1/6$ spleen cells	CPM in cultures with irradiated DBA/2 spleen cells
Day-7		
0 mg	3,486	9,944
1.5 mg	3,446	12,097
3.0 mg	3,554	6,181

Percent spleen 125 IUDR uptake in lethal BFD_1 hybrids 4 days after $C_{57}B1/6$ spleen cell injection

Treatment of donors	Treatment of recipients	
	None	Cycloheximide
No treatment	.22	.34
BCG d-7 0.75 mg	.19	.32
1.5 mg	.19	.82
3.0 mg	.30	.66

The next step was to try to eliminate suppressor cells (Figure 5) by chemotherapy. We have demonstrated (37) that they could be destroyed with methotrexate (Table 8), while Polack and Turk showed that they could be killed by cyclophosphamide (38). There are other reasons brought out by experimental data for combining chemotherapy and immunotherapy: a) chemotherapy is known to work mainly on cells in the cycle, while we showed with Olsson that immunotherapy works mainly on cells in Go or in G1 phases (Figure 6) (39); b) chemotherapy may not be efficient in immunodepressed animals (Figure 7) (40) and some forms are immunodepressive (41); hence it is reasonable to attempt to restore immunity between chemotherapy cycles; c) BCG stimulates hematorestoration after chemotherapy (Figure 8) (42) and may shorten the intervals between two chemotherapy cycles.

Interspersion of BCG or BCG, cells and chemotherapy has been shown to be superior to the same chemotherapy applied alone in acute myeloid leukemia in a historical control trial (43) and in many randomized trials (44,

533

Table 7—EFFECT OF ACUTE VERSUS CHRONIC ADMINISTRATION OF BCG ON IMMUNE RESPONSES IN MICE

Immune Responses		Control	BCG Treatment°				
			0.2 mg 1X	0.2 mg 5X	1 mg 1X	1 mg 5X	5 mg 1X
Plaque-forming cell responses	TNP-POL	+	+	++	++++	+++	+++
	TNP-KLH	+	++	+++	++++	++	++++
Peritoneal macrophage cytostatic activity		−	+	+++	+++	+++	+++
Mitogen responsiveness	T-cell mitogen	+++	++	+	±	−	−
	B-cell mitogen	++	++	+++	+++	++	++
Suppressor cells	Macrophages	−	±	+	+	+	+
	T-cells	−	−	±	−	±	++

° Schedule of i.v. BCG treatment

BCG   BCG   BCG   BCG   BCG   BCG   BCG

↔ 1 week

In vitro testing

Figure 6—PERCENTAGE DISTRIBUTION OF ASCITIC TUMOR-CELLS AS A FUNCTION OF SINGLE-CELL DNA-CONTENT AT VARIOUS TIMES AFTER INOCULATION I.P. OF 10^5 TUMOR-CELLS

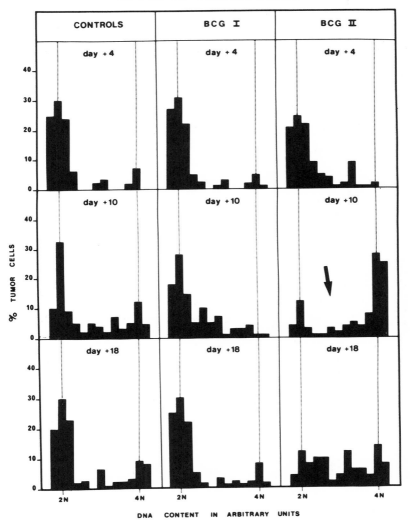

2N indicates the mean DNA-content of G1 cells, and 4N the mean DNA-content of mitoses (and G_2-phase cells).

Each value is the mean of 3-5 times.

BCG I : BCG treated mice with tumor load and tumor-cell mitotic activity no different from controls.

BCG II: BCG-treated mice with a lower tumor-cell number and a higher tumor-cell mitotic activity than controls.

535

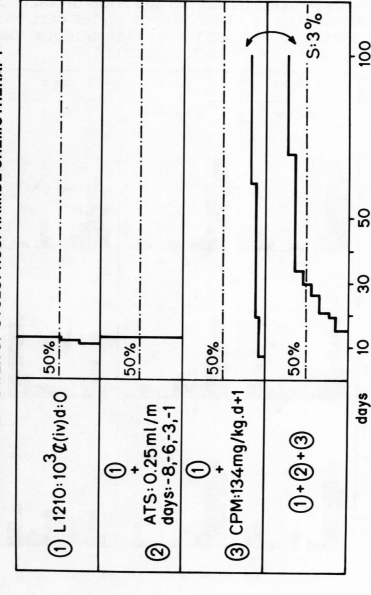

Figure 7—EFFECT OF ANTI-THYMOCYTE SERUM INDUCED IMMUNODEPRESSION IN THE ONCOSTATIC POWER OF CYCLOPHOSPHAMIDE CHEMOTHERAPY

Results are expressed in percentage of cumulative mortality of leukemia-bearing mice. Statistical significance is calculated by Wilcoxon's non-parametric test.

Figure 8—EFFECT OF BCG ON LYMPHOID STEM CELLS

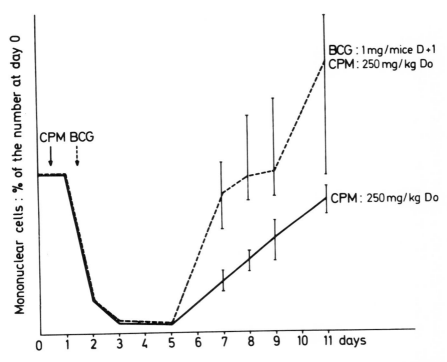

The restoration of blood lymphocyte number after cyclophosphamide aplasia is faster when BCG is administered one day after cytostatics.

45, 46, 47, 48, 49), in melanoma (23, 50), and in ovarian carcinoma (51, 52). Similarly, interspersion of immunotherapy using cells treated with neuraminidase (53) or tumor extracted antigen (54), and chemotherapy was shown to be superior to the same chemotherapy in acute myeloid leukemia (53) and in carcinoma of the bronchus (54), respectively. Not all trials of chemotherapy-immunotherapy interspersion gave a significant benefit (17). Experimentally, by applying several cycles of interspersed cyclophosphamide and of BCG in L1210 leukemia, we obtained a result which was inferior compared to the use of one cycle alone consisting of cyclophosphamide→ (CPM) followed by BCG (55). As the sequence cyclophosphamide BCG is more efficient than CPM or BCG alone, we questioned whether the reversed sequence BCG→CPM might not be the cause for this deterioration, which was subsequently demonstrated to be the case (Figure 9) (28). We have shown in an allogeneic skin graft experiment

537

Table 8—POSSIBLE EFFECT OF CHEMOTHERAPY ON SUPPRESSOR CELLS PHA RESPONSIVENESS OF LYMPHOID CELLS AFTER METHOTREXATE INJECTION

	5×10^5 Cells Cultivated	
	Alone	With PHA
Controls	549 ± 196	13 408 ± 710
Methotrexate day -5	2 799 ± 531	27 246 ± 2 559
BCG 3mg day -14	5 588 ± 722	7 831 ± 987
BCG 3mg day -14 Methotrexate day -5	3 855 ± 45	20 052 ± 1 672

Enhancement of the PHA reactivity (measured by the H3 thymidine incorporation in culture) of spleen cells from mice injected 5 days before the test with 0.5mg methotrexate. The suppressed response of cells from BCG injected animals is enhanced as much as the normal one.

Table 9—THE MAIN IMMUNOLOGICAL ACTIONS OF BCG AND OF THE SECOND GENERATION OF IMMUNITY ADJUVANTS†

Immunological Parameters	BCG	C. Parvum	Polynucleotides		Polysaccharides
			Poly I: C	Poly A: U	(ex: *Krestin*)
Delayed Hypersensitivity	↑	↑			↑
Humoral Responses	↑↑	↑↑	↑↑	↑	?
Suppressor Cells	↑↑	↑↑	↑↑	↑	?
K-Cells	↑↑	↑↑	↑↑		↑↑
Macrophage Activation	↑	↑↑	↑	↑	?
Interferon Induction			+	?	

†Those in italics are the object of trials presented in this meeting

Figure 9—SURVIVAL OF MICE CARRYING L1210 LEUKEMIA

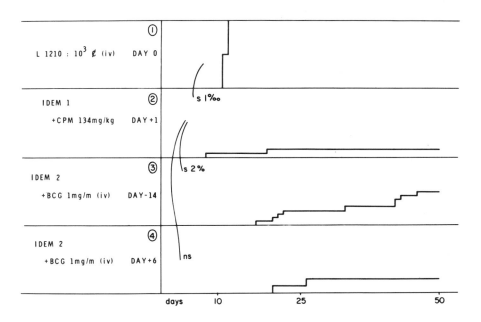

Deterioration by BCG given before 134MG/KG of cyclophosphamide on its antileukemic effect

that such a sequence can be strongly immunosuppressive, and we explained it by the fact that BCG pushes lymphocytes into the cycle which makes them more sensitive to the cytostatic effect of CPM, a phase dependent agent (56). But, although this is true for CPM, it is not valid for some sugar derivatives of nitrosoureas (57). The combination of RFCNU with BCG, even in the sequence BCG → RFCNU, is more efficient than the cytostatic alone or BCG alone (Figure 10) (58). Thus the choice of cytostatic in chemotherapy-immunotherapy interspersion is determinant. The choice of the immunity adjuvant may also be crucial. As seen in Table 9,BCG acts on all populations of cells exerting a role in immune reactions, including suppressor cells.

II: Among other adjuvants of the second generation (those already submitted to clinical trials), *C. parvum* is one of the most active, but it exerts inhibition of some T-cell reactions (59) probably via a stimulating action on suppressor cells. This could explain why this adjuvant has given the only randomized trial in which a deteriorating effect has been significant (60). Among interesting adjuvants which have been the object of much work

539

Figure 10

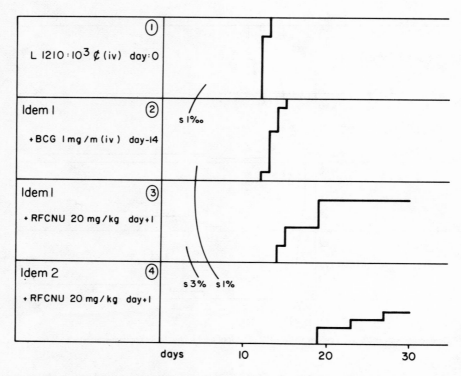

The sequence BCG-RFCNU (a non-immunosuppressive drug at the dose used) enhances the effect of both agents (contrary to the sequence of BCG-cyclophosphamide), an immunosuppressive agent

are the polynucleotides, poly I: poly C (61) and poly A: poly U (62). These are immunostimulants of T-lymphocytes and of macrophages, poly A : poly U probably via T-lymphocytes, and under some conditions via induction of interferon which, in itself, stimulates macrophages (Table 9) (63) and has, itself, given promising results in osteosarcoma (64). Several polysaccharides such as krestin (65) may also act as adjuvants, mainly stimulating macrophages, and the preliminary results in gastric cancer are encouraging (65) (Table 1).

One of the most interesting agents is levamisole. For years, we were unable to detect any of its effect, contrary to Renoux & Renoux (66), probably because we were working with 3 month old mice. Recently, searching for agents able to restore T-cell depleted old mice, we observed an immuno-restorative effect of levamisole (Table 10) (67), and noticed that

540

mice given this adjuvant developed less spontaneous tumors than non-treated animals, while BCG applied to another group not only did not restore the immune functions, but increased the incidence of spontaneous tumors (Figure 11) (67). The effect of levamisole was demonstrated in human acute lymphoid leukemia by Pavlovsky, et al., (68), in breast cancer (69), bronchus carcinoma (70), head and neck tumors (71) and in melanoma (72).

Table 10—EFFECT OF ACUTE AND CHRONIC ADMINISTRATION OF LEVAMISOLE TO TWELVE-MONTH-OLD MICE

Immune Response Tested (at the age of eighteen months)		Acute Treatment[1]	Chronic Treatment[1]
Spleen cell response to:	PHA	1.24[2] →	0.43 ↘
	DS	1.00 →	1.41 ↗
T-cell (nylon-non-adherent cell) response to:	PHA	0.85 →	0.88 →
Test for suppressor cell detection:			
Mitogen response of normal spleen cells co-cultivated with:			
Unfractionated levamisole-treated cells	PHA	1.43 ↗ (—)	0.67 ↘ (+)
	DS	0.91 → (—)	1.33 ↗ (—)
Nylon-non-adherent levamilsole-treated cells	PHA	0.86 → (—)	1.04 → (—)
	DS	0.87 → (—)	1.34 ↗ (—)
Macrophage cytostatic activity *in vitro* % inhibition of tumor cell proliferation		0%	Not tested
Antibody response to SRBC		1.54 ↗	2.57 ↗

[1]The chronic treatment consisted in weekly i.p. injections of 75 µg levamisole over a period of six months.

The acute treatment consisted in a single i.p.; injection of 75µg levamisole at the same time as the last injection of the chronic treatment.

Tests were performed 15 days after the last injection.

[2]Response of levamisole-treated mice
 Response of control mice

Figure 11—INCIDENCE OF SPONTANEOUS TUMORS WHICH APPEARED IN THREE GROUPS OF (DBA/2 x $C_{57}B1_{10}$)F1 AGED MICE SUBMITTED RESPECTIVELY TO LEVAMISOLE, BCG, OR NOT TREATED

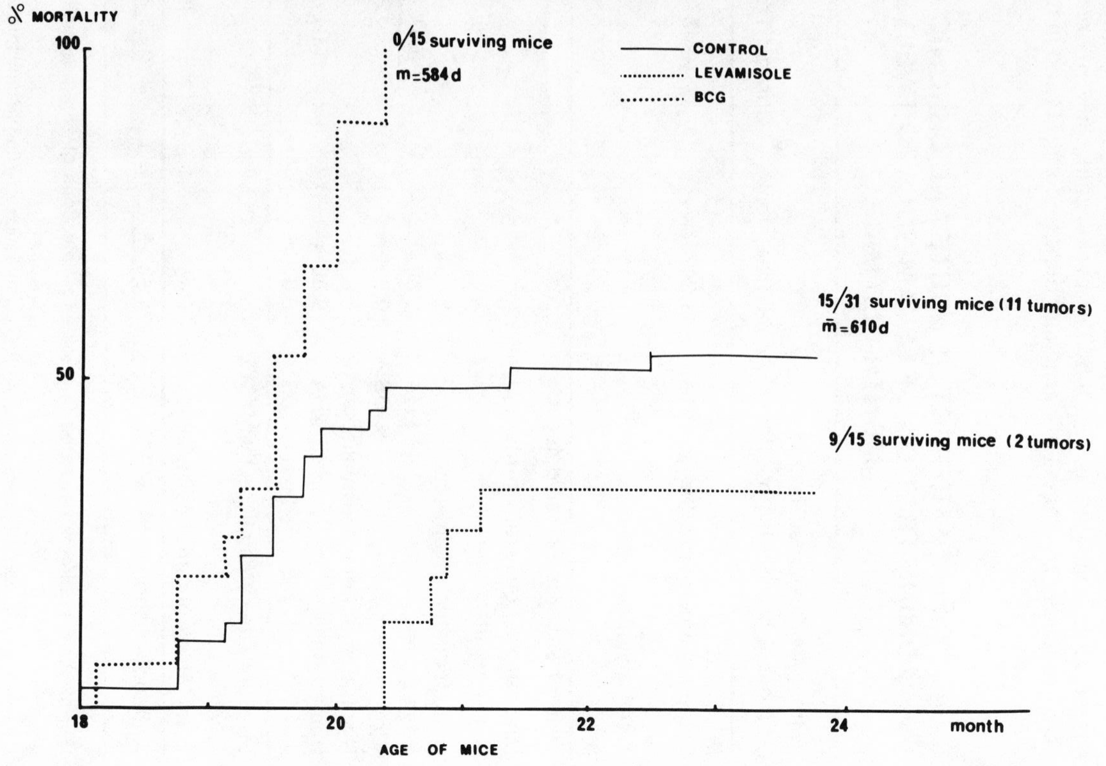

542

To summarize this first section: a) active immunotherapy has now been the object of a reasonable number of trials in a variety of tumors and the beneficial effect shown is significant not only in leukemias and lymphosarcoma but also in solid tumors (Table 1); b) we know at least two reasons for explaining BCG negative trials: not applying enough or administering too much BCG, which induces suppressor cells; c) the parameters which have been shown to determine the effect of BCG have to be studied for other adjuvants which have already given significant beneficial results; d) this underlines clearly the need for a valuable monitoring; at the present time only the increase of null cells has been found significant (73). The demonstration of monocyte decrease (73) and the suppressor cell appearance in some conditions (74) may also prove to be important modifications.

III: We shall now deal with new agents which can be considered as the third generation of systemic immunity adjuvants. We postulated that it will include agents which share the following characteristics: 1) they will be, preferentially, well defined chemical compounds, or at least well quantifiable agents; 2) their action will be limited to stimulation of one or few populations of cells; 3) they will not induce suppressor cells; 4) their side effects will be minimal. We think that after taking into account their respective mode of action, these adjuvants may be combined judiciously in such a way that a maximal antitumoral effect could be obtained without stimulation of suppressor cells. We shall discuss some agents which on the basis of experimental results fulfill at least some of the criteria described.

Thymosin, as shown in Table 11, when chronically administered to age-immunodepressed mice, restored their antibody response to a thymus-dependent antigen (sheep red blood cells, SRBC) and induced macrophage activation presumably by the intermediary of T lymphocyte stimulation. Examination of spleen cell mitogen responsiveness allowed us to demonstrate that no suppressor cells were induced by thymosin administration (75). Chretien (76) recently reported that thymosin in combination with chemotherapy increased survival of patients with oat cell lung carcinoma, but only if they were immunodepressed.

Bestatin, an antibiotic isolated by Umezawa et al., (77) from actinomycetes and which exhibited immunostimulating properties (78) was also examined for its ability to restore the immune capacity of aged mice. Results summarized in Table 12 demonstrated that T-cell functions were potentiated by the repeated administration of this compound. Small doses (10 μg per injection) were more effective in restoring humoral response to SRBC rather than delayed-type hypersensitivity reaction whereas larger doses (100 μg per injection) acted in the opposite way. Macrophage activation was observed only after treatment with the large doses suggesting that it resulted from a T-cell mediated immune response. No suppressor

Table 11—EFFECTS OF A CHRONIC ADMINISTRATION OF THYMOSIN TO 6-MONTH-OLD MICE UNTIL THE 15th MONTH

Immune Response Tested	Duration of Thymosin Treatment (1) : 9 Months	
Spleen cell response to:		
PHA	0.28 [2]	
Con A	0.40	
DS	1.23	
LPS	0.71	
T-cell (nylon-non-adherent cell) response to:		
PHA	0.72	
Con A	0.73	
Test for suppressor cell detection:		
Mitogen response of normal spleen cells cocultivated with thymosin-treated cells:		
PHA	1.08	(—)
Con A	0.97	(—)
Antibody response to SRBC	3.21	
Macrophage cytostatic activity *in vitro*. % inhibition of tumor cell proliferation	85%	

[1]Mice were given weekly injections of 100 µg thymosin i.p.

[2]$\dfrac{\text{Response of thymosin-treated mice}}{\text{Response of untreated mice}}$

cells were induced. Antibody-dependent cell cytotoxic activity of spleen cells against antibody-coated chick erythrocytes, which was markedly increased in non-treated aged mice when compared to young adult mice, returned to this normal value after bestatin treatment.

A new aziridine derivative, 2-[2-cyanaziridinyl-(1)-]-propane (Boehringer Mannheim: BM 12 531) (79), was tested for its immunostimulating properties in young adult mice. As shown in Table 13, it selectively potentiated immune responses involving T lymphocytes; delayed hypersensitivity to oxazolone (80) and antibody response to a thymus-dependent antigen

544

Table 12—EFFECTS OF A CHRONIC ADMINISTRATION OF BESTATIN TO 14-MONTH-OLD MICE UNTIL THE 20th MONTH

Immune Response Tested		Dose of Bestatin Per Injection[1]	
		10 µg	100 µg
Spleen cell response to:	PHA	1.16[2]→	1.33↗
	DS	1.52↗	1.72↗
T-cell (nylon-non-adherent cell) response to:	PHA	1.37↗	1.48↗
Test for suppressor cell detection:			
Mitogen response of spleen cells from 2-month-old mice cocultivated with:			
Unfractionated Bestatin-treated cells	PHA	0.80→(—)	0.78→(—)
	DS	1.81↗(—)	1.48↗(—)
Nylon-non-adherent Bestatin-treated cells	PHA	1.46↗(—)	0.91→(—)
	DS	1.09→(—)	1.11→(—)
Plastic-adherent Bestatin-treated cells	PHA	1.45↗(—)	1.35↗(—)
	DS	1.09→(—)	1.29↗(—)
Macrophage cytostatic activity % inhibition tumor cell proliferation		4%→	83%↗
Antibody response to SRBC		2.40↗	1.34→
Delayed-type hypersensitivity reaction to oxazolone		0.40↗	2.17↗
Antibody-dependent cell-mediated cytotoxicity % specific lysis effector cell to target cell ratio 1:100		70%↗	65%↗
Antibody dilution 1:2000		aged controls 86% young controls 65%	

[1]Mice were given weekly injections of 10 or 100 µg of Bestatin
[2]Response of Bestatin-treated mice
 Response of untreated mice

545

(trinitrophenyl-hemocyanin: TNP-KLH). Macrophage cytostatic activity for tumor cells was detected only after preceding evidence of a stimulation of T lymphocyte functions suggesting that these latter cells played a role in macrophage activation. Antibody response to a thymus-independent antigen (trinitrophenyl-polymerized flagellin: TNP-POL) was not potentiated and suppressor cells were not detected in the spleen of the animals whatever the time of BM 12 531 administration. Recently, Bicker demonstrated that BM 12 531 induced leucocytosis in normal rats and restored cyclophosphamide-induced leukopenia (81). Thus, an action of BM 12 531 on hematopoietic stem cells may be expected.

Table 13—EFFECT OF 2-[2-CYANAZIRIDINYL-(1)]-[2-CARBAMOYLAZIRIDINYL-(1)]-PROPANE (OR BM 12531) ON IMMUNE RESPONSES OF TWO-MONTH-OLD MICE

		Day of BM 12531 Administration[1]			
		0	-3	-7	-10
Spleen cell response to:	PHA	NT	1.00[2]	0.47	0.47
	Con A	NT	1.03	0.74	0.40
	LPS	NT	0.53	0.85	0.55
T-cell (nylon-non-adherent cell) response to:	PHA	NT	1.29	1.20	1.33
	Con A	NT	1.05	1.09	1.03
Test for suppressor cell detection: Mitogen responses of normal spleen cell co-cultivated with BM-treated cells	PHA	NT	1.19 (—)	1.09 (—)	1.98 (—)
	Con A	NT	0.88 (—)	1.49 (—)	1.45 (—)
	LPS	NT	1.40 (—)	0.98 (—)	1.52 (—)
Delayed-type hypersensitivity Reaction to oxazolone		1.6	1.3	1.0	1.1
Antibody response to	TNP-KLH	1.2	1.4	1.1	0.9
	TNP-POL	1.0	0.9	1.0	0.8
Macrophage cytostatic activity % inhibition of tumor cell proliferation		NT	0%	50%	65%

[1]BM 12531 was given i.v. at the dose of 25mg/kg.
[2]Response of BM 12531-treated mice / Response of untreated mice

Table 14—EFFECT OF HEAT-KILLED *PSEUDOMONAS AERUGINOSA* ON IMMUNE RESPONSES OF 2-MONTH-OLD MICE

Immune Response Tested	Day of *Pseudomonas* Administration[1]			
	3		7	
Spleen cell response to:				
PHA	0.92[2]		0.59	
DS	5.74		2.48	
T-cell (nylon-non-adherent cell) response to:				
PHA	1.07		1.03	
Test for suppressor cell detection Mitogen response of normal spleen cell cocultivated with:				
Unfractionated *Pseudomonas*-treated cells:				
PHA	1.50	(—)	1.04	(—)
DS	1.64	(—)	1.37	(—)
Nylon-non-adherent *Pseudomonas*-treated cells:				
PHA	0.97	(—)	0.92	(—)
DS	0.86	(—)	0.86	(—)
Macrophage cytostatic activity:				
% inhibition tumor cell proliferation	35%		36%	
Antibody responses to:				
TNP-KLH	1.17		0.99	
TNP-POL	1.53		1.98	
Delayed-type hypersensitivity reaction to oxazolone	0.85		0.78	
Antibody-dependent cell-mediated cytotoxicity				
% specific lysis	27.5%		33.5%	
(Effector cell to target cell ratio 1:100, antibody dilution 1:40,000e)	control: 40.2%		control: 31.2%	

[1]Mice were given 10[8] heat-killed organisms i.v. 3 or 7 days before testing.

[2]$\dfrac{\text{Response of } Pseudomonas\text{-treated mice}}{\text{Response of control mice}}$

With a preparation of *Pseudomonas aeruginosa* (mixture of 10 serotypes of bacteria, Pasteur Institute, Paris), we think we have at our disposal an adjuvant which mainly acts on B lymphocytes (Table 14) (82).

547

Table 15—EFFECT OF VARIOUS SYSTEMIC ADJUVANTS ON MACROPHAGE ACTIVATION IN MICE

Adjuvant	Day	Dose	Maximal Cytostatic Activity* % maximal inhibition of tumor cell proliferation
BCG	14	0.2 mg	33%
		1 mg	93%
		5 mg	99%
Levamisole	3	75 µg	0%
	7		
	14		
Pseudomonas Aeruginosa	3	10⁸ organisms	36%
	7		
Bestatin	7	100 µg	44 %
BM 12 531	7	500 µg	65 %
	14		
Glucan	7	500 µg	93 %
Tuftsine	7	400 µg	97 %

* % inhibition = $100 - \left[\dfrac{^{3}\text{H-TdR uptake by tumor cells incubated on treated macrophages}}{^{3}\text{H-TdR uptake by tumor cells incubated on normal macrophages}} \right] \times 100$

The conditions of administration (day and dose) were those inducing maximal macrophage activation.

Indeed, potentiation of antibody response to TNP-POL *in vivo* and stimulation of lymphocyte response to a B-cell mitogen (destran sulfate: DS) *in vitro,* were observed after injection of 10^8 heat-killed bacteria. In contrast, antibody formation against TNP-KLH and contact hypersensitivity reaction to oxazolone were not influenced by this adjuvant. Macrophage cytostatic activity for tumor cells was only slightly increased. Antibody-dependent cell-mediated cytotoxicity against antibody-coated chick erythrocytes was depressed 3 days after *Pseudomonas* injection. This adjuvant was capable of delaying the development of L1210 lymphoid leukemia in an immunoprophylaxis trial but the antitumoral effect is strongly dependent upon the number of bacteria injected and the time of administration (83). In clinical trials, *Pseudomonas aeruginosa* restored delayed-type hypersensitivity reactions in 50% of anergic cancer patients (84). It was reported by Oettgen (85) that lipopolysaccharide (LPS) from *Pseudomonas aeruginosa,* when administered before remission induction in patients with acute myeloid leukemia, prolonged the duration of the remission.

Since activated macrophages seem to play a major role in defense against neoplasia, we compared some of the new agents to BCG and levamisole for their capacity to render macrophages cytostatic for tumor cells. In addition to *Pseudomonas,* BM 12 531, we have tested bestatin, glucan (β-1-3 polyglucose extracted from yeast wall) (86) and tuftsine, a basic tetrapeptide synthetized by Martinez et al., (87). As shown in Table 15, glucan and tuftsine were as effective as BCG in inducing macrophage activation, whereas levamisole did not render macrophages cytostatic whatever the time of its administration. *Pseudomonas,* BM 12 531 and bestatin gave an intermediary level of macrophage activation.

Finally, among the adjuvants with cell specific action, muramyl dipeptide (MDP) (Table 16) (88) is the one which appears to amplify most the K cell functions (89).

IV: Thus, at the present time, we have in our hands various adjuvants which act rather selectively on one type of cell involved in immune responses (Table 17). We can attempt to combine these adjuvants with the aim of obtaining additional, if not synergistic immunostimulating effects because they are more cell population specific in their stimulatory activities than BCG and hence they might not result in suppressor cell induction. Should suppressor cells still be stimulated, we will search for such modalities of combinations which hopefully will be able to dissociate the respective kinetics of the different cell populations and then attempt to apply chemotherapy capable of neutralizing the suppressor cells (37). There are several other ways in which one could, at least theoretically, deal with this problem: a) thymectomy in order to eliminate short lived T suppressor cells; b) application of antibodies directed against cell surface antigens of suppressor cells as demonstrated in the sera of patients with active juvenile

Table 16—ANTIBODY-DEPENDENT-CELLULAR CYTOTOXICITY (1) AGAINST ^{51}Cr LABELLED CHICK-ERYTHROCYTES (CRBC) OF SPLEEN CELLS FROM MICE INJECTED I.V. WITH 100 μg MURAMYL DIPEPTIDE (MDP) AT DIFFERENT TIME PRIOR TESTING (DAY 0)

Day of M.D.P. Administration	Number of Spleen Cells Giving a 50% Specific Lysis (2) = 1 Lytic Unit (L.U.) of 10^4 target cells	Number of Nucleated cells per Spleen	Number of L.U. Per spleen
Day-1	38.10^4	9.9×10^7	260
Day-3	36.10^4	8.8×10^7	244
Day-7	36.10^4	10.1×10^7	280
Day-14	34.10^4	12.3×10^7	362
Control Group	76×10^4	8.4×10^7	110

[1]Cytoxicity was expressed as a function of effector: target cell ratio and anti CRBC serum was added at a constant dilution (1:80000)

[2] % specific lysis = $\dfrac{\text{Experimental} - \text{spontaneous release}}{\text{Maximal} \quad - \text{spontaneous release}} \times 100$

Table 17—IMMUNITY ADJUVANTS WITH A PREDOMINANT TARGET IMMUNOCOMPETENT CELL CLASSIFICATION ACCORDING TO THIS TARGET FOR SUGGESTION OF COMBINATIONS

Immunological state of the host	T Lymphocytes	B Lymphocytes	K cells	Macrophages
Immunocompetent	Aziridine Derivative (BM 12 531)	Pseudomonas Aeruginosa	MDP	Glucan Krestin Tuftsine
Immunodepressed	Thymosin Levamisole Bestatin			

Table 18—EFFECT OF A TREATMENT BY BCG AND *PSEUDOMONAS AERUGINOSA* ON THE GROWTH OF A METHYLCHOLANTHRENE-INDUCED FIBROSARCOMA (Mc C3-2) TRANSPLANTED S.C. IN C57BL/6 MICE

Treatment	Mean tumor diameter ± S.D. (mm) at day 22[1]	p value[2]	Mean tumor diameter ± S.D. (mm) at day 28	p value
Group 1 (control): 10 mice, 4.10^5 tumor cells s.c. day 0	11,32 ± 2,76		15,11 ± 3,01	
Group 2: 8 mice, idem control + BCG 1 mg i.v. day 1	10, 74 ± 3,41	N.S.	15,93 ± 4,05	N.S.
Group 3: 8 mice, idem control + *Pseudomonas* 0,01 ml i.v. day 14	12,08 ± 2,81	N.S.	17,83 ± 3,49	0,05 p 0.1 N.S.
Group 4: 10 mice, idem control + BCG day 1 and *Pseudomonas* day 14	9,14 ± 1,27	0,02<p<0,05	11,81 ± 1,62	0,001<p<0,01

[1]The mean tumor diameter is calculated from measurements of two tumor dimensions at right angles to each other.
[2]The significance of the differences between each group and the control group was assessed by Student's "t"-test.

Figure 12—EFFECTS OF TUMOR NECROSIS FACTOR (TNF) ON P815 MASTOCYTOMA

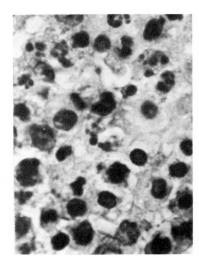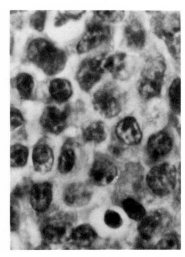

On the left, marked necrosis of the tumor in the animal treated with TNF serum (0.5ml i.v.) obtained from mice given BCG (1mg i.v.) followed 14 days later by *pseudomonas aeruginosa* (5.10⁸ bacilli). On the right, same tumor treated with a normal serum.

rheumatoid arthritis (90); c) potential use of thymic hormones for differentiation of immature T-cells shown to exert a suppressive activity which can be converted in this way into mature antitumoral effector T-cells (91). This latter hypothesis has been partially supported by Patt's observation (92) of inhibition by thymosin of suppressor cell induction in cancer patients; however, in our own experiments thymosin was not able to neutralize suppressor cells induced by BCG.

Combinations of adjuvants may also be envisaged with the objective of stimulating a particular mechanism of antitumoral activity. Carswell et al., (93) described, in the serum of mice given sequentially, BCG, or other macrophage activating agents, and then LPS, a factor which induced necrosis of some experimental tumors (tumor necrosis factor, TNF). Since LPS is strongly toxic, we have tried to induce TNF by injection of entire bacilli which are better tolerated in man (84) than in LPS (94). We have observed necrosis of P815 mastocytoma in mice given serum from animals injected with BCG followed by *Pseudomonas aeruginosa* (Figure 12). In another experiment, mice grafted with a chemically induced fibrosarcoma were directly treated with BCG and *Pseudomonas*. As shown in Table 18, a

553

significant reduction of the tumor size was observed in animals receiving both BCG and *Pseudomonas*. BCG alone was ineffective and *Pseudomonas* alone enhanced tumor growth in this particular experiment. This interesting adjuvant combination could serve as an example of potentially advantageous use of multiple adjuvants in the therapy of cancer.

REFERENCES

1. Le Pecq, J.B., Dat-Xuong, N., Gosse, C. and Paoletti, C., "A New Antitumoral Agent: 9 Hydroxyellipticine. Possibility of a Rational Design of Anticancerous Drugs in the Series of DNA Intercalating Drugs." *Proc. Nat. Acad. Sci.* 71:5078, 1974.

2. Frei, E. III, Bickers, J.N., Hewlett, J.S., et al., "Dose Schedule and Antitumor Studies of Arabinosyl Cytosine (NSC-63878)." *Cancer Res.* 29:1325, 1969.

3. Skipper, H.E., Schabel, F.M. and Wilcox, W.S., "Experimental Evaluation of Potential Anticancer Agents. XIII. On the Criteria and Kinetics Associated with Curability of Experimental Leukemia." *Cancer Chemoth. Rep.* 35:1, 1964.

4. Skipper, H.E., Schabel, F.M. and Wilcox, W.S., "Experimental Evaluation of Potential Anticancer Agents. XIV. Further Study of Certain Basic Concepts Underlying Chemotherapy of Leukemia." *Cancer Chemoth. Rep.* 45:5, 1966.

5. Skipper, H.E., Schabel, F.M. and Wilsox, W.S., "Experimental Evaluation of Potential Anticancer Agents. XXI. Scheduling of Arabinosylcytosine to take Advantage of its S-Phase Specificity Against Leukaemic Cells." *Cancer Chemoth. Rep.* 51:125, 1967.

6. Frei, E. III, Jaffe, N., Skipper, H.E. and Gero, M.G., "Adjuvant Chemotherapy of Osteogenic Sarcoma: Progress and Perspectiveness." 49 in *Adjuvant Therapy of Cancer*. Edited by Salmon, S.E. and Jones, S.J., Elsevier North Holland Biomedical Press, Amsterdam, 49, 1977.

7. Rossi, A., Valagussa, P. and Bonadonna, G., "Combined Modality Management of Operable Breast Cancer." In *Adjuvant Therapies and Markers of Post-Surgical Minimal Residual Disease*. Edited by Bonadonna, G., Mathé, G. and Salmon, S.E., Springer verlag, Heidelberg-New York, 1978. In press.

8. Jaffe, N., in "Third Annual Meeting of the Medical Oncology Society." Nice 4-6 December, 1977.

9. Salmon, S.E., "Kinetics Rationale for Adjuvant Chemotherapy of Cancer." In *Adjuvant Therapy of Cancer*. Edited by Salmon, S.E., Jones, S.J., Elsevier North Holland Biomedical Press, Amsterdam, 15, 1977.

10. Mathé, G., "Immunothérapie Active de la Leucémie L1210 Appliquée après la Greffe Tumorale." *Rev. Franç. Et. Clin. Biol., 13,* 881, 1968.

11. Mathé, G., Pouillart, P. and Lapeyraque, F., "Active Immunotherapy of L1210 Leukaemia Applied After the Graft of Tumor Cells." *Brit. J. Cancer* 23:814, 1969.

12. Mathé, G., "Active immunotherapy of Cancer. Immunoprophylaxis and immunorestoration. An introduction." 1st ed., Heidelberg-New York, 1976, Springer verlag.

13. Mathé, G., Amiel, J.L., Schwarzenberg, L., et al., "Active Immunotherapy for Acute Lymphoblastic Leukaemia." *Lancet* 1:697, 1969.

14. Mathé, G., Amiel, J.L., Schwarzenberg, L., et al., "Follow-up of the First (1962) Pilot Study on Active Immunotherapy of Acute Lymphoid Leukaemia: A Critical Discussion." *Biomedicine* 24:29, 1977.

15. Mathé, G., De Vassal, F., Schwarzenberg, L., et al., "Preliminary Results of Three Protocols for the Treatment of Acute Lymphoid Leukaemia of Children: Distinction of Two Groups of Patients According to Predictable Prognosis." *Medical Pediatr. Oncol.* 4:17, 1978.

16. Hemopathies Working Party of E.O.R.T.C. (P. Strychmans). "A Randomized Trial Comparing Immunotherapy and Chemotherapy as Maintenance Treatment of Acute Lymphoblastic Leukemia." In *2nd International Symposium on Therapy of Acute Leukemias,* p. 129, Rome, 1977.

17. Terry, W.D. and Windhorst, D., Editors, "Immunotherapy of Cancer: Present Status of Trials in Man." Raven Press, New York, 1978.

18. Hoerni, B., Chauvergne, J., Hoerni-Simon, G., et al., "BCG in the Immunotherapy of Hodgkin's Disease and Non-Hodgkin's Lymphomas. Results of a Controlled Trial Including 60 Patients." *Cancer Immunol. Immunoth.* 1:109, 1976.
19. Cabanillas, F., Rodriguez, V. and Bodey, G.P., "The Impact of Intensive Chemotherapy on the Duration of Remission and Survival of Patients (PTS) with Nodular Malignant Lymphomas (NML)." *Proc. Amer. Assoc. Soc. Clin. Oncol.* 19:abstract C-16, 1978.
20. Pouillart, P., Mathé, G., Palangie, T., et al., "Trial of BCG Immunotherapy in the Treatment of Resectable Squamous Cell Carcinoma on the Bronchus (stages I and II)." *Cancer Immunol. Immunoth.* 1:271, 1976.
21. McKneally, M.F., Maver, C.H. and Kausel, H.W., "Intrapleural BCG Immuno-Stimulation in Lung Cancer." *Lancet* 1:1003, 1977.
22. Ikonopisov, R.L., "The Use of BCG in the Combined Treatment of Malignant Melanoma." *Behring Inst. Mitt.* 56:206, 1975.
23. Kaufman, S.D., Carey, R.W., Cosimi, A.B. and Wood, W.C., "Randomized Trial of Adjuvant Therapy of high risk Primary Malignant Melanoma." *Proc. Amer. Soc. Clin. Oncol.* 9:374, 1978.
24. Paterson, A.H.G., Watson, M., Willimans, D. and McPherson, T.A., "Bacille Calmette-Guérin (BCG) Immunotherapy in Stage I Clark's Level (CL) 3-5 Malignant Melanoma." *Proc. Amer. Soc. Clin. Oncol.* 19:389, 1978.
25. Kiger, N., Olsson, L., Florentin, I. and Mathé, G., "Specific Active Immunotherapy of EAkR Leukaemia." In preparation.
26. Olsson, L., Ebbessen, P., Kiger, N., et al., "The Antileukemic Effect of Systemic Non-Specific BCG Immunostimulation With Irradiated Isogenic Leukemic Cells." *Europ. J. Cancer* 14:355, 1978.
27. Martyre, M.C., Weiner, R. and Halle-Pannenko, O., "The *in vivo* Activity of Soluble Extract Obtained from RC19 Leukemia: The Effect of the Method of Extraction. In *Investigation and Stimulation of Immunity in Cancer Patients.* Edited by Mathé, G. and Weiner, R., Springer verlag, Heidelberg-New York, p. 405, 1974.
28. Mathé, G., Halle-Pannenko, O. and Bourut, C., "Immune Manipulation by BCG Administered Before or After Cyclophosphamide for Chemo-Immunotherapy of L1210 Leukaemia." *Europ. J. Cancer* 10:661, 1974.
29. Mathé, G., Halle-Pannenko, O. and Bourut, C., "BCG in Cancer Immunotherapy. II. Results Obtained with Various BCG Preparations in a Screening Study for Systemic Adjuvants Applicable to Cancer Immunoprophylaxis or Immunotherapy." *Natl. Cancer Inst.* Monograph 39:107, 1973.
30. Martin, M., Bourut, C., Halle-Pannenko, O. and Mathé, G., "Routes Other Than I.V. Injection to Mice for BCG Administration in Active Immunotherapy of L1210 Leukemia." *Biomedicine* 23:339, 1975.
31. Economides, F., Bruley-Rosset, M. and Mathé, G., "Effect of Pre-Surgical Active BCG Immunotherapies on Murine EAkR Lymphosarcoma." *Biomedicine* 25:372, 1976.
32. Economides, F., Bruley-Rosset, M. and Mathé, G., "Treatment of the B16 Melanoma with Tumerectomy Combined or not with Adnectomy, Systemic or/and Regional BCG Immunotherapy." *Medical Oncology* 3:S34, 1977.
33. Mathé, G., "Side Effects and Possible Harmful Action of Immunomanipulation." In *The Prediction of Chronic Toxicity From Short Term Studies,* p. 67, 1975. *Excerpta Medica,* Amsterdam.
34. Khalil, A., Bourut, C., Halle-Pannenko, O., et al., "Histological Reactions of the Thymus, Spleen, Liver and Lymphnodes to Intravenous and Subcutaneous BCG Injections." *Biomedicine* 22:112, 1975.
35. Geffard, M. and Orbach-Arbouys, S., "Enhancement of T-Suppressor Activity in Mice by High Doses of BCG." *Cancer Immunol. Immunoth.* 1:41, 1976.

556

36. Kiger, N., Bruley-Rosset, M., Florentin, I., et al., "Effect of Acute Versus Chronic Administration of BCG on Immune Responses in Mice." In preparation.

37. Orbach-Arbouys, S., Castes, M. and Berardet, M., "Enhancement of Immunological Responses by Methotrexate Pretreatment as a Result of an Eventual Elimination of Suppressor Cells." In *Experimental Hematology Today*. Springer verlag, Heidelberg-New York, 1978. In press.

38. Polak, L. and Turk, J.L., "Reversal of Immunological Tolerance by Cyclophosphamide Through Inhibition of Suppressor Cell Activity," *Nature* 249:654, 1974.

39. Olsson, L. and Mathé, G., "A Cytokinetic Analysis of Bacillus Calmette-Guérin Induced Growth Control of Murine Leukemia." *Cancer Res.* 37:1743, 1977.

40. Mathé, G., Halle-Pannenko, O. and Bourut, C., "Effectiveness of Murine Leukemia Chemotherapy According to the Immune State. Reconsideration of Correlations Between Chemotherapy Tumor Cell Killing and Survival Time." *Cancer Immunol. Immunoth.* 2:139, 1977.

41. Clarysse, A., Kenis, Y. and Mathé, G., *Cancer Chemotherapy*. "Its Role in the Treatment Strategy of Hematologic Malignancies and Solid Tumors." Springer verlag, Heidelberg-New York, 1976.

42. Mathé, G., "Prevention of Chemotherapy Complications: Time, Toxicity, Pharmacokinetic and Logistic Factors." In *Complications of Cancer Chemotherapy*. Edited by Mathé, G. and Oldham, R.K., Springer verlag, Heidelberg-New York, p. 124, 1974.

43. Gutterman, J.U., Rodriguez, V., Mavligit, G., et al., "Chemo-Immunotherapy of Adult Acute Leukaemia Prolongation of Remission in Myeloblastic Leukaemia with BCG." *Lancet* 2:1405, 1974.

44. Powles, R.L., Crowther, D., Bateman, C.J.T., et al., "Immunotherapy for Acute Myelogenous Leukaemia." *Brit. J. Cancer* 28:365, 1973.

45. Udem, A.M., Lindemalm, C., Pauli, C., et al., "Effects of Immunotherapy and Chemotherapy on Immunocompetence. A Study of Patients with Acute Myeloblastic Leukemia in Remission." *Cancer Immunol. Immunoth.* 1978. In press.

46. Reizenstein, P., Brenning, G., Endstedt, L., et al., "Effect of Immunotherapy on Survival and Remission Duration in Acute Non-Lymphatic Leukaemia." In *Immunotherapy of Cancer: Present Status of Trials in Man*. Edited by Terry, W.D. and Windhorst, D., Raven Press, New York, p. 329, 1978.

47. Vogler, W.R. and Chan, Y.K., "Prolonging Remission in Myeloblastic Leukaemia by Tice-Strain Bacillus Calmette-Guérin." *Lancet* 2:128, 1974.

48. Vogler, W.R., Bartolucci, A.A., Omura, G.A., et al., "A Randomized Clinical Trial of BCG in Myeloblastic Leukemia Conducted by the Southeastern Cancer Study Group." In *Immunotherapy of Cancer: Present Status of Trials in Man*. Edited by Terry, W.D. and Windhorst, D., Raven Press, New York, p. 365, 1978.

49. Whittaker, J.A. and Slater, A.J., "The Immunotherapy of Acute Myelogenous Leukaemia Using Intravenous BCG." In *Immunotherapy of Cancer: Present Status of Trials in Man*. Edited by Terry, W.D. and Windhorst, D., Raven Press, New York, p. 393, 1978.

50. Jacquillat, C., Banzet, P., Civatte, J., et al., "Adjuvant Chemotherapy or Immunotherapy in the Management of Primary Melanoma of Level III, IV or V." In *Adjuvant Therapies, and Markers of Post-surgical Minimal Residual Diseases*. Edited by Bonadonna, G., Mathe , G. and Salmon, S.E., Springer verlag, Heidelberg-New York, 1978.

51. Hudson, C.N., Levin, L., McHardy, J.E., et al., "Active Specific Immunotherapy for Ovarian Cancer." *Lancet* 2:877, 1976.

52. Alberts, D.S., "Adjuvant Immunotherapy With BCG of Advanced Ovarian Cancer: A Preliminary Report." In *Adjuvant Therapy of Cancer*. Edited by Salmon, S.E. and Jones, S.E., Elsevier North Holland Biomedical Press, Amsterdam, p. 327, 1977.

53. Bekesi, J.G. and Holland, J.F., "Active Immunotherapy in Leukaemia With Neuraminidase Modified Leukaemic Cells." In *Tactics and Strategy in Cancer Treatment*.

Edited by Mathé, G., Springer verlag, Heidelberg-New York, p. 78, 1977.

54. Stewart, T.H.M., Hollinshead, A.C., Harris, J.E., et al., "Survival Study of Im- munochemotherapy in Lung Cancer." In *Immunotherapy of Cancer: Present Status of Trials in Man.* Edited by Terry, W.D. and Windhorst, D., Raven Press, New York, p. 203, 1978.

55. Mathé, G., Halle-Pannenko, O. and Bourut, C., "Interspersion of Cyclophosphamide and BCG in the Treatment of L1210 Leukaemia and Lewis Tumour." *Europ. J. Cancer* 13:1095, 1977.

56. Mathé, G., Halle-Pannenko, O. and Bourut, C., "Potentiation of a Cyclophosphamide Induced Immunodepression by the Administration of BCG." *Transplant. Proc.* 6:431, 1974.

57. Imbach, J.L., Montero, J.L., Moruzzi, A., et al., "The Oncostatic and Immunosuppressive Action of New Nitrosourea Derivatives Containing Sugar Radicals." *Biomedicine* 23:410, 1975.

58. Bruley-Rosset, M., Florentin, I., Kiger, N. and Mathé, G., "Comparative Experimental Immunopharmacology of Three Nitrosources: RFCNU, RPCNU and Chlorozotocin." In prepara- tion.

59. Scott, M.T., "Depression of Delayed-Type Hypersensitivity by *Corynebacterium parvum*: Mandatory Role of the Spleen." *Cell. Immunol.* 13:251, 1974.

60. Fortner, J.G., "Management of Recurrent Malignant Melanoma." In *3rd International Symposium on Oncology,* Abstract n °21. Teheran, March 1978.

61. Mathé, G., Hayat, M., Sakouhi, M. and Choay, J., "L'Action Immuno-Adjuvante du Poly I:C Chez la Souris et son Application au Traitement de la L1210." *C.R. Acad. Sci.* 272:170, 1971.

62. Lacour, F., Lacour, J. and Spira, A., "Poly A-poly U as an Adjunct to Surgery in the Treatment of Spontaneous Murine Mammary Adenocarcinoma." In *Investigation and Stimulation of Immunity in Cancer Patients.* Edited by Mathé, G. and Weiner, R., Springer verlag, Heidelberg-New York, p. 352, 1974.

63. Schultz, R.M., Chirigos, M.A., Pavlidis, N. and Stylos, W., "Cytotoxic Activity of Interferon Treated Macrophages Studied by Various Inhibitors." In *Immune Modulation and Control of Neoplasia by Adjuvant Therapy.* Edited by Chirigos, M.A., *Cancer Therapy Report,* 1978. In press.

64. Strander, H., "The Interferon System and its Possible Use in the Treatment of Neoplastic Disease." In *The Role of Non-Specific Immunity in the Prevention and Treatment of Cancer. Study Week Pontifical Academy of Sciences,* Vatican City, October, 1977. In press.

65. Taguchi, T., "Experimental and Clinical Studies on Krestin." In *Immune Modulation and Control of Neoplasia by Adjuvant Therapy.* Edited by Chirigos, M.A., *Cancer Therapy Report,* 1978. In press.

66. Renoux, G. and Renoux, M., "Levamisole Inhibits and Cures a Solid Malignant Tumor and its Pulmonary Metastases in Mice." *Nature New Biol.* 240:217, 1972.

67. Bruley-Rosset, M., Florentin, I., Kiger, N., et al., "Comparisons of the Effects of BCG and Levamisole Administration in Young Adult and Aged Mice." In *Immune Modulation and Control of Neoplasia by Adjuvant Therapy.* Edited by Chirigos, M.A., *Cancer Therapy Report,* 1978. In press.

68. Pavlovsky, S., Garay, G., Giraud, C., et al., "Chemo-Immunotherapy with Levamisole (LMS) in Acute Lymphocytic Leukemia (ALL)." *Proc. Amer. Assoc. Cancer Res.* 19:204, 1978.

69. Rojas, A.F., Feierstein, J.N., Glait, H.M. and Olivari, A.J., "Levamisole Action in Breast Cancer Stage III." In *Immunotherapy of Cancer: Present Status of Trials in Man.* Edited by Terry, W.D. and Windhorst, D., Raven Press, New York, p. 663, 1978.

70. Amery, W., "Final Results of a Multicenter Placebo Controlled Levamisole Study of Resectable Lung Cancer." In *Immune Modulation and Control of Neoplasia by Adjuvant Therapy*. Edited by Chirigos, M.A., *Cancer Therapy Report*, 1978. In press.

71. Wanebe, H.J., Hilal, E., Strong, E.W., et al., "Randomized Trial of Levamisole in Patients with Squamous Cell Carcinoma of the Head and Neck." In *Immune Modulation and Control of Neoplasia by Adjuvant Therapy*. Edited by Chirigos, M.A., *Cancer Therapy Report*, 1978. In press.

72. Gonzalez, R. and Spitler, L., "Effect of Levamisole as a Surgical Adjuvant Therapy on Malignant Melanoma. In *Immune Modulation and Control of Neoplasia by Adjuvant Therapy*. Edited by Chirigos, M.A., *Cancer Therapy Report*, 1978. In press.

73. Belpomme, D., Joseph, R. and Lelarge, N., "Increased Null Cells in Patients Submitted to Long-Term Active Immunotherapy." *Cancer Immunol. Immunoth.* 1:113, 1976.

74. Orbach-Arbouys, S., Unpublished data.

75. Bruley-Rosset, M., Florentin, I., Kiger, N., et al., "Prevention of Aged-Induced Immunodepression in Mice By Chronic Treatment With Thymosin and Systemic Adjuvants of Immunity." *Cancer Immunol. Immunoth.* 1978. In press.

76. Chretien, P., "Thymosin as Adjuvant in Treating Human Carcinomas. In *Immune Modulation and Control of Neoplasia by Adjuvant Therapy*. Edited by Chirigos, M.A., *Cancer Therapy Report*, 1978. In press.

77. Umezawa, H., Aoyagi, T., Suda, H., "Bestatin, a New Amino-Peptidase B Inhibitors Produced by Actinomycetes." *J. Antibiotics* 29:97, 1976.

78. Umezawa, H., Ishisuka, M., Aoyagi, T. and Takeuchi, T., "Enhancement of Delayed-Type Hypersensitivity by Bestatin, an Inhibitor of Amino-Peptidase B and Leucine Aminopeptidase." *J. Antibiotics*, 29:857, 1976.

79. Bicker, O., Ziegler, B.E. and Hebold, G., "2-2-Cyanaziridinyl-(1)-2-2-Carbamoyl Aziridinyl-(1) -Propane BM 12 531. A New Substance With Immune Stimulating Action." *IR.S.C. Med. Sci.* 5:299, 1977.

80. Schulz, J.I., Florentin, I., Bourut, C., et al., "Delayed-Type Hypersensitivity Response and Humoral Antibody Formation in Mice Treated. A New Immunostimulant 2-2-Cyanaziridinyl-(1)-2-2-Carbamoyl Aziridinyl-(1) -Propane BM 12 531." *I.R.S.C. Med. Sci.* 6:215, 1978.

81. Bicker, U., Hebold, G., Ziegler, A.E. and Maus, W., "Animal Experiments on the Compensation of the Immunosuppressive Action of Cyclophosphamide by 2-2-Cyanaziridinyl-(1)-2-2-Carbamoyl Aziridinyl-(1) -Propane BM 12 531." In preparation.

82. Florentin, I., Kiger, N., Bruley-Rosset, M., et al., "Effect of Seven Immunomodulators on Different Types of Immune Responses in Mice." In *Human Lymphocyte Differentiation: Its Application to Human Cancer*. Edited by Serrou, B. and Rosenfeld, C., Elsevier/North-Holland Biomedical Press, Amsterdam, p. 299, 1978.

83. Mathé, G., Florentin, I., Bruley-Rosset, M., et al., "Heat-Killed *Pseudomonas Aeruginosa* as a Systemic Adjuvant in Cancer Immunotherapy." *Biomedicine* 27:368, 1977.

84. Mathé, G., De Vassal, F., Gouveia, J., et al., "Comparison of the Restoration Effect of *Pseudomonas Aeruginosa*, BCG and Poly I:Poly C on Cancer Patients non Responsive to Recall Antigen Delayed Hypersensitivity." *Biomedicine* 27:328, 1977.

85. Oettgen, H.F., "Effects of Endotoxin and Endotoxin-Induced Mediators on Cancer and on the Immune System." In *The Role of Nonspecific Immunity in the Prevention and Treatment of Cancer. Study Week of the Pontifical Academcy of Sciences*, Vatican City, October 1977. 1978. In press.

86. Diluzio, N. "An Overview of Glucan Activity." In *Immune Modulation and Control of Neoplasia by Adjuvant Therapy*. Edited by Chirigos, M.A., *Cancer Therapy Report*, 1978. In Press.

87. Martinez, J., Winternitz, F. and Vindel, J., "Nouvelles Synthèses et Propriétés de la Tuftsine." *Eur. J. Med. Chem.* 1978. In press.

88. Chedid, L., Audibert, F. and Johnson, A.G., "Biological Studies of Muramyl Dipeptide, a Synthetic Glycopeptide Analogous to Bacterial Immunoregulating Agents." *Progess in Allergy* 25:63, 1978.

89. Kiger, N. et al. In preparation.

90. Strelkauskas, A.J., Schauf, V., Wilson, B.S. et al., "Isolation and Characterization of Naturally Occurring Subclasses of Human Peripheral Blood T Cells with Regulatory Functions." *J. Immunol.* 120:1278, 1978.

91. Trainin, N., Small, M. and Gabizon, A., "Thymic Humoral Factor (THF) as Modulator of T-Cell Differentiation Involved in Antitumor Reactivity." In *Human Lymphocyte Differentiation: Its Application to Human Cancer.* Edited by Serrou, B. and Rosenfeld, C., Elsevier/North-Holland Biomedical Press, Amsterdam, 1978.

92. Patt, Y.Z., Hersh, E.M., Goldman, R. and Washington, M., "Suppressor cells in Cancer Patients and Possible Effects of Thymic Hormone." In *Immune Modulation and Control of Neoplasias by Adjuvant Therapy.* Edited by Chirigos, M.A., *Cancer Therapy Report,* 1978. In press.

93. Carswell, E.A., Old, L.J., Kassel, R.L. et al., "An Endotoxin-Induced Serum Factor that Causes Necrosis of Tumors." *Proc. Nat. Acad. Sci.* 72:3666, 1975.

94. Hortobagyi, G.N., Gutterman, J.U., Richman, S.P. and Hersh, E.M., "*Pseudomonas Aeruginosa* Vaccine: A Phase I Evaluation for Cancer Immunotherapy." *Cancer Immunol. Immunoth.* 1978. In Press.

Chairman: Evan M. Hersh

Unidentified Speaker: Dr. Bundy, what would you consider the biological significance of NK activity since there is very little correlation with other functional assays?

Bonita Bundy: We believe that it is a primitive assay and that the effector cell that mediates natural killing may be a very primitive form of immune function. We can see it in patients with profoundly deficient immune function in other assays.

Evan Hersh: Would Dr. Bundy like to comment on the suggestion that has been made in the literature that the NK cell is interacting through natural antibody on its FC receptor to antigens on the surface of the cultured cell lines which are apparently widely distributed in nature and to which many individuals seem to have natural reactivity?

Bundy: There does seem to be some specificity involved in natural killing. As for the reports by other investigators that they can rearm Tripsinized defector cells with serum from normal individuals, we have been unable to repeat these experiments. I'm not sure what the difference is. They use different target cells. Whether this is involved or whether they are actually measuring an ADCC type of reaction, we are unsure.

Hersh: I observed in some of your tables that the range of natural killing was extremely wide, from 10% to 60% among normal individuals. Have you identified any characteristics of these individuals which would explain this range and is this the type of range reactivity you see with other target cell lines?

Bundy: Similar work done in other targets has shown that there is a clustering about a certain mean, and, even in our work, most normals were clustered around the mean. In those patients that were significantly different from the normal mean, we found no HLA type of correlation. But, in our particular assays, it may be because we had such a small number of normals to measure. It is known that HLA A3B7 is associated with low natural killing activity and it's possible that we just have not had any patients of this particular type to measure to be able to make a correlation like that.

Malcolm Mitchell: Dr. Bundy, about the nature of a target cell in NK activity. One thing that disturbs me and is something that you can't be faulted for because everyone uses the same type of culture line—has anyone used fresh cells as a target? What I'm wondering is, that since the fresh cells are apparently present, and since the killer activity is present, if it's not the target cell that is responsible for the presence of lysis throughout. That is, would anything lyse these things because they are so sensitive to even exquisitely small lytic influences?

Bundy: There is a large degree of difference between susceptibility and

561

different target cells. Some target cells are susceptible to natural killing and others are not susceptible.

Mitchell: But are these fresh cells being used on cultured lines?

Bundy: I am not sure if anyone has used fresh cells. Recently, Pross and Baines reported that they could remove the reactivity of effector cells for natural target cells by incubating the target cells with enzymes such as trypsin and pronase. Then the reactivity against these target cells is subsequently regenerated overnight after culture in normal human serum. It doesn't seem to be tied to the fact that these target cell lines are grown in fetal calf's serum which was, at one time, thought to be the reason that natural killing occurred.

Hersh: It is an extremely interesting point the Dr. Mitchell is alluding to. Dr. Zarling has just reminded me that fresh leukemia cells are not killed by allogeneic normal lymphocytes. Therefore, you would have to raise the question as to whether this NK activity that we are all interested in, including my own laboratory, really has any *in vivo* biological relevance. If freshly collected tumor cells from the patient are not killed, but the cell lines that have been sitting around in culture for 5 years are killed, it may be that natural killing is a phenomenon related to a tissue culture artifact.

Marius Teodorescu: You can find important differences between subpopulations of lymphocytes in contact with the cells, so it looks like this function is more prominent than that particular function, although it is distributed more or less like the others. It appears that the peripheral blood lymphocytes as a whole are much poorer killers than the subset of cells that are called T4, they are natural killers. Another thing is that as long as we leave the T4 cells by themselves, they will kill allogeneic lymphocytes, any allogeneic lymphcyte including autologous lymphocytes. In other words, I am talking about fresh cells. So it seems that this function exists there. I don't know if it has any clinical relevance because in cancer patients we find dramatic changes in the T1, T2 population. The T1, T2 population is partially wiped out, but the T4 population is not changed. We don't see any different in the T4 population, which is a natural killer, in patients doing really bad or really good. I don't know if it has any clinical significance and I think that correlates with what Dr. Bundy said.

Hersh: Since you mentioned your different subpopulations, have you looked at them in ADCC assays of any kind?

Teodorescu: We did not look at that. We know only that T4 population contains gamma T-cells. We did not look at ADCC yet.

Joyce Zarling: In mice and in rats we know that natural killer cell activity can be detected and after the animals are ten weeks old, it declines. Several people, mostly in Herberman's lab, have shown that presumably natural killer activity can be reactivated by tumor cells, viruses, BCG, *C. parvum*— many things can induce interferon. I am not sure it's fair to conclude that natural killer cells don't play a role in immune surveillance against cancer because fresh tumor cells aren't killed. If we are measuring natural killer activity in adults, it could be that when you are young you have natural killer activity against targets associated with malignant cells. Then this declines and it may be able to be reactivated again. I have been looking at natural killer activity against fresh leukemia cells. I, as well as other people, generally do not detect natural killer activity against fresh leukemia cells. However, if human lymphocytes are treated even for one hour, I've been using purified human fiberglass interferon from Dr. Carter at Roswell Park, these lymphocytes will kill allogeneic fresh leukemia cells. We haven't yet gotten to asking whether they will kill autologous cells. It could be that when we are young we have natrual killer activity against primary tumors and that this can be reactivated. In other words, natural killer cells may play a role.

Bundy: We are not discounting the possibility that there may be some sort of an acute crisis in the patient's natural killing that accounts for them developing a malignancy or that there may be a defect in natural killing in some organ other than the peripheral blood.

Hersh: This difference between old and young individuals may be a very important point. Have you looked at peripheral blood lymphocytes from young individuals to see if they do have natural killing? Evolution may have played a trick on us. Since most of the cancers we see are in older people and if it turns out that older people do not have this natural killer activity, then we could say perhaps that natural killer cells have a very important function in immune surveillance.

David Salkin: About six months ago at Bethesda, the Richmond Virginia Group gave some very exciting reports on their experiments with polymers. Has anyone on the panel used them?

Hersh: You mean the pyran-polymers?

Salkin: Yes.

Hersh: I think the question to the panel is has anyone worked with pyran-polymers? I'm glad you made that point because this is a class of immunotherapeutic agents which wasn't mentioned during this meeting and I think has great potential. The pyran-polymers are very potent macrophage activators and interferon inducers. Now pyran-polymers of defined molecular weight with limited toxicity and with good biological activity are going to become available. Their advantage is that they can be given systemically. It's my opinion that systemic administration of immunotherapeutic agents is the wave of the future in addition to the second generation material concept that Dr. Mathé advanced. That is, more defined agents, which can be given systemically and have effect all over the body.

Brahma Sharma: Going back to natural killing, most of the studies done on natural killing are with Ficoll-Hypaque purified lymphocytes? Is it possible that the cells which are killing are really the cells which somehow got sensitized with natural antigen, like bacterial antigen, and may really be sensitized lymphocytes and not natural killer cells?

Bundy: Well, many differences are seen in killing between the natural killer cells and immune T cells. We begin seeing natural killing in an hour's time, where as primary and even secondary T immune cytotoxicity generally requires sensitization for several days before you can see a cytotoxic reaction. Also, in mice it is found that the NK activity is generally insensitive to treatment with anti-theta and compliment which certainly wouldn't be the case with immune T cell factors.

Sharma: Have you isolated T lymphocytes and then tested the killing?

Bundy: Yes, we have. We have recently shown that when T gamma cells are isolated they do mediate natural cytotoxicity. We believe that this probably is a function of their interaction with the NK effector cell and that the killing is actually being done by the natural killer cells, the FC positive cell that is E-rosette negative.

Mitchell: Dr. Hersh, you said before that you would speak about the different strains of BCG and their effect.

Hersh: I think your question is related to the comments Dr. Mokyr made regarding variability in her results with BCG depending upon the lot of BCG, that is, the strain. This has been an area of major interest and I think that Prof. Mathé was the first one to point out that some BCG preparations were active in immunotherapy, while others were not. In this country, Mackaness and his group pointed out that it was not only the strain of BCG which was active, but also the viability and the amount of free soluble antigen. There is a number of published experiments in animal systems indicating that different types of BCG, that is BCG from different sources or BCG preparations with different viabilities, have varying immunotherapeutic activity. Perhaps Prof. Mathé would like to comment on this point further because I think it may also influence the subfractions of BCG and the source of BCG can cause those subfractions.

George Mathé: Yes, I think that variance is one factor and there may be other factors. One is richness in bacteria. We showed that for 1 mg. per mouse IV the Pasteur fresh was more active than the Glaxco vaccine. Baldwin showed that for a similar number of bacteria it was still true; but in Montreal they had two phenotypes from the original Pasteur strain, one rich in tuberculin activity and poor in adjuvant activity and the other rich in adjuvant activity and poor in tuberculin activity. So, I think that there is some genetic role for composition and this could be important.

Mitchell: One thing the Mackaness Group did show was that there was a correlation, when testing a variety of strains, between the immunogenicity of the BCG preparation and its ability to invoke an immune response to

564

itself and its adjuvancy. Dr. Mokyr and I saw some evidence of this in *in vitro* experiments, too. One must make a reaction to the BCG as an antigen, a requirement for making a response to BCG as an effective adjuvant.

Sharma: This is a question for Dr. Mathé. Is it now fashionable to do most of the immunotherapies with BCG? You mentioned using *pseudomonas.* We have been trying different bacterial antigens like salmonella, candida, and *pseudomonas pertussis.* Some of them can induce the killer lymphocyte against the allogeneic, the syngeneic and the autologous tumor target. Are there any investigators who are testing other bacteria besides BCG as a potential immunotherapeutic agent?

Mathé: In humans?

Sharma: Yes.

Mathé: I don't know. The Houston Group is working with LPS of *pseudomonas* and we are working with the microorganism itself. We have gotten some results in resectable disease and we have ongoing trials in both post operative and resectable disease. One interesting thing is to give BCG followed by *pseudomonas.* This could be a very exciting new field in immunotherapy. While I have the microphone, can I ask Dr. Zarling if she would advise for specific immunotherapy to give pooled cells or single donor cells? I think the T cells don't have any determinants to mix tumorous cells and lymphocytes from a pool of normal donors. Could you separate from your *in vitro* results to some *in vivo* imagination?

Zarling: I feel that before doing either *in vivo* three cell experiments or immunizing with a pool that we would want to know what is going to happen in mice. We have started experiments immunizing mice with pooled allogeneic cells.

Mathé: Of pooled allogeneic leukemia cells?

Zarling: No, pooled allogeneic normal cells. Pooled allogeneic normal cells can sensitize both mouse and human lymphocytes to kill autologous leukemia cells. One thing I might be concerned about, although we don't have any *in vitro* reason to be, is whether immunization with a pool will induce any kind of an auto immune response. We know that pooled sensitized cells kill autologous or syngeneic abnormal cells and not normal cells, but our normal cells have only been lymphocytes. Whether we might have some target antigen on another organ that could be cross-reacted with alloantigen, I don't know. Before considering any *in vivo* human experience, I think it would be wise to see the results of the animal experiments. I think my ultimate goal would be to immunize humans with remission lymphocytes instead of a pool. Sensitize the lymphocytes with a pool, then grow a large number of these cytotoxic lymphocytes in condition media with T cell growth factor and then give these cells back to the patient, rather than immunizing with a pool. Now we can show that the cells do kill *in vitro*. We don't have to worry about multiple immunizations with a pool inducing suppressor cells and so forth.

Hersh: Thank you. I would like to call on Dr. Crispen to make the closing comments. While he is approaching the microphone, I'd like to thank him very much on the part of all the speakers and the audience for a very interesting and stimulating meeting and a very hospitable welcome to Chicago. Thank you very much, Ray, we all enjoyed it.

Ray Crispen: Thank you Dr. Hersh. I want to express my thanks to all of you for attending the meeting. It has been very exciting and the speakers have been outstanding. We have over the last three days developed a great deal of information that is going to take us some time to assimilate. I'm sure many of us are going back to our institutions with renewed enthusiasm and vigor to try to attack some of these problems. I want to thank, again, all the speakers for this outstanding program. I'll look forward to seeing you next year. Thank you.

Index